PROCEEDINGS OF THE Vᴛʜ WORLD CONGRESS ON PAIN

Pain Research and Clinical Management

Volume 3

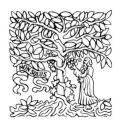

ELSEVIER
AMSTERDAM · NEW YORK · OXFORD

Proceedings of the Vth World Congress on Pain

Edited by

RONALD DUBNER

Neurobiology and Anesthesiology Branch, National Institute of Dental Research, National Institutes of Health, Bethesda, Maryland, USA

GERALD F. GEBHART

Department of Pharmacology, College of Medicine, University of Iowa, Iowa City, Iowa, USA

MICHAEL R. BOND

Department of Psychological Medicine, University of Glasgow, Glasgow, Scotland, UK

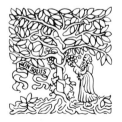

1988
ELSEVIER
AMSTERDAM · NEW YORK · OXFORD

ISBN volume: 0-444-80967-8
ISSN series: 0921-3287

Published by:
Elsevier Science Publishers B.V. (Biomedical Division)
P.O. Box 211
1000 AE Amsterdam
The Netherlands

Sole distributors for the USA and Canada:
Elsevier Science Publishing Company, Inc.
52 Vanderbilt Avenue
New York, NY 10017
USA

Library of Congress Cataloging-in-Publication Data

World Congress on Pain (5th: 1987: Hamburg, Germany)
    Proceedings of the Vth World Congress on Pain.

    (Pain research and clinical management, ISSN 0921-
3287; v. 3)
    Congress held in Hamburg on 2–7 August 1987.
    Includes index.
    1. Pain--Congresses. I. Dubner, Ronald. II. Gebhart,
Gerald F. III. Bond, Michael R. IV. Title. V. Title:
Proceedings of the Fifth World Congress on Pain.
VI. Title: Proceedings of the 5th World Congress on Pain.
VII. Series. [DNLM: 1. Pain--congresses. WL 704 W927
1987p]
RB127.W67   1987   616′.0472   88-11004
ISBN 0-444-80967-8 (U.S.)

Printed in The Netherlands

Contents

Preface

One can rightly ask whether an update on progress in pain research is necessary every three years. Did the Vth World Congress on Pain, in Hamburg, reveal significant advances in our knowledge? The answer is clearly an affirmative one based on the papers presented in this volume. Research has moved in important new directions that hold promise for future advances in the management of acute and chronic pain conditions. We have organized the contents of the volume to reflect these new findings.

Since the very first international symposium on pain in 1973 that preceded the formation of the International Association for the Study of Pain, research advances have focused primarily on an understanding of the transmission of signals related to transient tissue damage and the endogenous control systems in the brain that modify such signals. As a result, our understanding of acute pain and its control has increased in exciting ways. Ronald Melzack in his President's Address discusses the importance of eliminating needless pain throughout the world by educating health practitioners in the proper management of acute pain. The present volume, however, demonstrates a change in research emphasis towards understanding alterations in nervous system function following more persistent peripheral tissue and nerve injury. The John Bonica Distinguished Lecture presented by Patrick Wall draws our attention to this new research focus that will hopefully increase our understanding of chronic pain problems and lead to more effective therapeutic management.

A major section of this volume presents new findings on the role of the nervous system in peripheral inflammation. The release of chemicals from peripheral nerve endings during the inflammatory process and their interaction with humoral mediators are areas of intense study. We are also beginning to recognize that central nervous system changes occur soon after tissue and nerve injury. This neural plasticity associated with injury mimics, in part, changes that occur during development and learning, and thus has broad significance to our understanding of the nervous system. The major section on neuropathy pain points out the expansion of research interest in changes in the peripheral and central nervous system following peripheral neuropathies. We are now aware that abnormal impulse discharge from peripheral neural sites is insufficient and possibly not necessary to explain persistent pains associated with nerve damage. Research workers, therefore, are examining central nervous system changes associated with these injuries. It appears that there are multiple types of painful neuropathies with different etiologies and pathophysiological mechanisms. Some are mediated by nerve impulses originating in nociceptors, whereas others involve the activation of other types of peripheral receptors.

This volume also marks the first proceedings in which a major section is devoted to research on pain signals from other than cutaneous tissues. Considerable research has focused on visceral, musculoskeletal and vascular pains. The processing of signals arising from the viscera appears to be distinct in the dorsal horn from that arising from cutaneous tissues. We still know very little about mechanisms of musculoskeletal pain. Hopefully, the greater attention paid to the clinical characteristics of these conditions will foster basic research on their pathophysiology.

A very exciting aspect of the Vth World Congress was the numerous papers presented on pain in children. A number of these are published here. They point out the special problems of pain assessment in young people and present innovative approaches to solving them. Pain assessment in the adult, including the elderly, continues to receive great attention. This includes the development of new verbal report methods as well as the assessment of nonverbal behaviors.

We also see the initiation of research on the epidemiology of pain, a very neglected, but extremely important field. As scientists concentrate on the mechanisms of chronic pain conditions, they will benefit from clinical studies that describe their prevalence and signs and symptoms.

Finally, we take note of new advances in our knowledge of nociceptive mechanisms and their modulation. Novel classes of nociceptors are being discovered, new ascending projection pathways have been described and the chemical circuitry of these systems is being studied in greater detail.

The 1970s saw such major advances in pain research that we have tended to be disappointed with the significance of new discoveries in the 1980s. We believe that careful reading of this volume will dispel that notion. We believe we are at the threshold of discoveries that should reveal the mysteries of chronic pain conditions and reduce our inadequacies in managing them.

RONALD DUBNER
GERALD F. GEBHART
MICHAEL R. BOND
December, 1987

Acknowledgements

The editors of this volume and the officers and members of the Council of the International Association for the Study of Pain wish to express their appreciation to the many individuals whose efforts were so important to the success of the Vth World Congress on Pain and this book.

We first want to thank our colleagues on the Scientific Program Committee, Robert A. Boas, James N. Campbell, Kenneth L. Casey, Kenneth D. Craig, Howard L. Fields, Gisele Guilbaud, Jan Gybels, Ulf Lindblom, Carlo A. Pagni, Maryann Ruda, Barry J. Sessle, Horoshi Takagi, Toshikatsu Yokota and Manfred Zimmermann, who worked so diligently to produce an excellent program that was diversified in its content and format. Special thanks should go to Richard Gracely and Maryann Ruda who worked with Ronald Dubner and Gerald Gebhart in reviewing the abstracts, in organizing the free communication sessions and in selecting the short papers included in this volume. The fine work Maryann Ruda did in organizing the luncheon sessions at the Congress also deserves special recognition. Ms. Edith Welty, secretary to Ronald Dubner, deserves notice for her untiring work on behalf of the Scientific Program Committee.

We wish to offer our special thanks to Manfred Zimmermann and his colleagues on the local Arrangements Committee, Burkhart Bromm, Hermann O. Handwerker, Albert Herz, Dietrich Jungck, Klaus Kunze and Hanne Seemann, who worked so hard to insure that the myriad of small organizational details at the Congress were looked after. Their efforts helped assure the success of the Congress. Special thanks are also due to Mr. Matthias Rieger and Mrs. Marianne Winther and their staff in the Congress Organization Department of the Hamburg Messe and Congress GmbH, Mr. Walter Rosin, who managed the commercial exhibits and Mr. Volker Schnurrbusch, who ran the press room during the Congress. We are grateful for their hard work on our behalf.

The editors of this volume and the officers and members of the IASP Council would like to express their deepest appreciation to our Associate Editor, Louisa E. Jones, whose extraordinary efforts from the earliest planning stages of the Congress have been essential for the success of the Congress and the ultimate publication of these proceedings.

On behalf of the Council and members of the IASP, the editors also acknowledge and express their special appreciation for the financial support given the Vth World Congress by the following:

Deutsche Forschungsgemeinschaft
Freie und Hansestadt Hamburg
Gesellschaft zum Studium des Schmerzes für Deutschland, Österreich und Die Schweiz
Grünenthal GmbH (*FRG*)
Hoechst Pharma Deutschland (*FRG*)
Medtronic Inc., Neuro Division (*USA*)
E. Merck (*FRG*)
National Institute of Drug Abuse (*USA*)
(Grant No. 1 R13 DA04575-1)
Shiley Infusaid, Inc. (*USA*)
Syntex International Ltd. (*USA*)
. . . . .
Astra Alab AB (*Sweden*)
Astra Chemical GmbH (*FRG*)
Bayer AG (*FRG*)
Bristol-Myers Company (*USA*)
Ciba-Geigy AG (*Switzerland*)
Ciba-Geigy Canada Ltd. (*Canada*)

Eli Lilly and Company (*USA*)
Goedecke AG (*FRG*)
Hoffmann-La Roche Co. AG (*Switzerland*)
Imperial Chemical Industries, PLC (*UK*)
Johnson & Johnson (*USA*)
Medtronic GmbH (*FRG*)
G.D. Searle & Co. (*USA*)

. . . . .

Beecham Pharmaceuticals (*UK*)
Boehringer & Sohn GmbH (*FRG*)
Cascan (*FRG*)

Ciba-Geigy GmbH (*FRG*)
Hoffmann-La Roche Inc. (*USA*)
Janssen GmbH (*FRG*)
3 M Company (*USA*)
Much AG (*FRG*)
Roche Products Pty. Ltd. (*Australia*)
Sandoz AG (*FRG*)
Sandoz Pharmaceuticals (*USA*)
The Upjohn Company (*USA*)
Winthrop GmbH (*FRG*)

Introductory Remarks

Charmides' work of Pain

Prof. Dr. Klaus Michael Meyer-Abich

Senator, City-State of Hamburg, Hamburger Strasse 37,
2000 Hamburg 76, Federal Republic of Germany

Mr. President, Mr. Chairman, Ladies and Gentlemen, Dear Colleagues,

It is a pleasure for me to welcome you to Hamburg on behalf of the Senate as well as the citizens of Hamburg. We hope that you will enjoy your stay and that not only your heads will be fed with thoughts and information but also your hearts with what we need beyond science, also showing us what is worth knowing in human affairs. This may be particularly important when speaking about pain.

To those who came from abroad, perhaps I should mention that Hamburg is a city and a state at the same time, being one of the states which constitute our Federal Republic. The state government is called the Senate and the ministers are called senators; I am the senator in charge of science.

Up to this century Hamburg was mainly a city of trade, particularly of international trade, but by now it has become also a center of science. Our university hospital is about one hundred years old and many of its well-known scholars have an international reputation. Today it is appropriate to mention only Professor Bromm in pain research. We appreciate very much that Hamburg has been chosen to be the site of the Vth World Congress on Pain. Professor Bonica's presence has been especially noted. We welcome him not only as a pioneer in medicine but as a scholar who has given the medical profession great insight into pain and its control.

Following medicine beyond modern medicine, I would like to remind you of what Socrates thought about pain. In his dialogue *'Charmides'* Plato tells us how Socrates once was introduced to a young man, Charmides. Charmides was inflicted by some pain, namely by a headache, and Socrates was introduced to him as a physician. Charmides then expected to be cured, made healthy, and asked for a suitable herb as a medication. Socrates replied that he should certainly get a drug for the headache, but that the one he knew and could recommend worked only if the physical treatment of the body was complemented by an intellectual treatment of the mind.

This is, Socrates explained to Charmides, because the drug does not only cure the head but works as described by good physicians: when somebody's eyes are inflicted and he wants to be cured, they reply that the eyes cannot be treated separately but that the head must be taken as a whole to cure the eyes; and again that a medical treatment of the head alone does not work, but that the whole body has to be considered. This, however, Socrates added, is not yet the last step, but I am going still one step further, namely, the body again cannot be cured separately without considering the soul, because everything originates from the soul, health as well as disease. And the soul can be treated by discourse or reasoning. The drug, therefore, must be complemented by (philosophical) reasoning.

Now this was not exactly what Charmides had expected as necessary to get rid of his headache, but he liked Socrates and agreed to start the treatment. The dialogue then proceeds from self-awareness in pain to self-recognition, or to the Delphian Know-thyself (gnôthi seauthón). This is Plato's idea of working out pain, or Schmerzarbeit. I wish that also this Congress may develop as a discourse not only on medication, but beyond medication, and reasonably consider the mind as well. This could also be an important service to other fields of medicine. If you are lucky, some modern Socrates among you might provide insights. I wish you all the best.

Welcoming address on the occasion of the Vth World Congress on Pain

The Meaning of Pain

Dr. theol. Peter Fischer-Appelt

President, University of Hamburg

Professor Melzack, Professor Bonica, Ladies and Gentlemen!

I should like to express my gratitude for having the privilege of addressing you on the occasion of the Vth World Congress on Pain. It is by four reasons that I recognize with appreciation the possibility of underlining the importance of your Congress.

First of all, the well-known and yet unknown phenomenon of pain draws our attention to the fact that the focus of human experience, the origins of conceptual thought, derive not from contemplation, but from human practice. I may quote here Ernst Cassirer, a German philosopher who taught at Hamburg University during its first decade from 1919 to 1933, who said in his book *'Language and Myth'* (1946): "Humanity really attains its insight into objective reality only through the medium of its own activity." That is to say, if curiosity is the beginning of all research, then the desire to ease the burdens of mankind will be its justification. To help people, to meet their needs, to find solutions from their problems and thus contribute to satisfying the 'conditio humana', the necessary conditions for human life, is indeed the final purpose of scientific work.

Secondly, medicine ranks very high if we consider the fields that try to serve people. Patients throughout the ages consulted doctors, medicine men or others experienced in medical matters to find help and cure from their pains.

Pain is certainly the father of all diagnosis. Therefore, it is hard to understand that pain research has not found more attention in basic scientific work in the past. It is therefore a relief to recognize that the International Association for the Study of Pain is dedicated to the investigation of the mechanisms and syndromes of pain and to improve the management of patients with acute and chronic pain. For millions of people who suffer from undiagnosed pain, it is of great importance that basic scientists, physicians and other health professionals devote their research interest and practical cooperation to the elucidation of a problem which many feel to be a scourge of their lives. Anyone who has been exposed to life crises caused by continuous strong pain will support the urgent appeal to enlarge and continue pain research programs sponsored by national and international research agencies.

Nevertheless, and that is my third point, pain is like a key which opens both the internal and the external world to our experience. It seems to stimulate the progress of learning, the capacity to integrate and to share the essence and the significance of compassion. As the Greek poet Menander said: "learn of your own pain; thus you shall acquire the compassion of other people."

If pain is one of the human conditions of life, we can also better understand the universal meaning of knowledge: that knowledge attains its real significance and vivid creativity only through compassion and that it includes virtually the participation of all.

Fourthly, to conclude, I would like to state with satisfaction that pain research in Hamburg is conducted on a broad scale, particularly in the Department of Neurophysiology in our School of Medicine. I can also underline that the work of this Department has developed in close cooperation with some of our clinics and other institutes, as the causes of pain are numerous and successful research can only show results if an interdisciplinary approach is pursued.

It might be of interest that it was Ernst von der Porten, who conducted pain research here in the 1920s, then Arthur Jones, Professor of Internal Diseases and Endocrinology until 1967, who introduced psychosomatic aspects into his work on pain, and that the first Chair for Anesthesiology in our country was established at the University Hospital (Eppendorf) in 1966 and filled by Professor Karl Horatz.

Ladies and Gentlemen, I should like to thank you that you have accepted the invitation to come to Hamburg for your meeting. I wish you, our guests and colleagues, a favorable stay in Hamburg, and I hope that this Congress will open new scientific insights and personal friendships for all of you.

R. Dubner, G.F. Gebhart & M.R. Bond (Eds.)
Proceedings of the Vth World Congress on Pain
© 1988 Elsevier Science Publishers BV (Biomedical Division)

CHAPTER 1

IASP President's Address
The tragedy of needless pain: a call for social action

Ronald Melzack

Department of Psychology, McGill University, 1205 Dr. Penfield Avenue, Montreal, Quebec, Canada H3A 1B1

This Vth World Congress provides exciting evidence that great strides have been made in pain therapy. But many pain syndromes are still beyond our control. Low back pain is the most common kind of pain and millions of sufferers continually seek help. Sometimes they obtain temporary relief, but most continue to suffer. Migraine and tension headaches similarly plague millions of people. New drugs and psychological techniques provide help for some, but the pains persist in the majority. Perhaps the most terrible of all pains are those suffered by some cancer patients in the terminal phases of the disease.

We do not understand the causes of low back pain in most people and the causes of migraine continue to elude us. So, too, are we perplexed by the causes of a variety of muscle pains as well as abdominal pains in children and adults. Pelvic pains in women often appear unexpectedly and persist in the absence of any apparent organic or psychological cause. All of these pains have ruined many lives and put terrible strains on spouses and other family members. Physicians, psychologists and other health-care professionals try every known kind of therapy, often without success. We stand by helplessly and hope fervently that more research will bring an answer.

There are also, of course, many pains whose causes are clear but for which we do not have an adequate treatment. These include severe osteo- and rheumatoid arthritis, pains due to lesions of nerves and portions of the central nervous system, phantom limb pain, and, of course, pain associated with some kinds of cancer. We have an armamentarium of drugs as well as sensory and psychological techniques which help up to a point; but beyond that we can only hope that future breakthroughs will soon bring us new drugs or other ways to abolish these pains. That we can do nothing because these problems are beyond the state of our knowledge is understandable and forgivable.

But then there are the pains which we *are* able to control and fail to do so because of ignorance. My brother-in-law, whom I loved very much, had cancer and died in terrible pain. For months he suffered not only pain but something just as frightening – the loss of his personal dignity by having to weep and plead for the next injection of morphine. His narcotic was carefully doled out because his physician was convinced that if she gave it to him in larger doses or more often he would develop tolerance to it and in the final days, when the pain would be at its worst, he would die in uncontrolled pain. We now know – thanks to Cicely Saunders, Robert Twycross, Balfour Mount and others – that this was a wrong assumption. There is overwhelming, convincing evidence that significant tolerance and addiction rarely occur when narcotics are taken for pain. Yet millions of people throughout the world continue to die in needless pain. Despite all the evidence we are still haunted by the fears of addiction and tolerance. Why? As we shall soon see, it is largely because the patient-in-pain is mistaken for the street addict. Understandably, law-enforcement agencies are confused and poor teaching in medicine, nursing and other health-care and graduate schools has kept us in ignorance so that morphine and its related compounds still hold a special terror. Patients are just as perplexed and believe that they will become addicts and social outcasts if they take narcotics for their pain and often insist on suffering needless pain. The fact is that when morphine and other narcotics are given to *people in pain*, tolerance is minimal and addiction is rare.

Because of understandable fears about addiction in psychologically disturbed people, the governments of many countries have enacted stringent laws to prevent narcotic drugs from reaching street addicts. As a result, it is difficult for physicians to obtain these drugs for their patients, and nurses feel intimidated about administering them. As a result, innocent patients are penalized by laws aimed at criminals and mentally ill people.

The plague of needless pain

The needless pain that plagues the people of the world – in rich and poor nations alike – is appalling. We now know that the intelligent use of morphine can virtually abolish pain in 80–90% of cancer patients, but the drug is essentially unobtainable by millions of people with cancer pain in Asia, Africa and even in some countries in Europe and South America. The pain produced by changes in dressings in burn patients, the pains of punctures of the spine or bone taps, pain after major surgery – all of these can be blocked or at least diminished by the use of one or more of many kinds of techniques that are now available. Yet many health professionals fail to provide adequate relief.

Pain in children

Anyone who has watched a child suffer pain, whether due to minor diseases or major ones such as cancer, feels anguish and a sense of helplessness. Children are so vulnerable that it 'hurts' to watch a child suffer. We like to think that the health professionals who look after children do everything they can to prevent pain or to relieve it as much as possible. It comes as a shock, then, to find out that our ideas about pain in children are dominated by the myth that young children do not feel pain as intensely as adults and therefore require fewer analgesics or none at all (McGrath and Unruh, 1987). In one study (Eland and Anderson, 1977), more than 50% of children who underwent major surgery – including limb amputation, excision of a cancerous neck mass and heart surgery – were not given any analgesics, and the remainder received inadequate doses. Statistics such as these are found in virtually every study that examines the treatment of severe pain in children. Older children and adolescents are the butt of another myth – that they will become drug addicts if they are given narcotic drugs for severe pain – and do not fare much better.

Recent studies, using the assessment tools available to us, indicate that children experience the same qualities and intensities of pain felt by adults (Jeans, 1983; McGrath and Unruh, 1987). But they are horribly undermedicated. In Eland and Anderson's study (1977) cited above, only half the children were given any analgesics. But even more revealing is that when 18 of these children were matched with 18 adults who had had similar operations, the children were given a total of 24 doses of analgesic drugs while the adults received 372 narcotic and 299 non-narcotic doses of analgesics. Similarly, Beyer et al. (1983) followed 50 children and 50 adults after heart surgery. Children received 30% of the analgesic doses compared to 70% given to adults. Six children received no analgesics during the first 3 post-operative days. Another study (Schecter et al., 1986) examined random samples of 90 children and 90 adults matched for medical problems (appendectomies, hernias, fractures and burns) and found that, depending on the diagnostic category, children received a half to a third of the number of doses of narcotic drugs given to the adults.

Postoperative pain

Postoperative pain is not managed as well as it should be (Bonica, 1983; Melzack, 1987; Melzack et al., 1987). Patients with post-surgical pain are often undermedicated even though the importance of pain control for optimal recovery has been repeatedly emphasized. Although the pain decreases rapidly in most patients during the three or four days following surgery, the high levels of pain during the first few days have led to studies of the causes. The most obvious cause is that inadequate doses of drugs are prescribed. In a recent study, Donovan et al. (1987) examined 353 medical-surgical inpatients who reported experiencing pain during their hospitalization. They found that '58% of these patients experienced excruciating pain. Fewer than half of the patients with pain had a member of the health care team ask them about their pain or note the pain in the patient record. ... As in earlier studies, the dose of analgesic administered over a 24-h period was less than a quarter of the amount ordered.' The unfounded fear of addiction lies at the heart of the problem, so that physicians and nurses tend to prescribe and administer doses at the low end of the range (Bonica, 1983).

A recent study (Melzack et al., 1987) has shown that surgical wards contain two populations: a young group that recovers quickly and a group of older patients whose pain lingers on at high levels for many days beyond the expected 3–4-day recovery period. Despite the persistent, high level of pain in these older patients (presumably due to complications after surgery), they do not receive larger doses of drugs. Indeed, they receive smaller doses at shorter intervals, but this strategy evidently fails to reduce pain adequately. These patients comprise about 30% of the patients on a surgical ward at any time and therefore represent a substantial number of people who suffer needlessly high levels of pain.

Burn pain

It is easy to imagine the severe pain of a burn, par-
ticularly when a large surface of the body has received third-degree burns that destroy all the layers of the skin. The pain suffered by these patients is extremely high (Choiniere, 1988). In addition to this pain, there are daily sessions in which bandages and dead tissue are removed – the painful process of debridement. Although such pains are well-controlled in some burn units, they are not controlled at all in others. Even in excellent burn units, with highly capable, compassionate physicians, nurses, physiotherapists and others, the pain levels are very high. A study of 30 consecutive patients during debridement and physiotherapy shows that in the first two weeks 23% suffer severe pain, and 30% have extremely severe pain. Even at rest, 13% of patients suffer severe pain and another 20% suffer extremely severe pain. These data, by the way, were obtained in patients who were already medicated according to standard textbook recommendations.

Research is needed to determine the most effective drugs and doses, and, equally important, the best time to carry out these procedures after administration of the drug. Sometimes a drug is given and debridement is started immediately, when in fact it may take an hour before the drug has its optimal analgesic effect.

Cancer pain

This still remains the most frightening kind of pain that can befall any of us. The hospice (Saunders, 1978) and Palliative Care Service (Mount, 1976) approaches to pain control are the best of all possibilities. Unfortunately, there are not nearly enough specialized services of these kinds. So people suffer and the suffering can be tremendous. Bonica (1980), in an excellent review of several surveys, concludes that 'moderate to severe pain is experienced by about 40% of patients with intermediate stages of the disease, and by 60 to 80% of the patients with advanced cancer' (p. 336).

The causes of most types of cancer pain are well known (Bonica, 1980) and most of the pain can be controlled by the extraordinarily simple procedure of providing adequate doses of narcotics. Beginning with a reasonable level, such as 10 mg of morphine in water ingested orally every 4 hours (or 3 hours if necessary), the dose is increased gradually until pain is brought under control. Twycross, Saunders, Mount, Foley and many others have shown that once pain control has been achieved, a patient can continue on the same dose for weeks, months, even years without developing any significant tolerance. Increased pain is almost invariably due to a progression in the disease. Satisfactory treatment which produces a reduction of the pathology is often accompanied by the patient's request to decrease the dosage. Patients on high doses of morphine over a period of years can have their drug diminished in large jumps over a 3 or 4 day period until reduced to zero, yet show no signs of withdrawal.

Those of us at this Congress are aware of the power of oral morphine. And many know too that 'breakthrough' pains can be helped with nitrous oxide, TENS and other expedients. Tragically, there still remains a residual group with intolerable, uncontrolled pain but, fortunately, it is relatively small, perhaps not more than 10–20% (Melzack et al., 1976; Mount et al., 1976). It is the 80–90% that is of concern here. Their pain can be controlled but the vast majority of patients fail to receive the elixir of morphine that could relieve their pain. This happens in rich countries and in poor ones. Ignorance is pervasive. But it is not ignorance alone. Inadequate treatment is also due to a tragic misconception about narcotic drugs. They have been misunderstood and damned for so long that they are not prescribed in adequate doses.

People who face such pain should be aware of the help that is available. Morphine can be administered through various routes – orally, intravenously, by slow drip into a brain ventricle or onto the spinal cord. If given orally, by far the preferred route, it should be 'titrated upward' in gradually increasing doses until a dose is found which maintains continuous pain relief (Twycross and Lack, 1983). The goal is to keep the patient pain-free at all times. With some kinds of cancer, patients still

have sharply rising 'breakthrough' pains which are not kept under control by morphine. In these instances, nitrous oxide can rapidly be made available by using a small tank and mask; the patient breathes the nitrous oxide/oxygen mixture until the pains are gone. Even with this, about 10% of people still have serious pain, which underscores the need for more research.

The myth of narcotic addiction and tolerance in pain patients

We are confronted with a dilemma. The traditional textbook story tells us that 'narcotic drugs' (used here as a general term to refer to all opiate and opioid drugs) are dangerous: that they give rise rapidly to addiction and tolerance, that withdrawal symptoms are severe when they are discontinued, and that they should be avoided or given in the smallest amounts possible. Narcotics are described as forbidden fruit – so desirable as analgesics yet so terrifying as addictive substances.

In contrast, another picture has been emerging for the past 25 years or more: that narcotic drugs, when given to *people in pain*, do not have the undesirable effects found in the textbooks. Tolerance rarely occurs; small increases in dosage may be needed during the first few days but, once an optimal dose range is found, it remains effective for months or years. Withdrawal symptoms are rarely seen: patients, after months or years of ingestion of narcotics, can be given a series of decreasing doses for 3 or 4 days and then taken off the drug entirely with little or no adverse psychological effect. The management of physical dependence, in other words, is not difficult (Saunders, 1978; Twycross and Lack, 1983).

How do we reconcile these two radically opposing views? This is no academic debate, because narcotic drugs are extremely powerful, come in a multitude of variations which are virtually tailor-made to diminish specific undesirable side-effects, and are cheap and easy to obtain. The poorest countries can afford to make them available, and the World

Health Organization recommends the use of morphine for cancer pain in whatever doses are necessary to control the pain. So why this double-faceted picture: heaven on one side, hell on the other?

The answer seems to the quite simple: we have persistently confused the *street addict* who is psychologically sick and takes narcotic drugs for psychopathological needs and the *patient in pain* who is psychologically healthy and takes the drugs only as long as they are needed. Law enforcement agencies and our whole health-care system have confused these two fundamentally different kinds of people: one kind seeks drugs to achieve oblivion – a psychological escape or release from fears, terrors, depression, horrible anxiety; the other kind seeks freedom from pain and, in fact, dislikes the psychological clouding, loss of affect and other feelings that come from narcotic drugs. The confusion is depicted in Fig. 1.

Government drug-control agencies are rightly concerned with the effects of narcotics on street addicts. These people, it must be kept in mind, are usually mentally ill and it is the illness that leads to narcotic addiction rather than the other way around. Our negative social attitudes to street addicts have become generalized to people-in-pain

who take drugs. As a result, physicians usually prescribe low ranges of the drugs, nurses tend to administer on the low side of the range, the patient suffers, the family suffers, and quite often society in general suffers because long-lasting pain means hospitalization and an economic burden to society.

Government drug-control agencies, like most of society, usually have a difficult time maintaining a balanced understanding of these two completely different kinds of people. Similarly, medical and nursing school training and health-care practice reflect our general failure to distinguish between street addicts and people-in-pain. Street addicts show 'psychological dependence' (Portenoy and Foley, 1986, p. 182): 'a set of aberrant behaviors marked by drug craving, efforts to secure its supply, interference with physical health or psychosocial function, and recidivism after detoxification.' People in pain who receive narcotics for their pain show none of these characteristics.

Studies with people in pain

The evidence is growing rapidly to show that psychologically healthy people do not become addicts when exposed to narcotics. Portenoy and Foley (1986, p. 183) have recently reviewed the evidence on use and abuse of narcotics by general medical patients: 'Porter and Jick (1980) reported that abuse occurred in only 4 of 11 882 patients without a history of drug dependence who were treated with opioids in the hospital. In only one instance was this abuse considered major. A survey of analgesic use in units specializing in burn pain failed to reveal a single case of iatrogenic addiction in over 10 000 patients without prior opioid abuse who received these medications while hospitalized (Perry and Heidrich, 1982). A review (Medina and Diamond, 1977) of 2369 patients with chronic headache uncovered 3 abusing opioids, including 2 taking codeine and 1 propoxyphene. These studies do not support the view that opioids begun for legitimate medical purposes are used inappropriately by a significant proportion of patients.'

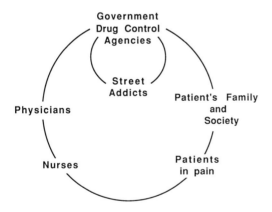

Fig. 1. The legal and medical concepts of drug addiction and tolerance, which are based on the behaviour of 'street addicts', are generalized to the whole population. Physicians, nurses and other health professionals are influenced in the way they treat patients who suffer severe pain. Inevitably, the patients' families are also affected by the suffering of people they love.

Another example is a survey of the consequences of injections of narcotics given to the many thousands of Israeli casualties in the Yom Kippur War. Not a single case of narcotic addiction was found among these men in spite of the fact that most were in the age range most commonly at risk for social addiction (Wall, personal communication, 1982).

Still further evidence comes from studies that use a special machine which allows the patient to give himself regulated small doses of morphine at short intervals (Keeri-Szanto, 1979). When these methods were introduced, there was considerable fear that the patient would abuse the drug. Instead, it soon became clear that patients do not push their drug intake to the highest permitted dose. On the contrary, they bring their pain down to a bearable level at which they do not have mental clouding. Then they continue to give themselves the narcotic at the doses required to maintain this desired state. The overall result is that the patient gives himself no more (and sometimes less) than the medical staff would administer.

In contrast to this evidence, consider the sad story of a patient seen recently at our Pain Clinic at the Montreal General Hospital. Here was a 50-year-old man in severe pain from abdominal cancer that had metastasized so that tumor tissue was literally pushing through his skin. He was able to work but was in terrible pain. He slept badly and his moans prevented his wife and children from sleeping. His family was in a state of misery and dejection, watching him suffer. Yet this man, who was highly moral, felt it was wrong for him to take a narcotic because the newspapers and other media made it clear that he would become an addict, a 'junky', and he would rather die in pain than become a social outcast. His family doctor turned to our Pain Clinic in desperation, and it took ten pain specialists to eventually convince this good man that he would not become an addict, that taking narcotics is not a sin and in fact the quality of life would improve not only for himself but for his family as well. Fortunately, we persuaded him. Here we touch on religion and need help from all religious clergy who wish to prevent needless suffering.

Studies with animals

The observations made with psychologically healthy people have been confirmed in many animal studies in my laboratory. We used the formalin test, which produces a moderately severe pain for about 90 minutes, and which has been shown to be a reasonable animal model of pain in people. In our studies (Abbott et al., 1981, 1982a,b), there was no evidence of tolerance to successive injections of morphine at analgesia-producing levels. This was in sharp contrast to use of the drug in the tail-flick test: a very mild, brief pain accompanied by a spinally mediated reflex which requires increasingly large doses of morphine. This led us to conclude (Abbott et al., 1981, 1982; Abbott and Melzack, 1983) that different neural systems are involved in different kinds of pain, and the system involved in intense, prolonged pain does not show tolerance to repeated doses of morphine. Similar results have been obtained by Colpaert et al. (1978). Abbott, Cohen and I (Abbott et al., 1981; Abbott and Melzack, 1982; Cohen et al., 1984; Cohen and Melzack, 1985, 1986) went on to show that higher brain systems are involved in morphine analgesia, in contrast to the spinal systems, which appear to show rapid tolerance. With studies such as these, we can begin to investigate why some people become 'street addicts' while the vast majority of people do not.

By avoiding simple-minded generalizations, we learn more about the neural mechanisms of analgesia and find a rationale for providing better pain relief to large numbers of people. The laws of our governments must become increasingly flexible to accommodate our newer knowledge and our new approaches to the control of severe, prolonged pain.

The consequences of needless pain

John Bonica has argued often and eloquently that severe, prolonged pain has serious consequences. If we cannot help a sufferer because the state of knowledge in our field is not up to it, then we must turn to our research and pray for a breakthrough. But my concern here is the pain that *can* be controlled but still exists because the care-giver or the patient are ignorant of the facts.

Prolonged, severe post-surgical pain can also have terrible consequences. Bonica (1983) and Cousins (1988) have reviewed the serious, negative effects of postoperative pain on respiratory and gastrointestinal functions, particularly in elderly patients. And, as we have seen, these are the people in whom postoperative pain is most poorly controlled.

Uncontrolled, persistent postsurgical pain, burn pain and other kinds of pain have serious consequences for people whose lives are at risk from other physical problems, such as respiratory or cardiac problems. Pain can further impede the adequate ventilation and circulation necessary to provide the oxygen and nutrition for recovery. Pain can therefore have a major impact on morbidity and mortality in these patients. In short, it can mean the difference between life and death.

Pain is also a source of stress and there is now a powerful, convincing literature on the damaging effects of stress on the immune response. Several excellent studies by Shavit and his colleagues (Shavit et al., 1984, 1985) have looked at pain-induced stress – prolonged, intermittent, inescapable foot-shock in the rat – on the body's ability to resist the effects of implanted tumor tissue. The frightening conclusion is that animals which received 'foot-shock prior to tumor implantation had reduced median survival time and percent survival compared to non-stressed controls.' These data are part of a larger body of evidence showing that stress suppresses immune function generally. The evidence in rats is powerful; the data with humans (though more difficult to obtain and assess) are consistent with it. Taken together, the results suggest that severe, prolonged pain can have serious, health-threatening consequences; and because it occurs more often in older people who are likelier to have more severe postoperative and other kinds of pain, pain can no longer be brushed aside as 'well, it's just

pain; it can't kill you.' The evidence, especially on tumor suppression, suggests that it is possible.

A final word on needless pain. Besides its capacity to destroy life itself, it destroys the quality of life. S. Weir Mitchell (1872) stated it well: 'Perhaps few persons who are not physicians can realize the influence which long-continued and unendurable pain may have upon both body and mind... Under such torments the temper changes, the most amiable grow irritable, the soldier becomes a coward, and the strongest man is scarcely less nervous than the most hysterical girl.' Prolonged pain destroys the will to live. It drives people to suicide. It often prevents weakened, older people from obtaining the nourishment necessary for life.

Control of chronic non-cancer pain

I have not yet mentioned the most pervasive of all the pains – the chronic pains which we understand so poorly, such as low-back pain, migraine headaches, the awful neuralgic pains and atypical facial pains. They perplex us as scientists and healers; they grind sufferers into the ground. They have all the characteristics – prolonged, severe, intermittent and beyond control – necessary to produce the stress that can harm us. Our careful weighing of risks and benefits – in view of what we now know about pain, stress and immunosuppression – must be re-evaluated. Risks we might not have considered before must now be entertained. It was once unthinkable to give narcotics to patients with chronic pain not attributable to cancer. But it is being done, and it can be effective. A pervasive argument was that these patients abuse drugs; but that might well be due to such low doses that they were almost useless and patients begged for more. Because of our prejudices about narcotics, the lowest possible doses are prescribed and they are often ineffective, or at least fail to act for sufficiently long periods of time. Angell's (1982) description of the effects of inadequate medication for cancer pain is also true for chronic non-cancer pain: 'we are left, then, with the image of a patient who can anticipate severe pain toward the end of each three- or four-hour period, who counts the minutes until the end of the interval, and desperately hopes that a nurse will be nearby and promptly give him his dose of narcotics when it is time. To such a patient, the medical profession's attention to pain must seem confined to limiting relief from it. To doctors and nurses, on the other hand, the patient's anxiety and clock watching may seem to indicate growing dependence on the drug, not inadequate relief of pain. I believe there is a tendency for an adversarial relationship to develop in which the doctor or nurse ascribes to the patient the motivations and impulsions of an addict. He is seen to be obsessed with drugs – not pain – and too weak to stop himself.'

There is now a growing body of evidence that narcotic drugs can be used effectively in patients with chronic pain *who do not have psychological problems or a history of drug abuse*. Portenoy and Foley (1986, pp. 178–179) have summarized this literature. 'Taub (1982) described 313 personally treated patients with refractory pain who were maintained on opioid analgesics for up to 6 years. Only 13 presented serious management problems, all of whom had prior histories of substance abuse. Escalation of dose and toxicity were not encountered and all patients appeared to benefit from the therapy. Tennant and Uelman (1983) reported 22 patients who had been maintained on opioids after failing treatment at pain clinics. Two-thirds returned to work and all reduced medical visits. Finally, France et al. (1984) described 16 patients who chronically received low-dose opioids as part of a comprehensive pain-management program. Patient function was improved and neither side-effects nor clinically significant tolerance developed.'

Portenoy and Foley (1986) carried out a study with 38 patients who were maintained on opioid analgesics for non-cancer pain. About 60% obtained satisfactory pain relief. Management became a problem in only 2 patients, both with a history of prior drug abuse. Portenoy and Foley conclude that 'opioid maintenance therapy can be a safe, salutary and more humane alternative to the options of surgery or no treatment in those patients with intractable non-malignant pain and no history of drug abuse.'

None of the above investigators is suggesting that narcotic drugs be prescribed indiscriminately to all sufferers of chronic pain. On the contrary: they approach the problem with great caution. Portenoy and Foley (1986) note the satisfactory results but, at the same time, provide careful guidelines for such treatment programs and point out the problems that may accompany opioid maintenance therapy. Nevertheless, these papers represent a phenomenon akin to 'breaking the sound barrier'. Our attitudes to narcotics for pain relief are influenced by unfounded prejudice based on street addicts, and these studies represent a breakthrough to a reasoned, unbiased study of the effectiveness of narcotic drugs in patients who normally would never be considered for such therapy. Yet it appears to help a substantial number of people who have not been helped by any other kind of therapy. Except for those patients with drug-abuse problems (who can be screened out by careful psychological investigation), the patients who were helped received a genuinely new lease on life. The evidence from these patients, like those with cancer pain, is that most *patients in pain* exposed to narcotics do not become drug abusers.

This approach is highly controversial. Sternbach (1987) and others fear that patients will receive a prescription for a narcotic and will never receive the advantages of a multidisciplinary approach to pain. Portenoy and Foley (1986) feel that both approaches to pain relief are compatible. We need to acquire data in well-controlled studies, which will take time, and Rose (1987) fears that government agencies may harm the atmosphere for dispassionate scientific evaluation. Let us hope this does not happen. We must continue to experiment and think about this hitherto unthinkable problem with the hope of saving lives that have been ruined by pain.

The need for education

Many people, beginning with Weir Mitchell (1872),

have recognized that prolonged, severe pain can be so devastating that people would sooner be dead than have to live with such dreadful suffering. Relentless pain grinds people down; it destroys them. There is nothing uplifting, nothing do be gained from continual pain. A few religious zealots have argued that pain is good for the soul, that it somehow cleanses it of evil. But there is not a shred of evidence that we become better human beings when we suffer relentlessly. On the contrary, moral religious systems demand that we help one another, that we allay one another's pains and torments.

Albert Schweitzer (1953) has stated it beautifully for all of us: 'We must all die. But that I can save [a person] from days of torture, that is what I feel as my great and ever-new privilege. Pain is a more terrible lord of mankind than even death himself.'

Marcia Angell (1982) has put it another way in relation to needless cancer pain: 'Pain is soul-destroying. No patient should have to endure intense pain unnecessarily. The quality of mercy is essential to the practice of medicine; here, of all places, it should not be strained.'

The solution to needless pain is education in all its facets: congresses like this one; an excellent journal that evaluates new research and ideas and publishes the best of it for people to read throughout the world; refresher courses to keep us abreast of what is new in clinical practice. We urgently need a wider distribution of books and pamphlets to everyone who is involved in research and therapy in the field of pain. We pride ourselves that we have 3000 members in IASP, but there are several thousand times that number of people who practise the healing arts throughout the world. And, tragically, many of them practise it badly. The World Health Organization (1986) is aware of just how bad it is – particularly in third-world countries. In many parts of Asia and Africa people with cancer die in agony with no medication whatever. *Nothing!* Hundreds of thousands of health-care-givers have to be taught that a few pennies worth of morphine each day can bring relief from the most terrible suffering.

The Canadian, British and American governments have produced some outstanding booklets on the care of cancer pain, written for care-givers and for patients. More of this kind of informational material is needed and it is essential that it really be distributed, read, understood and practised. It is easy to talk about our desire to help third-world countries; it comes as a shock, therefore, to find that very large numbers of our colleagues, many of them associated with the teaching hospitals of some of the best universities in the western world, still believe that morphine must be given PRN and insist that addiction and tolerance inevitably occur. Ask for the sources of their information and they cite textbooks and lectures of 20 or 30 years ago. Ignorance is not limited to students; it is also found among teachers and then it is dangerous because misinformation spreads like a plague and the consequences are awful.

The International Pain Foundation, which has its origins in IASP and is now an independent fund-raising organization, has enormous potential in helping us achieve our tasks. Educational materials and their appropriate distribution, exchanges of scientists and clinicians among countries, refresher courses, audiovisual learning materials – all these things cost money. And the purpose of IPF is to raise the money to 'spread the word' – that our salvation from pain lies in better research, more enlightened therapy and educational measures that are able to bring about a revolution in the management of pain.

Every one of us must become involved in this process of educating the world. Pain is still a plague. It ruins lives, it devastates whole families. It calls for political and social action. The alarm bells went off when AIDS made its appearance. But nothing of the sort happened when Bonica and a few other prophets among us told the world that tens of millions of people are suffering terribly, that their lives and families' lives are devastated, that the cost to society is in the billions of dollars. There is money for research on cancer and neurosurgical procedures; but there is very little money for research on cancer pain and post-surgical pain.

At whom do we aim our efforts of re-education?

The answer is: at everyone – at physicians and all health-care givers, at patients, and at politicians who can help us in this battle against misinformation, ignorance and needless suffering.

We have a mission – all of us – to rectify the existing situation, for cancer pain as well as for post-surgical pain, in adults and in children, and for any kind of severe pain which can be helped by sensible administration of narcotic drugs. In addition to educating one another in current pain research and therapy, as we do at this congress, we must promote education on the treatment of pain for medical students and for physicians and nurses. We must also teach patients to communicate better about their pain, and inform them that they have a right to freedom from pain, that each suffering human being deserves the best that science has to offer. We must also get our message to those in government that pain is a major plague that saps the strength of society, that funds for research and therapy are urgently needed, that regulations regarding the supply of drugs must be modified (where necessary) to meet the needs of people in pain, not just the misdeeds of street addicts. If we can pursue these goals together – as scientists and therapists, as members of the full range of the scientific and health professions – we can hope to meet the goal we all strive for: to help our fellow human beings who suffer needless pain.

Acknowledgement

Supported by grant A7891 from the Natural Sciences and Engineering Research Council of Canada.

References

Abbott, F.V. and Melzack, R. (1983) Dissociation of the mechanisms of stimulation-produced analgesia in tests of tonic and phasic pain. In J.J. Bonica et al. (Eds.), Advances in Pain Research and Therapy, Vol. 5, Raven Press, New York, pp. 401–409.

Abbott, F.V., Franklin, K.B.J., Ludwick, R.J. and Melzack, R. (1981) Apparent lack of tolerance in the formalin test suggests difference mechanisms for morphine analgesia in different types of pain. Pharmacol. Biochem. Behav., 15: 637–640.

Abbott, F.V., Melzack, R. and Leber, B.F. (1982a) Morphine analgesia and tolerance in the tail-flick and formalin tests: dose-response relationships. Pharmacol. Biochem. Behav., 17: 1213–1219.

Abbott, F.V., Melzack, R. and Samuel, C. (1982b) Morphine analgesia in the tail-flick and formalin pain tests is mediated by different neural systems. Exp. Neurol., 75: 644–651.

Angell, M. (1982) The quality of mercy. N. Engl. J. Med., 306: 98–99.

Beyer, J., DeGood, D.E., Ashley, L.C. and Russell, G.A. (1983) Patterns of postoperative analgesic use with adults and children. Pain, 17: 71–81.

Bonica, J.J. (1980) Cancer pain. In J.J. Bonica (Ed.), Pain, Raven Press, New York, pp. 335–362.

Bonica, J.J. (1983) Current status of postoperative pain therapy. In T. Yokota and R. Dubner (Eds.), Current Topics in Pain Research and Therapy, Excerpta Medica, Amsterdam, pp. 169–189.

Choinière, M. (1988) Burn pain. In P.D. Wall and R. Melzack (Eds.), Textbook of Pain, Churchill Livingstone, Edinburgh, in press.

Cohen, S.R., Abbott, F.V. and Melzack, R. (1984) Unilateral analgesia produced by intraventricular morphine. Brain Res., 303: 277–287.

Cohen, S.R. and Melzack, R. (1985) Morphine injected into the habenula and dorsal posteromedial thalamus produces analgesia in the formalin test. Brain Res., 359: 131–139.

Cohen, S.R. and Melzack, R. (1986) Habenular stimulation produced analgesia in the formalin test. Neurosci. Lett., 70: 165–169.

Colpaert, F.C., Niemegeers, C.R.E. and Janssen, P.A.J. (1978) Nociceptive stimulation prevents development of tolerance to narcotic analgesia. Eur. J. Pharmacol., 49: 335–336.

Cousins, M.J. (1988) Acute and postoperative pain. In P.D. Wall and R. Melzack (Eds.), Textbook of Pain, Churchill Livingstone, Edinburgh, in press.

Donovan, M., Dillon, P. and McGuire, L. (1987) Incidence and characteristics of pain in a sample of medical-surgical inpatients. Pain, 30, 69–78.

Eland, J.M. and Anderson, J.E. (1977) The experience of pain in children. In A.K. Jacox (Ed.), Pain: A Sourcebook for Nurses and Other Health Professionals, Little Brown, Boston, pp. 453–473.

France, R.D., Urban, B.J. and Keefe, F.J. (1984) Long-term use of narcotic analgesics in chronic pain. Soc. Sci. Med., 19: 1379–1382.

Jeans, M.E. (1983) The measurement of pain in children. In R. Melzack (Ed.), Pain Measurement and Assessment, Raven Press, New York, pp. 183–189.

Keeri-Szanto, M. (1979) Drugs or drums: what relieves post-operative pain? Pain, 6: 217–230.

McGrath, P.J. and Unruh, A.M. (1987) Pain in Children and Adolescents, Elsevier, Amsterdam.

Medina, J.L. and Diamond, S. (1977) Drug dependency in patients with chronic headache. Headache, 17: 12–14.

Melzack, R. (1987) The Short-Form McGill Pain Questionnaire. Pain, 30:191–197.

Melzack, R., Abbott, F.V., Zackon, W., Mulder, D.S. and Davis, M.W.L. (1987) Pain on a surgical ward: a survey of the duration and intensity of pain and the effectiveness of medication. Pain, 29: 67–72.

Melzack, R., Ofiesh, J.G. and Mount, B.M. (1976) The Brompton Mixture: effects on pain in cancer patients. Canad. Med. Assoc. J., 115: 125–129.

Mitchell, S.W. (1872) Injuries of Nerves and their Consequences, Lippincott, Philadelphia.

Mount, B.M. (1976) The Palliative Care Unit as a possible solution. Canad. Med. Assoc. J., 115: 119–121.

Mount, B.M., Ajemian, I. and Scott, J.F. (1976) Use of the Brompton Mixture in treating the chronic pain of malignant disease. Canad. Med. Assoc. J., 115: 122–124.

Perry, S. and Heidrich, G. (1982) Management of pain during debridement: a survey of U.S. burn units. Pain, 13: 267–280.

Portenoy, R.K. and Foley, K.M. (1986) Chronic use of opioid analgesics in non-malignant pain: report of 38 cases. Pain, 25: 171–186.

Portenoy, R.K. and Foley, K.M. (1987) Letter to the Editor in reply to R.A. Sternbach. Pain, 29: 259–261.

Porter, J. and Jick, H. (1980) Addiction rate in patients treated with narcotics. N. Engl. J. Med., 302: 123.

Rose, H.L. (1987) Letter to the Editor re article by Portenoy and Foley. Pain, 29: 261–262.

Saunders, C.M. (1978) The Management of Terminal Disease, Edward Arnold, London.

Schecter, N.L., Allen, D.A. and Hanson, K. (1986) The status of pediatric pain control: a comparison of hospital analgesic usage in children and adults. Pediatrics, 77: 11–15.

Schweitzer, A. (1953) On the Edge of the Primeval Forest, Adam and Charles Black, London, p. 70.

Shavit, Y., Lewis, J.W., Terman, G.W., Gale, R.P. and Liebeskind, J.C. (1984) Opioid peptides mediate the suppressive effect of stress on natural killer cell cytotoxicity. Science, 223: 188–190.

Shavit, Y., Terman, G.W., Martin, F.C., Lewis, J.W., Liebeskind, J.C. and Gale, R.P. (1985) Stress, opioid peptides, the immune system, and cancer. J. Immunol., 135 Suppl., 834S–837S.

Sternbach, R.A. (1987) Letter to the Editor re article by Portenoy and Foley. Pain, 29: 257–258.

Taub, A. (1982) Opioid analgesics in the treatment of chronic intractable pain in non-neoplastic origin. In L.M. Kitahata and D. Collins (Eds.), Narcotic Analgesics in Anesthesiology, Williams and Wilkins, Baltimore.

Tennant, F.S. and Rawson, R.A. (1982) Outpatient treatment of prescription opioid dependence. Arch. Int. Med., 142: 1845–1847.

Twycross, R.G. and Lack, S.A. (1983) Symptom Control in Far-Advanced Cancer, Vol. 1, Pain Relief, Pitman Books, New York.

World Health Organization (1986) Cancer Pain Relief, World Health Organization, Geneva.

R. Dubner, G.F. Gebhart & M.R. Bond (Eds.)
Proceedings of the Vth World Congress on Pain
© 1988 Elsevier Science Publishers BV (Biomedical Division)

CHAPTER 2

The John J. Bonica Distinguished Lecture
Stability and instability of central pain mechanisms

Patrick D. Wall

Department of Anatomy, University College London, Gower Street, London WC1E 6BT, England

It is entirely natural and proper to honour Professor John J. Bonica, because he has been a teacher for all of us. It is he who has insisted from the beginning that we must study the patient and his pain and not be misled into forcing the patient to express pain in terms of an academic fantasy.

Neuroscientists are, in general, an orderly lot with a passion for classification. They, in common with the rest of mankind, are faced with a disorderly mess and wish to extract regularity from chaos by identifying classes, categories and laws of cause and effect. In attempts to identify pain mechanisms, the dorsal horn has been a particular target for classification since it is interposed between the periphery, where afferents detect noxious events, and the rest of the central nervous system, which generates reactions to noxious events.

There are many different guesses (hypotheses) as to which features are significant in linking observable properties of dorsal horn cells to pain mechanisms. These guesses in turn depend on the overall model of pain mechanisms which is favoured by the proponent. The simplest hypothesis, specificity theory, proposes that pain is the unique consequence of excitation of nociceptive afferents. If this were true and a special class of peripheral nerve fibres contained all the necessary properties for detecting all those events which result in pain, then it would be reasonable to expect that specific cells would be found in the dorsal horn. These cells would specialize in transmitting the unique infor-

mation encoded by the nociceptive afferent nerve fibres. Such a system would be the equivalent of a burglar or fire alarm. It would have a single, dedicated, hard-wired function. Its working would be independent of other functions of the overall structure. It would reliably report its activation to a central monitor (sensation). After the report, a separate process would decide on the appropriate reaction (mental perception). The proposal is simple and therefore attractive. It is the basis of the chapters on sensation and pain in the most popular textbook of neuroscience of our time (Kandel and Schwartz, 1985) and is described in the following three section headings:

Stimulus quality is encoded by a labelled line code.

Pain is mediated by nociceptors.

Primary pain afferents terminate in the dorsal horn of the spinal cord.

In only slightly more cautious terms, one of the major contributors to the subject states 'In my view, selective nocireceptive projections have much to do with both the recognition and localization of tissue-damaging stimuli as pain sensation' (Perl, 1985).

I regret that the expectation of a hard-wired, labelled line fits neither the phenomena of pain in general nor the observed facts of the dorsal horn in particular. We should therefore turn to the systems of categorization which have been used and inspect them openly for their usefulness in identifying pain mechanisms. Six systems have been used. While all have their validity and usefulness and do not contradict each other, I will propose the last as the one most likely to reveal pain mechanisms in a useful way with respect to the future.

Classification (1): cell bodies organized in laminae

An investigation of cell body size, shape, orientation and packing (Rexed, 1952) showed them to be organized in 6 laminae within the dorsal horn. There is also a cylindrical zone of cells around the central canal, lamina 10, which should be included. The two most dorsal laminae 1 and 2 make up the clear area, substantia gelatinosa.

The importance of this laminar organization has been emphasized by the discovery that the afferent fibre classes distribute themselves to fit the laminae. Of the nociceptive afferents, the small myelinated A delta afferents terminate mainly in laminae 1, 2 and 5, while the unmyelinated C afferents end mainly in laminae 1 and 2.

Physiological investigation supports the coincident laminar organization of cell bodies and afferent terminals. High concentrations of cells responding to A delta and C afferents are found in laminae 1 and 2 (Christensen and Perl, 1970; Fitzgerald and Wall, 1980; McMahon and Wall, 1983). Lamina 4 cells tend to respond to low-threshold mechanoreceptors (Wall, 1967) and lamina 5 cells respond to a wide range of low- and high-threshold mechanoreceptors. Lamina 6 cells respond to low-threshold muscle mechanoreceptors. Accompanying this dorsoventral separation of afferent terminations and physiological responses, there is a mediolateral somatotopic organization of terminals and of receptive fields (Wall, 1967). Lateral parts of the laminae receive afferents from the proximal parts of the dermatome, while the medial region receives from distal areas. A comparable organization of afferents, cells and physiological properties exists within the trigeminal nuclei (Gobel and Hockfield 1977).

Critique
The matching of afferents, cell bodies and physio-

logical responses in a laminar organization is a major discovery and simplification. However, it is crucial that the reader does not oversimplify and view the laminae as precise and stable and monopolized by single functions for the following reasons:

A. Laminae contain more than one type of cell
Within any particular lamina, cells differ in their morphology (Brown, 1981; Woolf and Fitzgerald, 1983; Egger et al., 1986; Gobel and Hockfield, 1977; Schoenen, 1982), in their chemistry, in the destination of their axons and in their physiology.

B. Laminar borders are not precise The lines drawn by Rexed (1952) were never intended to mark an abrupt change from one type of cell to another. There is a considerable overlap of cell types. Even the border of grey and white matter is not absolute. For example, many lamina 1 type neurons are found in the white matter of the dorsal columns (Fitzgerald and Woolf, 1982). Much more important than the question of cell body location is the distribution of the dendrites of these cells. It has been clear since the use of the Golgi technique by Cajal that dendritic trees spread very widely. Now, with the introduction of single-cell staining techniques, it is possible to define the full extent of dendrites in physiologically identified cells. In some lamina 1 cells, the dendrites are in a flattened disc restricted to lamina 1. However, this is a unique example and even this only applies to cat and is not seen in such cells in rat, monkey and man (Beal, 1979; Coimbra et al., 1974; Schoenen, 1982). Similarly, the staining of the full extent of the termination of single identified afferents shows many to spread widely beyond the boundaries of particular laminae (Brown, 1981; Light and Perl, 1979).

C. The inputs and the responses of cells are not fixed
See classification 6.

Classification (2): the morphology of cells

Since the time of Cajal with the Golgi technique, it has been possible to observe the entire shape of single cells. More recently it has become possible to place a microelectrode in single cells and to record their physiological function and then to fill the cell with a marker such as horseradish peroxidase (Brown, 1981). It was reasonably expected that a correlation between form and function would e-merge. While beautiful pictures appear, the expected correlation is minimal or absent.

Critique
Studies in cat dorsal horn have failed to reveal clear associations between somadendritic morphology and receptive field properties of neurons in laminae 3, 4 and 5 (Bennett et al., 1984; Maxwell et al., 1983; Brown and Fyffe, 1981; Egger et al., 1986; Ritz and Greenspan, 1985) and in rat deep dorsal horn (Renehan et al., 1986; Woolf and King, 1987). Even in the most superficial laminae no relationship was found in cat (Light and Perl, 1979) or in rat (Woolf and Fitzgerald, 1983). The only possible exception to this litany of negative results is in the identification of a single characteristically shaped interneuron in lamina 2, the islet cell (Bennett et al., 1980). Even the location of the receptive field on the skin only very roughly matches the distribution of afferent terminals and the spread of the dendrites. There are two reasons why one should not be surprised by the failure of this classification. First, synapses may be relatively ineffective (Wall, 1977). Second, the properties of a cell depend not only on its monosynaptic contacts with afferents but also on its contact with polysynaptic chains of interneurons. We know little of the details of the relevant microcircuitry within the cord.

Classification (3): the chemistry of cells

The greatest efforts are being expended at the present time on this subject. The reasons are excellent, since they offer a bridge between the older disciplines of cellular and systems biology with the tremendous analytic power of modern molecular biology. Furthermore they promise the practical consequence of a rational pharmacology able to manipulate particular functions. The particular targets have been:

(1) Classical fast transmitters (amino acids, cate-cholamines, etc.).

(2) Peptides and their precursors (substance P etc.).

(3) Enzymes, particularly those concerned with transmitters.

(4) Receptors.

(5) Surface markers.

The future of this approach is undoubtedly bright. Exciting as the results are, they have not yet led to a precise identification of pain mechanisms in chemical terms for the reasons we will now describe.

Critique
(1) The same neurotransmitters are released at synapses in systems which have entirely different functions. The specificity of the system is provided not by the synaptic transmitters but by the anatomical inputs and outputs.

(2) The peptides. *A.* We do not really know the function of any peptide in the spinal cord. The biological or pathological circumstances of their release are largely unknown. Their action, once released, on postsynaptic structures is still under investigation. There are indications that their action can be dissociated from that of the fast transmitters (Wall and Woolf, 1986). They may be responsible for the long-latency, long-duration changes of excitability which influence activity triggered by fast neurotransmitters.

B. The problems of assigning a role to any one peptide are complicated by the discovery of multiple peptides and neurotransmitters within single cells and terminals. The solution may be that their individual function will be revealed by examining their activity-dependent and target-dependent changes over periods of minutes, hours and days.

C. There have been embarrassingly simplistic and premature assignments of function to particular peptides. For example, the chain of sentences 'C fibres are pain fibres. C fibres contain substance P. Therefore substance P is the pain transmitter' collapses completely on investigation, although this does not mean that C fibres and substance P are not involved in pain mechanisms (Wall and Fitzgerald, 1982).

The most intriguing of these assignations has followed the discovery of the endogenous opioids and their receptors. It seemed reasonable to propose that the location of endogenous opiates and their receptors would label pain mechanisms. This proposal is no longer tenable and even our understanding of the role of endogenous opiates in pain control is in chaos (Woolf and Wall, 1983).

(3) Receptors. Since no clear functional labels have appeared from studies of the distribution of neurotransmitters and peptides, it might be hoped that specificity would be achieved by the discovery of a functional restricted localization of their receptors. The opposite has been the case, with receptors being very widely and diffusely distributed. Some improvement may be expected as receptors are subdivided into subclasses, as is happening with opiate and substance P receptors. One reason for the widespread distribution of receptors may be that they are not necessarily functional but are simply included innocently in the structure of cell membranes. An example might be the presence of opiate receptors on dorsal root ganglion cells which are many millimetres from the nearest synapse. Sympathetic ganglia contain GABA receptors but no known source of GABA. The presence of these ectopic receptors produces two problems of interest. First, it remains possible that, in addition to the precise synapse such as the neuromuscular junction with its controlled microcosm of source and receptor of the transmitter, there are synaptic actions at greater and greater distances from the source. The extreme of distance would be hormonal action with the substances transmitted by the blood stream, but there may be intermediate distances where substances diffuse in the extracellular space. The other problem is that if a naturally occurring compound is administered systemically or by local application, it may produce a physiological action in a location which never receives that compound from an endogenous source.

Classification (4): the destination of axons

This very logical method of subdividing cells is fully described elsewhere (Willis, 1985; Yaksh, 1986).

Critique
While there is no doubt about the factual nature of this method of subdivision and its usefulness, there are certain cautions which are necessary in correlating destination and pain mechanisms.
(1) Destination is usually interpreted as long-range destinations. However, one should remember the experiment of Schiff repeated by Basbaum (1973) in which bilateral hemisection of the cord separated by 3 segments does not abolish evoked pain behaviour. This shows that some forms of pain may be triggered by multisynaptic short axon chains of neurons when all the known long-running tracts have been cut, as emphasized by Noordenbos (1959).
(2) There has been a particular emphasis on the neospinothalamic tract as the main transmitter of pain triggering impulses. This emphasis comes from the questionable assumption that the crucial fibres cut in a ventral cordotomy are the spinothalamic tract. It ignores the chronic return of sensitivity after section (Vierck and Luck, 1979) and the disastrous effect of cutting the tract in the midbrain. It originates from the classical assumption that thalamus and cortex are the structures required for pain perception and ignores the chronic failure of surgery to eliminate pain by excisions in these areas.
(3) Many fibres branch and supply more than one destination. This is now becoming apparent with double labelling methods. For example, axons of cells in the dorsal horn destined for the dorsal column nuclei also supply the lateral cervical nucleus (Nishikawa et al., 1983; but see Brown et al., 1986) even though these are thought to be very separate functional systems.

Classification (5): the brief response of cells to brief stimuli

Microelectrode recording permits an examination of the response properties of single cells. Five classes have been described in the dorsal horn. All respond to ipsilateral natural and electrical stimuli.

(1) Low-threshold mechanoreceptive cells. These cells are found in all laminae but are concentrated particularly in lamina 4 (Wall, 1967). They are excited by A beta afferents.

(2) Thermoreceptive cells. These cells respond to warming (35–43°C) or to cooling (35–20°C). They are concentrated in lamina 1 and to a lesser extent in layers 3–5 (Price and Dubner, 1977).

(3) Movement-detection cells. These cells respond to gentle movement of joints and to stretch of muscles and to electrical stimulation of the large diameter afferents from muscle. They are found in lamina 6 and more ventrally (Wall, 1967).

(4) Nociceptive specific neurons. These cells respond only to heavy pressure and to pinch and to noxious chemicals and to heat above 45°C (Christensen and Perl, 1970; Willis, 1985; Perl, 1985). These cells have obviously received particular attention from those interested in pain mechanisms and who expect to find specific cells which would link injury to pain. They respond to electrical stimulation of A delta and C fibres and a few to C fibres only. They are found in lamina 1 and to a lesser extent in laminae 4 and 5.

A particular group of lamina 1 neurons has been intensively studied in rat (Menetrey et al., 1982; McMahon and Wall, 1983; 1984; MacMahon et al., 1984) which also exists in cat and monkey (Jones et al., 1984; 1985). 43% of such cells responded to pressure and not to smaller stimuli and 14% responded only to C-fibre stimulation. They project mainly into the contralateral dorsolateral funiculus of the spinal cord and terminate in the midbrain and thalamus.

(5) Wide-dynamic-range neurons: by far the commonest type of neuron in the dorsal horn, first described in 1960 (Wall, 1960) and subsequently by many others (see Price and Dubner, 1977; Willis and Coggeshall, 1978; Yaksh, 1986, for reviews). They respond to light brush, touch, pressure, pinch, heat and chemicals. Electrical stimulation shows that excitatory A beta, A delta and C afferents converge on them. They are the commonest cell in every lamina.

The receptive fields of these cells are highly structured (Hillman and Wall, 1969). In the centre, all types of stimuli produce excitation with a rising response as the stimulus rises. Towards the edge of the excitatory receptive field, the threshold rises and the cells respond only to intense stimuli. There is also an elaborate inhibitory component of their receptive fields which will be discussed below.

Perhaps the greatest surprise in terms of non-specificity has been the failure to discover neurons specific to visceral inputs. Cells responding to visceral stimulation have been found to have associated cutaneous receptive fields excited by myelinated afferents (Pomeranz et al., 1968; Gokin et al., 1977; Takahashi and Yokota, 1983; Cervero, 1983).

Critique

(1) Individual cells change their input-output categories

This sentence, which we will now justify, abolishes at a stroke the concept of a hard-wired, dedicated, modality-specific system. At the same time, it opens the way to questioning the circumstances under which cells change their input-output functions. The answer to that question leads to classification 6, which I support. This critique does not cast doubt on the many published observations of single cells. It proposes that they represent snapshots of cells in one of the modes of operation contained in their repertoire.

A. Comparison of individual cells in the decerebrate or spinal state   Since the time of Sherrington and Sowton (1915) it has been known that there is a steady descending barrage from the brain stem to the spinal cord. They showed that if the spinal cord is cut to prevent the descending volleys reaching the lumbar cord, there is an exaggeration of cutaneous reflexes and a decrease of proprioceptive reflexes. With the introduction of single-cell recording (Kolmodin, 1957) and of reversible blocks to the cord (Wall, 1967), this phenomenon has been repeatedly examined.

Lamina 1 cells include a particularly high proportion of nociceptive-specific cells (Christensen and Perl, 1970; McMahon and Wall, 1983). However, the modality of a particular cell depends crucially on the circumstances under which it is observed. The overall tonic effect of blocking descending impulses is to decrease the excitability of such cells. A cell which is a wide-dynamic-range cell in the decerebrate state becomes nociceptive-specific with a small receptive field in the spinal state. Lamina 3–5 cells have their cutaneous input affected in the opposite direction from lamina 1 cells, i.e., they are continuously inhibited in the decerebrate state (Wall, 1967; Hillman and Wall, 1969). Lamina 5 wide-dynamic-range cells have small excitatory receptive fields with a marked inhibitory surround in the decerebrate state. This inhibitory surround extends over the entire animal and is the basis of the diffuse noxious inhibitory control DNIC (Le Bars et al., 1979). When the cord is blocked, excitability rises, receptive fields expand and inhibition is markedly weakened. This effect is so profound that bradykinin, a powerful pain-producing substance, has no effect on these cells in their decerebrate state but produces intense excitation in the spinal state. Lamina 6 cells show particularly dramatic shifts of modality in the two states. They are dominated by muscle stretch afferents in the decerebrate and by cutaneous afferents in the spinal state.

B. A comparison of cells in the presence and absence of anaesthetics The dorsal horn of the freely moving animal is characterized by a high degree of inhibition (Wall et al., 1967). Light anaesthesia can decrease some of this inhibition so that nociceptive-specific cells become wide-dynamic-range cells (Collins and Ren, 1987). Further anaesthesia may again decrease the effective input so that cells which are wide-dynamic-range under light anaesthesia be-

come nociceptor-specific under conditions of medium anaesthesia (Dickhaus et al., 1985).

C. Effect of attenuation and training Cells have been studied in the medullary dorsal horn of awake performing monkeys following stimuli to the face (Hoffman et al., 1981; Dubner et al., 1981). The responses of these cells change radically depending on the state of alertness and the area of the face to which attention is directed. Most dramatically, when the animal is fully trained, cells respond not only to their cutaneous receptive field but also to the visual alerting stimulus and again preceding the motor response to achieve reward.

(2) Painful behaviour fails to relate to the discharge of nociceptive specific cells
Even if we accept this type of classification, at face value, the prediction of the classical school (Perl, 1985) that nociceptive specific cell discharge relates to the sensation of pain is not supported by observation. Price (1986) summarizes the considerable evidence which he and others have collected to show that wide-dynamic-range cell discharges in man and animals appear to be the input signal associated with pain. Using quite different reasons, Le Bars et al. (1986) come to the same conclusions. The most direct evidence comes from Bushnell et al. (1984), who show that monkey nociceptive-specific cells are too insensitive to explain aversive behaviour to high-temperature stimuli, while wide-dynamic-range neurons show a well-correlated change of discharge which relates to behaviour.

Classification (6): contingent classification dependent on context

The reasons for this classification are:
(1) There is no fixed relationship between excitation of particular afferent categories and the sensory or behavioural outcome (Wall and McMahon, 1985).
(2) There is no fixed relationship between the input and output of individual dorsal horn cells (see critique of classification 5).

These two strong and negative statements demand the creation of an ordered input-output scheme even though the order changes with time and with the situation. Such a scheme recognizes the inherent plasticity of the adult nervous system, which is a crucial aspect of pain mechanisms. The variation of the painful response to injury is not random nor is it to be attributed only to mental processes. The arrival of an afferent barrage in the dorsal horn is followed by the processing of the new information by dorsal horn cells in the context of other inputs from the periphery and from the brain. These different ways of processing the same information change in at least three different time epochs.

(1) Rapid (milliseconds–seconds) Gate Control.

(2) Slow (minutes–hours) Sensitivity Control.

(3) Prolonged (days–months) Connectivity Control.

These three time epochs of change should be considered in relation to three phases of pain mechanisms.

(1) The highly variable relationship of injury to pain at the time of injury depending on other events in progress and on the set of the central nervous system.

(2) The spreading tenderness, hyperalgesia, allodynia and reorganized reflex and motor patterns which develop slowly after injury.

(3) The chronic changes of sensitivity particularly apparent after peripheral nerve and root damage.

We will now examine the contingent changes in the response of dorsal horn cells at various times after injury, remembering that these cells are only the beginning of chains of neurons leading to overall response patterns and that modulations must certainly occur at each of the subsequent stages.

(1) Rapid control: Gate Control

A. By peripheral inputs

(1) Inhibition. Coincident activation of large diameter low-threshold mechanoreceptors inhibits the response of all dorsal horn cells to nociceptive inputs. This discovery (Wall and Cronly-Dillon, 1960) has been investigated repeatedly (see Willis and Coggeshall, 1979; Yaksh, 1986, for review). It

led to the introduction of transcutaneous electrical nerve stimulation, TENS (Wall and Sweet, 1967) and to dorsal column stimulation, since the antidromic activation of these fibres in the dorsal columns produces the same dorsal horn inhibition as is produced by peripheral stimulation (Hillman and Wall, 1969). Part of the inhibition is presynaptic (Wall, 1964) and part postsynaptic (Hongo et al., 1968). The pharmacology of this effect has been studied (Yaksh, 1986).

Distant intense stimulation inhibits the response of wide-dynamic-range cells to local noxious inputs (Le Bars et al., 1979). Part of this DNIC inhibition is produced by a loop circuit to the brain stem and back to the cord (Le Bars et al., 1979) and part by local segmental inhibitory mechanisms (Fitzgerald, 1982).

(2) Facilitation. Activation of high-threshold afferents is followed by facilitation or wind-up (Mendell, 1966; Mendell and Wall, 1965). This rapid-onset facilitation is followed by a longer-latency facilitation (Woolf, 1983), to be discussed below.

B. By descending control

In the decerebrate animal, a tonic barrage descends from the brain stem which facilitates nociceptive responses in lamina 1 cell (McMahon and Wall, 1988) and inhibits nociceptive responses in deeper cells (Wall, 1967; Hillman and Wall, 1969). The nature and origin of these descending inhibitory controls have been extensively studied (Willis, 1985; Yaksh, 1986). They form the basis of some aspects of stimulation-induced analgesia and of narcotic analgesia.

(2) Slow sensitivity control

A. By peripheral inputs

When C fibres from muscle and joint are stimulated, 1 Hz, 20 s, in the decerebrate spinal rat there is a fast rise of excitability in the spinal cord which drops by 5 min followed by a second rise which lasts over 1 h (Wall and Woolf, 1984). When C fibers from skin are stimulated only the early 5 min excitation occurs. The long-latency, long-duration facilitation affects cells in lamina 1 and in the deeper laminae (Cook et al., 1987). It produces a very large expansion of receptive fields and can convert nociceptive-specific cells to cells which respond to light stimulation as well as to intense stimuli (Cook et al., 1987). It affects cells with receptive fields distant from the area subserved by the stimulated nerve. The facilitation is triggered by the arrival of impulses in C fibres from deep tissue but it is sustained by an intrinsic spinal cord process (Woolf and Wall, 1986b). C fibres which have been chronically cut in the periphery change their peptide content but, while they are still able to excite dorsal horn cells rapidly, they are no longer able to evoke the prolonged facilitation (Wall and Woolf, 1986). This result shows that the transmitters for rapid excitation differ from those responsible for the long-lasting effects. Peptides may be the compounds responsible for the prolonged changes, a suggestion reinforced by the sensitivity of the facilitation to peptides. The prolonged facilitation is increased by the local application of substance P and CGRP (Woolf and Wiesenfeld-Hallin, 1986) and abolished by narcotics (Woolf and Wall, 1986a). The entire phenomenon is very reminiscent of the widespreading slow-onset tenderness which spreads far beyond the region of a deep injury.

B. By descending systems

The action of descending systems on dorsal horn cells has been extensively studied. It has been common for physiologists to examine cells for only a few hundred milliseconds after the arrival of an input. However, it now becomes apparent that after this classical period, there may by very prolonged changes which have been missed in the usual method of study. For example, lamina 1 cells are commonly briefly inhibited for 1–200 ms by activation of descending volleys in the dorsolateral funiculus. However, if no further stimuli are given, it is observed that many cells become markedly facilitated with a large expansion of their receptive fields and a movement away from being nociceptive-specific to responding to light stimuli (McMahon and Wall, 1988).

In summary, it is evident that the arrival in the dorsal horn of afferent volleys or of descending volleys can trigger very prolonged changes of receptive field and modality by mechanisms which differ from the fast inhibitions and excitations which have been the subject of most studies.

(3) Prolonged connectivity control

A. By peripheral inputs

When peripheral nerves are cut and, even more strikingly, if roots are cut, a cascade of slow changes sweeps centrally from the lesion and involves the cells on which the afferents terminate. The immediate effect of cutting afferents is obviously to abolish the receptive fields of cells which are normally excited by the cut afferents (Devor and Wall, 1978, 1981, Hylden et al., 1987; Wall and Devor, 1981). After some days, there is a collapse of the presynaptic and postsynaptic inhibitory mechanisms associated with the deafferented cells. There is a resulting marked rise in the excitability of the cells. For some cells, this increased excitability is sufficient for them to begin to respond to afferents which were previously ineffective. The result is that the cells adopt a new receptive field activated by the nearest intact afferents. The appearance of new receptive fields in deafferented cells has been seen in lamina 1 and in deeper cells in the dorsal horn and in the trigeminal nuclei and the dorsal column nuclei. It is therefore inevitable that such changes are found in thalamus and cortex, which are supplied by the cells with new receptive fields.

The mechanism by which the slow changes are triggered is not dependent on nerve impulses, since they are not produced by prolonged block of afferents by TTX (Wall et al., 1982b). A change in transported chemical substances is therefore likely. A continuous supply of nerve growth factor prevents many of the changes from occurring (Fitzgerald et al., 1985). The C-fibre afferents are suspected of being particularly important in producing the central effects, since most of them occur if only the C fibres in a peripheral nerve are affected by capsaicin poisoning (Wall et al., 1982a). The signal which produces the central changes is subtle and is not simply dependent on the contact of the afferents with the target tissue. For example, crush lesions of peripheral nerves do not produce the central effects produced by nerve section (Devor and Wall, 1981). Furthermore the peptide content of C fibres depends on the target tissue they contact, as shown by cross-anastomosis experiments (McMahon and Gibson, unpublished observations). The prolonged central effects of stimulation of C fibres similarly depends on the tissue from which the afferents originate and change appropriately if peripheral nerves are cross-anastomosed from skin to muscle and vice versa.

B. By descending systems

Since the discovery of slow central changes induced by peripheral lesions is relatively recent, work on the effect of descending controls on this plasticity is only beginning. If the feet of rats are made anaesthetic by section and ligation of the sciatic and saphenous nerves, the rats begin to attack the anaesthetic foot after a delay of some three weeks (Wall et al., 1979). However, if the dorsolateral funiculus of the spinal cord on the opposite side to the sectioned nerves has been cut, the attack begins in some three days. The acceleration of the attack, autotomy, also occurs if the tract has been cut ipsilateral to the sectioned nerves. The probable significance of this release phenomenon is that the contralateral funiculus contains the ascending fibres from lamina 1 and the ipsilateral tract contains the bulk of the descending inhibitory controls. The effect of cutting either side of this loop may be to abolish the ability of the animal to control the tendency of the deafferented segments to become hyperexcitable.

Consequences

It is obvious that the discovery of at least three classes of control system which profoundly change the response of dorsal horn cells abolishes the validity of the classical expectation of hard-wired dedicated systems monopolized in the service of a single sen-

sation. It means that it is no longer sufficient to define the stimulus. It means that it is also necessary to define the setting of the central nervous system which receives the afferent volley generated by the stimulus.

The 'normal' setting Trained human subjects are in a similar setting to trained monkeys (Dubner et al., 1981). They have had considerable experience of the stimulus and the situation and know that, far from being damaged by the stimulus, they will be rewarded for responding to it. We know that the monkey dorsal horn cells have adopted a firing pattern peculiar and specific to the situation as well as to the stimulus. There is no reason to doubt that the same applies in the human cord. The animal has the neural equipment to change its dorsal horn cells as well as most other parts of its nervous system to respond appropriately to the situation. It is therefore to be expected that the response of dorsal horn cells to noxious stimuli will differ in standard physiological preparations whether they are lightly or deeply anaesthetized or decerebrate or spinal or even in vitro. The observations in the various situations are all 'correct' and are not contradictory. In these preparations, the physiologist records a fraction of the repertoire through which the cell can move under various biological behavioural circumstances. The repertoire is not infinite and, in that sense, a particular cell is limited to a range of input-output functions. It can be locked into one mode of its repertoire and made to appear specific by locking the setting. That may be real science but it is not real life.

The pathological setting The classical assumption has been that pain would only continue so long as there was a continuous source of nociceptive impulses in the periphery. With the discovery of at least three different types of central control system, it is necessary to consider the possibility that peripheral pathology could trigger an abnormal resetting of the central controls so that pain persists after the original peripheral signal has ceased. In this situation, the source of the pain would have migrated from the periphery to the central nervous system. The original trigger could be the injury discharge itself or the chemical change induced in the afferent fibres. We have shown that afferent barrages in unmyelinated afferents from deep tissue can trigger very prolonged increases of excitability of dorsal horn cells. This could be the basis of the widespread prolonged tenderness which follows lesions to deep tissue. It is not known whether these abnormal excitabilities simply drift back to their normal setting or whether there are active central processes which force the setting back toward normal. The answers to these questions have considerable therapeutic importance. Peripheral nerve and dorsal root lesions, by way of transport mechanisms, unmask normally ineffective central circuits with a loss of inhibition. This mechanism appears the most likely basis for the deafferentation pains. It is clearly of the greatest therapeutic importance to identify the abnormal chemistry which is responsible for the switching.

Idiopathic setting We have stressed the existence of powerful and elaborate control systems at each synaptic region. The best-known biological controls are homeostatic. The deafferentation syndromes could be described in terms of the reaction of a homeostatic regulation. In the normal state, the system receives an input and regulates the output. If the input fails, the regulatory controls move the system into a state of maximal amplification. We are familiar with a number of neurally operated control systems which regulate the steady states of blood pressure, temperature, appetite, etc., by generating an appropriate output for variable inputs. However, we also know that, for each of these systems, there are rare idiopathic diseases in which the system moves to some grossly pathological set point. If that occurs in these controlled systems and if pain mechanisms operate on the same general principles, we may ask the question 'Are there examples of idiopathic disease related to pain where the central controls move to some grossly abnormal set point?' Such diseases might be particularly likely when the control systems are powerful and when in normal circumstances they move the system to its extreme. The spectacular analgesia which can occur in emergencies and widespread allodynia and hyperalgesia where innocuous stimuli to undamaged stimuli produce pain are examples of the power of the central control systems. An obvious possible candidate for an idiopathic setting of control systems is congenital analgesia with no associated morphological abnormality. But are there conditions in which the system moves into a state of maximal amplification? In trigeminal neuralgia and in migraine, there is no evidence in most cases for any morphological abnormality or for any abnormal input. It may be reasonable to propose that control systems within small areas of the trigeminal nuclei have drifted to such a state of enhancement that activity commences and that innocuous stimuli to normal peripheral tissue are grossly amplified by the abnormal setting of trigeminal control systems. These are speculations but it is certain that we must consider the lability of central transmission pathways as well as seeking peripheral pathology in all painful conditions.

References

Basbaum, A.I. (1973) Conduction of the effects of noxious stimulation of short fibre systems in the spinal cord of rat. Exp. Neurol., 40: 699–716.

Beal, J.A. (1979) The ventral dendritic arbor of marginal (lamina I) neurons in the adult primate spinal cord. Neurosci. Lett., 14: 201–206.

Bennett, G.J., Abdelmoumene, M., Hayashi, H. and Dubner, R. (1980) Physiology and morphology of substantia gelatinosa neurons intracellularly stained with horseradish peroxidase. J. Comp. Neurol., 194: 809–827.

Bennett, G.J., Nishikawa, N., Lu, G.U., Hoffert, M.J. and Dubner, R. (1984) The morphology of dorsal column postsynaptic spinomedullary neurons in the cat. J. Comp. Neurol., 224: 568–578.

Brown, A.G. (1981) Organization in the Spinal Cord, Springer Verlag, Berlin.

Brown, A.G. and Fyffe, R.E.W. (1981) Form and function of dorsal horn neurons with axons ascending the dorsal columns in the cat. J. Physiol., 381: 333–349.

Brown, A.G., Noble, R. and Riddell, J.S. (1986) Relations between spinocervical and post-synaptic dorsal column neurones in the cat. J. Physiol., 381: 333–349.

Bushnell, M.C., Duncan, G.H., Dubner, R. and Lian Fang He, J. (1984) Activity of trigeminothalamic neurons in medullary dorsal horn of awake monkeys trained in a thermal discrimination task. J. Neurophysiol., 52: 170–187.

Cervero, F. (1983) Somatic and visceral inputs to the thoracic spinal cord of the cat. J. Physiol., 337: 51–67.

Christensen, B.N. and Perl, E.R. (1970) Spinal neurons specifically excited by noxious or thermal stimuli: marginal zone of the dorsal horn. J. Neurophysiol., 33: 293–307.

Coimbra, A., Sodre-Borges, B.P. and Magahaed, M.M. (1974) SG of the rat: fine structure cytochemistry and changes after dorsal root section. J. Neurocytol., 3: 199–217.

Collins, J.G. and Ren, K. (1987) WDR response profiles of spinal dorsal horn neurons may be unmasked by barbiturate anaesthesia. Pain, 28: 369–378.

Cook, A.J., Woolf, C.J., Wall, P.D. and McMahon, S.B. (1987) Dynamic receptive field plasticity in rat spinal cord dorsal horn following C-primary afferent input. Nature, 325: 151–153.

Devor, M. and Wall, P.D. (1978) Reorganisation of spinal cord sensory map after peripheral nerve injury. Nature, 275: 75–76.

Devor, M. and Wall, P.D. (1981) The effect of peripheral nerve injury on receptive fields of cells in the cat spinal cord. J. Comp. Neurol., 199: 277–291.

Dickhaus, H., Pauser, G. and Zimmerman, M. (1985) Tonic descending inhibition affects intensity coding of nociceptive responses in spinal dorsal horn neurones in the cat. Pain, 23: 145–158.

Dubner, R., Hoffman, D.S. and Hayes, R.L. (1981) Neuronal activity in medullary dorsal horn of awake monkeys trained in a thermal dicrimination task. III. Task-related responses and their functional role. J. Neurophysiol., 46: 444–464.

Egger, M.D., Freeman, N.C.G., Jacquin, M., Proshansky, E. and Semba, K. (1986) Dorsal horn cells in the cat responding to stimulation of the plantar cushion. Brain Res., 383: 68–82.

Fitzgerald, M. (1982) The contralateral input to the dorsal horn of the spinal cord in the decerebrate spinal rat. Brain Res., 236: 275–287.

Fitzgerald, M. and Wall, P.D. (1980) The laminar organization of dorsal horn cells responding to peripheral C fibre stimulation. Exp. Brain Res., 41: 36–44.

Fitzgerald, M., Wall, P.D., Goedert, M. and Emson, P.C. (1985) Nerve growth factor counteracts the neurophysiological and neurochemical effects of chronic sciatic nerve injury. Brain Res., 232: 131–141.

Gobel, S. and Hockfield, S. (1977) An anatomical analysis of the synaptic circuitry of layers I, II and III of trigeminal nucleus caudalis in the cat. In D.J. Anderson, and B. Matthews (Eds.), Pain in the Trigeminal Region, Elsevier, Amsterdam, pp. 203–211.

Gokin, A.P., Kostyuk, P.G. and Preobrazhensky, N.N. (1977) Neuronal mechanisms of interactions of high threshold visceral and somatic afferent influences in spinal cord and medulla. J. Physiol. (Paris), 73: 319–333.

Hillman, P. and Wall, P.D. (1969) Inhibitory and excitatory factors controlling lamina 5 cells. Exp. Brain Res., 9: 284–306.

Hoffman, D.S., Dubner, R., Hayes, R.L. and Medlin, T. (1981) Neuronal activity in medullary dorsal horn of awake monkeys trained in a thermal discrimination task. I. Responses to innocuous and noxious thermal stimuli. J. Neurophysiol., 46: 409–427.

Hongo, T., Jankowska, E. and Lundberg, A. (1968) Postsynaptic excitation and inhibition from primary afferents in neurons of the spinocervical tract. J. Physiol., 199: 569–592.

Hylden, J.L.K., Nahin, R.L. and Dubner, R. (1987) Altered responses of nociceptive cat lamina I spinal dorsal horn neurons after chronic sciatic neuroma formation. Brain Res., 411: 341–350.

Jones, M.W., Hodge, C.J., Apkorian, A.V. and Stevens, R.T. (1985a) A dorsolateral spinothalamic pathway in the cat. Brain Res., 335: 188–193.

Jones, M.W., Apkorian, A.V., Stevens, R.T. and Hodge, C.J. (1985b) A dorsolateral spinothalamic pathway. Soc. Neurosci. Abstr., 11: 577.

Kandel, E.R. and Schwartz, J.H. (1985) Principles of Neural Science, 2nd edn., Elsevier, New York.

Kolmodin, G.M. (1957) Integrative processes in single spinal interneurons with proprioceptive connections. Acta Physiol. Scand., 40 Suppl. 139: 1–89.

Le Bars, D., Dickenson, A.H. and Besson, J.M. (1979) Diffuse noxious inhibitory controls DNIC. Effects on dorsal horn convergent neurones in the rat. Pain, 6: 283–304.

Light, A.R. and Perl, E.R. (1979) Spinal terminations of functionally identified primary afferent neurons with slowly conducting myelinated fibres. J. Comp. Neurol., 186: 133–150.

Maxwell, D.J., Fyffe, R.E.W. and Rethelyi, M. (1983) Morphological properties of physiologically identified lamina 3 neurons in the cat spinal cord. Neuroscience, 10: 1–22.

McMahon, S.B. and Wall, P.D. (1983) A system of rat spinal cord lamina 1 cells projecting through the contralateral dorsolateral funiculus. J. Comp. Neurol., 214: 217–223.

McMahon, S.B. and Wall, P.D. (1984) Receptive fields of rat lamina I projection cells move to incorporate a nearby region of injury. Pain, 19: 235–247.

McMahon, S.B. and Wall, P.D. (1988) Descending inhibition and excitation of spinal cord lamina I projection neurones. J. Neurophysiol., in press.

McMahon, S.B., Wall, P.D., Granum, S. and Webster, K.E. (1984) The chronic effects of capsaicin applied to peripheral nerves on responses of a group of lamina I cells in rats. J. Comp. Neurol., 227: 393–400.

Mendell, L.M. (1966) Physiological properties of unmyelinated fibre projection to the spinal cord. Exp. Neurol., 16: 316–332.

Mendell, L.M. and Wall, P.D. (1965) Responses of single dorsal cord cells to peripheral cutaneous unmyelinated fibres. Nature, 206: 97–99.

Menetery, D., Chaouch, A., Binder, D. and Besson, J.M. (1982) The origin of the spinomesencephalic tract in the rat: an anatomical study using the retrograde transport of horseradish peroxidase. J. Comp. Neurol., 206: 193–207.

Nishikawa, N., Bennett, G.J., Ruda, M.A., Lu, G.W. and Dubner, R. (1983) Serotoninergic innervation of dorsal column postsynaptic neurons in the cat and monkey. Neuroscience, 10: 1333–1340.

Noordenbos, W. (1959) Pain, Elsevier/North-Holland, Amsterdam.

Perl, E.R. (1985) Unravelling the story of pain. In H.L. Fields et al. (Eds.), Advances in Pain Research and Therapy, Vol. 9, Raven Press, New York.

Pomeranz, B., Wall, P.D. and Weber, W.V. (1968) Cord cells responding to fine myelinated afferents from viscera, muscle and skin. J. Physiol., 199: 511–532.

Price, D.D. (1986) The question of how the dorsal horn encodes sensory information. In T.H. Yaksh (Ed.), Spinal Afferent Processing, Plenum, New York, pp. 445–468.

Price, D.D. and Dubner, R. (1977) Neurons that subserve the sensory-discriminative aspects of pain. Pain, 3: 307–338.

Price, D.D., Dubner, R. and Hu, J.W. (1976) Trigeminothalamic neurons in nucleus caudalis responsive to tactile thermal and nociceptive stimulation of monkey's face. J. Neurophysiol., 39: 936–953.

Renehan, W.E., Jacquin, M.F., Mooney, R.D. and Rhoades, R.W. (1986) Structure function relationships in rat medullary and cervical dorsal horns. J. Neurophysiol., 55: 1187–1201.

Rexed, B. (1952) The cytoarchitectonic organization of the spinal cord in the cat. J. Comp. Neurol., 96: 415–495.

Ritz, L.A. and Greenspan, J.D. (1985) Morphological features of lamina 5 neurons receiving nociceptive input in cat sacrocaudal spinal cord. J. Comp. Neurol., 238: 440–452.

Schoenen, J. (1982) The dendritic organization of the human spinal cord in the dorsal horn. Neuroscience, 7: 2057–2088.

Sherrington, C.S. and Sowton, S.C.M. (1915) Observations on reflex responses to single break shocks. J. Physiol., 49: 331–343.

Takahashi, M. and Yokota, T. (1983) Convergence of cardiac and cutaneous afferents onto neurons in the dorsal horn of cat spinal cord. Neurosci. Lett., 38: 251–256.

Vierck, C.J. and Luck, M.M. (1979) Loss and recovery of reactivity to noxious stimuli in monkeys with primary spinothalamic cordotomies. Brain, 102: 233–248.

Wall, P.D. (1964) Presynaptic control of impulses at the first central synapse in the cutaneous pathway. In Physiology of spinal neurons, Progress in Brain Research, Vol 12, Elsevier, Amsterdam, pp. 92–118.

Wall, P.D. (1967) The laminar organization of dorsal horn and effects of descending impulses. J. Physiol., 188: 403–423.

Wall, P.D. (1977) The presence of ineffective synapses and the circumstances which unmask them. Phil. Trans. R. Soc. Lond. B, 278: 361–372.

Wall, P.D. and Cronly Dillon, J.R. (1960) Pain, itch and vibration. Arch. Neurol., 2: 365–375.

Wall, P.D. and Devor, M. (1981) The effect on peripheral nerve injury on dorsal root potentials and on transmission of afferent signals into the spinal cord. Brain Res., 209: 95–111.

Wall, P.D. and Fitzgerald, M. (1982) If substance P fails to fulfill the criteria as a neurotransmitter in somatosensory afferents, what might be its function? In: Substance P in the nervous system, CIBA Foundation Symposium 91. Pitman, London.

Wall, P.D. and McMahon, S.B. (1985) Microneuronography and its relation to perceived sensation. Pain, 21: 209–229.

Wall, P.D. and Sweet, W.H. (1967) Temporary abolition of pain in man. Science, 155: 108–109.

Wall, P.D. and Woolf, C.J. (1984) Muscle but not cutaneous C-afferent input produces prolonged increases in the excitability of the flexion reflex in the rat. J. Physiol., 356: 443–458.

Wall, P.D. and Woolf, C.J. (1985) The brief and the prolonged facilitatory effects of unmyelinated afferent input on the rat spinal cord are independently influenced by peripheral nerve injury. Neuroscience, 17: 1199–1206.

Wall, P.D., Freeman, J. and Major, D. (1967) Dorsal horn cells in spinal and in freely moving rats. Exp. Neurol., 19: 519–529.

Wall, P.D., Devor, M., Inbal, R., Scadding, J.W. Schonfeld, D., Seltzer, Z. and Tomkiewicz, M.M. (1979) Autotomy following peripheral nerve lesions; experimental anaesthesia dolorosa. Pain, 7: 103–113.

Wall, P.D., Fitzgerald, M. and Woolf C.J. (1982a) Effects of capsaicin on receptive fields and on inhibitions in rat spinal cord. Exp. Neurol., 78: 425–436.

Wall, P.D., Mills, R., Fitzgerald, M. and Gibson, S.J. (1982b) Chronic blockade of sciatic nerve transmission by tetrodotoxin does not produce central changes in the dorsal horn of the spinal cord of the rat. Neurosci. Lett., 30: 315–320.

Willis, W.D. (1985) The Pain System. In: Pain and Headache, Vol. 8, Karger, Basel.

Willis, W.D. and Coggeshall, R.E. (1978) Sensory Mechanisms in the Spinal Cord, Plenum, New York.

Woolf, C.J. (1983) Evidence for a central component of post-injury pain hypersensitivity. Nature, 306: 686–688.

Woolf, C.J. and Fitzgerald, M. (1983) The properties of neurons recorded in the superficial dorsal horn in the rat spinal cord. J. Comp. Neurol., 221: 313–328.

Woolf, C.J. and King, A.E. (1987) Physiology and morphology of multireceptive neurons with C-afferent fibre inputs in the deep dorsal horn of the rat lumbar spinal cord. J. Neurophysiol. 58.

Woolf, C.J. and Wall, P.D. (1983) Endogenous opioid peptides and pain mechanisms: a complex relationship. Nature, 306: 739–740.

Woolf, C.J. and Wall, P.D. (1986a) Morphine-sensitive and morphine-insensitive actions of C-fibre input on the rat spinal cord. Neurosci. Lett., 64: 221–225.

Woolf, C.J. and Wall, P.D. (1986b) The relative effectiveness of C-primary afferents of different origins in evoking a prolonged facilitation on the flexor reflex in the rat. J. Neurosci., 6: 1433–1442.

Woolf, C.J. and Wiesenfeld-Hallin, Z. (1986) Substance P and CGRP synergistically modulate the gain of the nociceptive flexor reflex in the rat. Neurosci. Lett., 66: 226–230.

Yaksh, T.L. (1986) Spinal Afferent Processing, Plenum, New York.

R. Dubner, G.F. Gebhart & M.R. Bond (Eds.)
Proceedings of the Vth World Congress on Pain
© 1988 Elsevier Science Publishers BV (Biomedical Division)

CHAPTER 3

Pain and suffering in art

Paolo Procacci

Cattedra di Terapia Medica Sistematica, Servizio di Algologia, Università di Firenze, Viale G.B. Morgagni 85, 50134 Firenze, Italy

When we consider the expressions of pain and suffering in figurative art, first of all we must observe that in many cases it is difficult to distinguish the physical pain from the psychic pain. The two conditions, always intertwined in life, are often joined in art, defined as fantastic intuition. Pain itself is often only one expression of the different passions of the soul. It is intermingled, as we shall see, with fear, desperation, anxiety.

In the history of art, there are periods in which these different expressions (happiness, pain, fear and so on) are well represented. In other periods man is represented without any passion in a more or less abstract manner. Of course, the abstraction is related to a different perception of the world (*Weltanschauung*), as we can see in Egyptian art, in old Chinese art and in Byzantine art.

If we consider Egyptian art and classical Greek art of the fifth and fourth centuries B.C., we do not find expressions of pain even when pain is surely present, for example in a wound on the field of battle. This is true also for the Etruscan art of this period, which is in part related to Greek art and also to the Punic art of Carthage, a city that had many political, religious and artistic relationships with the Etruscans. However, we must remember that in late Etruscan art we find different expressions which pass in Roman art with the beginning of true portraiture in sculpture.

When we come to Hellenistic art, developed initially in the great School of Pergamum and later in the rest of the Hellenistic world, the passions of the soul are often present. This period has been called 'the Baroque of Greek art', making a comparison between Renaissance art and Baroque art. The first typical example of pain and suffering is the '*Galata moriens*' (Galatian warrior dying), a Roman copy of a bronze statue placed on the acropolis of Pergamum in honor of Attalus I to celebrate his victory over the Galatians. In the marble, now in the Muse-

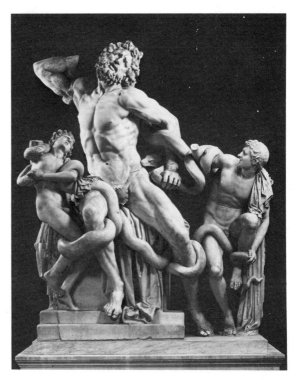

Fig. 1. Unknown artist (School of Rhodes): *The Laocoon*.

um Capitolinum in Rome, the face of the warrior shows an intense expression of pain. Of the same period is the marble representing Hercules killing the centaur Nessus, in which again physical pain is expressed in the face of the centaur. Two centuries later, we have the famous Laocoon (Fig. 1), an original Greek marble of the School of Rhodes, found in good condition during the Renaissance, in 1506, in the ruins of Nero's Domus Aurea. Here the suffering of Laocoon and of the two sons is complex: physical pain, fear, impotence, desperation. In Roman times and in the Renaissance this group was admired by all artists: a famous copy by Baccio Bandinelli is in the Uffizi Gallery in Florence. In modern times some scholars have found an excess of emphasis in this work.

In Roman art, both styles, that of man devoid of passion and also that of the true portrait of the face and of the body, are present and intermingle. The first style is found in many of the copies of classical Greek statues and is present in Roman art both in the classical period (*Ara pacis Augustae*) and during the period of the Emperor Adrian (second century A.D.). The second style, in which passions are represented, is found above all in marble portraits from the Republican period through to the second century A.D. Their derivation from Etruscan and Hellenistic art is evident. We have not found in this period a true expression of pain and suffering. In late Roman art, from Constantine to the fall of the Western Empire (476 A.D.), we can see a return to the schematization of the face and of the body without the expression shown in the classical Roman period. The fragments of the statues and the mosaics of that time are a proof of this return to an abstract approach to art.

In Byzantine art, the absolute schematization of man and absence of any expression of pain and suffering is the rule. This attitude lasts for nearly one thousand years. The first representations of the Crucifixion, painted in different parts of Europe, represent the '*Christus vivens*' (Christ living), without any expression of suffering. The turning point is in the Romanesque sculptures of Italy and of the South of France and even more so in Gothic art

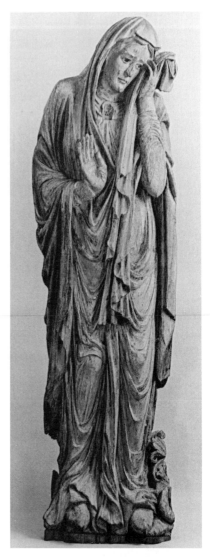

Fig. 2. Unknown artist: The Virgin in the group of *the Triumph of the Cross* of Naumburg.

from all over Europe. Christ is represented as suffering ('*Christus patiens*'): the Crucifix of Cimabue is the best example of this trend. At the same time, in Germany, a great unknown artist shows an intense suffering in the figure of the Virgin in the group of the 'Triumph of the Cross' in Naumburg (Fig. 2). This trend is fully developed in Giotto's frescos e.g., the pain of the Passion and other events. The death of Saint Francis, painted by Giotto in the Basilica of Santa Croce in Florence,

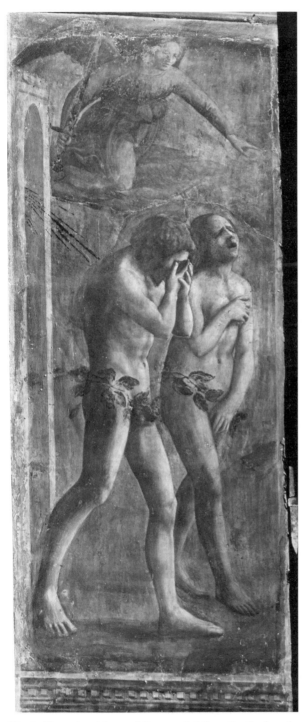

is a fully represented expression of suffering and desperation. Giotto's followers in Italy and the Gothic School in Europe attempted to represent suffering and pain: the most classical examples are the Universal Judgements in which the damned are represented suffering the tortures of the devils.

The Renaissance period begins with one of the most tragic expressions of suffering: Masaccio's fresco of Adam and Eve expelled from the Garden of Eden (Fig. 3). In sculpture, Niccolò dall'Arca shows the intense desperation and suffering of the Holy Women of Christ.

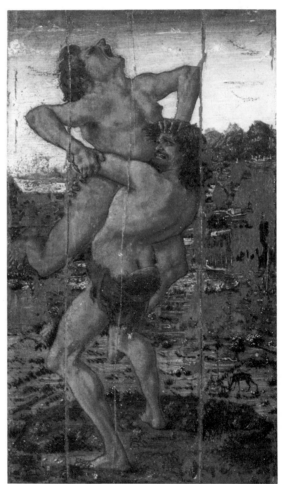

Fig. 3. Masaccio: *Adam and Eve expelled from the Garden of Eden.*

Fig. 4. Antonio del Pollaiolo: *Hercules killing Anteus.*

For about one thousand years art in the West was devoted only to religious themes. In Florence, at the time of the first Medici, from Cosimo to Laurent the Magnificent, we have a return to non-religious themes, generally inspired by classical mythology, as in the Birth of Venus and in Pallas and the Centaur of Botticelli.

In this period we have a marvellous representation of true physical pain in 'Hercules killing Anteus' by Antonio del Pollaiolo (Fig. 4): the expression of Anteus, constricted by the strong arms of Hercules, is really a vivid portrayal of intense suffering.

Proceeding on through the Renaissance, we come to the great German artist, Dürer. The famous drawing in which he indicates his left hypochondrium as the site of his pain in a letter sent to his physician is the first anatomical representation of pain. Recently, some authors have suggested that, rather than true pain, Dürer was indicating a state of melancholia or hypochondria.

An extremely interesting piece of German sculpture is the wooden statue of Christ suffering by Hans Leinberger (ca. 1530), now in the Dahlem Museum in Berlin (Fig. 5). In the representation of intense pain we can see the synthesis of the experience of German and Italian art of the first Renaissance.

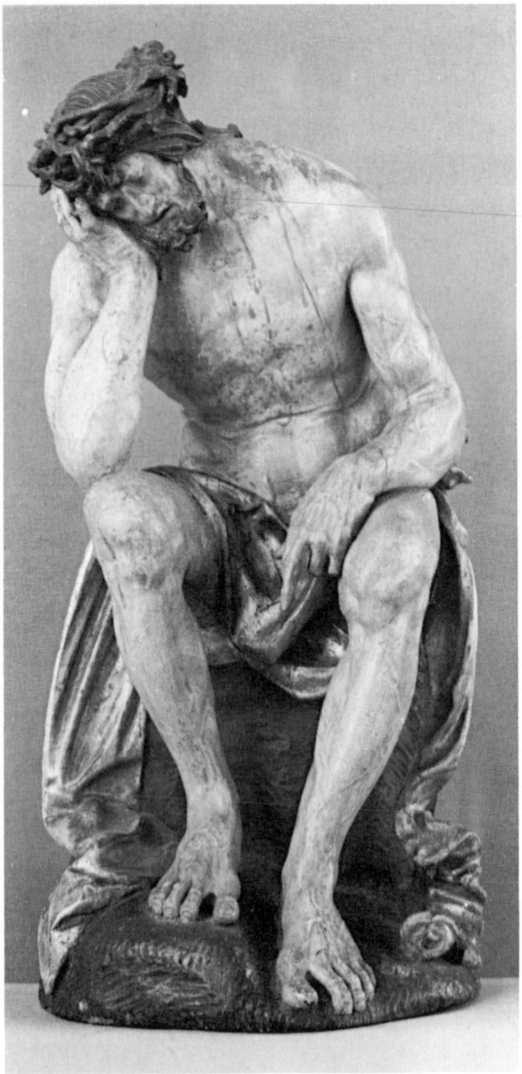

Fig. 5. Hans Leinberger: *Christ suffering*.

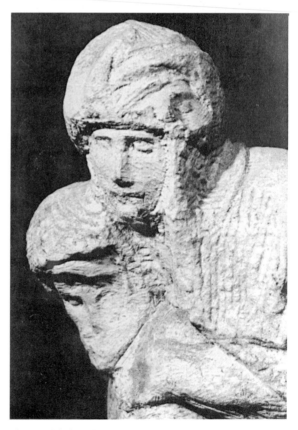

Fig. 6. Michelangelo: *Pietà Rondanini* (detail).

If we examine the work of Michelangelo, perhaps the greatest artist in the whole of the history of art, we have many expressions of desperation and pain, from the 'Struggle of Centaurs and Lapithae', a bas-relief made when he was seventeen years old, and the damned of the 'Universal Judgement' in the Sistine Chapel, to the 'Pietà Rondanini' (Fig. 6), unfinished because of the death of the artist.

In Flemish art, an extremely interesting painting is from the School of Peter Bruegel, representing a 'pain clinic' of that period.

In the latest Renaissance, with Mannerism the expressions of pain are frequent: the 'Saint Sebastian' by Guido Reni shows suffering and ecstasy at the same time; the Death of Cleopatra shows suffering and desperation. Then, at the end of the Renaissance, in the work of Michelangelo da Caravaggio, we find many examples of pain. A classic example is the 'Deposition'; and a new trend in painting is represented by 'a boy bitten by a green lizard' (Fig. 7) and by the 'Toothdrawer'.

With Baroque art, a full expression of pain and suffering can be observed in the art issuing from every part of Europe. Baroque developed to its peak in Rome, the South of Italy and in Germany. 'Christ in prison' by G. Groninger, now in Cologne (Fig. 8), is one of the best examples of the representation of pain in Baroque art. Interesting, as an example of Northern art, is a Swedish painting of the seventeenth century showing a surgeon who makes an incision on the head of a patient who shows intense suffering.

In the eighteenth century, between the various trends, a period of classical representation, without suffering and pain, is prevalent. In the nineteenth century many trends began to overlap. In the academic Schools we have representations of pain in daily life, but here often what is lacking is not pain but art. The most interesting examples of representation of pain in this period are some 'caricatures': one by Cruikshank shows little devils torturing a man with migraine; a French lithograph, a copy of

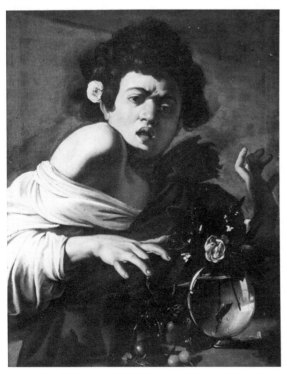

Fig. 7. Caravaggio: *The boy bitten by a green lizard.*

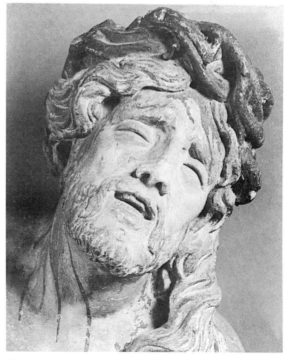

Fig. 8. G. Groninger: *Christ in prison.*

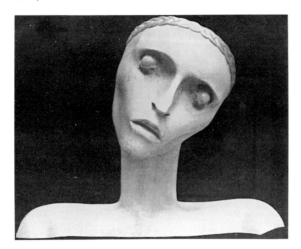

Fig. 9. A. Wildt: *Head of woman.*

a familiar painting, shows a woman with a head-ache attack. Of interest in this period also are some Japanese wood-cut prints: a woman with abdominal pain, possibly biliary cholic; and a skin grafting without anesthesia, in which the face of the man does not show any expression of pain, but a strong expression of a voluntary effort to tolerate pain without showing it.

In the twentieth century, new trends of art must be considered. Pain and suffering and perhaps desperation are present in the 'Cry' by Munch. A special consideration must be given to Wildt, an Italian artist of German ancestry. Here, suffering and pain are expressed in a dramatic fashion. Most of the

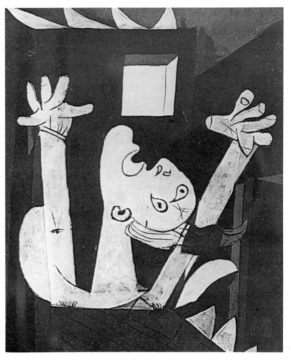

Fig. 10. P. Picasso: *Guernica* (detail).

works were made during the First World War, as in the face of the 'Head of Woman' (Fig. 9) in which the artist represented the intense suffering of that period. I think that this short discussion on pain and suffering in art can well be concluded by reference to Picasso's well known painting 'Guernica' (Fig. 10), in which once again the passions of the soul are expressed in such a dramatic manner.

Inflammation and Pain

R. Dubner, G.F. Gebhart & M.R. Bond (Eds.)
Proceedings of the Vth World Congress on Pain
© 1988 Elsevier Science Publishers BV (Biomedical Division)

CHAPTER 4

The peripheral nervous system and the inflammatory process

Jon D. Levine[1, 2, 5], Terence J. Coderre[1, 5] and Alan I. Basbaum[3, 4, 5]

Departments of [1]Medicine, [2]Oral and Maxillofacial Surgery, [3]Anatomy and [4]Physiology, and [5]Program in Neurosciences, University of California, San Francisco, CA 94143, USA

Inflammation

Inflammation is a complex biological process involving interactions between immunocompetent cells (e.g., lymphocytes, macrophages, polymorphonuclear leukocytes and mast cells) that lead to the production of various humoral mediators of inflammation, including kinins, prostaglandins, leukotrienes and interleukins. Inflammation presumably evolved as a healing process, to repair tissues following injury, but it may also contribute to tissue injury, as occurs in so-called inflammatory diseases. The differences that determine which of these two opposing outcomes will occur, tissue repair or tissue injury, are not well understood.

Inflammation can be easily recognized by the presence of its five cardinal features: rubor (redness), calor (heat), tumor (swelling), dolor (pain) and functio lassae (loss of function). These clinical features of inflammation can be accounted for by a relatively small number of physiological changes: vasodilatation produces redness and heat, increased plasma extravasation and migration of cells from the vascular space produces edema or swelling, sensitization of primary afferent nociceptors produces hyperalgesia and, taken together, all three contribute to loss of function. Any mechanistic explanation of the inflammatory process must account for these clinical features.

Unmyelinated primary afferents

The sources of the humoral mediators of inflammation are remarkably diverse. Of particular interest is evidence that the peripheral terminals of primary afferent nociceptors not only respond to noxious stimuli, to produce pain (Bessou and Perl, 1969), but are also the source of inflammatory mediators that are released when these neurons are activated (Buck et al., 1982; Leeman and Gamse, 1981). Based on his classic axon reflex experiments, Lewis attributed the neurally evoked cutaneous wheal and flare response to substances released from the peripheral terminals of a group of 'nocifensor' nerves. Antidromic activation of peripheral nerves produces vasodilatation and plasma extravasation in the innervated tissue (Lembeck and Holzer, 1979; Morton and Chahl, 1980; Jancso et al., 1967) and prior treatment with capsaicin, a neurotoxin which is selective for neuropeptide-containing small-diameter afferents, prevents this form of neurogenic inflammation.

The best-studied proinflammatory factor released from primary afferents is the undecapeptide neurotransmitter, substance P (SP). Up to 90% of the SP synthesized by dorsal root ganglion cells is transported from the cell body to the peripheral terminals, from which it can be released. Significantly, many of the physiological changes associated with acute inflammation, including vasodilatation, increased vascular permeability (Jancso et al., 1967; Lembeck and Holzer, 1979) pavementing of leukocytes in venules, stimulation of phagocytosis by polymorphonuclear leukocytes and mast cell degranulation, can be produced by introducing synthetic SP directly into peripheral tissues (Foreman et al., 1982; Lembeck et al., 1977) or by electrically stimulating peripheral nerves at the same intensities that release SP (Jancso et al., 1967; Bill et al., 1979; Blinn et al., 1980; Brodin et al., 1981; Schumacher, 1975). Finally, destruction of unmyelinated afferent axons with capsaicin, which significantly attenuates the inflammatory response produced by injection of noxious substances or nerve stimulation (Blinn et al., 1980; Bill et al., 1979), also depletes SP (Jancso et al., 1981). The primary afferent neuron thus serves a dual function. It transmits neural stimuli centrally and releases neuromediators of inflammation peripherally into stimulated tissues.

One possible target of SP is the mast cell, which is found in close proximity to peripheral nerve terminals (Wiesner-Menzel et al., 1981; Kruger et al., 1985; Newson et al., 1983). Micromolar concentrations of SP stimulate the release of histamine from mast cells (Foreman et al., 1982; Theoharides and Douglas, 1981; Fitzgerald, 1983) which, in turn, increases vascular permeability (Fox et al., 1980). Although it has been argued that this effect of SP on mast cells is analogous to that of other chemically basic peptides which stimulate mast cells at high concentrations (Baxter and Adamik, 1978; Brindley et al., 1983), SP also stimulates the synthesis and release of unstored mediators, such as leukotrienes (Goetzl et al., 1986). Somatostatin activates mast cells only minimally, which indicates that there is a degree of peptide specificity to this effect. Importantly, plasma extravasation and vasodilatation produced by antidromic peripheral nerve stimulation or by injection of SP are blocked by H_1-antagonists (Foreman and Jordan, 1984; Lembeck and Holzer, 1979) or by prior treatment with the mast cell degranulator, compound 48/80 (Lembeck and Holzer, 1979; Arvier et al., 1977). Taken together, these studies suggest a simple neuroimmunological

circuit. Proinflammatory factors released from small-diameter primary afferents act on mast cells to release other mediators of inflammation, such as histamine, serotonin and leukotrienes. These mast cell factors, in turn, act on the vascular system to produce vasodilatation and increased vascular permeability. Likely targets of the inflammatory mediators released from mast cells include the microvessels and/or the peripheral terminals of the sympathetic postganglionic neuron. Histamine receptors have been described on both of these targets and we, in fact, have recently shown that the sympathetic postganglionic nerve terminal is a key element in the circuit that produces increases in vascular permeability in response to activation of primary afferents and mast cells (Coderre et al., 1987).

Nervous system in arthritis

Rheumatoid arthritis (RA) is a common disease which produces significant morbidity in a majority of patients, causing pain and contributing significantly to medical care costs and loss of work hours. The prevalence of RA is approximately 1% of the world population (O'Sullivan and Cathcart, 1972). Important diagnostic features in RA are a dramatic symmetry in distribution of joints involved and a distal-to-proximal gradient of severity of joint involvement; more peripheral joints are more severely affected.

The existence of an experimentally induceable arthritis (EA) in animals with clinical manifestations that mimic those of RA in humans provides an excellent model for investigating the contribution of the nervous system in arthritis (Pearson, 1963). This animal model is similar to RA with regard to symmetric and distal (i.e., high- and low-risk) joint involvement, acute and subacute synovitis, invasion of joint and bone by pannus (vascular granulation tissue composed of proliferating fibroblasts, numerous small blood vessels, and various numbers of inflammatory cells, considered the most important destructive element in RA) and response to anti-inflammatory and remittive therapies (Tsukano et al.,

1983; Lewis et al., 1985; Billingham and Davis, 1979). The presence of symmetrical involvement is particularly helpful in studying a neural contribution, since it permits specific investigation of the pathogenic contribution of the individual components of the neural innervation. In addition, comparison of joints at low (i.e., knee) and high (i.e., ankle) risk of developing EA can be used to determine the correlation between severity of arthritis and specific neurobiology of the low- and high-risk joints.

Contribution of primary afferents

Several features of the innervation of joints by SP-containing neurons are consistent with a contribution of their peptides to arthritis (Levine et al., 1984, 1986a). First, distal joints (ankles), which are at greater risk of developing more severe arthritis, are more densely innervated by nociceptive afferent neurons. High-risk joints in normal rats also have significantly lower nociceptive thresholds than do low-risk (knee) joints, an observation expected from the differences in innervation density. Second, the concentration of substance P is highest in the high-risk joints of normal rats, i.e. prior to the onset of arthritis. This is also consistent with the differential innervation density. Neonatal administration of the neurotoxin capsaicin increases the nociceptive threshold in the high-risk joint, to a level not significantly different from the nociceptive threshold normally found in the low-risk joint. Like prior denervation of the joint (Courtright and Kuzzel, 1965), the C-fiber neurotoxin capsaicin markedly decreased the concentration of SP in both high- and low-risk joints. Thus, the difference in the concentration of SP in high- and low-risk joints reflects differences in small-fiber intraneuronal content of SP.

These observations provided the foundation for the hypothesis that modification of the level of SP in joints would alter the severity of joint injury in arthritis. The effect of capsaicin-induced depletion of SP on severity of arthritis in high-risk joints was first examined. Colpaert and colleagues had already shown that pretreatment of peripheral nerve with capsaicin produced a significant reduction in hind-paw swelling and hyperalgesia in adjuvant arthritic rats (Colpaert et al., 1983). Using skeletal X-rays as a quantitative index of joint injury, we subsequently demonstrated that neonatal treatment with capsaicin reduces the severity of joint injury in arthritic rats (Levine et al., 1984, 1985).

Neonatal capsaicin, of course, destroys most unmyelinated afferents (Fitzgerald, 1983; Gamse and Saria, 1984) and, because unmyelinated fibers in peripheral nerves release other inflammatory mediators, these data do not directly implicate SP. Therefore, to avoid the complexity of interpretation inherent in the loss of other neurally derived inflammatory factors, we studied the effect of direct infusion of SP into a low-risk joint on joint injury. The intra-articular injection of SP, in fact, significantly increased the severity of arthritis. Taken together, these experiments suggest that there are significant neurobiological differences between the innervation of joints which develop mild and severe arthritis in rat experimental models, and that continuing release of intraneuronal SP into joints contributes to the severity of joint injury in arthritis.

As described previously, substance P is not the only peptide found in the small-diameter unmyelinated sensory neurons (Gamse and Saria, 1984; Gazelius et al., 1981; Hokfelt et al., 1980). Of the more recently discovered neuropeptides, the two tachykinins, neurokinin A and neurokinin B, and calitonin gene-related peptide (CGRP) are of particular interest with regard to the mechanism of neurogenic inflammation. Neurokinin A and neurokinin B are chemically related to substance P and have similar physiological properties. Each produces vasodilatation and increased vascular permeability. Conversely, calcitonin gene-related peptide has a very different profile of physiological effects (Gazelius et al., 1985; Gibson et al., 1984; Goodman and Iversen, 1986; Struthers et al., 1986; Rosenfeld et al., 1983). It is several-fold more potent than SP as a vasodilator. Intradermal injection of femtomole doses of CGRP increases local blood flow for several hours (Brain et al., 1986a,b). However, CGRP does not produce anywhere near as potent an increase in vascular permeability as SP. Since SP-containing dorsal root ganglion cells are a subpopulation of the calcitonin gene-related peptide-containing sensory neurons (Gibbons et al., 1985; Lundberg et al., 1985), it is of interest that injection of the combination of either substance P, neurokinin A or neurokinin B along with calcitonin gene-related peptide potentiates the plasma protein leakage induced by the tachykinin component of the combination (Gazelius et al., 1985), probably because of the increased vasodilatation.

Further evidence for a contribution of the peripheral nervous system to arthritis comes from an electron microscopic study of the effect of gold on the ultrastructure of the saphenous nerve. We studied the density of myelinated and unmyelinated axons in the saphenous nerve of rats which were treated for two months with systemic gold sodium thiomalate, at a dose known to attenuate adjuvant arthritis (Levine et al., 1985). The number and density of unmyelinated axons in the saphenous nerves of gold-treated rats were significantly reduced (by 23%) compared to normal rats, without a significant change in the density of the myelinated axons. These anatomic data, which are consistent with the results of several other studies of neuropathic effects of gold therapy, including a polyneuropathy (Endtz, 1958; Meyer et al., 1978), demonstrate that gold selectively destroys unmyelinated axons in the peripheral nervous system of the rat.

Contribution of sympathetic efferents

In addition to unmyelinated afferent and mast cell effects, there is evidence that the peripheral limb of the sympathetic nervous system (SNS) contributes to neurogenic inflammation. Linde et al., 1974 demonstrated an increase in vascular permeability following sympathetic nerve stimulation, and Engel (Engel, 1941, 1978) has shown that lumbosacral sympathectomy substantially reduces baseline plasma extravasation. Also, chemical sympathectomy

potently inhibits plasma extravasation evoked by intradermal injection of the mast cell degranulator compound 48/80, or by injection of substances found in mast cell granules, such as histamine and serotonin (Helme and Andrews, 1985; Gozsy and Kato, 1966). The edema or swelling induced by intradermal injection of carrageenan, dextran or formalin is also significantly reduced in sympathectomized rats (Arntzen and Briseid, 1973; Arrigoni-Martelli et al., 1967; Brown et al., 1968; Lenfeld et al., 1973; Nilsson and Folkow, 1982). These observations suggested that sympathetic efferents, as well as the primary afferent components of the peripheral nervous system, contribute to joint inflammation and injury in experimentally induced arthritis (EA).

To test this hypothesis, rats were sympathectomized with 6 weeks of daily injections of guanethidine. This regimen depletes catecholamines by selectively destroying the sympathetic postganglionic neurons. Another group of rats received daily subcutaneous injections of the catecholamine depleter reserpine, starting 2 days before induction of arthritis and continuing through the duration of the study. In both protocols, the chemical sympathectomy significantly decreased the radiographically demonstrated severity of joint injury in the hindlimbs (Levine et al., 1986a).

The relationship between sustained release of catecholamines and the severity of joint injury in EA was also examined in rats with *increased* sympathetic activity. Arthritis was induced in spontaneously hypertensive rats, which exhibit increased tonic sympathetic activity compared to that of the parent, Wistar-Kyoto, normotensive strain (Nilsson and Folkow, 1982; Okamoto et al., 1967). The severity of EA in the hindlimbs of the spontaneously hypertensive rat was found to be significantly greater than in the parent strain.

One possible explanation for the reduction in arthritis produced by sympathectomy is that it results from a decrease in facilitation of peripheral interactions between primary afferent nociceptors and sympathetic efferent neurons. For example, there is evidence that activity in sympathetic efferents excites sensory afferents in experimentally induced neuromas (Devor and Janig, 1981; Wall and Gutnick, 1974) and in heat-responsive afferents (Roberts and Elardo, 1985). Activation of nociceptive afferents also elicits spinal cord reflexes that markedly increase the activity of postganglionic sympathetic efferents (Blinn et al., 1980; Beacham and Perl, 1964; Koisumi et al., 1970). The interaction between primary afferents and sympathetic efferents can also increase local tissue production of prostaglandins, which, of course, are potent mediators of inflammation (Levine et al., 1986b).

A contribution of large-diameter primary afferents

The attenuating effects of treatment with capsaicin (Colpaert et al., 1983) are consistent with the hypothesis that the peripheral terminals of sensory afferent fibers contribute to the process of inflammation. Neonatal capsaicin treatment, however, destroys cells of the dorsal root ganglia and thus eliminates *both* the central and the peripheral branches of primary afferent fibers. To selectively eliminate the central connections of joint afferents, while leaving peripheral connections intact, a group of rats underwent a unilateral deafferentation of the hindlimb, by dorsal rhizotomy; 7 days later arthritis was induced. To our surprise onset of arthritis was *earlier* in the deafferented limb and maximal severity was also reached earlier in that limb. The non-deafferented limb eventually caught up, so that by day 28, when the rats were X-rayed, no differences were present. Since normal rats develop less severe arthritis in the forepaw than in the hindpaw, we felt that the exacerbation of arthritis might be best studied in the forelimbs. Therefore, a separate group of rats underwent unilateral cervical rhizotomy and 7 days later arthritis was induced. In contrast to the attenuation of arthritis seen in rats with peripheral nerve section (Courtright and Kuzzel, 1965) or in rats which had been neonatally treated with capsaicin, and consistent with the results from the hindlimb study, arthritis in the deafferentated forelimb (cervical rhizotomy) was significantly *worse*

than in the neurologically intact, contralateral forelimb and the difference persisted until the rats were X-rayed on day 28.

Since capsaicin destruction of small-diameter primary afferents *decreased* the arthritis, it appeared that the increased arthritis produced by rhizotomy might have resulted from *enhanced* activity in the unmyelinated peripheral afferent terminals of the joint. We reasoned, for example, that some type of neuroma might have formed on the cut dorsal roots. Hyperactivity in such a neuroma would generate increased antidromic activity in C-fibers which could increase the release of inflammatory mediators in the joint. This would be analogous to the development of neuromas on cut peripheral nerve (Wall and Gutnick, 1974). If this hypothesis were true, then the effect of dorsal rhizotomy would disappear in capsaicin-treated rats. To test the hypothesis we evaluated the effect of dorsal rhizotomy on the severity of joint injury in rats pretreated with capsaicin; some rats were treated prior to deafferentation with guanethidine. As expected, there was an attenuation of the absolute severity of arthritis in the neonatal capsaicin-treated group but there was *still* an asymmetric arthritis. That is, dorsal rhizotomy still exacerbated arthritis in the absence of small fibers. In contrast, there was no significant difference in the severity of joint injury of the intact and rhizotomized limbs in sympathectomized rats. We believe that these data are indicative of an additional contribution of large-diameter primary afferents, which are known to tonically inhibit certain classes of spinal cord neurons. Specifically, we propose that the effect of dorsal rhizotomy is secondary to an increase in activity in sympathetic efferents following the loss of large-fiber inhibition of the sympathetic preganglionic neurons of the spinal cord.

To test the hypothesis that rhizotomy results in increased activity in sympathetic neurons, we measured the norepinephrine content of peripheral nerves in rhizotomized rats. We found that the norepinephrine level of the sciatic nerve was significantly higher in rhizotomized than in control rats (unpublished observations). Finally, we evaluated the effect of central sympatholytic therapy on experimental arthritis. Specifically, we studied the effect of intracerebroventricular morphine, which acts centrally to inhibit the preganglionic sympathetic outflow (Karoum et al., 1982), on the severity of joint injury. Morphine (5 μg), when injected every 2 h for 72 h, significantly attenuated joint injury in EA measured 28 days later. Infusion of saline had no effect on arthritis severity. Thus, the conclusion that dorsal rhizotomy increases arthritic severity by removal of inhibitory controls on sympathetic neurons is consistent with the decrease in severity of arthritis that was produced by activating descending inhibitory controls with intracerebroventricular injection of morphine.

In summary, we believe that there are four major components of the neural circuitry controlling experimental arthritis in the rat: C-fiber afferents, sympathetic pre- and postganglionic neurons, large-diameter primary afferents and descending brainstem controls (see Fig. 1). The critical question, of course, is whether this holds true for inflammatory diseases in humans.

Clinical associations between neurological states and rheumatoid arthritis have, in fact, been reported. Some neurological abnormalities appear early in the course of the disease, but these have not been systematically explored. Some patients with RA have autonomic dysfunction, even without clinical evidence of neuropathy (Bennet and Scott, 1965; Leden et al., 1983). Perhaps more importantly, focal neurological lesions, from various causes, can dramatically alter the bilateral symmetry of joint involvement. Patients who sustain paralysing lesions of the central or peripheral nervous system, prior to developing RA, all manifest less or no joint inflammation, erosions or formation of rheumatoid nodules in paretic limbs (Glick, 1967; Thompson and Bywaters, 1962). A sparing effect of neurological lesions on the expression of arthritis is not restricted to RA. There are reports of patients developing Heberden's nodes only on the side unaffected by a stroke (Bonelli et al., 1983). Gout is also less common on a paretic side (Glynn and Clayton, 1976).

Although the sparing effect of neurological le-

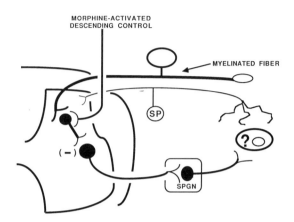

Fig. 1. Schematic representation of the neural circuitry involved in the control of experimental arthritis in the rat. Joint injury is exacerbated when pro-inflammatory mediators, including substance P (SP), are released from the peripheral terminals of SP-containing unmyelinated afferents and/or sympathetic postganglionic neurons (SPGNs) in response to axon and somato-sympathetic reflexes. The pro-inflammatory effect of sympathetic activity is subject to morphine-activatable descending inhibitory controls, as well as to inhibition from large myelinated afferent fibers. The peripheral target(s) of the mediators released from peripheral nerves is unknown.

sions on arthritis has usually been attributed to decreased use of these joints, attempts to correlate the use of joints with the severity of arthritic involvement have failed. In fact, decreased use does *not* significantly reduce joint injury (Glick, 1967). An alternative hypothesis for the decreased arthritis in the paralysed limb is that blood flow is reduced in paretic extremities. Little information is available on use-related alteration in blood flow in the synovial capsule; however, phenosulfophthalein clearance time from the skin is similar in normal and hemiplegic limbs in patients with RA who have sustained a cerebrovascular accident (Mizushima and Yamara, 1969).

There is also clinical evidence suggesting that the peripheral limb of the sympathetic nervous system contributes to inflammation in the synovium. For example, patients with the syndrome of reflex sympathetic dystrophy, in whom there is marked sympathetic hyperactivity, experience pain and inflammation of synovial joints (Kozin et al., 1976). In these patients, regional sympathetic blockade with guanethidine (Bonica, 1979; Hannington-Kiff, 1977; Loh and Nathan, 1978) or other sympatholytic agents (Benzon et al., 1980) can reduce the inflammation. Further evidence of a contribution of altered autonomic function to the severity of arthritis is the observation that stress-induced hyperactivity of the autonomic nervous system can trigger flares of RA (Baker, 1982). Twin studies also indicate that an increase in life stress may precede the onset of arthritis (Meyerowitz et al., 1968). The benefits of prolonged hospitalization, once commonly prescribed for active RA patients as a way to reduce the use of joints, may, in fact, be due to a reduction in stress and a consequent reduction in sympathetic outflow (Short et al., 1957).

The mechanisms through which stress could enhance arthritis are obviously not understood. In addition to increasing sympathetic activity, stress has variable effects on the immune system. These depend on what type of stress is examined, what immune function is measured, and which animal is used (Riley, 1981; Stein et al., 1976). Stress-induced depressive effects on immune function which are independent of corticosteroid production have, in fact, been demonstrated (Kozin et al., 1976), but those observations do not appear to explain even transient alterations in the chronic inflammatory process seen in joints of patients with RA.

Pain-induced morbidity

Although pain is a common feature in arthritis, it is not generally considered to be a critical factor in the morbidity and outcome of the disease. Instead, the deterioration in the health of the patients with arthritis is usually attributed to the disease process itself. Chronic pain, however, is often associated with poor overall health, including decreased activity, weight loss and sleep disturbances (Colpaert et al., 1980, 1982; Costa et al., 1985). It follows that the morbidity of patients with arthritis might result, in part, from the pain that is experienced. In fact, the degree of pain reported by patients with RA correlates highly with physical and psychological disability and with the amount of medication required (Bar-Shavit et al., 1980; Kazis et al., 1983). Most significantly, the current pain level of patients with RA, rather than current disability, is the best predictor of future physical and psychological disability (Kazis et al., 1983).

We have studied the contribution of pain to morbidity in the disease model of experimental arthritis in the rat (Levine et al., 1986c). Rats with arthritis typically lose weight and are considerably less active than are normal rats (Colpaert et al., 1980, 1982, 1983; Costa et al., 1985). Although both of these signs of the morbidity of chronic illness may be directly related to the severity of the inflammatory disease, we hypothesized that morbidity was, in part, *secondary* to the pain experienced by the rats. To test the hypothesis that pain contributes to general morbidity in EA, we examined the effects of interruption of the major ascending nociceptive transmission pathways of the spinal cord on weight loss and decrease in activity in rats with EA.

The rostral transmission of nociceptive information from the hindpaws was eliminated by bilaterally sectioning the spinothalamic and spinoreticulothalamic pathways in the ventrolateral funiculus (VLF) of the spinal cord. To measure changes in health status in EA, we compared weight and activity in operated arthritic and nonoperated arthritic rats. Bilateral lesions of the VLF in nonarthritic rats did not alter weight or level of activity, the measures of morbidity. Cutting the VLF in rats with EA, however, significantly attenuated weight loss and the decrease in activity. Importantly, the severity of the joint disease, inflammation and tissue destruction was *not* affected by the cord lesion.

The results of this study provide strong evidence that the pain which accompanies various disease states makes an important contribution to morbidity. Since pain is a prominent feature of most forms of arthritis in humans, it follows that morbidity in these patients might, in part, be derived from the chronic tenderness and pain of affected joints. This may be particularly important in clinical decision-making. Although it may not always be possible to arrest the primary disease process, there is a wide range of therapies available for the treatment of pain.

Clinical studies

Encouraged by the animal data and because sympatholytic therapy is used for painful conditions, such as reflex sympathetic dystrophy, we have performed a trial of regional intravenous guanethidine (Levine et al., 1986) in patients with longstanding RA and active disease. In this randomized double-blind short-term (14 day) study, we evaluated the effect of therapy on subjective responses (change in pain, stiffness and morning stiffness) and on objective responses (change in pinch strength, grip strength and joint tenderness). Compared to placebo, a single treatment with guanethidine (10 mg, i.v.) produced a decrease in pain and an increase in pinch strength over the 2 week duration of the study. These data demonstrate that in RA, as well as in experimental arthritis, interruption of sympathetic postganglionic function can ameliorate signs and symptoms in patients with RA.

In summary, some clinical features of rheumatoid arthritis, for example, preferential joint involvement and bilateral symmetry, taken together with the strong evidence of neurogenic inflammatory processes, suggest that the nervous system contributes to the inflammatory component of RA and other types of arthritis. We propose that the increased risk and severity of disease in particular joints reflects a greater innervation of those joints, by unmyelinated afferent and sympathetic efferent fibers. Release of the proinflammatory peptide, substance P, from the peripheral terminals of nociceptive joint afferent fibers, through interactions with many non-neuronal cells, exacerbates the inflammatory process. Release of mediators from sympathetic efferents (including norepinephrine) also contributes to the inflammation, either through an independent mechanism, or by acting in concert with the nociceptive afferent-derived substances. Therapies directed at interruption of the nervous system contribution to the pathophysiology of these diseases should offer a new direction for treatment.

References

Arntzen, F.C. and Briseid, K. (1973) Inhibition of carrageenin-induced paw oedema by catecholamines and aminedepleting drugs. Acta Pharmacol. Toxicol., 32: 193–204.

Arrigoni-Martelli, E., Toth, E., Segre, A.D. and Corsico, N. (1967) Mechanism of inhibition of experimental inflammation by antidepressant drugs. Eur. J. Pharmacol., 2: 229–233.

Arvier, P.T., Chahl, L.A. and Ladd, R.J. (1977) Modification by capsaicin and compound 48/80 of dye leakage induced by irritants in the rat. Br. J. Pharmacol., 59: 61–68.

Baker, G.H.B. (1982) Life events before the onset of rheumatoid arthritis. Psychother. Psychosom., 38: 173–177.

Bar-Shavit, Z., Goldman, R., Stabinsky, Y., Gottlieb, P., Fridkin, M., Teichberg, V.I. and Blumberg, S. (1980) Enhancement of phagocytosis–a newly found activity of substance P residing in its N-terminal tetropeptide sequence. Biochem. Biophys. Res. Commun., 94: 1445–1451.

Baxter, J.H. and Adamik, R. (1978) Differences in requirements and actions of various histamine-releasing agents. Biochem. Pharmacol., 27: 497–503.

Beacham, W. and Perl, E.R. (1964) Characteristics of a spinal sympathetic reflex. J. Physiol. (Lond.), 173: 431–448.

Bennett, P.H. and Scott, J.T. (1965) Autonomic neuropathy in rheumatoid arthritis. Ann. Rheum. Dis., 24: 161–168.

Benzon, H.T., Chomka, C.M. and Bruner, E.A. (1980) Treatment of reflex sympathetic dystrophy with regional intravenous guanethidine. Anesth. Analg. 59: 500–502.

Bessou, P. and Perl, E.R. (1969) Response of cutaneous units with unmyelinated fibers to noxious stimuli. J. Neurophysiol., 32: 1025–1043.

Bill, A., Stjernschantz, J., Mandahl, A., Brodin, E. and Nilsson, G. (1979) Substance P: release on trigeminal stimulation, effects in the eye. Acta Physiol. Scand., 101: 371–373.

Billingham, M.E.J. and Davis, G.E. (1979) Experimental models of arthritis in animals as screening tests for drugs to treat arthritis in man. In J.R. Vane and S.H. Ferreira (Eds.), Handbook of Experimental Pharmacology, Vol. 50/II, Springer-Verlag, Berlin, pp. 108–144.

Blinn, G., Heinz, G. and Jurna, I. (1980) Effects of substantia nigra stimulation on suralis-evoked spinal reflex activity: comparison with the effects of morphine and stimulation in the periaqueductal gray matter. Neuropharmacology 19: 75–85.

Bonelli, S., Conoscente, F., Movilia, P.G., Restelli, L. Francucci, B. and Grossi, E. (1983) Regional intravenous guanethidine versus stellate ganglion block in reflex sympathetic dystrophies: A randomized trial. Pain 16: 297–307.

Bonica, J.J. (1979) Causalgia and other reflex sympathetic dystrophies. In Proceedings of the Second World Congress on Pain (Advances in Pain Research and Therapy, Vol. 3), Raven Press, New York, pp. 141–166.

Brain, S.D., MacIntyre, I. and Williams, T.J. (1986a) A second form of human calcitonin gene-related peptide which is a potent vasodilator. Eur. J. Pharmacol., 124: 349–352.

Brain, S.D., William, T.J., Tippins, Morris, H.R. and MacIntyre, I. (1986b) Calcitonin gene-related peptide is a potent vasodilator. Nature, 313: 54–56.

Brindley, L.L., Sweet, J.M. and Goetzl, E.J. (1983) Stimulation of histamine release from human basophils by human platelet factor 4. J. Clin. Invest., 72: 1218–1223.

Brodin, E., Gazelins, B., Olgart, L. and Nilsson, G. (1981) Tissue concentration and release of substance P-like immunoreactivity in the dental pulp. Acta Physiol. Scand., 113: 141–149.

Brown, J.H., Mackey, H.R., Riggilo, D.A. and Schwartz, N.L. (1968) Studies on the acute inflammatory response. II. Influence of antihistaminics and catecholamines on formaldehyde-induced edema. J. Pharmacol. Exp. Ther., 160: 243–248.

Buck, S.H., Walsh, J.H., Yamamura, H.T., et al. (1982) Neuropeptides in sensory neurons. Life Sci., 30: 1857–1866.

Coderre, T.J., Basbaum, A.I. and Levine, J.D. (1987) Interactions between primary afferents, mast cells and sympathetic efferents in the control of synovial vascular permeability. (Submitted)

Colpaert, F.C., DeWitte, P., Maroli, A.N., Awouters, F., Niemegeers, C.J.E. and Janssen, P.A.J. (1980) Self-administration of the analgesic suprofen in arthritic rats: evidence of *Mycobacterium butyricum*-induced arthritis as an experimental model of chronic pain. Life Sci., 27: 921–928.

Colpaert, F.C., Meert, T.H., DeWitte, P.H. and Schmitt, P. (1982) Further evidence validating adjuvant-induced arthritis as an experimental model of chronic pain in the rat. Life Sci., 31: 67–75.

Colpaert, F.C., Donnerer, J. and Lembeck, F. (1983) Effects of capsaicin on inflammation and on substance P content of nervous tissues in rats with adjuvant arthritis. Life Sci., 32: 1827–1834.

Costa, M.C., Sutter, P., Gybels, J. and VanHees, J. (1985) Adjuvant-induced arthritis in rats: a possible animal model of chronic pain. Pain, 10: 173–185.

Courtright, L.J. and Kuzzel, K.C. (1965) Sparing effect of neurological deficit and trauma on the course of adjuvant arthritis in the rat. Ann. Rheum. Dis., 24: 360–368.

Devor, M. and Janig, W. (1981) Activation of myelinated afferents ending in a neuroma by stimulation of the sympathetic supply in the rat. Neurosci. Lett., 24: 43–47.

Endtz, L.J. (1958) Complications nerveuse du traitment aurique. Rev. Neurol. (Paris), 99: 395–410.

Engel, D. (1941) The influence of the sympathetic nervous system on capillary permeability. J. Physiol., 99: 161–181.

Engel, D. (1978) The influence of the sympathetic nervous system on capillary permeability. Res. Exp. Med., 173: 1–8.

Fitzgerald, M. (1983) Capsaicin and sensory neurones—a review. Pain, 15: 109–130.

Foreman, J.C. and Jordan, C.C. (1984) Neurogenic inflammation. Trends Pharmacol. Sci., 116–119.

Foreman, J.C., Jordan, C.C. and Piotrowski, W. (1982) Interaction of neurotensin with the substance P receptor mediating histamine release from rat mast cells and the flare in human skin. Br. J. Pharmacol., 77: 531–539.

Fox, J., Galey, F. and Wayland, H. (1980) Action of histamine on the mesenteric microvasculature. Microvasc. Res., 19: 108–126.

Gamse, R. and Saria, A. (1984) Is substance P the only mediator of neurogenic inflammation? An analysis of extracts of spinal cord and roots. Neurosci. Lett., 18: 347–352.

Gazelius, B., Brodin, E. and Olgart, L. (1981) Evidence that substance P is a mediator of antidromic vasodilation using somatostatin as a release inhibitor. Acta Physiol. Scand., 113: 155–159.

Gazelius, B., Edwall, B., Lundberg, J.M., Fisher, J.A. and Hokfelt, J. (1985) Calcitonin gene-related peptide (CGRP), a potent vasodilator related to sensory nerves in the cat. Acta Physiol. Scand., 124 (Suppl. 542): 134.

Gibbins, I.L., Furness, J.B., Costa, M., MacIntyre, I., Hillyard, C.J. and Girgis, S. (1985) Co-localization of calcitonin gene related peptide-like immunoreactivity with substance P in cutaneous vascular and visceral sensory neurons of guinea pigs. Neurosci. Lett., 57: 125–130.

Gibson, S.J., Polak, J.M., Bloom, S.R., Sabate, I.M., Mulderry, P.M., Ghatei, M.A., McGregor, G.P., Morrison, J.F.B., Kelly, J.S., Evans, R.M. and Rosenfield, M.G. (1984) Calcitonin gene-related peptide immunoreactivity in the spinal cord of man and of eight other species. J. Neurosci., 4: 3101–3111.

Glick, E.N. (1967) Asymmetrical rheumatoid arthritis after poliomyelitis. Br. Med. J., 3: 26–29.

Glynn, J.J. and Clayton, M.L. (1976) Sparing effect of hemiplegia on tophaceous gout. Ann. Rheum. Dis., 35: 534–535.

Goodman, E.C. and Iversen, L.L. (1986) Calcitonin gene-related peptide: Novel neuropeptide. Life Sci., 38: 2169–2178.

Goetzl, E.J., Chernov-Rogan, T., Furuichi, K., et al. (1986) Neuromodulation of mast cell and basophil function. In Mast Cell Differentiation and Heterogeneity, Raven Press, New York, pp. 223–248.

Gozsy, B. and Kato, L. (1966) Role of norepinephrine and 5-hydroxytryptamine in the delayed phase of the inflammatory reaction in rats. Int. Arch. Allergy, 30: 553–560.

Hannington-Kiff, J.G. (1977) Relief of Sudeck's atrophy by regional intravenous guanethidine. Lancet, i: 1132–1133.

Helme, R.D. and Andrews, P.V. (1985) The effect of nerve lesions on the inflammatory response to injury. J. Neurosci. Res., 13: 453–459.

Hokfelt, T., Johansson, O., Ljungdahl, A., Lundbert, J.M. and Schulzberg, M. (1980) Peptidergic neurones. Nature, 284: 515–521.

Jancso, N., Jancso-Gabor, A. and Szolcsanyi, J. (1967) Direct evidence for direct neurogenic inflammation and its prevention by denervation and by pretreatment with capsaicin. Br. J. Pharmacol. Chemother., 31: 138.

Jancso, G., Hokfelt, T., Lundberg, J.M., Kiraly, E., Halasz, N., Nilsson, G., Terenius, L., Rehfeld, J., Steinbusch, H., Verhofstad, A., Elde, R., Said, S. and Brown, M. (1981) Immunohistochemical studies on the effect of capsaicin on spinal and medullary peptides and monoamine neurons using antisera to substance P, gastrin/CCK, somatostatin, VIP, enkephalin, neurotensin, and 5-hydroxytryptamine. J. Neurocytol., 10: 963–980.

Karoum, F., Commissiong, J. and Wyatt, R.J. (1982) Effects of morphine on norepinephrine turnover in various functional regions of rat spinal cord. Biochem. Pharmacol., 31: 3141–3143.

Kazis, L.E., Meenan, R.F. and Anderson, J.J. (1983) Pain in the rheumatic diseases: investigation of a key health status component. Arth. Rheum., 26: 1017–1022.

Koizumi, K., Collier, R., Kaufman, A. and Brook, M.C. (1970) Contribution of unmyelinated afferent excitation to sympathetic reflexes. Brain Res., 20: 99–106.

Kozin, F., McCarthy, D.J., Sims, J. and Genant, H. (1976) The reflex sympathetic dystrophy syndrome. I. Clinical and histological studies: evidence for bilaterality, response to corticosteroids and articular involvement. Am. J. Med., 60: 321–331.

Kruger, L., Sampogna, S.L., Rodin, B.E., Clague, J. and Yeh, Y. (1985) Thin-fiber cutaneous innervation and its intraepidermal contribution studied by labeling methods and neurotoxin treatment in rats. Somatosens. Res., 2: 335–356.

Leden, O., Eriksson, A., Lilja, B., Sturfelt, G. and Sundkvist, G. (1983) Autonomic nerve function in rheumatoid arthritis of varying severity. Scand. J. Rheumatol., 12: 166–170.

Leeman, S.E. and Gamse, R. (1981) Substance P in sensory neurons. Trends Pharmacol. Sci., 2: 119–121.

Lembeck, F. and Holzer, P. (1979) Substance P as neurogenic mediator of antidromic vasodilation and neurogenic plasma extravasation. Naunyn-Schmiedeberg's Arch. Pharmacol., 310: 175–183.

Lembeck, F., Gamse, R. and Juan, H. (1977) Substance P and sensory nerve endings. In von Euler vs. Pernow, B. (Eds.): Substance P (37th Noble Symposium, Stockholm, 1976). New York, Raven Press, 1976, p. 169–181.

Lenfeld, J., Marek, J. and Tikal, K. (1973) The influence of sympatholytics, ganglioplegics and cocaine on the anti-inflammatory effect of reserpine in experimental rats. Acta Univ. Palak. Olomu. Tom., 66: 161–167.

Levine, J.D., Clark, R., Devor, M., Helms, C., Moskowitz, M.A. and Basbaum, A.I. (1984) Intraneuronal substance P

contributes to the severity of experimental arthritis. Science, 226: 547–549.

Levine, J.D., Moskowitz, M.A. and Basbaum, A.I. (1985) The contribution of neurogenic inflammation in experimental arthritis. J. Immunol., 135: 843s–847s.

Levine, J.D., Dardick, S.J., Roizen, M.S., Helms, C. and Basbaum, A.I. (1986a) Contribution of sensory afferents and sympathetic efferents to joint injury in experimental arthritis. J. Neurosci., 6: 3423–3429.

Levine, J.D., Taiwo, Y.O., Collins, S.D. and Tam, J.K. (1986b) Noradrenaline hyperalgesia is mediated through interaction with sympathetic postganglionic neurone terminals rather than activation of primary afferent nociceptors. Nature, 323: 158–160.

Levine, J.D., Fye, K., Heller, P., Basbaum, A.I. and Whiting-O'Keefe (1986c) Clinical response to regional intravenous guanethidine in patients with rheumatoid arthritis. J. Rheumatol., 13: 1040–1043.

Lewis, A.J., Carlson, R.P. and Change, J. (1985) Experimental models of inflammation. In I.L. Bonta, M.A. Bray and M.J. Parnham (Eds.), Handbook of Inflammation, Vol. 5, Elsevier, Amsterdam, pp. 371–397.

Linde, B., Chisholm, G. and Rosell, S. (1974) The influence of sympathetic activity and histamine on the blood-tissue exchange of solutes in canine adipose tissue. Acta Physiol. Scand., 92: 145–155.

Loh, L. and Nathan, P.W. (1978) Painful peripheral nerve states and sympathetic blocks. J. Neurol. Neurosurg. Psychiatry, 41: 664–671.

Lundberg, J.M., Franco-Cereceda, A., Hua, X., Hokfelt, T. and Fischer, J.A. (1985) Co-existence of substance P and calcitonin gene-related peptide-like immunoreactivities in sensory nerves in relation to cardiovascular and bronchoconstrictor effects of capsaicin. Eur. J. Pharmacol., 108: 315–319.

Meyer, H., Haecki, M., Ziegler, W., Forster, W. and Schiller, H.H. (1978) Autonomic dysfunction and nyokima in gold neuropathy. In Peripheral Neuropathy. Elsevier, Amsterdam, pp. 475–480.

Meyerowitz, S., Jacox, R.F. and Hess, D.W. (1968) Monozygotic twins discordant for rheumatoid arthritis: a genetic clinical and psychologic study of eight sets. Arth. Rheum., 11: 1–21.

Mikkelsen, W.M., Dodge, H.J., Duff, I.F. and Kato, I.H. (1967) Estimates of the prevalence of rheumatic diseases in the population of Tecumseh Michigan, 1959–1960. J. Chronic Dis., 20: 351–369.

Mizushima, Y. and Yamara, M. (1969) Arthropathy and inflammation reaction in hemiplegic patients. Acta. Rheum. Scand., 15: 297–304.

Morton, C.R. and Chahl, L.A. (1980) Pharmacology of the neurogenic oedema response to electrical stimulation of the saphenous nerve in the rat. Naunyn-Schmiedeberg's Arch. Pharmacol., 314: 271–276.

Nagy, J.I., Iversen, L.L., Goedert, M., Chapman, D. and Hunt, S.P. (1983) Dose-dependent effects of capsaicin on primary sensory neurons in the neonatal rat. J. Neurosci., 3: 399–406.

Newson, B., Dahlstrom, A., Enerback, L. and Ahlman, H. (1983) Suggestive evidence for a direct innervation of mucosal mast cells. Neuroscience, 10: 565–570.

Nilsson, H. and Folkow, B. (1982) Vasoconstrictor nerve influence on isolated mesenteric resistance vessels from normotensive and spontaneously hypertensive rats. Acta Physiol. Scand., 116: 205–208.

Okamoto, K.S., Nosaka, S., Yomori, Y. and Matsumoto, M. (1967) Participation of neural factor in the pathogenesis of hypertension in the spontaneously hypertensive rat. Jpn Heart J., 8: 168–180.

O'Sullivan, J.B. and Cathcart, E.S. (1972) The prevalence of rheumatoid arthritis. Ann. Intern. Med., 76: 573–577.

Pearson, C.M. (1963) Experimental joint disease. J. Chronic Dis., 16: 863.

Riley, V. (1981) Psychoneuroendocrine influences on immunocompetence and neoplasia. Science, 212: 1100–1115.

Roberts, W.J. and Elardo, S.M. (1985) Sympathetic activation of A-delta nociceptors. Somatosensory Res., 3: 33–44.

Rosenfeld, M.G., Mermod, J., Amara, S.G., Swanson, L.W., Sawchenko, P.E., Rivier, J., Vale, W.W. and Evans, R.M. (1983) Production of a novel neuropeptide encoded by the calcitonin gene via tissue-specific RNA processing. Nature, 304: 129–135.

Schumacher, H.R. (1975) Synovial membrane fluid morphologic alterations in early rheumatoid arthritis: microvascular injury and virus-like particles. Ann. N.Y. Acad. Sci., 256: 39–64.

Short, C.L., Bauer, W. and Reynolds, W.L. (1957) Rheumatoid Arthritis, Harvard University Press, Cambridge, MA, p. 480.

Stein, M., Schiavi, R.C. and Camerino, M. (1976) Influence of brain and behavior on the immune system. Science, 191: 435–440.

Struthers, A.D., Brown, M.J., McDonald, D.W.R., Beacham, J.L., Stevenson, J.C., Morris, H.R. and MacIntyre, I. (1986) Human calcitonin gene-related peptide: a potent endogenous vasodilator in man. Clin. Sci., 70: 389–393.

Theoharides, T.C. and Douglas, W.W. (1981) Mast cell histamine secretion in response to somatostatin analogues: structural considerations. Eur. J. Pharmacol., 73: 131–136.

Tsukano, M., Nawa, Y. and Kotani, M. (1983) Characterization of low dose-induced suppressor cells in adjuvant induced arthritis in rats. Clin. Exp. Immunol., 53: 60–66.

Wall, P.D. and Gutnick, M. (1974) Ongoing activity in peripheral nerves: the physiology and pharmacology of impulses originating from a neuroma. Exp. Neurol., 43: 580–593.

Wiesner-Menzel, L., Schulz, B., Vakilzadeh, F. and Czarnetzki, B.M. (1981) Electron microscopical evidence for a direct contact between nerve fibres and mast cells. Acta Dermatol., 61: 465–469.

R. Dubner, G.F. Gebhart & M.R. Bond (Eds.)
Proceedings of the Vth World Congress on Pain
© 1988 Elsevier Science Publishers BV (Biomedical Division)

CHAPTER 5

Direct observation of the sensitization of articular afferents during an experimental arthritis

H.-G. Schaible and R.F. Schmidt

Physiologisches Institut der Universität Würzburg, Röntgenring 9, D-8700 Würzburg, FRG

Summary

The changes in response properties of fine afferent units in the medial articular nerve of cat knee joint were studied while an acute experimental arthritis developed in this joint. The arthritis led to sensitization of high-threshold units and to induction of mechanosensitivity in units which were unresponsive to mechanical stimuli to the normal joint. In addition, some of the low-threshold afferents showed enhanced responsiveness during arthritis. From the time course of the sensitization of the articular units we conclude that the time course of hyperalgesia and pain during developing arthritis is matched best by that of the sensitization of high-threshold afferents and that of the induction of mechanosensitivity in afferent units which are unresponsive in the normal joint.

Introduction

Comparisons between the responses to passive movements in populations of afferent units from normal and inflamed joints led us to conclude that an inflammatory lesion of the joint causes sensitization of high-threshold (nociceptive) afferents, sensi-tization of low-threshold (non-nociceptive) afferents and induction of mechanosensitivity in units without mechanical excitability in the normal joint (Schaible and Schmidt, 1985; Grigg et al., 1986). The appearance or increase of resting discharges was noted as a second major consequence of arthritis. The movement-evoked activity and the additional resting discharges were discussed as the afferent correlate of the arthritic movement-evoked and resting pain (Schaible and Schmidt, 1985; Grigg et al., 1986).

Due to the diverse types of afferent unit in the nerves of the normal joint (Schaible and Schmidt, 1983a,b, 1984; Grigg et al., 1986), the comparison of two populations yields only indirect and incomplete evidence for the inflammation-induced changes, and it does not allow a determination of the time course of the alteration of response properties. We now report experiments where the inflammation-induced changes of the discharge of single articular afferent fibers were observed directly by long-time recordings beginning prior to and lasting several hours after induction of an acute experimental inflammation.

The background of this study is formed by our recent work on ascending spinal cord neurons with articular input (Schaible et al., 1986, 1987a,b). Some of these neurons were also recorded during a developing arthritis. Ascending wide-dynamic-range neurons increased their responses to movements in the working range of the joint, and ascending no-

Correspondence: Privatdozent Dr. med. Hans-Georg Schaible, Physiologisches Institut der Universität Würzburg, Röntgenring 9, D-8700 Würzburg, F.R.G.

ciceptive-specific neurons began to respond to those movements. The major changes started within the second hour after injection of the inflammatory compounds into the knee, with a further enhancement of the neuronal changes within the following two to four hours (Schaible et al., 1987b). In alpha and gamma motoneurons, such a developing arthritis induced characteristic changes of reflexes with a similar time course (He et al., 1987). In both cases the time course of the sensitization of spinal cord neurons was similar to the time course of behavioral 'pain reactions' which were observed in animals during a developing experimental monoarthritis (references in Schaible et al., 1987b).

Methods

The experiments were done on anesthetized cats. The narcosis was initiated with an intramuscular injection of 15–25 mg/kg ketamine hydrochloride (Ketanest) and continued with chloralose administered intravenously at an initial dose of 60 mg/kg. Additional chloralose was injected in doses of 20 mg/kg to maintain a deep level of anesthesia throughout the experiment. Depth of narcosis was judged from the size of the pupils, which had to be completely closed. To allow artificial respiration, the animal was tracheotomized and immobilized with pancuronium bromide (Pancuronium, Organon), 0.6 mg/h, intravenously. Blood pressure (measured in one carotid artery), end-expiratory CO_2 and body temperature were kept at physiological levels.

The recordings were performed on afferent fibres in the medial articular nerve (MAN) from the right knee joint. The set-up was described previously in detail (Schaible and Schmidt, 1983a,b, 1985; Kanaka et al., 1985; Heppelmann et al., 1985).

Single units originating from MAN were isolated in saphenous nerve using as a search stimulus electrical stimulation of MAN suprathreshold for all unmyelinated fibres. The axonal conduction velocity and the receptive field(s) in the joint were determined. Movements were performed to characterize the unit according to its responses to innocuous and noxious movements (Schaible and Schmidt 1983b, 1984). If a unit had a response to innocuous movements in the working range, this response was quantified by applying defined test movements. Resting activity, if present, was recorded for 10 min. Units unresponsive to local mechanical stimulation and movements were tested for a response to close intraarterial injection of a KCl solution (twice isotonic, 0.3 ml). Such an injection of KCl discriminates well between afferent units (responding with a short burst of impulses) and efferent sympathetic units (no response) (Schaible et al., 1983a; Kanaka et al., 1985; Grigg et al., 1986).

After isolation and identification of one to several nerve strands containing single units, an experimental inflammation was induced by injecting kaolin (4%, 0.4 ml) and thereafter carrageenan (2%, 0.3 ml) into the knee joint cavity. Slow rhythmic flexion and extension movements for 15 and 5 min followed, respectively, to distribute the compounds within the joint space. In each experiment one of the selected afferents was observed during this procedure, to record the effects evoked by the injection itself and the subsequent movements. Then the fine nerve strands were recorded alternately (for periods of 5–120 min) to study the units during the developing arthritis. Spontaneous discharges and movement-evoked impulses were counted (most often the leg was flexed or extended starting from a midflexed position of the knee; the flexed or extended position was maintained for 15–30s before returning to the resting position). In some cases (see Results) the local mechanosensitivity of a unit in the joint was also repeatedly checked. The repeated electrical stimulation of MAN confirmed that the observed units were the same as those identified prior to induction of arthritis.

Results

In all experiments the injection of kaolin and carrageenan induced an inflammation with swelling and edematous deformation of the joint structures.

This inflammatory reaction was accompanied by marked changes in the receptive properties of non-nociceptive, nociceptive and mechanically inexcitable afferent units.

Non-nociceptive afferent units
Sixteen group II units (conduction velocity 21–47 m/s), 11 group III fibres (c.v. 2.5–20 m/s) and 3 group IV units (c.v. less than 2.5 m/s) were classified as non-nociceptive afferents because they responded to movements in the working range of the normal joint (prior to inflammation). All of them were excited by supination and/or pronation and some of them also responded to extension and/or flexion of the knee.

Group II units Typical inflammation-induced changes in group II fibres are exemplified in the unit shown in Fig. 1. This unit had initially phasic responses to extension (Fig. 1A) and to flexion (Fig. 1B). About 30 min after injection of kaolin (and carrageenan) the fibre was again put on the recording electrode. The responses to extension and flexion were already enhanced, having a higher peak discharge and a tonic response component. Further increase in reactions to flexion and extension were found in the second to sixth hour after kaolin.

In 12 of the 16 low-threshold units we noted such changes in responses in the early stage of inflammation. In six of seven units which in the normal joint had no response to flexion, this movement led to excitation during development of arthritis. In five units responsive to flexion in the control period this response was enhanced during inflammation (see example in Fig. 1B). In these twelve low-threshold units, a response to extension was absent in five units prior to inflammation but developed in the course of arthritis. In five afferents, extension

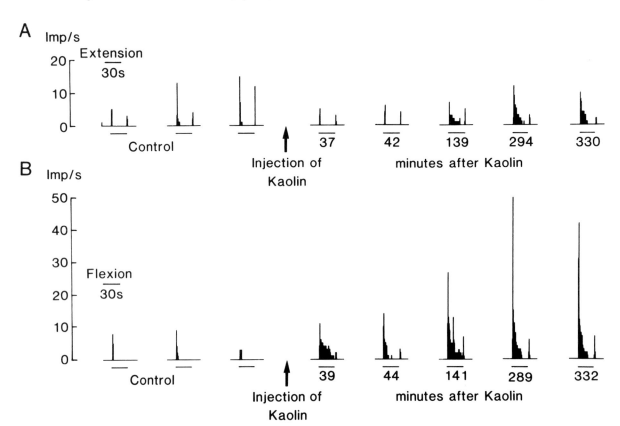

Fig. 1. Responses of a low-threshold group II unit to movements of the knee before and during arthritis (details in text).

activated the unit prior to inflammation and the response was enhanced during arthritis (see unit in Fig. 1A). In two units a response to extension declined following inflammation whereas the response to flexion increased. There were 4 group II units in which no change or only a decrease of responses was noted.

Resting activity was only induced in 1 previously silent unit, and in another 3 units previous ongoing discharges were enhanced. The remaining twelve units did not develop resting discharges.

As in the typical case shown in Fig. 1, the first change in the response of group II units was observed within the first hour after injection of kaolin and carrageenan. In units recorded during the injection itself, initial effects were mostly found immediately after this injection. From then on most afferents continued to develop higher responses within the next hours. A few afferents, after an initial increase of movement-evoked activity after the injection, first showed a decrease to the control value and then began to develop a stable increase of the response to flexion and extension.

Group III units Ten low-threshold group III units were tested. All showed changes in their responses to movements during inflammation similar to those observed in the group II units. Resting activity was induced in 5 of 7 units which were previously silent or showed some single impulses in the control period. In 4 units, inflammation led to an increase in previous resting activity.

Group IV units In one of three units a response to flexion and extension and resting activity were induced. One further unit was not altered and in the third one ongoing discharges were enhanced.

Nociceptive afferent units
One group II, 14 group III and 9 group IV units were classified as nociceptive because in the normal joint (prior to inflammation) they responded only to noxious supination and/or pronation whereas movements in the working range (e.g. flexion and extension) were ineffective. None of them had resting discharges prior to inflammation. Two of the group III and one of the group IV units had no detectable receptive field in the knee.

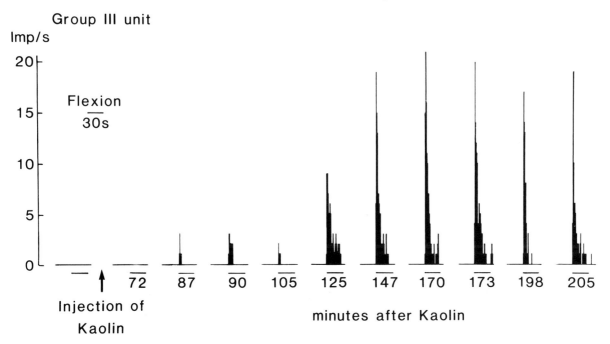

Fig. 2. Responses of a high-threshold group III unit to flexion before and during arthritis (details in text).

Within 3 h after induction of the experimental arthritis movements in the working range induced responses in the group II unit, in 10 group III units and in 3 group IV units. The sensitization of these units usually started to develop in the second hour after injection of kaolin. A typical example of the sensitization of a high-threshold group III unit is shown in Fig. 2. This unit reacted in the control period only to noxious rotations and not to flexion and extension. The inflammation led to the appearance of responses to flexion (Fig. 2) and to extension (not shown) within the second hour after induction of inflammation and a further enhancement thereafter.

Resting activity was induced in 9 group III and in 4 group IV units. It consisted of irregular (some-times frequent) discharges or single impulses.

No change of the (nociceptive) response character was found in 4 group III units and in 2 group IV units within the observation time (however, in 2 of the group III and one of the group IV units resting discharges were induced). In another 4 group IV units the responses to noxious movements were reduced (i.e., they showed desensitization in the course of inflammation).

Units which did not respond to movements in the normal joint

The sample of these units could be divided into three groups: (a) units having a receptive field and a response to KCl but no response to any movement (1 group III, 2 group IV units); (b) units lack-

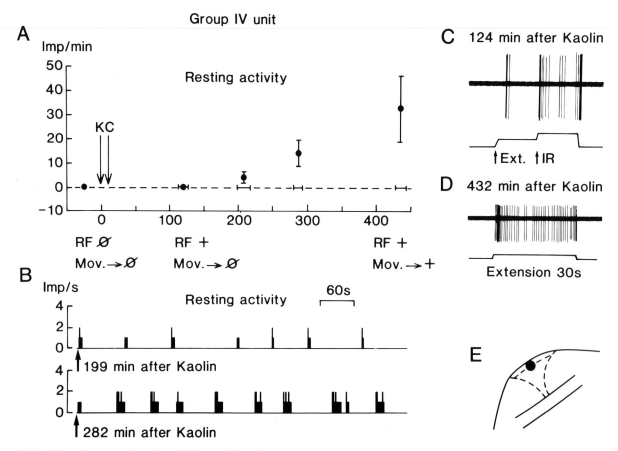

Fig. 3. Effect of an experimental arthritis on a silent afferent group IV unit. A. Mean and standard deviation of resting discharges quantified during the indicated times (bars). B. Peristimulus time histograms. C and D. Responses to movements in the inflamed state; Ext., extension; IR, pronation. E. Receptive field (dot).

ing a detectable receptive field or a response to innocuous or noxious movements, but exhibiting a response to KCl (2 group III, 16 group IV units); and (c) units without any sensitivity to local or movement stimuli and without a clear response to KCl (8 group IV units).

During inflammation, none of the units described in (a) developed responses to movements or resting activity. In the 18 fibres described in (b) the major finding was the induction of afferent activity in 11 of them. Inflammation led to a detectable receptive field in 9 units, to resting discharges in 10 units and to a response to movements in 10 units. An example is displayed in Fig. 3. In the control period this group IV unit had no resting discharges; a receptive field could not be found and movements (even noxious ones) did not excite the unit (Fig. 3A). At the end of the second hour after injection of kaolin a receptive field could be demonstrated in the patellar region (Fig. 3E). Extension evoked only a few impulses in the unit whereas pronation elicited a clear response (Fig. 3C). Within the following hours the unit started to be active without intentional stimulation (Fig. 3A and B) and extension evoked a clear reaction (Fig. 3D). Typically, the sensitization in these units started at the earliest within the second hour.

The units described in (c) showed no change within several hours (with one exception, where a receptive field became detectable and resting discharges were noted). These units were probably sympathetic efferents.

Discussion

The present results illustrate the way in which an acute (developing) experimental arthritis in the knee joint of the cat changes the response properties of afferent units in the medial articular nerve. High-threshold (nociceptive) group II, III and IV units were sensitized to respond during inflammation to movements in the working range of the joint. In units which could be excited by neither local mechanical stimulation nor movements in the normal joint (most of them were group IV units), mechanosensitivity was induced during arthritis, i.e., they began to respond to movements and to palpation of the joint. In addition, and to our surprise, some of the non-nociceptive afferents (low-threshold group II, III and IV units) also showed increased responsiveness to movements in the working range of the joint during inflammation.

Resting activity was induced or enhanced in many non-nociceptive, nociceptive and non-responsive group III and IV units, whereas group II units did not develop activity in most cases.

Presumed efferent units, i.e., fibres without mechanosensitivity and without response to KCl during the normal period, remained unresponsive and silent during inflammation. The time course of the changes in afferent discharges showed characteristic differences between the various classes of afferent units. The low-threshold units were affected first, often showing enhanced responses within the first hour of the developing inflammation (or immediately after the intraarticular injections). On the other hand, high-threshold units typically became sensitized within the second and third hours. Mechanosensitivity in previously non-responsive units appeared even later.

Our data correlate well with behavioural experiments in which an acute monoarthritis was induced and possible signs of hyperalgesia and pain were observed thereafter (references in Schaible et al., 1987b, and own unpublished observations). In several species (including the cat), signs of hyperalgesia or pain appeared within the second to fourth hours of crystal- (kaolin, urate) or carrageenan-induced inflammation. At this time most nociceptive units in the present experiments began to respond to movements in the working range of the joint, indicating sensitization. Thus, this sensitization of high-threshold (nociceptive) groups III and IV units is probably crucial for the development of hyperalgesia and pain. Presumably the recruitment of originally non-responsive afferent units (mainly group IV fibres) leads to a massive enhancement of the total nociceptive afferent inflow determining intensity and quality of hyperalgesia and pain (e.g. resting pain).

There is no clear evidence that the enhanced activity in low-threshold (presumably non-nociceptive) units contributes to hyperalgesia and pain. In these units, increased responsiveness appeared very early, at a time when in behavioural experiments no signs of hyperalgesia or pain are observable. But their discharges may induce the appearance of hyperalgesia and pain by converging on the wide-dynamic-range spinal neurons with ascending axons (see Introduction).

Several factors may contribute to the sensitization of the afferents. Crystals and carrageenan evoke release and synthesis of mediators eliciting the local inflammatory reaction (Moncada et al., 1979). Group III and IV articular afferents are chemosensitive to these mediators; their increased mechanosensitivity may be caused by chemical sensitization (Heppelman et al., 1987; see also Guilbaud et al., 1987). The early effects observed in some units immediately after the injection of the compounds suggest that mechanical factors may also contribute to sensitization. During developing inflammation, the tissue becomes edematous and infiltrated and intraarticular pressure may increase (Schumacher et al., 1974). Such mechanical factors are probably responsible for the sensitization of group II units which are not chemosensitive (Kanaka et al., 1985) and they may add to the presumed chemical sensitization of group III and IV units.

Acknowledgements

The authors thank Maria Ludwig, Margit Schulze, Volker Neugebauer and Thomas Heinicke for their excellent assistance. This work was supported by the Deutsche Forschungsgemeinschaft.

References

Grigg, P., Schaible, H.-G. and Schmidt, R.F. (1986) Mechanical sensitivity of group III and IV afferents from posterior articular nerve in normal and inflamed cat knee. J. Neurophysiol., 55: 635–643.

Guilbaud, G., Benoist, J.M., Kayser, V. and Neil, A. (1987) Responses of ventrobasal thalamic neurones to carrageenan-induced inflammation in the rat. In R.F. Schmidt, H.-G. Schaible and C. Vahle-Hinz (Eds.), Fine Afferent Nerve Fibers and Pain, VCH Verlagsgemeinschaft, Weinheim, pp. 411–425.

He., X., Proske, U., Schaible, H.-G. and Schmidt, R.F. (1988) Changes in reflex excitability of flexor motoneurones evoked by acute inflammation of the knee joint in the cat. J. Neurophysiol. in press.

Heppelmann, B., Herbert, M.K., Schaible, H.-G. and Schmidt, R.F. (1987) Morphological and physiological characteristics of the innervation of cat's normal and arthritic knee joint. In L.M. Pubols and B.J. Sessle (Eds.), Effects of Injury on Trigeminal and Spinal Somatosensory Systems, Alan R. Liss, New York, pp. 19–27.

Heppelmann, B., Schaible, H.-G. and Schmidt, R.F. (1985) Effects of prostaglandins E_1 and E_2 on the mechanosensitivity of group III afferents from normal and inflamed cat knee joints. In H.L. Fields, R. Dubner and F. Cervero (Eds.), Advances in Pain Research and Therapy, Vol. 9, Raven, New York, pp. 91–101.

Kanaka, R., Schaible, H.-G. and Schmidt, R.F. (1985) Activation of fine articular afferent units by bradykinin. Brain Res., 327: 81–90.

Moncada, S., Ferreira, S.H. and Vane, J.R. (1979) Pain and inflammatory mediators. In J.R. Vane and S.H. Ferreira (Eds.), Handbook of Experimental Pharmacology, Vol. 50, Part I: Inflammation, Springer, Berlin, pp. 588–616.

Schaible, H.-G. and Schmidt, R.F. (1983a) Activation of group III and IV sensory units in medial articular nerve by local mechanical stimulation of knee joint. J. Neurophysiol., 49: 35–44.

Schaible, H.-G. and Schmidt, R.F. (1983b) Responses of fine medial articular nerve afferents to passive movements of knee joint. J. Neurophysiol., 49: 1118–1126.

Schaible, H.-G. and Schmidt, R.F. (1985) Effects of an experimental arthritis on the sensory properties of fine articular afferent units. J. Neurophysiol., 54: 1109–1122.

Schaible, H.-G., Schmidt, R.F. and Willis, W.D. (1986) Responses of spinal cord neurones to stimulation of articular afferent fibres in the cat. J. Physiol., 372: 575–593.

Schaible, H.-G., Schmidt, R.F. and Willis, W.D. (1987a) Convergent inputs from articular, cutaneous and muscle receptors onto ascending tract cells in the cat spinal cord. Exp. Brain Res., 66: 479–488.

Schaible, H.-G., Schmidt, R.F. and Willis, W.D. (1987b) Enhancement of the responses of ascending tract cells in the cat spinal cord by acute inflammation of the knee joint. Exp. Brain Res., 66: 489–499.

Schumacher, H.R., Phelps, P. and Agudelo, C.A. (1974) Urate crystal induced inflammation in dog joints: sequence of synovial changes. J. Rheumatol., 1: 102–113.

R. Dubner, G.F. Gebhart & M.R. Bond (Eds.)
Proceedings of the Vth World Congress on Pain
© 1988 Elsevier Science Publishers BV (Biomedical Division)

CHAPTER 6

Peripheral release of substance P from primary afferents

Tony L. Yaksh[1], Jane Bailey[2], Diane R. Roddy[2] and Gail J. Harty[1]

[1]*Section of Neurosurgical Research and* [2]*GI Hormone Research Laboratory, Mayo Clinic, Rochester, MN 55905, USA*

Summary

Substance P (sP) is contained in the peripheral terminals of primary afferents. In the present study, we show that the levels of sP in the perfusate of knee joint, skin bleb or in the lymph can be elevated by antidromic stimulation of the sciatic nerve. This release is also evoked by locally applied capsaicin, which subsequently blocks antidromic-evoked release.

Introduction

Substance P (sP) synthesized in dorsal root ganglion (Hokfelt et al., 1975) is transported both centrally and peripherally to the distant terminals (Brimijoin et al., 1980). Ample evidence exists to suggest that the spinal sP exists within a releasable fraction by virtue of the ability to evoke an increase in the extracellar levels by orthodromic stimulation of small but not large somatic afferents (Yaksh et al., 1980; Go and Yaksh, 1987). Significantly, this release is Ca^+-dependent and subject to modulation by several populations of receptors (opioid, α_2; Yaksh et al., 1980; Pang and Vasko, 1986; Go and Yaksh, 1987; Kuraishi et al., 1985). The disposition

of sP in the peripheral terminals is less well characterized, though it has long been appreciated that antidromic activity releases a material with physiological properties similar to those of sP (see Pernow, 1983). There is evidence for peripheral secretion of sP from tooth pulp and eye, released by antidromic stimulation of the trigeminal nerve (Brodin et al., 1981; Mandahl et al., 1984), and from the skin by antidromic stimulation of the sciatic nerve in the rat (White and Helme, 1985). These data suggest that the pools of sP in peripheral terminals can be released by antidromic activity. In the present studies we endeavored to characterize the effects of antidromic stimulation on the peripheral release of sP into the synovial joint and from the skin in the cat.

Methods

Artificially ventilated, halothane-anesthetized (1%) cats were prepared for perfusion of the synovial joint and skin blebs. To perfuse the synovial joint, 23-gauge needles were inserted on either side of the patella. Perfusion of a modified Krebs solution containing bacitracin (30 μg/ml) was initiated (100 μl/min) using a two-channel peristaltic pump in an infusion withdrawal mode. To perfuse the skin, a bleb was formed by the injection of 1 ml of a Krebs solution subdermally with a 30-gauge needle. The bleb was penetrated with a 25-gauge needle for infusion

---

Correspondence: Tony L. Yaksh, Ph.D., Mayo Clinic, Rochester, MN 55905, U.S.A.

(50 μl/min) and a 22-gauge needle for passive out-flow. Typically, knee joint and skin blebs were pre-pared bilaterally. Alternatively, in some experi-ments, the saphenous lymph duct was catheterized using PE-10 just below the popliteal fossa to collect lymph drainage from the foot.

All perfusate samples were collected for 20-min intervals in polyethylene tubes with 50 μl of acetic acid. Perfusate was then frozen, lyophilized and stored at $-70°C$ until assay. The sP assay was car-ried out using antibody No. 4892 (1:15000). The li-gand was ^{125}I-Tyr^8-sP. Bound and free were sepa-rated by immunoprecipitation. Details of the assay are reported elsewhere (Go and Yaksh, 1987). Ab-solute sensitivity of the assay was 1 pg/tube. Inter- and intra-assay reliability was 11% and 5%, respec-tively.

The assay shows less sensitivity following reduc-tion of either the amino- or the carboxy terminus and essentially no cross-reactivity at 100 pg/ml with substance K, bombesin, cholecystokinin octapept-ide, neurotensin, somatostatin, methionine enke-phalin, vasoactive intestinal polypeptide, physalae-min or calcitonin gene-related peptide.

To antidromically activate peripheral terminals, the sciatic nerve was exposed bilaterally at the level of the ischeal notch and locally ligated and cut pro-ximal to the spinal cord. The nerves were then placed on hook electrodes; the incision was filled with vegetable oil, and loosely closed. To establish a stimulation threshold, the minimum stimulation intensity necessary for evoking a detectable twitch of the hindlimb was assessed. All stimulation was carried out at 3-times or 30-times the minimum mo-tor threshold (MMT). Previous studies have shown these intensities to reliably activate fibers which conduct at >50 m/s and also fibers which conduct as slowly as 0.5–1 m/s, respectively (Go and Yaksh, 1987). After determining these thresholds, the ani-mal was given pancuronium to achieve ventilatory control.

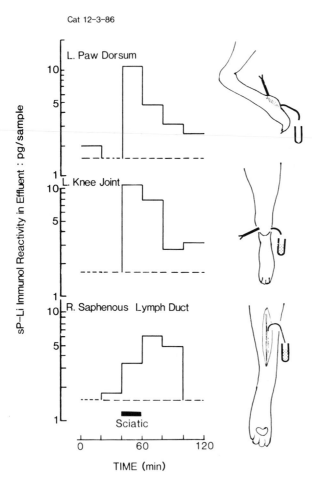

Cat 12-3-86

Fig. 1. Levels of sP-like immunoreactivity (pg/sample) measured concurrently in a single cat in the skin bleb perfusate of the left paw (top), left knee joint (middle) and the drainage from the right saphenous lymph duct (bottom). At the time indicated by the black bar, the peripheral segments of the left and right sciatic nerves were stimulated at 30× minimum motor threshold (see text for other details).

Results

As shown in the results from a single experiment (Fig. 1), under resting conditions, little or no sP-like immunoreactivity (sP-LI) was detected in the knee joint (KJ) or skin bleb (SB) perfusates. As indicated in Table I, under these conditions, we were unable to measure sP-LI in 12 of 18 SB or 18 of 24 KJ per-fusates or in 5 of 6 lymph studies (< 1 pg/20 min). Stimulation of the sciatic nerves (50 Hz; 0.1 ms stimulus pulse, 30× MMT; 1 s pulse trains; 0.5 Hz

TABLE I

Levels of substance P-like immunoreactivity in perfusates of synovial joint and skin bleb during resting and periods of sciatic nerve stimulation or the addition of capsaicin to the perfusate

| | Levels of sP-LI in the perfusates (pg/sample) | | | | | |
	Skin bleb	*n*	Synovial	*n*	Lymph	*n*
Control	–[a]	18	–[b]	24	–[c]	6
Sciatic stimulation (30 × MMT)	11 ± 5[d]	8	15 ± 9[d]	12	22 ± 11	6
Capsaicin (100 μM)	18 ± 9[d]	10	22 ± 7[d]	12	–	–

[a]Below assay sensitivity of 12 of 18 experiments.
[b]Below assay sensitivity in 18 of 24 experiments.
[c]Below assay sensitivity in 5 of 6 experiments.
[d]All above assay sensitivity.
n = number of experiments.

train rate) resulted in a clear stimulus-dependent increase in the levels of sP-LI in the left KJ and SB perfusates and in the lymph collected from the right saphenous lymph duct.

As shown in Fig. 1, the rise of sP-LI measured in KJ and SB perfusates was maximal in the sample collected during stimulation. In contrast, lymph sP was commonly observed to be maximal in the sample collected after the brief interval of stimulation. Table I shows the mean increase in sP-LI activity over baseline during stimulation.

To determine whether the release of sP with stimulation was dependent upon primary afferent terminals, animals were prepared as described for KJ perfusion. After the control period, capsaicin (10^{-4} M) was added to the perfusate of the left knee. Capsaicin and sciatic nerve stimulation both resulted in a prominent release of sP-LI similar to that displayed in Table I. After 60 min, both sciatic nerves were stimulated and a prominent increase in KJ-sP secretion was observed in the right KJ but not the left (the one previously receiving capsaicin).

In preliminary experiments, we addressed the question of whether the peripheral release of sP was a function of activity in small- or large-diameter afferents. To accomplish this, the sciatic nerve was stimulated initially at an intensity of 3 × MMT and

followed three samples later by stimulation at 30 × MMT. 3 × MMT stimulation had no effect on the resting levels of sP-LI in the KJ (4 of 4 remained below assay sensitivity). In contrast, the subsequent stimulation at 30 × MMT resulted in KJ perfusate levels of sP-LI similar to those shown in Table I (17 ± 4 pg/sample; $p < 0.01$; $n = 4$).

Discussion

These results indicate that sP-LI is secreted into the KJ and the skin secondary to antidromic activity in somatic nerve. Based on the thresholds of stimulation required to evoke the release and the ability of capsaicin to attenuate the antidromically evoked release, it is reasonable to conclude that the secretion is secondary to activity in small-diameter primary afferents. Capsaicin has been shown to depolarize the terminals of slowly conducting primary afferents and this leads to a subsequent desensitization (see Fitzgerald, 1983). The prominent release evoked by capsaicin in these studies is consistent with that interpretation.

These observations regarding the peripheral secretion of sP suggest that the peripheral afferent terminals may possess physiological and pharmacological properties comparable to those of the central terminals. Thus, both terminals secrete sP following depolarization and both are stimulated and desensitized by capsaicin (see Go and Yaksh, 1987). In recent studies we observed that the peripheral release evoked by sciatic nerve stimulation was diminished by the local perfusion of sufentanil and this effect was antagonized by naloxone (Yaksh, unpublished observations). Such results are comparable to reports where the depletion of sP in tooth pulp by antidromic stimulation is diminished by morphine (Brodin et al., 1983). Given that opioid binding substance is synthesized in the cell body and then transported peripherally in primary afferents (Laduron, 1984), such observations are consistent with the presence of opioid receptors on the peripheral terminals coupled to the release process.

The role of peripherally secreted sP is not known, but there is accumulating evidence that sensory innervation of the joint by capsaicin-sensitive fibers may be responsible for the trophic changes in joints observed during adjuvant arthritis (Levine et al., 1985). The present studies suggest that antidromic activation of the sensory nerve, or a local stimulus (such as capsaicin), may evoke that secretion. The ability of opiates to diminish the peripheral release of sP and to block the spontaneous activity observed in afferents innervating an inflamed KJ (Russell et al., 1987) is particularly interesting. sP can evoke the degranulation of mast cells (releasing serotonin and histamine: Fewtrell et al., 1982) and perhaps increase prostanoid formation (see Jonsson et al., 1986). The idea that such peripheral secretion plays complex roles in the peripheral tissues therefore appears certain to be correct.

Acknowledgements

This work was supported in part by the Mayo Foundation and by NIH grant AM-34988. We would like to thank Ms. Gail Harty for helping carry out the perfusion experiments.

References

Brimijoin, S., Lundberg, J.M., Brodin, E., Hokfelt, T. and Nilsson, G. (1980) Axonal transport of substance P in the vagus and sciatic nerves of the guinea-pig. Brain Res., 191: 443–457.

Brodin, E., Gazelius, B., Olgart, L. and Nilsson, G. (1981) Tissue concentration and release of substance P-like immunoreactivity in the dental pulp. Acta Physiol. Scand., 111: 141–149.

Brodin, E., Gazelius, B., Panopoulos, P. and Olgart, L. (1983) Morphine inhibits substance P release from peripheral sensory nerve endings. Acta Physiol. Scand., 117: 567–570.

Fewtrell, C.M.S., Foreman, J.C., Jordan, C.C., Oehme, P., Renner, H. and Stewart, J.M. (1982) The effects of substance P on histamine and 5-hydroxytryptamine release in rat. J. Physiol., 330: 393–411.

Fitzgerald, M. (1983) Capsaicin and sensory neurones – review. Pain, 15: 109–130.

Go, V.L.W. and Yaksh, T.L. (1987) Release of substance P from the cat spinal cord. J. Physiol., 383: in press.

Hokfelt, T., Kellerth, J.O., Nilsson, G. and Pernow, B. (1975) Experimental immunohistochemical studies on the localization and distribution of substance P in cat primary sensory neurons. Brain Res., 100: 235–252.

Jonsson, C.-E., Brodin, E., Dalsgaard, C.-J. and Haegerstrand, A. (1986) Release of substance-P-like immunoreactivity in dog paw lymph after scalding injury. Acta Physiol. Scand., 126: 21–24.

Kuraishi, Y., Hirota, N., Sato, Y., Kaneko, S., Satoh, M. and Takagi, H. (1985) Noradrenergic inhibition of the substance P-containing sensory primary afferents in the rabbit dorsal horn. Brain Res., 359: 177–182.

Laduron, P.M. (1984) Axonal transport of opiate receptors in capsaicin-sensitive neurones. Brain Res., 294: 157–160.

Levine, J.D., Moskowitz, M.A. and Basbaum, A.I. (1985) The contribution of neurogenic inflammation in experimental arthritis. J. Immunol., 15: 843S–847S.

Mandahl, A., Brodin, E. and Bill, A. (1984) Hypertonic KCl, NaCl and capsaicin intracamerally causes release of substance P-like immunoreactive material into the aqueous humour in rabbits. Acta Physiol. Scand., 120: 579–584.

Pang, I.-H. and Vasko, M.R. (1986) Morphine and norepinephrine but not 5-hydroxytryptamine and γ-aminobutyric acid inhibit the potassium-stimulated release of substance P from rat spinal cord slices. Brain Res., 376: 268–279.

Pernow, B. (1983) Substance P – A putative mediator of antidromic vasodilation. Gen. Pharmac., 14: 13–16.

Russell, N.J.W., Schaible, H.-G. and Schmidt, R.F. (1987) Opiates inhibit the discharges of fine afferent units from inflamed knee joint of the cat. Neurosci. Lett., 76: 107–112.

White, D.M. and Helme, R.D. (1985) Release of substance P from peripheral terminal nerve terminals following electrical stimulation of the sciatic nerve. Brain Res., 336: 27–31.

Yaksh, T.L., Jessell, T.M., Gamse, R., Mudge, A.W. and Leeman, S.E. (1980) Intrathecal morphine inhibits substance P release from mammalian spinal cord in vivo. Nature, 286: 155–156.

R. Dubner, G.F. Gebhart & M.R. Bond (Eds.)
Proceedings of the Vth World Congress on Pain
© 1988 Elsevier Science Publishers BV (Biomedical Division)

CHAPTER 7

Peripheral actions of opiates in the blockade of carrageenan-induced inflammation

Kenneth M. Hargreaves, Ronald Dubner and Jean Joris

*Neurobiology and Anesthesiology Branch, National Institute of Dental Research, National Institutes of Health,
Bethesda, MD, USA*

Introduction

Several lines of evidence indicate that opiates produce effects through activation of receptors located in the central nervous system (CNS) at both spinal and supraspinal levels (for review see Dubner and Bennett, 1983; Basbaum and Fields, 1983). However, opiates may also possess peripheral activity. Opioid receptors have been demonstrated on primary afferent nerve fibers, where they undergo transport towards the periphery (Fields et al., 1980; Young et al., 1980; Laduron, 1984). It is not known whether these peripheral receptors contribute to the analgesic activity of opiates and opioid peptides.

One peripheral effect of opiate agonists has been suggested using a model of sensitization induced by the administration of exogenous prostaglandins (Ferreira and Nakamura, 1979). In an actual model of inflammation, it has been reported that opiate antagonists possess peripheral agonist-like analgesic activity (Rios and Jacob, 1983). However, the pharmacological specificity of opiate agonists at peripheral sites of inflammation is unknown. A second peripheral effect of opiates is inhibition of the plasma extravasation that occurs after electrical stimulation of peripheral nerves (Lembeck and

Holzer, 1979; Smith and Buchan, 1984). However, the effect of opiates on inhibiting the plasma extravasation that occurs with actual tissue injury is unknown.

In the present study, we used carrageenan (CARRA) to produce a model of inflammation which is highly predictive of analgesic drug activity in human inflammatory pain (Otterness and Bliven, 1985). We report here that opiates administered locally into a site of inflammation at doses which have no systemic effect produce analgesia restricted to the injected area. In addition, systemic administration of morphine suppresses the plasma extravasation and edema that occurs during carrageenan-evoked inflammation.

Methods

For evaluating the peripheral analgesic effects of opiates, rats were placed beneath an inverted clear plastic chamber on a glass floor. After a 5-min habituation period, the plantar surface of their paws was exposed to radiant heat; paw-withdrawal latency (PWL) was taken as an index of the nociceptive threshold. Previous studies have demonstrated that organized intentional behaviors from which pain and analgesia can be inferred are correlated with withdrawal latency in this model (Hargreaves et al., 1987a).

Correspondence: Dr. Kenneth Hargreaves, NAB, NIDR, NIH, Bldg. 10, Room 1A-09, Bethesda, MD 20892, U.S.A.

In an initial study, the peripheral effect of the kappa agonist EKC (Sterling Winthrop Res. Inst., NY) was assessed. One group ($n = 7$) received initial injections (0.1 ml) of saline (SAL) into the plantar surface of both hind paws at time 0, and 90 min later received injections of SAL into both paws and subcutaneously (s.c.) into the neck. Three other groups ($n = 7$-10) received initial injections (0.1 ml) of 2 mg of lambda CARRA into both paws. Ninety minutes later, one CARRA group received an injection of 10 μg EKC into one inflamed paw; SAL was injected into the other inflamed paw and also s.c. into the neck. At the same time, another CARRA group received SAL injections into both paws and the same dose of EKC (10 μg) injected s.c. into the neck. The last CARRA group received SAL injections in both paws and the neck. Rats were tested once at baseline and 2, 3 and 4 h after the initial paw injections.

In the next experiment, the dose-response relationship and the stereoselectivity of the peripheral opiate effect were determined using a mu agonist, levorphanol (Hoffman-La Roche Inc., NJ), and its inactive dextrorotatory isomer, dextrorphan (Hoffman-La Roche Inc., NJ). CARRA ($n = 6$) was injected into both paws and 90 min later SAL was injected into one hind paw, while the other inflamed paw was injected with either levorphanol (20, 40, 80 or 160 μg) or dextrorphan (160 μg). Rats were tested once at baseline and at 2 h after the CARRA injections.

For evaluating the effect of morphine on plasma extravasation, male Sprague-Dawley rats had catheters implanted in the left jugular vein under pentobarbital anesthesia. Two days after surgery, one hindpaw was injected s.c. in the plantar surface with 2 mg (in 0.1 ml saline) of lambda CARRA (Sigma Co., St. Louis), while the other hindpaw received 0.1 ml of saline. Ninety minutes later, rats were injected i.v. with either 2 mg/kg morphine sulfate ($n = 12$) or saline ($n = 11$); 15 min later, all animals received an i.v. injection of Evans blue dye (33 mg/kg). Dorsal-plantar paw thickness was measured to the nearest 0.1 mm at 120 min using a caliper. Edema was calculated by measuring the difference between the thickness of the control saline-injected paws and the thickness of the carrageenan-injected paws. The animals were then killed and a 6-mm punch biopsy of hindpaw skin (Baker Cummins, Fl.) was taken. The punch was positioned just proximal to the two distal callous pads on the plantar surface of the hind paw (see Fig. 3 insert). Since Evans blue binds to plasma proteins normally restricted to the vascular compartment, its presence in s.c. tissue is a standard marker for plasma extravasation (Lembeck and Holzer, 1979). The dye was

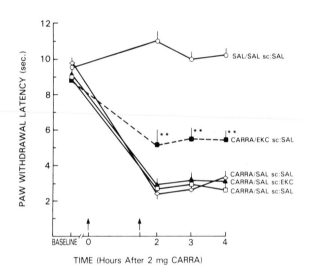

Fig. 1. Peripheral analgesic effect of ethylketocyclazocine (EKC, 10 μg). One group received initial injections of saline (SAL) into the plantar surface of both hindpaws at time 0 (first arrow) and 90 min later (second arrow) received injections of SAL into both hindpaws and subcutaneously (s.c.) into the neck (SAL/SAL sc:SAL, open circles). The three other groups received initial hindpaw injections of carrageenan (CARRA). Ninety minutes later, one CARRA group received an s.c. injection of SAL into the neck and EKC (10 μg) into one inflamed paw (CARRA/EKC sc:SAL, filled squares) and SAL into the other inflamed paw (CARRA/SAL sc:SAL, open squares). At the same time, another CARRA group received SAL injections into both paws and the same dose of EKC injected into the neck (CARRA/SAL sc:EKC, filled triangles). The last CARRA group (CARRA/SAL sc:SAL, open diamonds) received SAL into the paws and the neck. The circles, the triangles and the diamonds represent the mean latencies of both hindpaws which had received the same treatment. ** = $P < 0.01$ as compared to the contralateral, saline-treated inflamed paw (open squares). Error bars depict SEM. From Joris et al. (1987) Anesthesia and Analgesia, 66: 1277–1281.

extracted from the tissue samples for 3 days by the addition of 2 ml of formamide. The optical density (620 nm) of the samples was converted to µg of dye by comparison of a standard curve of Evans blue dye in formamide.

For all studies, data were collected by an observer unaware of treatment allocation and analysed by analysis of variance (ANOVA) for repeated measures followed by Duncan's multiple range test (Winer, 1975). To determine a dose-response relationship for levorphanol-treated paws, a linear regression ANOVA tested the zero-slope hypothesis (Winer, 1975).

Results

Fig. 1 shows the peripheral analgesic effects of EKC. Administration of CARRA into both paws followed by SAL injections resulted in a sustained hyperalgesia ($P < 0.01$) as compared to rats administered SAL only. In the group receiving CARRA followed by a peripheral opiate injection into one paw, 10 µg of EKC produced a significant peripheral analgesia ($F[1,9] = 13.6$; $P < 0.01$) as compared to contralateral inflamed paws injected with SAL (Fig. 1). This effect persisted for more than 2 h. In contrast, EKC had no effect when administered systemically.

Administration of levorphanol into an inflamed paw produced a peripheral, dose-related analgesia ($F[1,20] = 11.9$; $P < 0.005$) as compared to the inflamed contralateral paw injected with SAL (Fig. 2). The analgesic effect was most clearly evident with the 40 µg ($P < 0.05$), 80 µg ($P < 0.01$) and 160 µg ($P < 0.01$) doses. This peripheral analgesic effect was stereoselective, since administration of 160 µg of dextrorphan did not alter the nociceptive threshold (Fig. 2). Levorphanol at these doses had no systemic effect, since the contralateral saline-injected paws exhibited neither a significant difference between any groups nor a dose-response relationship.

As compared to the contralateral control paws, the inflamed hind paws had significantly ($F[1,21]=91.0$; $P < 0.001$) greater plasma extrava-

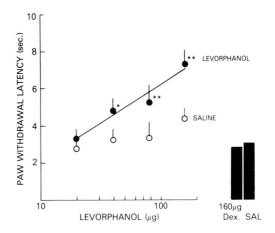

Fig. 2. Dose-response relationship and stereoselectivity for the peripheral analgesic effects of levorphanol ($n=6$/group). CARRA was injected into both hindpaws and 90 min later saline was injected into one hindpaw while the other hindpaw was injected with either levorphanol (20, 40, 80 or 160 µg) or dextrorphan (160 µg). Rats were tested 3 h after the CARRA injection. The asterisks denote significant differences between the paw-withdrawal latencies of the levorphanol-treated paws (filled circles) and the contralateral, saline-treated paws (corresponding open circles) with * = $P < 0.05$ and ** = $P < 0.01$. There was no significant difference for the paw-withdrawal latency between dextrorphan (filled histogram) and the contralateral saline-treated paws (open histogram). Error bars depict SEM. From Joris et al. (1987) Anesthesia and Analgesia, 66: 1277–1281.

sation, as indicated by an accumulation of Evans blue dye in the subcutaneous tissue (Fig. 3). However, the carrageenan-induced plasma extravasation was significantly ($F[1,21]=6.47$; $P < 0.01$) inhibited by administration of morphine; there were no differences between the saline-treated paws (Fig. 3).

Morphine also produced a significant ($F[1,21]=7.9$; $P < 0.01$) reduction of carrageenan-induced edema (Fig. 4). The carrageenan-treated paws of rats given i.v. morphine had significantly less edema ($P < 0.01$) as compared to rats given i.v. saline (Fig. 4).

Discussion

We have demonstrated that local administration of EKC and levorphanol into an inflamed paw produ-

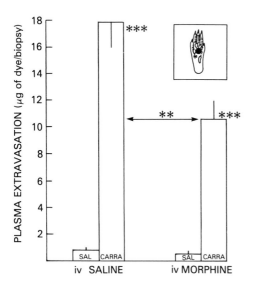

Fig. 3. Effect of systemic morphine on carrageenan-induced plasma extravasation. Rats had one hindpaw injected with 2 mg carrageenan (CARRA) while the other hindpaw was injected with saline (SAL). The animals were divided into two groups and 90 min later were administered i.v. 2 mg/kg morphine ($n = 12$) or saline ($n = 11$). The rats received i.v. Evans blue (33 mg/kg) 15 min later. Rats were then killed and 6 mm punch biopsies of the inflamed and saline-treated paws were collected. Evans blue dye was extracted from the tissue samples with formamide and quantitated by comparison to a standard curve at 620 nm. Inset: plantar surface of a rat hindpaw illustrating the position of the 6-mm punch biopsy. **$P < 0.01$ vs. the CARRA-injected paw of the i.v. saline group. ***$P < 0.001$ vs. the contralateral saline-injected paw. Error bars depict the SEM.

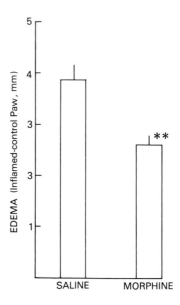

Fig. 4. Effect of systemic morphine (2 mg/kg) on carrageenan-induced edema. The treatment groups are the same as those described in Fig. 3. The dorsal-plantar paw thickness was measured by a caliper to 0.1 mm. Edema was calculated by measuring the difference between the thickness of the saline-injected paws and the thickness of the contralateral carrageenan-injected paws. The thickness of the saline-injected paws did not differ for rats given i.v. saline (5.0 + 0.1 mm) or i.v. morphine (5.1 + 0.1 mm). **$P < 0.01$. Error bars depict the SEM.

ces a dose-related analgesia restricted to the injected paw. These effects are opioid receptor-specific, since levorphanol is analgesic while its dextrorotatory isomer, dextrorphan, is inactive. An additional test to determine opioid specificity, naloxone challenge, was contraindicated because of naloxone's reported agonist-like effects in this model of inflammation (Rios and Jacob, 1983). In addition, morphine suppresses plasma extravasation by 41% and inhibits edema by 32% in CARRA-evoked inflammation.

If opiates acted only in the central nervous system to produce analgesia, then a bilateral analgesic effect should have been observed in both inflamed hind paws, regardless of the site of administration.

However, systemic administration of this low dose of EKC had no effect, while peripheral administration into an inflamed paw produced localized analgesia. Additional evidence for lack of a systemic opiate effect is the similar latencies of the SAL-injected contralateral paws of the group receiving local opiate and for the CARRA group receiving no opiate. Finally, the latencies of the SAL-treated paws of the four levorphanol groups were statistically indistinguishable, despite the dose-related analgesia observed in the opiate-treated paws. We interpret these results to indicate that opiate-induced analgesia is due to a peripheral as well as to its well-recognized central mechanism of action. The peripheral analgesic effect is observed with both kappa and mu agonists.

These results raise the question of the mechanism of this peripheral opiate effect. Since plasma extravasation is a fundamental step in the development of inflammation, the blockade of edema and hyper-algesia by opiates may be related to an initial opiate blockade of plasma extravasation. The two most likely targets are peripheral terminals of primary afferents and leukocytes, both of which are known to possess opioid receptors (Fields et al., 1980; Young et al., 1980; Laduron, 1984; Wybran, 1985). An opioid effect on the nerve terminals may be direct, by modulating nociceptive transmission (Jurna and Grossman, 1977; Russell et al., 1987) or may be indirect, by an anti-inflammatory effect (Lembeck and Holzer, 1979; Smith and Buchan, 1984). This last issue is pertinent, since carrageenan-evoked inflammation has a significant neurogenic component (Joris et al., 1987). An alternative hypothesis is that the opiate effect on edema and plasma extravasation is due to a CNS alteration of efferent outflow. Since morphine was administered systemically, it remains to be determined whether the suppression of plasma extravasation and edema are related to the peripheral effects of opiates or to their systemic effects.

The existence of a peripheral site of action for opiate-induced analgesia provides a potential target for circulating opioid peptides. Numerous studies have demonstrated that blood-borne levels of opioid peptides increase significantly under conditions of stress (Mueller, 1980) and inflammatory pain (Hargreaves et al., 1986; Joris et al., 1986). However, their physiological role is unclear. The potential role of pituitary β-endorphin (β-END) in modulating pain has been evaluated under conditions designed to stimulate its release and activate endogenous pain suppression systems (Amir and Amit, 1978a,b: Marek et al., 1983). These observations may be clinically relevant, since patients pretreated with low doses of dexamethasone have lower levels of circulating β-endorphin and significantly greater levels of post-operative pain as compared to patients treated with placebo (Hargreaves et al., 1987b). Recent studies have extended these findings by administration of corticotropin-releasing factor (CRF) to post-operative patients. CRF is the endogenous signal for evoking the release of pituitary β-END in response to stressors such as surgery or post-operative pain (Vale et al., 1981). Administration of CRF was found to stimulate β-END secretion and significantly reduce post-operative pain in patients following extraction of impacted third molars (Hargreaves et al., 1987c). Results from the present study suggest that one potential target for these circulating opioids is the peripheral modulation of nociception secondary to inflammation.

References

Amir, S. and Amit, Z. (1978a) Endogenous opioid ligands may mediate stress-induced changes in the affective properties of pain related behavior in rats. Life Sci., 23: 1143–1152.

Amir, S. and Amit, Z. (1978b) The pituitary gland mediates acute and chronic pain responsiveness in stressed and non-stressed rats. Life Sci., 24: 439–448.

Basbaum, A. and Fields, H. (1984) Endogenous pain control systems; brainstem spinal pathways and endorphin circuitry. Annu. Rev. Neurosci., 7: 309–338.

Dubner, R. and Bennett, G. (1983) Spinal and trigeminal mechanisms of nociception. Annu. Rev. Neurosci., 6: 381–418.

Ferreira, S. and Nakamura, M. (1979) Prostaglandin hyperalgesia, II: the peripheral analgesic activity of morphine, enkephalins and opioids antagonists. Prostaglandins, 23: 53–60.

Fields, H., Emson, P., Leigh, B., Gilbert, R. and Iversen, L. (1980) Multiple opiate receptor site on primary afferent fibers. Nature, 284: 351–353.

Hargreaves, K., Dionne, R., Mueller, G., Goldstein, D. and Dubner, R. (1986) Naloxone, fentanyl and diazepam modify plasma beta-endorphin levels during surgery. Clin. Pharmacol. Ther., 40: 165–171.

Hargreaves, K., Dubner, R., Brown, F., Flores, C. and Joris, J. (1987a) A new and sensitive method for measuring thermal nociception in cutaneous hyperalgesia. Pain, in press.

Hargreaves, K., Schmidt, E., Mueller, G. and Dionne, R. (1987b) Dexamethasone alters plasma levels of beta-endorphin and post-operative pain. Clin. Pharm. Ther., 42: 601–607.

Hargreaves, K., Mueller, G., Dubner, R., Goldstein, D. and Dionne, R. (1987c) Corticotropin releasing factor (CRF) produces analgesia in humans and rats. Brain Res., 422: 154–157.

Joris, J., Dubner, R., Brown, F., Flores C. and Hargreaves, K. (1986) Behavioral and endocrine correlates of thermal nociception in carrageenan-induced cutaneous hyperalgesia. Abstr. Soc. Neurosci., 12: 374.

Joris, J., Dubner, R. and Hargreaves, K. (1987) Involvement of the peripheral nervous system in carrageenan-induced inflammation. Abstr. Soc. Neurosci., 13: 1017.

Jurna, I. and Grossman, W. (1977) The effect of morphine on mammalian nerve fibers. Eur. J. Pharmacol., 44: 339–348.

Laduron, P. (1984) Axonal transport of opiate receptors in the capsaicin sensitive neurones. Brain Res., 294: 157–160.

Lembeck, F. and Holzer, P. (1979) Substance P as a neurogenic mediator of antidromic vasodilation and neurogenic plasma extravasation. Arch. Pharmacol., 310: 175–183.

Marek, P., Panocka, I. and Hartman, G. (1983) Dexamethasone reverses adrenalectomy enhancement of footshock-induced analgesia in mice. Pharmacol. Biochem. Behav., 18: 167–169.

Mueller, G. (1981) Beta endorphin immunoreactivity in rat plasma: variations in response to different physical stimuli. Life Sci., 29: 1669–1674.

Otterness, I. and Bliven, M. (1985) Laboratory models for testing non-steroidal anti-inflammatory drugs. In J. Lombardino (Ed.), Nonsteroidal Anti-inflammatory Drugs, Wiley, New York, pp. 112–252.

Rios, L. and Jacobs, J. (1983) Local inhibition of inflammatory pain by naloxone and its N-methyl quaternary analog. Eur. J. Pharmacol., 96: 277–283.

Russell, N., Schaible, H. and Schmidt, R. (1987) Opiates inhibit the discharge of fine afferent units from inflamed knee joint of the cat. Neurosci. Lett., 76: 107–112.

Smith, T. and Buchan, P. (1984) Peripheral opioid receptors located on the rat saphenous nerve. Neuropeptides, 5: 217–220.

Vale, W., Spiess, J., River, C. and Rivier, J. (1981) Characterization of a 41-residue ovine hypothalamic peptide that stimulates secretion of corticotropin and beta-endorphin. Science, 213: 1394–1397.

Winer, B. (1975) Statistical Principles in Experimental Designs, MacGraw-Hill, New York.

Wybran, J. (1985) Enkephalins and endorphins as modifiers of the immune system: present and future. Fed. Proc., 44: 92–94.

Young, W., Wamsley, J., Zaren, M. and Kuhar, M. (1980) Opioid receptors undergo axonal flow. Science, 210: 76–78.

R. Dubner, G.F. Gebhart & M.R. Bond (Eds.)
Proceedings of the Vth World Congress on Pain
© 1988 Elsevier Science Publishers BV (Biomedical Division)

CHAPTER 8

Enhanced dynorphin gene expression in spinal cord dorsal horn neurons during peripheral inflammation: behavioral, neuropeptide, immunocytochemical and mRNA studies

Michael J. Iadarola[1], M.A. Ruda[1], Leslie V. Cohen[1], Christopher M. Flores[1] and Jose R. Naranjo[2]

[1]*Neurobiology and Anesthesiology Branch, National Institute of Dental Research, Bethesda, MD 20892, USA, and* [2]*Department of Molecular Neurobiology, The S. Ramon y Cajal Institute, C.S.I.C., c/Velazquez 144, Madrid 28006, Spain*

Summary

Peripheral inflammation produced by several different inflammatory agents caused edema, hyperalgesia and an increase in dynorphin A 1–8 peptide and dynorphin mRNA content in the dorsal horn of the spinal cord. The changes in dynorphin biosynthesis could be localized by both immunocytochemistry and in situ hybridization to two neuronal populations in the dorsal horn: cells in laminae I–II and cells in laminae V–VI. These data indicate that the elevation of dynorphin is a CNS consequence common to peripheral inflammatory processes and suggest an increased demand for dynorphin peptide in spinal dorsal horn nociceptive circuitry.

Introduction

Recent neurochemical research has suggested that, in spinal cord, biosynthesis of opioid peptides, in

Correspondence: Dr. Michael J. Iadarola, Bldg. 10, Rm 1A09, NIH, NIDR, Bethesda, MD 20892, U.S.A.

particular those of the dynorphin family (Goldstein et al., 1979) may be activated in response to an acute peripheral inflammatory process (Iadarola et al., 1985, 1986b, 1988a; Ruda et al., 1988) or a more chronic polyarthritis (Hollt et al., 1987; Millan et al., 1985, 1987). Dynorphin neuropeptides are derived from post-translational enzymatic processing of the prodynorphin protein precursor. The precursor is synthesized by transcription of the dynorphin gene and translation of the preprodynorphin mRNA. A second family of opioid peptides, the enkephalins, occurs in the spinal cord and a similar synthetic process underlies the formation of these peptides. Our original observation, using an acute unilateral adjuvant-induced inflammation model, was of a pronounced increase in the content of the prodynorphin-derived peptide dynorphin A 1–8 in the dorsal spinal cord ipsilateral to the affected hind limb (Iadarola et al., 1985). One explanation for this observation was that spinal cord dynorphin neurons were making more peptide in order to meet an increased demand placed upon them as a consequence of the peripheral inflammation. However, other explanations are possible. For example, the increase might be a consequence of neuronal inhibition whereby accumulation of peptide occurs because cell activity is suppressed while synthesis still proceeds. Assessment of additional parameters associated with neuropeptide biosynthesis, such as mRNA levels, would provide insight into mechanisms underlying the increase and a new perspective from which to interpret the physiological meaning of the increase (for review see Schwartz and Costa, 1986).

We have addressed these possibilities by measuring the content of preprodynorphin mRNA using a cloned genomic DNA fragment complementary to rat preprodynorphin mRNA (Civelli et al., 1985) in dorsal spinal cord during acute adjuvant-induced inflammation. We have also extended these biochemical observations to the anatomical level using the techniques of (a) in situ hybridization with a synthetic oligodeoxynucleotide probe and (b) immunocytochemistry with an antiserum directed against dynorphin A 1–8. Not only do these results confirm our biochemical observations, but, by identifying the cells involved, we can make some inferences about the neural circuitry that may be modulated by the dynorphin-containing neurons.

The above studies employed complete Freund's adjuvant (CFA) as the inflammatory stimulus (e.g. Iadarola et al., 1985, 1986b, 1988a). This is the same agent used in polyarthritic models (e.g. Millan et al., 1985, 1987). However, we have modified the procedure to produce only an acute inflammation. In order to avoid confusion between the two models, we have termed our model adjuvant-induced inflammation, as opposed to adjuvant-induced arthritis. We have also evaluated the ability of other known inflammatory agents to induce an elevation in spinal cord dynorphin. The temporal relationship between the increase in dynorphin and several physiological (edema) and behavioral (hyperalgesia) manifestations of the inflammation produced by each agent have also been investigated. These studies show that the elevation in dynorphin is a common feature of peripheral inflammation and that only a relatively brief period of hyperalgesia is needed to trigger a long-lasting increase in dynorphin. Thus, the response of the spinal dynorphin

system is specific to inflammation but not necessarily to any one inflammatory agent.

Methods

Tissue dissection and treatments

Male Sprague-Dawley rats (300–400 g) were used throughout. Injections of all inflammatory substances were made into the plantar surface of one hind paw under ether anesthesia. The inflammatory substances and volume of the injection were: (1) phorbol ester (phorbol 12-myristate 13-acetate, PMA or TPA, Calbiochem) 80 nmol in 200 μl of saline, 2% dimethyl sulfoxide; (2) carrageenan (lambda carrageenan, Sigma type IV) 8 mg in 200 μl saline; (3) yeast extract, 200 μl of a 10% suspension in saline; and (4) a 1:1 emulsion of complete Freund's adjuvant and saline, 150 μl (a total of 75 μg of *Mycobactericum butyricum* dry cells, Calbiochem). The latter stimulus, which we have characterized previously, was used for further examination of the effects of inflammation on the dynorphin system using RNA blot analysis, in situ hybridization and immunocytochemical methods. The characteristics of the inflammation models (see results) were reviewed and approved by the NIDR Animal Care and Use Committee. The procedures also conform to the guidelines of the International Association for the Study of Pain (Zimmerman, 1983).

Survival times were between one and 14 days and are specified for each experiment. The lumbar spinal cord was removed as described (Iadarola et al., 1988a) and tissue was either frozen immediately on dry ice for in situ hybridization or, with the cords on ice, the lumbar enlargement was subdivided into dorsal/ventral and left/right quadrants which were frozen immediately on dry ice and stored at −80°C until extracted for RNA or peptides. Tissue used for immunocytochemistry was obtained from rats perfused intracardially with 4% paraformaldehyde (Ruda et al., 1988) under deep pentobarbital anesthesia. The better to visualize the dynorphin peptide accumulation with immunocytochemistry, rats were given an intrathecal injection of colchicine

(100 μg in 100 μl sterile saline) days after unilateral induction of inflammation and then killed after a further 2 days. A large volume was used to prevent possible artifacts caused by lateralization of the intrathecal catheter.

Radioimmunoassay and RNA blot analysis

The specificity of the dynorphin A 1–8 antiserum has been described, as has the RIA procedure (Iadarola et al., 1986a). The procedures for preprodynorphin mRNA analysis have also been described in detail elsewhere (Tang et al., 1983; Naranjo et al., 1987). Briefly, tissues were homogenized in 5 M guanidinium thiocyanate solution and total cellular RNA was isolated by centrifugation through a dense cesium chloride cushion (Chirgwin et al., 1979). Poly(A$^+$)RNA was selected by oligo(dT) cellulose affinity chromatography and was electrophoresed through a denaturing agarose gel and blotted to nitrocellulose. Hybridization to the dynorphin probe was performed overnight at 42°C; the probe was labelled by nick translation to a specific activity of $2-3 \times 10^5$ cpm/ng. After washing, the blots were exposed to X-ray film to produce an autoradiogram. The probes used were from plasmid sp64D1.7, which contains a 1.7 kilobase insert of genomic DNA corresponding to the entire coding region and 3′-nontranslated portion of rat preprodynorphin mRNA (kindly provided by Drs. J. Douglass and O. Civelli (Civelli et al., 1985)). After dehybridization, blots were probed a second time with plasmid pAc18.1, which contains an insert of genomic DNA corresponding to the mRNA for rat β-actin (kindly provided by Dr. U. Nudel (see Nudel et al., 1983)). Autoradiograms were quantitated by densitometry and peak integration; several scans through each band were made and the densitometric values were averaged.

Behavioral testing

After induction of inflammation, rats were tested for behavioral hyperalgesia with a radiant heat stimulus as previously described (Iadarola et al., 1988a; Hargreaves et al., 1988). Briefly, the rats were placed on a raised glass plate with a small plastic cage over them to form an enclosure. A box containing a projector lamp shining through a 3×5 mm aperture was positioned under the foot. A photocell directed through the aperture provided an automatic detection of paw withdrawal latency. The lamp intensity was set to produce a paw withdrawal latency of approximately 10 s in control rats; shorter latencies were taken as a measure of hyperalgesia. In these same rats edema was assessed by measuring the dorsal-plantar foot thickness with a caliper; weight gain was also monitored.

In situ hybridization histochemistry and immunocytochemistry

The procedure for in situ hybridization was essentially that of Young et al. (1986). A synthetic oligodeoxynucleotide probe of 48 nucleotides (48mer) complementary to bases 862–909 of rat preprodynorphin mRNA was labelled with adenosine 5′-[^{35}S]thiotriphosphate to a specific activity of $10-15 \times 10^3$ Ci/mmol using terminal deoxynucleotidyl transferase. The 48mer was hybridized to slide-mounted sections at 37°C for 18–24 h with $1-2 \times 10^6$ cpm of probe overnight. The sections were washed and the slides were coated with Kodak NTB3 emulsion (diluted 1:1) and exposed for 4–12 weeks at 4°C. After development and fixing the sections were stained with neutral red. Immunocytochemistry was performed using the peroxidase-antiperoxidase (PAP) method as previously described (Ruda et al., 1988). The peroxidase label was developed in 0.05% 3,3-diaminobenzidine HC1, 0.01% H_2O_2.

Statistics

Statistical tests used are noted in the figure legends. Criterion for significance in all cases was at a level of $P < 0.05$.

Results

All four inflammatory agents rapidly produced edema (Fig. 1) and hyperalgesia in our thermal test (Fig. 2). Significant ($P < 0.05$) decreases in paw

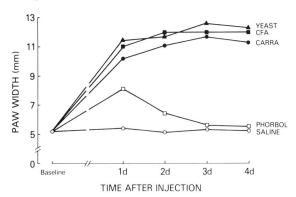

Fig. 1. Time course of edema induced by several inflammatory agents. A similar degree of inflammation was obtained with yeast, complete Freund's adjuvant and carrageenan when used as described in the text. The 80 nmol dose of phorbol ester produced the shortest-lasting effects of the four agents tested. Data are the mean values of 5 rats per group; standard errors were within 5% of the mean in all cases (Iadarola et al., 1988b).

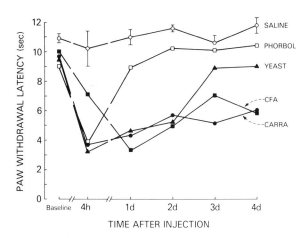

Fig. 2. Time course of hyperalgesia to a thermal stimulus. Radiant heat was applied to the plantar surface of the hindpaws while the rats were unrestrained, at rest, in a small enclosure (29 × 18 × 12.5 cm) on a glass plate. The latency to reflex withdrawal was recorded automatically. The data are the mean values of 5 rats per treatment; the standard error of the mean is shown for the saline controls but was similar for the other groups. The withdrawal latencies for yeast, CFA and carrageenan were significantly different from control for all four test days. The effects of phorbol ester were short-lived and only the 4 h time point is significantly different. Comparisons were made by analysis of variance with one repeated measure; significance at individual time points was determined with Duncan's multiple range test. Criterion for significance was $P < 0.05$ (Iadarola et al., 1988b).

withdrawal latencies were observed within 4 h of administration of CFA, yeast, phorbol ester and carrageenan. In general, maximal effects are observed at this time for all agents at these doses; the delayed peak effect of CFA in this experiment is somewhat unusual in our experience. The effect of phorbol ester resolved most rapidly and was nearly at control level by 24 h. The hyperalgesia associated with CFA and carrageenan treatments was the longest lasting; at 4 days, latencies were still 50% shorter than control. The effect of yeast was of intermediate duration; latencies were only 20% shorter than control by day 3. In the early stages there was a close parallel between the development of hyperalgesia and edema. The edema was rapid in onset with noticeable swelling by 4 h (e.g. paw widths of 5 mm were increased to 9 mm (CFA) and 9.9 mm (carrageenan) within 4 h). The rapid resolution of hyperalgesia seen with phorbol ester was paralleled by a rapid resolution of the edema. Also, the maintained hyperalgesia seen with carrageenan and CFA was accompanied by a maintained edema. A disparate time course between the two measures was only seen after treatment with yeast extract, where the edema outlasted the hyperalgesia. Although Figs. 1 and 2 depict data to the end of day 4, our preliminary studies found that the hyperalgesia and inflammation resolved completely by 14–15 days post-treatment in all cases.

Using weight gain as a monitor of feeding behavior, we observed a small (not more than 6%), but significant, weight loss with all of the unilateral inflammatory treatments (Fig. 3). The effect is clearly related to the severity of the inflammatory process as assessed by the edema and hyperalgesia measurements. The phorbol-induced weight loss was much less than that associated with the other three treatments. Similar to the data depicted in Figs. 1 and 2, only the early part of the inflammation is shown. However, as with the signs of inflammation, the decrease in feeding reverses with the resolution of the inflammation. The change we see in this parameter is much less than that reported to occur with the adjuvant-induced polyarthritis model (Millan et al., 1987), where weight loss amounts to as much as a

25% decrease compared to non-arthritic control rats. Other than the transient weight loss we did not observe alterations in locomotor activity. In contrast to the polyarthritis model, the rats maintained normal grooming behavior and exploratory behavior when placed in an unfamiliar cage. The rats did keep the inflamed limb elevated and guarded it from any disturbances. However, it is evident that the impact of these localized, transient inflammatory syndromes upon the animal's behavior is much less than that seen with polyarthritis models (Millan et al., 1985, 1987; Newbould, 1963).

A pronounced elevation in dorsal spinal cord dynorphin A 1–8 occurred with all 4 treatments (Fig. 4). By day 2 of inflammation, increases were just beginning to be apparent and reached statistical significance for CFA and phorbol ester. By day 4, a pronounced increase (between 3- and 4-fold) had occurred for CFA, carrageenan and yeast. The elevation for phorbol was comparatively less (2-fold), which may be a reflection of the comparatively short duration of inflammation associated with this treatment. The major and significant alteration in dynorphin A 1–8 content occurred in the dorsal spinal cord ipsilateral to the inflamed limb; no significant alteration occurred in the dorsal cord contralateral to the inflamed limb in comparison to saline controls.

RNA blot analysis was performed using dorsal spinal tissue from rats with adjuvant-induced inflammation. A significant increase (approximately 3-fold) in preprodynorphin mRNA was observed within 24 h after induction of inflammation (Fig. 5). The elevation was even more pronounced when the cord was sampled at day 5 of inflammation (Fig. 6). The autoradiagrams shown were obtained by hybridizing the blot for the preprodynorphin transcript first and then for the β-actin transcript (Fig. 6). The autoradiograms were scanned with a densitometer for quantitative comparison. The densitometric signal for dynorphin mRNA was normalized to that of β-actin (which does not change with inflammation) to precisely standardize each lane for the amount of RNA applied. The scan showed that an 8–9-fold increase in preprodynorphin mRNA occurred on the inflamed side compared to control untreated rats or to the contralateral side of the same animal. Not only was the effect lateralized but it was also confined to the lumbar cord; no alteration in the content of preprodynor-

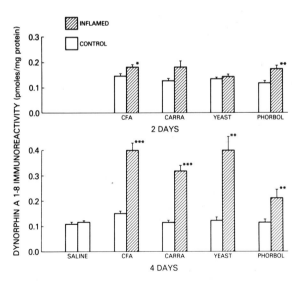

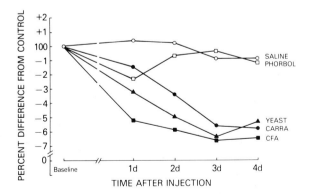

Fig. 3. Percent decrease in body weight during unilateral hindpaw inflammation. The maximal decrease was not more than 7% from the baseline body weight and not more than 6% compared to the control group. Note that the effects of phorbol ester were the shortest-lasting of the treatments (Iadarola et al., 1988b).

Fig. 4. Increase in dynorphin A 1–8 content of the lumbar dorsal spinal cord during hindpaw inflammation. By day two, measurable differences begin to appear and reach significance for the CFA and phorbol groups. By day four, all treatments produce significant increases. $n = 5$/group. Comparisons to the contralateral control side were made with a paired t-test. *$P < 0.05$, **$P < 0.01$, ***$P < 0.05$ (Iadarola et al., 1988b).

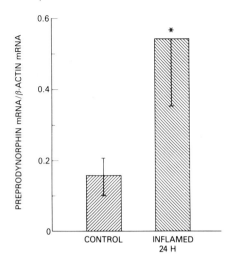

Fig. 5. RNA blot analysis of preprodynorphin mRNA after 24 h of inflammation. Results were obtained from three separate blots from three separate groups of animals. The blots were probed successively for dynorphin and β-actin transcripts (see Fig. 6 for an example). The latter mRNA does not change with inflammation and the densitometric scan of the β-actin autoradiogram is used to correct for any inequalities in the amount of RNA applied to the different lanes. The ordinate is, therefore, the ratio of dynorphin:β-actin peak areas from the densitometric scans. Comparisons were made by the Student t-test; *criterion for significance was $P < 0.05$ (from Iadarola et al., 1988b).

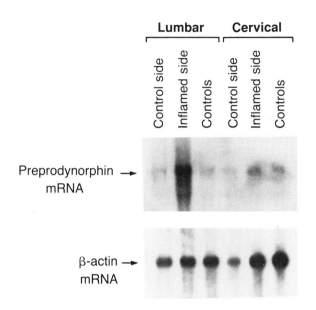

Fig. 6. RNA blot analysis of preprodynorphin mRNA. Poly(A+) RNA was prepared from the dorsal spinal cord from the lumbar and cervical regions of rats with a unilateral inflammation and from noninflamed control rats at day 5 of inflammation. Densitometric scans of the bands were used to construct preprodynorphin:β-actin mRNA ratios. These quantitative data showed that an 8–9-fold increase occurred on the side of the inflammation compared to either control or the contralateral side of the same animals (from Iadarola et al., 1988b).

phin mRNA was observed in dorsal cord tissue from the cervical segments.

Results obtained with in situ hybridization and immunocytochemistry extended the biochemical observations to the single cell level. (Ruda et al., 1988). As with the RNA blot experiments, these studies employed the adjuvant-induced inflammation model. Tissue was examined 4 days after induction of inflammation. In situ hybridization with the 48mer localized the increase in dynorphin mRNA to neurons in laminae I–II and laminae V–VI (Fig. 7). The densest accumulation of silver grains was associated with neurons in the superficial laminae. These neurons were found in the medial two-thirds of the dorsal horn, the region that somatotopically corresponds to the distribution of afferents from the distal portion of the limb. The neurons in laminae V–VI accumulated fewer silver grains than the superfical neurons. These neurons also contain the dynorphin peptide as shown by the

immunocytochemical technique (Fig. 8). The immunocytochemical staining of neurons in the superficial laminae is also very dark but is somewhat obscured by the dense terminal staining in this region. In order to ascertain further that treatment with colchicine did not interfere with the inflammation-induced elevation in dynorphin, we quantified the elevation in dynorphin A 1–8 in a separate group of rats ($n = 5$) by radioimmunoassay. The elevation in colchicine-treated rats was 335% of control, an increase similar that seen in non-colchicine-treated rats (Fig. 4).

Discussion

The present data demonstrate that an elevation of spinal cord dynorphin biosynthesis can be rapidly induced (within 1–2 days) by a variety of inflammatory stimuli. This elevation is preceded by prominent edema and hyperalgesia with minimal alteration of the animal's general behavior. Most of the changes in behavior were specifically associated with the inflamed limb and consisted mainly of guarding of the limb and persistent flexion. Thus, during locomotion the animals did not place weight on the foot. The main nonspecific effect was on feeding, where a small decrease in body weight was observed. However, this could not be attributed to an inability to move about, since the rats displayed normal exploratory behavior when placed in an unfamiliar cage.

The increase in dynorphin peptide content is pre-

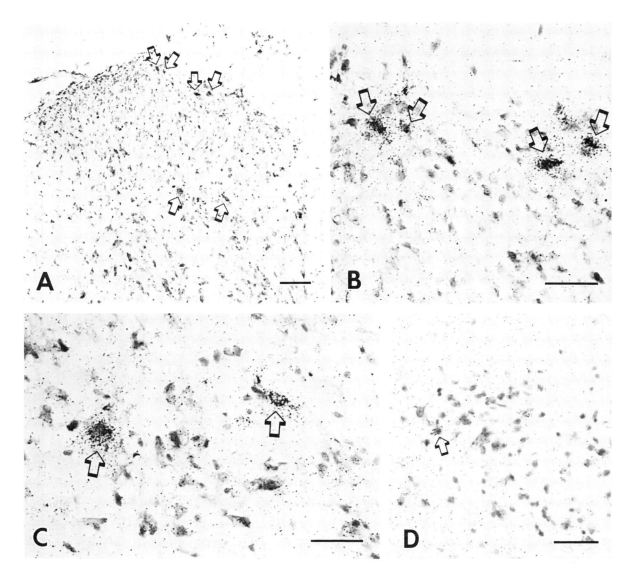

Fig. 7. In situ hybridization histochemical analysis of the spinal cord dorsal horn at day 4 of inflammation. (A) Inflamed side. In situ hybridization shows a marked labelling of cells (increase in the number of silver grains, see neurons indicated by arrows) in the superficial laminae of the dorsal horn and laminae V and VI. (B) A high magnification of the superficial dorsal horn neurons indicated by arrows in A. (C) Higher-magnification view of the neurons in lamina V, indicated by arrows in A. (D) Labelling of neurons on the non-inflamed side from the same animals is sparse. Scale bar = 100 μm. For more details see Ruda et al. (1988).

ceded by a prominent increase in preprodynorphin mRNA content. The mRNA and peptide increases occur in spinal cord dorsal horn neurons located in two distinct areas (laminae I–II and laminae V–VI) which are strategic in modulation of nociceptive information. Furthermore, the elevation in dynor- phin biosynthesis was confined to the side of the spinal cord ipsilateral to the site of inflammation and was segmentally specific. In addition, the dy- norphin neurons were located in the medial part of the dorsal horn receiving input from the inflamed portion of the limb. These data indicate a strong as-

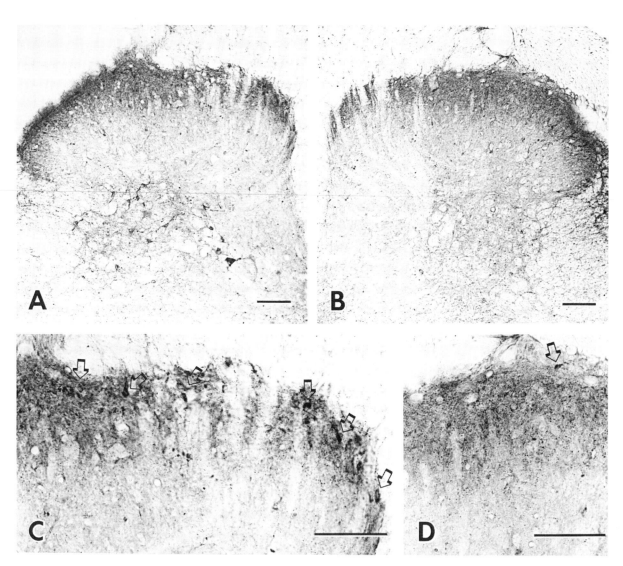

Fig. 8. Immunocytochemical analysis of dorsal horn stained for dynorphin A 1–8. Low-power views of (A) the inflamed side and (B) the control side of the same tissue section. With this technique the neurons in laminae V and VI exhibit an increased level of immunoreactivity on the side ipsilateral to the inflammation. The immunoreactive neurons in the superficial laminae tend to be some- what obscured by the dense terminal staining, but can be seen at higher magnification (arrows in C). As in laminae V and VI, more neurons are visible on the ipsilateral side (arrows in C) as compared to the contralateral (arrows in D) superficial dorsal horn. Scale bar = 100 μm. For more details see Ruda et al. (1988).

sociation between the elevation of dynorphin and abnormal sensory input arising from the site of inflammation. The strict regional localization of the increase within the spinal cord also indicates that the increase cannot be solely attributed to an effect of stress or a circulating hormone. If the latter case applied then both sides of the cord and/or other cord segments would be expected to show an alteration.

One of the most interesting observations concerns the stimulus requirements necessary for the induction of the increase in dynorphin biosynthesis. From previous studies in which a denervation was performed prior to induction of inflammation with CFA, we know that there is an absolute requirement for an intact peripheral nerve connection to observe an increase in spinal dynorphin. Thus, the initial trigger appears to come from the primary afferent input, be it either directly or indirectly on the dynorphin neurons. The short-lived hyperalgesia and edema produced by phorbol ester treatment suggests that the early time period is critical for induction of dynorphin, with no more than 24 h being necessary. By 24 h the hyperalgesia and edema are not substantially different from control; nevertheless, an elevation of peptide still occurs. One possible explanation is that the mRNA accumulation is a response that, once generated, will yield an increase in peptide even in the absence of continued peripheral signs of inflammation. However, a maintained stimulus causes a greater elevation in peptide content. Thus, in the case of carrageenan, CFA and yeast, where the inflammatory process is sustained, an elevated biosynthesis is sustained.

Despite the rapid increase in dynorphin mRNA at 24 h there is an appreciable delay before large amounts of dynorphin A 1–8 are accumulated. The peptide elevation is just beginning by day 2, consistently reaches significance (between 70 and 100% over control) by day 3 (not shown) and is massively increased by day 4. We can only speculate why an increase in peptide levels is not observed sooner. If the dynorphin neurons are being driven by the afferent input then it seems reasonable to hypothesize that a dynamic state exists between active release

and resupply via upregulation of biosynthesis. During the early phases (i.e. between days 1 and 2) the increase in biosynthesis may not be keeping pace with the release process, and the intracellular levels of peptide may not start to rise until biosynthesis has increased well beyond the need to support an increase in cellular activity. A somewhat analogous situation has been shown by Birnberg et al. (1983) to occur in the pituitary where, after adrenalectomy, proopiomelanocortin gene transcription and mRNA levels increase rapidly. A large ACTH increase occurs in tissue but it is delayed in comparison to the increase in mRNA. However, circulating hormone levels increase rapidly, with a time course similar to that seen for the mRNA. It is possible that extracelluar peptide levels (i.e. what is released) will give a more accurate picture of functional cellular activity than the total content of peptide in the tissue.

The elevation in spinal dynorphin biosynthesis that occurs in these acute inflammation models is much more rapid than that observed with adjuvant-induced polyarthritis models (Millan et al., 1985, 1987). This difference is probably related to the delayed appearance of disseminated inflammation processes in the polyarthritis model used by Millan et al., (1985, 1987). As employed in their polyarthritic studies, the adjuvant is injected into the tail and a disseminated inflammation does not occur for approximately 2 weeks. Thus, the elevation in dynorphin in this model may not be dependent upon a chronic process, per se, but simply reflect the delayed appearance of inflammation due to the route of administration and formulation of the adjuvant. Our data demonstrate that a delayed process is not necessary for the induction of dynorphin biosynthesis. The dynorphin neurons emerge as being much more dynamically responsive than might have been apparent from the polyarthritic model. The polyarthritic model also cannot take advantage of the anatomical specificity of the nervous system to control for possible hormonal and nonspecific effects.

The elevation in dynorphin biosynthesis was localized to two populations of neurons in laminae I–

II and laminae V–VI of the dorsal horn. The results showed a clear increase in labelling for the dynorphin peptide and mRNA in the two populations in comparison to the contralateral side and to non-inflamed controls. These results, as well as those from the RNA blot analysis, indicate that the increase is subserved by neurons whose cell bodies are in the dorsal spinal cord. Recent studies in rat (Nahin, 1987, 1988) and cat (Standaert et al., 1986) have shown that a small proportion of dynorphin-containing dorsal spinal cord neurons project to rostral brain sites; thus, a portion of the peptide increase may occur in these more distantly located synaptic sites.

The anatomical location of the involved cells suggests several functional implications for the role of dynorphin in the modulation of sensory input during inflammation. The dynorphin neurons which undergo an increase in biosynthesis are located in two regions of the spinal cord which contain neurons that project rostrally and convey nociceptive information. The dynorphin neurons may be either local circuit or projection neurons. It is possible that the output of neurons that convey nociceptive information to rostral CNS centers is modulated by an increase in the local release of dynorphin. The spinal dynorphin system may suppress the transmission of nociceptive information from the spinal cord to the brain, although alternative hypotheses are certainly possible. The net direction of the functional change has not been fully delineated but it may involve the control of hyperalgesia (Millan et al., 1986). It may be possible to use this response as an index of central nociception to screen the efficacy of peripherally acting antiinflammatory drugs and other analgesics.

References

Birnberg, N.C., Lissitzky, J.-C., Hinman, M. and Herbert E. (1983) Glucocorticoids regulate proopiomelanocortin gene expression in vivo at the levels of transcription and secretion. Proc. Natl. Acad. Sci. USA, 80: 6982–6986.

Chirgwin, J.M., Prybyla, A.E., MacDonald, R.J. and Rutter, W.J. (1979) Isolation of biologically active ribonucleic acid from sources enriched in ribonuclease. Biochemistry, 18: 5294–5299.

Civelli, O., Douglass, J., Goldstein, A. and Herbert, E. (1985) Sequence and expression of the rat prodynorphin gene. Proc. Natl. Acad. Sci. USA, 82: 4291–4295.

Goldstein, A., Tachibana, S., Lowney, L.I., Hunkapiller, M. and Hood, L. (1979) Dynorphin-(1–13), an extraordinarily potent opioid peptide. Proc. Natl. Acad. Sci. USA, 76: 6666–6670.

Hargreaves, K.H., Dubner, R., Brown, F., Flores, C.M. and Joris, J. (1988) A new and sensitive method for measuring thermal nociception in cutaneous hyperalgesia. Pain, 32: 77–88.

Hollt, V., Haarmann, I., Millan, M.J. and Herz, A. (1987) Prodynorphin gene expression is enhanced in the spinal cord of chronic arthritic rats. Neurosci. Lett., 73: 90–94.

Iadarola, M.J., Yang, H.-Y.T. and Costa, E. (1985) Increase in spinal cord dynorphin during an experimentally-induced inflammation of the rat hind limb. Fed. Proc., 44: 422.

Iadarola, M.J., Shin, C., McNamara, J.O. and Yang H.-Y.T. (1986a) Changes in dynorphin enkephalin and cholecystokinin content of hippocampus and substantia nigra after amygdaloid kindling. Brain Res., 365: 185–191.

Iadarola, M.J., Douglas, J., Civelli, O. and Naranjo, J.R. (1986b) Increased spinal cord dynorphin mRNA during peripheral inflammation. In J.W. Holaday, P.-Y. Law and A. Herz (Eds.), Progress in Opioid Research, NIDA Research Monographs, 75: 406–409.

Iadarola, M.J., Douglass, J., Civelli, O. and Naranjo, J.R. (1988a) Differential activation of spinal cord dynorphin and enkephalin neurons during hyperalgesia: evidence using cDNA hybridization. Brain Res., in press.

Iadarola, M.J., Brady, L.S., Draisci, G. and Dubner, R. (1988b) Enhancement of dynorphin gene expression following peripheral inflammation: stimulus specificity, behavioral parameters and opioid receptor binding. Pain, in press.

Millan, M.J., Millan, M.H., Pilcher, C.W.T., Czlonkowski, A., Herz, A. and Colpaert, F.C. (1985) Spinal cord dynorphin may modulate nociception via a κ-opioid receptor in chronic arthritic rats. Brain Res., 340: 156–159.

Millan, M.J., Czlonkowski, A., Pilcher, C.W.T., Almeida, O.F.X., Millan, M.H., Colpaert, F.C. and Herz, A. (1987) A model of chronic pain in the rat: functional correlates of alteration in the activity of opioid systems. J. Neurosci., 7: 77–87.

Naranjo, J.R., Mocchetti, I., Schwartz, J.P. and Costa, E. (1987) Permissive effect of dexamethasone on the increase of proenkephalin mRNA induced by depolarization of chromaffin cells. Proc. Natl. Acad. Sci. USA, 83: 1513–1517.

Nahin, R.L. (1987) Immunocytochemical identification of long ascending peptidergic neurons contribution to the spinoreticular tract in the rat. Neuroscience, 23: 859–869.

Nahin, R.L. (1988) Immunocytochemical identification of long ascending peptidergic lumbar spinal neurons terminating in either the medial or lateral thalamus in the rat. Brain Res., in press.

Newbould, B.B. (1963) Chemotherapy of arthritis induced in rats by mycobacterial adjuvant. Br. J. Pharmacol., 21: 127–136.

Nudel, U., Zakut, R., Neuman, S., Levy, Z. and Yaffe, D. (1983) The nucleotide sequence of the rat cytoplasmic β-actin gene. Nucleic Acids Res., 11: 1759–1771.

Ruda, M.A., Iadarola, M.J., Cohen, L.V. and Young, S.W. III (1988) In situ hybridization histochemistry and immunocytochemistry reveal an increase in spinal dynorphin biosynthesis in a rat model of peripheral inflammation and hyperalgesia. Proc. Natl. Acad. Sci. USA, 85: 622–626.

Schwartz, J.P. and Costa, E. (1986) Hybridization approaches to the study of neuropeptides. Annu. Rev. Neurosci., 9: 277–304.

Standaert, D.S., Watson, S.J., Houghten, R.A. and Saper, C.B. (1986) Opioid peptide immunoreactivity in spinal and trigeminal dorsal horn neurons projecting to the parabrachial nucleus in the rat. J. Neurosci., 6: 1220–1226.

Tang, F., Costa, E. and Schwartz, J.P. (1983) Increase of proenkephalin mRNA and enkephalin content of rat striatum after daily injection of haloperidol for 2 to 3 weeks. Proc. Natl. Acad. Sci. USA, 80: 3841–3844.

Young, W.S. III, Bonner, T.I. and Brann, M.R. (1986) Mesencephalic dopamine neurons regulate the expression of neuropeptide mRNAs in the rat forebrain. Proc. Natl. Acad. Sci. USA, 83: 9827–9831.

Zimmerman, M. (1983) IASP ethical guidelines. Pain, 16: 109–110.

R. Dubner, G.F. Gebhart & M.R. Bond (Eds.)
Proceedings of the Vth World Congress on Pain
© 1988 Elsevier Science Publishers BV (Biomedical Division)

CHAPTER 9

Paradoxical effects of low doses of morphine and naloxone in models of persistent pain (arthritic rats)

V. Kayser*, G. Guilbaud, J.M. Benoist, M. Gautron, A. Neil and J.M. Besson

Unité de Recherches de Neurophysiologie Pharmacologique, INSERM U. 161, 75014 Paris, France

Summary

In one model of persistent pain, Freund's adjuvant-induced arthritic rats, where morphine (100–1000 μg/kg i.v.) is highly effective in producing analgesia, the opiate receptor antagonist naloxone induced a bidirectional dose-dependent effect on the vocalization threshold to paw pressure: paradoxical analgesia with low doses (3–10 μg/kg i.v.) and hyperalgesia with high doses (1000 and 3000 μg/kg i.v.). The paradoxical analgesic effect almost disappeared in morphine-tolerant arthritic rats, while the hyperalgesic effect was not affected. In addition, a cross-tolerance between low analgesic doses of naloxone and morphine could be demonstrated in these animals.

Similarly, naloxone (3 μg/kg i.v.) was analgetic in a model of inflammatory pain having a more rapid onset, the carrageenan-induced paw edema model. In electrophysiological studies of ventrobasal thalamic neurons, naloxone depressed unit responses to stimulation of the inflamed paw.

We suggest that the paradoxical analgesic effect of naloxone could be due to the involvement of opiate receptors which presynaptically modulate the release of opioid peptides. According to this hypothesis, extremely low doses of morphine 3–10 μg/kg i.v.) would induce a hyperalgesic effect in arthritic rats.

---

* To whom correspondence should be addressed.

Introduction

In Freund's adjuvant-induced arthritic rats, we have previously shown that the opiate receptor antagonist naloxone induces a bidirectional, dose-dependent effect: hyperalgesia at high doses (1–3 mg/kg i.v.) and paradoxical analgesia at low doses, with maximum effects occurring at 3 μg/kg i.v. (mean peak value was 207 $\pm$ 6% of the control) (Kayser and Guilbaud, 1981, 1987a; Kayser et al., 1986a). An electrophysiological study paralleled these results, and showed that naloxone at comparable doses induced a rapid reduction in ventrobasal (VB) thalamic neuronal responses to mechanical stimulation of the inflamed joint (Guilbaud et al., 1982).

Since such effects of naloxone were not observed in normal animals, we hypothesized (Kayser et al., 1986a) that they were related to the fact that endogenous opioid systems are modified in these rats, which have been in a state of pain for 3 weeks. The objectives of the present study were, first, to determine whether this phenomenon also exists in another model of inflammatory pain, and how rapidly it develops. For this purpose we used the carrageenan-induced rat paw edema model of inflammatory pain (Winter et al., 1962; Vinegar et al., 1969; Di Rosa et al., 1971; Roch-Arveiller et al., 1977; Ferreira et al., 1978). The importance of this model is the rapid onset of a localized, hyperalgesic inflammatory state, the course of which can be followed for at least 24 h. Second, in an attempt to determine the mechanisms involved in these bidirectional effects of naloxone, we investigated the effects of naloxone on the pain reactivity of morphine-tolerant chronically arthritic rats. Thereafter, the results led us to examine the effects of extremely low doses of morphine in these arthritic animals.

Methods

Male Sprague-Dawley rats weighing 200–290 g were used. In some rats, hyperalgesia was produced by injecting carrageenan Lambda (Satia laboratory, Paris, France) (0.2 ml, 1% solution in saline) subcutaneously into the right plantar area of the hindpaw. The effects of naloxone (3 μg/kg i.v.) were gauged over two stages of the carrageenan-produced inflammation: an acute stage (1–4 h after injection of carrageenan) and a sub-acute stage (24 h after injection of carrageenan).

In other rats, Freund's adjuvant was injected at the base of the tail at the breeding center (Charles River) and the rats were used experimentally 21 days later, a time at which the arthritic lesions and concomitant humoral changes are maximal and stable (Gouret et al., 1976).

The effects of naloxone (1–3000 μg/kg i.v.) were determined in chronically arthritic rats pretreated twice daily for 4 days with either saline (control) or morphine (3000 μg/kg s.c.). Due to the inflammatory process that affected the tail in arthritic rats, repeated intravenous injections were ruled out, so morphine was administered by the subcutaneous route. The chronic morphine dose used induced analgesic effects roughly similar to those obtained in naive animals by 1000 μg/kg i.v. morphine (unpublished observations). It has been previously reported (Kayser et al., 1986b) that this morphine pretreatment renders arthritic animals tolerant to morphine. The effects of an acute i.v. injection of naloxone was evaluated in these animals 24 h after the last morphine or saline injection.

The effects of low doses of morphine (100–1000 μg/kg i.v.) were determined in chronically arthritic rats pretreated twice daily for 4 days with either naloxone (9 μg/kg s.c.) or Fixanal (a buffer solution with a pH equivalent to that of the naloxone solution). The naloxone dose used induced analgesic effects roughly similar to those obtained with 3 μg/kg i.v. in naive arthritic animals (unpublished observations) and will render arthritic animals 'tolerant to naloxone', since the analgesic effects of low doses of naloxone are strongly and dose-dependently reduced (Kayser and Guilbaud, 1987b).

As a nociceptive test, we determined the vocalization threshold to paw pressure using the Basile analgesimeter (Apelex). For each rat, preliminary threshold determinations at least 5 min apart were carried out, until two consecutive tests with thresholds varying by no more than 10% were obtained (the mean of these served as base-line). Thereafter, naloxone or morphine was injected intravenously into the tail vein and subsequent nociceptive pressure thresholds were measured every 5 min for at least 30 min. Thresholds were then expressed as a percentage of pre-drug control values. For each group of rats tested with naloxone or morphine, a mean curve of the overall effect of the drug was constructed. The areas under the curves obtained for each rat in each group were then calculated and plotted. Statistical analyses were performed on the data using the Student t-test and Fisher ANOVA. Differences were considered to be significant when P values were less than 0.05.

For electrophysiological studies in carrageenan-treated rats, previously described surgical and recording techniques were used (Guilbaud et al., 1986). Only neurons exclusively driven by intense mechanical stimulation of the hindpaw (e.g. pinch) were studied. At least two stable control responses (pinch by graduated forceps, 15 s duration, applied at intervals of 5 min) were recorded. Carrageenan was then injected subcutaneously in the plantar region of the hindpaw and modifications of the neuronal responses due to carrageenan were monitored every 10 min over 1–2 h. Naloxone was subsequently injected and neuronal responses to pinch were determined every 5 min for at least 30 min. In the second part of the study, we considered the effects of naloxone on VB thalamic responses recorded in the sub-acute stage of the inflammatory process (24 h after injection of carrageenan). We selected hyperalgesic rats for which the vocalization threshold for the injected paw was less than or equal to 84% of the control value (Kayser and Guilbaud, 1987a) as gauged prior to the recording session, and we studied neurons exclusively activated by mild stimulation of the inflamed ankle (mild lateral pressure delivered by calibrated forceps or movement such as flexion, extension). At least two stable control responses were determined, naloxone (3 μg/kg i.v.) was injected, and neuronal responses were determined every 5 min for at least 30 min. As a control, the effects of naloxone were tested on VB

neuronal responses induced by pinch in additional normal rats. For each neuron, the number of spikes in every test response was counted, including the after-discharge. The data were expressed as a percentage of the control values. The Student t-test was used for statistical analyses. Differences were considered to be significant when P values were less than 0.05.

Results

In non-morphine-tolerant chronically arthritic rats (Fig. 1), we first confirmed the bidirectional effect of naloxone (Kayser and Guilbaud, 1981, 1987b).

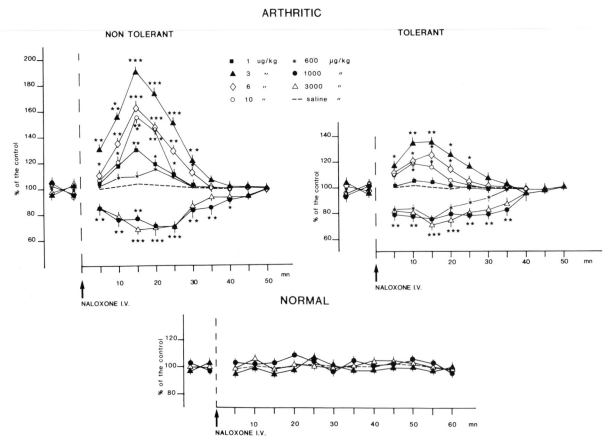

Fig. 1. Mean curves of the effects of naloxone upon the threshold for vocalization (mean ± S.E.M.) expressed as percentages of control in non-tolerant (saline-pretreated) and tolerant (morphine-pretreated) arthritic rats and in normal rats. Arthritic rats were pretreated twice daily over 4 days with either morphine (3000 μg/kg s.c.) or saline administered in the same volume. $n = 9$ in each group of arthritic rats; saline, $n = 5$. $n = 6$ in each group of normal rats. *$P < 0.05$, **$P < 0.01$, ***$P < 0.001$; Student's t-test.

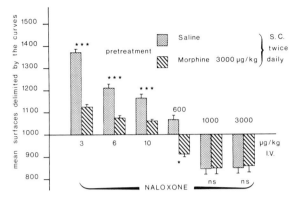

Fig. 2. Comparison between saline- and morphine-pretreated arthritic rats of the mean areas (mean ± S.E.M.) under the curves calculated for each dose of naloxone. Each mean area was calculated from the individual curves obtained for each group of rats. *$P<0.05$, ***$P<0.001$; Student's t-test (from Kayser and Guilbaud, 1987b).

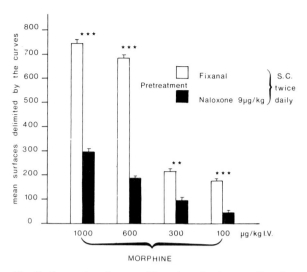

Fig. 3. Comparison between Fixanal- and naloxone- (9 μg/kg s.c. twice daily over 4 days) pretreated arthritic rats of the mean area (mean ± S.E.M.) under the curves calculated for each dose of morphine. Each mean area was calculated as in Fig. 2 from the individual curves obtained for each group of rats. $n=9$ in naloxone-pretreated and $n=6$ in Fixanal-pretreated rats. **$P<0.01$, ***$P<0.001$; Student's t-test.

The paradoxical analgesic effect peaked at 3 μg/kg. The mean elevation in the vocalization threshold 15 min after the injection was 190.5 ± 4.3% (expressed as a percentage of the control value, $n=9$; $P<0.001$). This was roughly comparable to the analgesic effect induced by morphine 1000 μg/kg i.v. in arthritic rats (Kayser and Guilbaud, 1983). The analgesic effect decreased with increasing doses, but was still significant at 10 μg/kg i.v. Hyperalgesia was observed at 1000 μg/kg i.v.; it was not significantly enhanced by increasing the dose to 3000 μg/kg.

In morphine-tolerant arthritic rats (Fig. 1), the bidirectional effect of naloxone was still present. However, the analgesic effect of low doses of naloxone was attenuated and of shorter duration than in saline-pretreated arthritic animals. The mean elevation in the vocalization threshold induced by 3 μg/kg naloxone dropped from 190% to 136% of the control values (Fig. 1); the analgesic effect of naloxone decreased in a dose-dependent manner (linear regression from 10 to 3 μg/kg i.v. naloxone, $r=0.97$, $n=27$, $P<0.001$) (Fig. 2). In contrast, by comparison with saline-pretreated rats, the hyperalgesic effect induced by greater doses of naloxone (1000 and 3000 μg/kg i.v.) remained roughly unmodified. In these morphine-pretreated rats, naloxone

did not precipitate withdrawal, although diarrhea was observed in some rats at the 1000 and 3000 μg/kg doses.

No significant modifications of the vocalization threshold were observed in non-arthritic control rats (Fig. 1).

We further evaluated the effects of low doses of morphine in naloxone-pretreated chronically arthritic rats. In these 'naloxone-tolerant' rats, the typically potent analgesic effect of morphine (100–1000 μg/kg i.v.) was profoundly and dose-dependently decreased (Fig. 3). The mean elevation in the vocalization threshold induced by 1000 μg/kg i.v. morphine dropped from 204.1 ± 9.3% to 144.6 ± 3.4% of the control values (linear regression for 100, 300, 1000 μg/kg i.v. morphine, $r=0.94$, $n=36$, $P<0.001$). Lesser doses of morphine were less efficacious and, paradoxically, produced significant hyperalgesia (Fig. 4). The maximum hyperalgesic effect was observed at 6 μg/kg; the mean vocalization threshold 20 min after injection of morphine was 62.7 ± 2.1% of control ($n=9$, $P<0.001$). Simultaneously with the decrease in vocalization threshold, we observed a clear modification of behavior, the animals being more reactive to manipulation and vocalizing when touched. This hyperalgesic effect was antagonized by naloxone (3 μg/kg i.v.) injected simultaneously with morphine.

The paradoxical analgesic effects of naloxone in the carrageenan-induced model of inflammation are presented in Fig. 5. This analgesic effect increased progressively over time following the injection of carrageenan. At 24 h after injection of carrageenan two groups of rats could be determined. Some rats were clearly hyperalgesic from their injected paw (n=21); the mean value for the vocalization threshold was decreased by 30% (Fig. 5B). In these animals, the analgesic effect of naloxone was

more potent than that observed in the group of rats tested 4 h after injection of carrageenan. The mean peak value was then 151.4 ± 5.5% of control (Fig. 5A). Fisher's analyses of variance, performed with vocalization threshold values expressed in grams, confirmed that the antinociceptive effects of naloxone were greater in rats tested 24 h than in those tested 4 h after the injection of carrageenan ($F(3,58)$ = 23.9, $P<0.001$). When the mean areas were calculated from the individual curves of naloxone's effects obtained for each group of rats (Fig. 5C), it appeared that the analgesic effect of naloxone was about 2 times greater in rats tested 24 h than in those tested 4 h after injection of carrageenan.

Some rats (n=13) tested 24 h after the injection of carrageenan were not clearly hyperalgesic, exhibiting a decrease in the vocalization threshold of less than 16% of control values when determined immediately before the administration of naloxone (Kayser and Guilbaud, 1987a). In these animals, the analgesic effect of naloxone was less than that observed in the group of hyperalgesic rats. The mean peak value was 117.9 ± 3.5% of the pre-naloxone control value. In fact, when all rats treated 24 h previously with carrageenan were pooled, a significant correlation between the degree of the analgesic effect of naloxone and the degree of the carrageenan-induced hyperalgesia was observed (Fig. 6).

Electrophysiological data paralleled the behavioral observations: naloxone (3 μg/kg i.v.) did not affect neuronal responses to pinch in normal rats or those tested 1 h after injection of carrageenan. However, naloxone depressed VB neuronal responses induced by mild stimulation of the joint by about 50% in rats 24 h after injection of carrageenan and selected as hyperalgesic just before the electrophysiological study (Fig. 7).

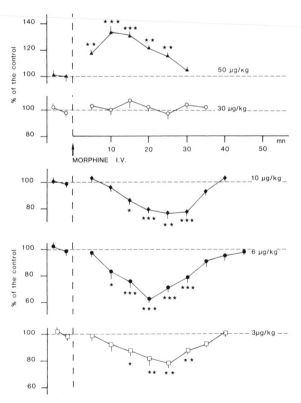

Fig. 4. Mean curves of the effects of various doses of morphine upon the threshold for vocalization (mean ± S.E.M.) in arthritic rats. Values are expressed as a percentage of the control. n=9 in each group of rats. *$P<0.05$, **$P<0.01$, ***$P<0.001$; Student's t-test (from Kayser et al., 1987).

Discussion

We have confirmed here the analgesic effect of low doses of naloxone described first in 1981 (Kayser and Guilbaud, 1981). This paradoxical effect was

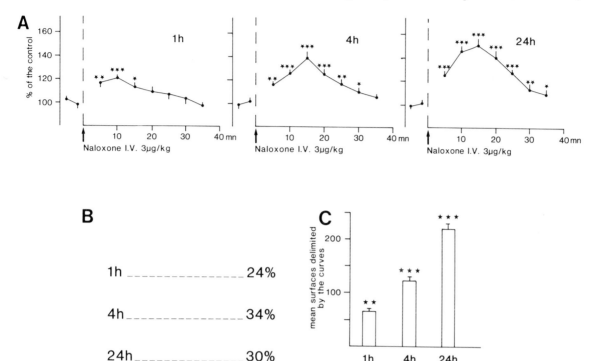

Fig. 5. A: mean curves of the effects of naloxone (3 μg/kg i.v.) in rats tested 1 h ($n=10$), 4 h ($n=10$) and 24 h ($n=21$) after injection of carrageenan. All rats exhibited a significant decrease in vocalization threshold to paw pressure by comparison with pre-carrageenan control values. B: mean decrease in vocalization threshold (expressed as percentage of the pre-carrageenan control value) in each group of rats. C: mean areas under the curve ($\pm$ S.E.M.) calculated from the individual curves obtained for each group of rats for naloxone 3 μg/kg i.v. *$P<0.05$, **$P<0.01$, ***$P<0.001$; Student's t-test.

observed only in arthritic rats, either chronically (Freund's adjuvant) or acutely (carrageenan) arthritic, and never in normal rats. Further, the carrageenan model of inflammatory pain clearly demonstrated that the analgesic effects of naloxone are related to the degree and duration of hyperalgesia. The electrophysiological study paralleled the behavioral observations. It precludes possible experimental bias in the behavioral studies, given that the experiments were not performed blind.

In chronically arthritic animals tolerant to morphine, the paradoxical analgesic effect of low doses of naloxone is significantly attenuated, as previously observed using massive doses of morphine to induce analgesic tolerance (Kayser et al., 1986). Furthermore, we have clearly demonstrated a cross-tolerance between naloxone and morphine at low

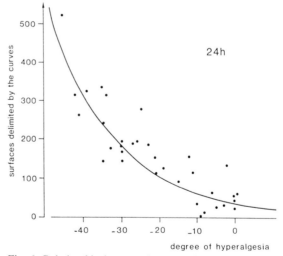

Fig. 6. Relationship between the analgesic effect of naloxone (areas under the curves obtained for each rat) and the degree of hyperalgesia observed in rats 24 h after injection of carrageenan. Each point represents an individual animal. $r=0.77$, $\alpha<0.01$, $n=34$.

doses: the potent analgesic effects of morphine were also strongly and dose-dependently reduced in arthritic animals 'tolerant to naloxone.'

These data indicate that the analgesic effect of naloxone in arthritic rats is mediated through binding sites sensitive to morphine. We suggested that this paradoxical 'agonist' effect may result from the interaction of naloxone with putative presynaptic opiate receptors specially sensitive to naloxone in arthritic rats and responsible for the continuing suppression of release of opioid peptide. Such a mechanism has been hypothesized in different studies (Kosterlitz and Hughes, 1975; Goldstein and Cox, 1977; Hagan and Hugues, 1984) and is com-

mon for other neuromediators (Langer, 1981; Starke, 1981; Arrang et al., 1983). Low doses of naloxone would presumably suppress this inhibitory control in arthritic rats and thus generate an analgesic effect. However, when arthritic rats are tolerant to morphine, the presynaptic receptors responsible for the control of enkephalin release would themselves be rendered tolerant and thus low doses of naloxone will have no effect at this presynaptic site. By contrast, the hyperalgesic effect induced by low doses of naloxone remained roughly unmodified in morphine-pretreated animals. This persistence, while the analgesic effect of low doses declined, emphasizes the involvement of opiate

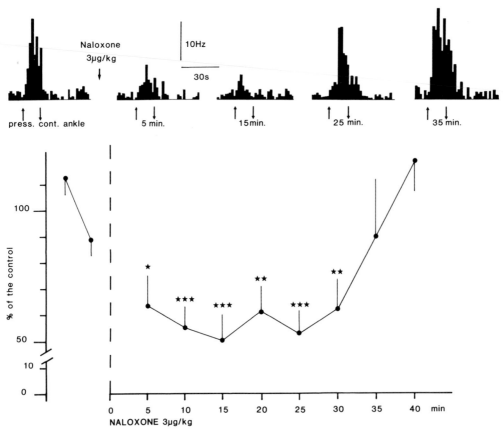

Fig. 7. Effect of naloxone (3 μg/kg i.v.) upon VB thalamic neuronal responses elicited by mild stimulation of the inflamed joints in rats 24 h after injection of carrageenan. Top: an individual example of a neuron activated by mild lateral pressure on the hindpaw, contralateral to the recording site. Stimulation duration is indicated between the two arrows. Bottom: mean curve of the depressive effect of naloxone on responses of 10 VB neurons comparable to that illustrated in the upper part of the figure. *P < 0.05, **P < 0.01, ***P < 0.001; Student's t-test.

receptors different in their sensitivity and/or in their functions in these two opposite effects of naloxone.

In addition, we have clearly demonstrated that in arthritic animals morphine administered in extremely low doses may induce a paradoxical hyperalgesia which is maximal at a dose of 6 μg/kg i.v. This paradoxical hyperalgesic effect of low doses of morphine is consistent with the hypothesis of a presynaptic modulation of opioid peptide release, which appears to be especially sensitive in animals which experience persistent pain.

Acknowledgements

The authors wish to thank Dr. A.H. Dickenson, Mrs. M. Gautron and Mr. E. Dehausse for technical assistance.

References

Arrang, J.M., Garbarg, M. and Schwartz, J.C. (1983) Auto-inhibition of brain histamine release mediated by a novel class (H3) of histamine receptors. Nature (Lond.), 302: 832–837.

Di Rosa, M., Giroud, J.P. and Willoughby, D.A. (1971) Studies of the mediators of the acute inflammatory response induced in rats in different sites by carrageenan and turpentine. J. Pathol., 104: 15–29.

Ferreira, S.H., Lorenzetti, B.B. and Correa, F.M.A. (1978) Central and peripheral antianalgesic action of aspirin-like drugs. Eur. J. Pharmacol., 53: 39–48.

Goldstein, A. and Cox, B.M. (1977) Opioid peptides (endorphins) in pituitary and brain. Psychoneuroendocrinology, 2: 11–16.

Gouret, C., Mocquet, G. and Raynaud, G. (1976) Use of Freund's adjuvant arthritis test in anti-inflammatory drug screening in the rat: value of animal selection and preparation at the breeding center. Lab Anim. Sci., 26: 281–287.

Guilbaud, G., Benoist, J.M., Gautron, M. and Kayser, V. (1982) Effects of systemic naloxone upon ventrobasal thalamus neuronal responses in arthritic rats. Brain Res., 243: 59–66.

Guilbaud, G., Kayser, V., Benoist, J.M. and Gautron, M. (1986) Modifications in the responsiveness of rat ventrobasal thalamic neurons at different stages of carrageenan-produced inflammation. Brain Res., 385: 86–98.

Hagan, R.M. and Hugues, I.E. (1984) Opioid receptor sub-types involved in the control of transmitter release in cortex of the brain of the rat. Neuropharmacology, 23: 491–495.

Kayser, V. and Guilbaud, G. (1981) Dose-dependent analgesic and hyperalgesic effects of systemic naloxone in arthritic rats. Brain Res., 226: 344–348.

Kayser, V. and Guilbaud, G. (1983) The analgesic effect of morphine, but not those of the enkephalinase inhibitor Thiorphan, are enhanced in arthritic rats. Brain Res., 267: 131–138.

Kayser, V. and Guilbaud, G. (1987a) Local and remote modifications of nociceptive sensitivity during carrageenan-induced inflammation in the rat. Pain, 28: 99–108.

Kayser, V. and Guilbaud, G. (1987b) Cross-tolerance between analgesic low doses of morphine and naloxone in arthritic rats. Brain Res., 405: 123–129.

Kayser, V., Besson, J.M. and Guilbaud, G. (1986a) Analgesia produced by low doses of the opiate antagonist naloxone in arthritic rats is reduced in morphine-tolerant animals. Brain Res., 371: 37–41.

Kayser, V., Neil, A. and Guilbaud, G. (1986b) Repeated low doses of morphine induce a rapid tolerance in arthritic rats but a potentiation of opiate analgesia in normal animals. Brain Res., 383: 392–396.

Kayser, V., Besson, J.M. and Guilbaud, G. (1987) Paradoxical hyperalgesic effect of exceedingly low doses of systemic morphine in an animal model of persistent pain (Freund's adjuvant-induced arthritic rats). Brain Res., 414: 155-157.

Kosterlitz, H.W. and Hugues, J. (1975) Some thoughts on the significance of enkephalin, the endogenous ligand. Life Sci., 17: 91–96.

Langer, S.Z. (1981) Presynaptic regulation of the release of catecholamine. Pharmacol. Rev., 32: 337–362.

Roch-Arveiller, M., Dunn, C.J. and Giroud, J.P. (1977) Comparison des properties inflammatories des fractions λ et k de carrageenine. J. Pharmacol. (Paris), 8: 461–476.

Starke, K. (1981) Presynaptic receptors. Annu. Rev. Pharmacol. Toxicol., 21: 7–30.

Vinegar, R., Schreiber, W. and Hugo, R. (1969) Biphasic development of carrageenan edema in rats. J. Pharmacol. Exp. Ther., 166: 96–103.

Winter, C.A., Risley, E.A. and Nuss, G.W. (1962) Carrageenan-induced edema in hindpaw of the rat as an assay for anti-inflammatory drugs. Proc. Soc. Exp. Biol. Med., 111: 544–547.

R. Dubner, G.F. Gebhart & M.R. Bond (Eds.)
Proceedings of the Vth World Congress on Pain
© 1988 Elsevier Science Publishers BV (Biomedical Division)

CHAPTER 10

New strategies for the use of anti-inflammatory agents

Thomas G. Kantor

Department of Medicine, New York University School of Medicine, New York City, USA

Except for the infectious arthridities, there are no known etiologies for most of the common connective tissue syndromes which cause musculo-skeletal and joint pain. Therefore, no rational treatments exist and relief of pain becomes the main therapeutic objective of the practitioner. The non-steroidal anti-inflammatory drugs (NSAIDs) including salicylates provide modest but significant pain relief. Until recently both relief of pain and anti-inflammatory effect were considered to be due to the same mechanism, namely inhibition of the enzyme cyclo-oxygenase by NSAIDs. This so-called Vane Hypothesis (Vane, 1972) showed that membrane disruption allowed lipid components to be acted upon by phospholipases to produce arachidonic acid. The latter in turn was enzymatically transformed by cyclo-oxygenase into endoperoxides which mediated the initial phases of inflammation. Further end-products include prostaglandins, PGE_2 and PGI_2 (prostacyclin) and thromboxane. These prostaglandins sensitize peripheral nerve endings to the further action of bradykinin and/or histamine and activate the neuronally mediated pain signal ascending to the spinal cord and thence to the central nervous system (Ferriera, 1972).

In addition to cyclo-oxygenase, at least five lipoxygenases also act on arachidonic acid. Each of these has separate effects on leukocytes, platelets and tissue sources and they produce various leukotrienes and hydroxyeicosatetraenoic acid derivatives (HPETE and HETEs) which are chemotactic for leukocytes and macrophages and are vasoactive, thus having a considerable role in inflammation. Few of the extant NSAIDs have an inhibitory effect on the lipoxygenase pathways and those that do inhibit only to a very small extent.

While the endoperoxides themselves are felt by some to be the true mediators of inflammation through the cyclooxygenase pathway (Kuehl et al., 1977), the mechanism by which they are converted to prostaglandins in various tissues is incompletely understood. It seems probable that the prostaglandins themselves are also important in mediating inflammation. Thus, inhibition of cyclo-oxygenase inhibits inflammation and pain. Since the Vane hypothesis was proposed, several problems with it have arisen.

1. Another of the end-products of cyclo-oxygenase action on arachidonic acid is PGE_1, which has clearly been found to be anti-inflammatory (Zurier and Quagliata, 1971). The inhibition of its production is obviously at cross-purposes with the proposed effects of NSAIDs.

2. There seems to be a ceiling to the dose of NSAIDs necessary to provide relief of pain beyond which no increment in dose confers further pain relief. The effect of this ceiling dose is usually well under 100% pain relief.

3. NSAIDs modify monocyte-macrophage, lymphocyte and neutrophile function. This may not necessarily be related to their function of inhibiting prostaglandin synthesis (Abramson et al., 1985).

Thus not only is inflammation affected by the NSAIDs, but immune events may be affected as well. Immune events have a great deal to do with most of the inflammatory arthritides. Therefore, simple inhibition of endperoxide and prostaglandin production is not the whole effect of the NSAIDs on inflammation.

4. Non-acetylated salicylates (e.g., diflunisal, disalcid, trilisate, Na$^+$-salicylate, etc.) do not inhibit the enzyme cyclo-oxygenase in vitro as do the other NSAIDs and aspirin. Aspirin destroys the enzyme by donation of its acetyl moeity (Roth et al., 1975). Despite this, non-acetylated salicylates are both anti-inflammatory and analgesic.

5. The drug acetaminophen (paracetamol) is known to mostly work peripherally as an analgetic but has only a very weak inhibitory effect on cyclo-oxygenase and is only weakly anti-inflammatory.

With respect to these objections, it has been shown that leukotriene B$_4$, a product of the enzyme lipoxygenase's effect on arachidonic acid, may substitute for PGE$_2$ and prostacyclin as a sensitizer of nociceptive peripheral nerve endings (Levine et al., 1984). The NSAIDs have little or no effect on lipoxygenase and the lack of inhibition of the production of leukotriene B$_4$ may account for the less than perfect analgesia of NSAIDs. In addition, Vane has recently shown an in vivo inhibition by non-acetylated salicylate on cyclooxygenase (Higgs et al., 1987). Finally, the modulation of inflammation and immune events by the white blood cells is, after all, the direct result of inhibition of prostaglandin production and may be considered to be an expansion of the Vane Hypothesis.

While there is therefore some question about explaining the effect of NSAIDs on inflammation on the basis of the hypothesis, the hypothesis has continued to hold up reasonably well with respect to the efficacy of NSAIDs as analgetics.

Adverse effect of NSAIDs

There is little if any question that inhibition of cyclo-oxygenase is an explanation for the adverse effects of NSAIDs. Prostaglandins are physiological substances with a variety of roles in the body. The presence of PGE$_2$ and prostacyclin in the gastric mucosa and the incoming blood supply of the kidney has profound effects on gastric physiology and cytoprotection of the gastric mucosa and in modulating the effect of pressor substances on the renal blood supply, respectively.

Gastropathy

Gastric mucosal prostaglandins increase the production of mucus and mucosal blood supply and reduce the production of free acid (Johannson et al., 1980). Inhibition of prostaglandin synthesis interferes with mucus production, depriving the stomach of one of its primary defenses against self-digestion. Reduction of mucosal blood supply and increased acid information added to the loss of the mucus barrier produce conditions for gastric irritation, erosion and peptic ulcer formation. In actual practice, there is an approximate 1–2% incidence of peptic ulcer in clinical trials of all NSAIDs and an approximate 20–30% incidence of gastro-intestinal (GI) symptoms as well (Emmanuel and Montgomery, 1971; Jick and Porter, 1978; Pemberton and Strand, 1979). About half of those patients find the drug intolerable because of these symptoms. Most disturbing is the fact that there seems to be little correlation between the gastroscopic appearance of the stomach and the symptoms produced (Lanza et al., 1975). The most dangerous feature of this is the gastroscopic appearance of large ulcerations which are completely asymptomatic (Roth and Boost, 1975). In the case of NSAIDs, these ulcerations are almost always on the pre-pyloric side of the stomach and the incidence is higher in elderly women (Levy and Dela Fuente, 1963). Since women over the age of 60 are the largest single users of NSAIDs, ulcer and massive active gastric bleeding are serious clinical problems (Davies-Caradoc, 1984).

There are several strategies open to the practitioner. He can simply switch from one NSAID to another in the often vain hope that the problem is related to an idiosyncratic effect of a particular drug. Differences in lipo- or hydrophilicity between the drugs give some hope in this regard because of their effects on absorption and access to the target tissues. When faced with the prior demonstration of an ulcer or an episode of hemetemesis, only an extraordinarily brave clinician would dare to simply switch drugs.

The situation is further complicated by the fact that a greater incidence of peptic ulcer disease has been found in patients with all sorts of chronic inflammatory disease (Donaldson, 1975). In addition, one British observer gave aspirin again shortly after an aspirin-related bout of hemetemesis to three hospitalized patients and was unable to show renewed bleeding (Parry and Wood, 1967). Mucosal adaptation does take place in the case of aspirin and presumably other NSAIDs. Gastroscopic examinations continually over a period of two weeks after daily high-dose aspirin therapy have shown large numbers of gastric erosions within a few days of the start of therapy, but complete or almost complete resolution within a week or so despite continuing dosage (Graham et al., 1983). Despite these possible encouragements, it would be dangerous to continue NSAID therapy in patients with bleeding or ulcers without at least some further therapeutic intervention.

Successful enteric coatings have now placed aspirin on a par with other NSAIDs as far as gastropathy is concerned (Orozco-Alcala and Baum, 1979). Aspirin, uncoated, not only inhibits cyclo-oxygenase in common with all NSAIDs, but also breaks the mucosal barrier by a direct effect in the stomach. Enteric coating greatly modifies this latter effect.

Antacid therapy does provide some protection, but interference with absorption of NSAIDs from the GI tract and an increase in the renal excretion of drug are consequences. The histamine-2 receptor blockers have been somewhat disappointing in reversing NSAID GI toxicity and are, in addition, expensive.

Recently, trials of sucralfate performed in patients taking NSAIDs have been encouraging and trials of synthetic prostaglandins are also showing positive protective results (Charlet et al., 1985).

Both of these strategies depend on augmenting the stomach's cytoprotective defenses, directly in the case of 15,15-dimethyl- and 16,16-dimethylprostaglandins and indirectly by promoting mucosal prostaglandin production in the case of sucralfate. It may be possible to incorporate such agents with a given dose of an NSAID in the same pill or capsule. Further research is badly needed in this important area.

Renal toxicity

The problem of renal toxicity resides in the passively protective effect of prostaglandins. PGE_2 and prostacyclin are not produced in the kidney unless renal blood supply is reduced by conditions such as dehydration or diuretics, liver, cardiac or other diseases which cause production of renin, angiotensins or catecholamine substances. These reduce renal perfusion by constriction of the arterial blood supply. When this occurs, prostaglandins are produced which modulate the pressor effect to maintain renal function (Dunn et al., 1983). In general, end-products of the cyclo-oxygenase pathway are vasodilatory. If this effect is lost, as in NSAID therapy, unopposed pressor influences cause salt and water retention and sometimes progressive renal failure. In addition, the effectiveness of salt-reducing diuretics may be lost. Regular monitoring of blood urea nitrogen and creatinine, especially under conditions where reduced blood volume is suspected, is necessary. As with any drug given chronically, a very few unfortunate patients will develop an idiosyncratic interstitial nephritis with potential for total and permanent renal failure.

The protective strategy here, in addition to vigilance, may lie in the use of so-called prodrugs. For example, sulindac and some others not available in the U.S.A. have no intrinsic pharmacological activity on their own, but are reduced in the liver to active compounds which inhibit cyclo-oxygenase. The parent inactive drug and the active sulfide, in the case of sulindac, then circulate in the blood in equilibrium with one another. In the kidney, however, it has been shown that the equilibrium becomes skewed in the direction of the inactive parent and there is therefore little if any effect on prostaglandins in the kidney (McGiff, 1980; Ciabattoni et al., 1987). While there are still some problems with renal failure associated with sulindac, various trials have shown reduced renal toxicity. Further drug development may produce safer drugs in this regard while maintaining effectiveness.

Gynecological effects

In the uterus, prostaglandins cause uterine contractions and have been shown to cause dysmenorrhea when present in excess. An extraordinarily successful use of NSAIDs is in the control of dysmenorrhea (Dawood, 1983). However, prostaglandins are also initiators of uterine contractions during parturition, and interference with their production at that time can lead to prolonged and unsuccessful labor. The strategy here is to simply suspend the use of NSAIDs in the last trimester of pregnancy. However, this feature may also inhibit the use of the synthetic prostaglandins for cytoprotection. While many of the natural prostaglandins are metabolized to inactive compounds in the liver and lung, the synthetics are not. Unwanted abortion might be attendant on their use as cytoprotective agents and it is possible to inhibit closure of patent ductus arteriosus in the fetus.

Other adverse effects

Hepatic and acute allergic responses to NSAIDs are extremely rare but are noted because of their potential severity.

It is not unusual for elevations in serum transaminase to be seen during the course of NSAID therapy. Not infrequently these return to normal despite continued therapy. However, if they exceed triple the normal range or are accompanied by an elevation in alkaline phosphatase, it is wise to discontinue therapy. Liver cell damage with bile plugs in the caniculi is a very rare event but one which must be remembered and monitored.

Another very rare but potentially serious event is an acute asthmatic attack. These are almost exclusively seen in individuals with a history of allergic reactions to aspirin consisting of hives and wheezing. These patients may also have nasal polyps. Patients with such a history will have cross-reactive sensitivity to all the NSAIDs and may die of an asthmatic attack if given an NSAID (Samter, 1973).

The mechanism for this is an apparent shift toward the lipoxygenase pathway of arachidonic metabolism causing suppression of leukotrienes C, D and E, which, as a complex, mediate bronchoconstriction and vasoconstriction (Hanson et al., 1983). This complex has been found to be identical to Slow-Reacting Substance A, which has similar properties. Why this expansion of the lipoxygenase pathway occurs and seems relegated to only a small population is as yet unexplained.

Patients will often say they are allergic to aspirin. This almost invariably means that aspirin upsets their stomach. Further questioning will determine whether hives and asthma accompany their 'allergy'. This is a very small but important population of patients.

Metabolism

All of the NSAIDs are metabolized to inactive compounds by conjugation in the liver. The prodrugs are an exception, of course. The conjugated compounds, mostly glucuronides, are then excreted by the kidney. Some of the drugs, such as sulindac, have an extensive biliary excretion, with the end-products appearing in the feces. The effect of hepatic or renal incompetence must thus be considered in the use and dosage of NSAIDs. Some NSAIDs are so extensively metabolized that even under conditions of reduced renal formation they may be considered safe. The makers of ketoprofen, for example, have made such a claim (Kantor, 1986). However, it is well known that septagenarians have about half the functioning nephrons of a thirty-year-old and, while liver function generally maintains a large reserve in the elderly, increased use of alcohol and smoking in the face of a previously damaged liver may take its toll.

In addition, the elderly have larger fat depots as compared to their lean body mass and a larger proportion of lipophilic drug may be stored in such depots. The serum albumin of the elderly is also lower than in younger individuals, providing fewer binding sites for these highly albumin-bound drugs. This may alter the ratio of free or pharmacologically active drug to bound or pharmacologically inactive drug and make the total biologic effect greater.

In general, NSAIDs with longer half-lives are a theoretical danger to the elderly because of the above. Unfortunately, NSAIDs with a long half-life which may be taken only once a day are a great convenience to the elderly who may for various good reasons be taking as many as six or seven different drugs with different dosing schedules daily. An NSAID with a very short half-life may have to be taken three or four times a day, but is rapidly metabolized and excreted. An NSAID with a long half-life such as piroxicam may have a considerably longer half-life in a patient in his eighties, who by ordinary measures of renal and hepatic function will appear to be normal. I have listed the various NSAIDs available in the U.S.A. in Table I along with their elimination half-lives, which have been derived from data on normal young individuals.

The clinician must be aware of these to properly advise and safe-guard his patients. The drug benoxaprofen, despite warnings in the literature (Halsey and Cardoe, 1982) prior to its introduction in the U.S.A. and the U.K., was given with fatal results to a number of patients over the age of 70. Its half-life is 51 h.

The future

Three-dimensional modelling has allowed pharmacologists to accurately determine the spatial characteristics of a drug which will inhibit the enzyme cyclo-oxygenase (Humes et al., 1981) and the same kind of effort is being applied to the lipoxygenases as well. There are at least 100 drugs which have some or all of the desired characteristics and less than half of these have gone through the review processes required for sale world-wide. There may be a number of these which will be shown to be at least as potent as the drugs now extant and, one hopes, some will have significantly reduced adverse effects.

Additionally, there is a recent preoccupation on the part of the pharmacologists with NSAIDs which have enantiomers. Whereas many drugs have dextro- or levorotatory configurations, some have a carbon atom which can rotate with its associated atoms around the plane of an attached phenyl group (see Fig. 1). With such enantiomers, which

TABLE I

A listing of NSAIDs and their elimination half-lives in hours

	Half-life (h)
Pyrazoles	
Oxphenbutazone	72–96
Phenylbutazone	84–96
Indoleacetic acids	
Indomethacin	3–4.5
Sulindac	13
Tolmetin	1
Phenylalkanoic Acids	
Fenoprofen	3
Ibuprofen	2–3
Ketoprofen	2–3
Naproxen	13
Naproxen Sodium	13
Fenamic acids	
Meclofenamate	2–5
Mefenamic acid	2–5
Oxicams	
Piroxicam	44–50
Salicylates	
Aspirin	Variable
Choline magnesium trisalicylate	7–18
Diflunisal	8
Magnesium salicylate	2–2.5
Salsalate	8

Benoxaprofen
Carprofen
Fenoprofen

Flurbiprofen

Ibuprofen
Indoprofen
Ketoprofen

Pirprofen

Suprofen

Tiaprofen

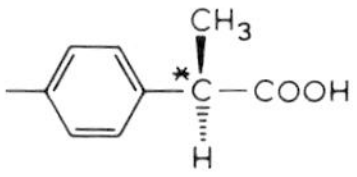

Fig. 1. Ketoprofen as an example of a drug with R and S enantiomers along with a list of other propionic acids having potential enantiomers.

are designated R and S forms, the S form contains all of the pharmacological activity (Rhone-Poulenc Canada files). Flurbiprofen, when separated into R and S forms, has most of its analgetic efficacy in the S form (Sunshine et al., 1987). As yet there has been too little drug available to evaluate such exciting possibilities as increased potency in one form or reduced adverse effects. The pure enantiomers may be too difficult to separate or commercially too expensive to manufacture, but the prospect of exploring this new universe is exciting. Thus far only the pro-

pionic acid group of NSAIDs is being explored in this way and not all of them have the proper chemical configuration. Naproxen, for example, does not, and exists only in the S form.

In addition, the R and S forms studied thus far may change from one to another in vivo, which would preclude any advantage of giving a pure form.

Summary

NSAIDs are the first line of defense against the pain of musculo-skeletal disease. Problems of toxicity limit their use in the very population most affected by these diseases, the elderly female. These problems may be inseparably interwoven with the main pharmacological effect of these drugs. However, there are some pharmacological strategies which may minimize the adverse effects while maintaining or augmenting the wanted effect.

The era of NSAIDs has not yet passed and may not even have peaked. They have provided a relatively safe and effective defense against extremely common pain syndromes.

References

Abramson, S., Korchak, H., Ludewig, R., Edelson, H., Haines, K., Levin, R.I., Herman, R., Rider, L., Kimmel, S. and Weissmann, G. (1985) Modes of action of aspirin-like drugs. Proc. Natl. Acad. Sci. USA, 82: 7227–7221.

Charlet, N., Gallo-Torres, H.E., Bournameaux, Y. and Wills, R.J. (1985) Prostaglandins and the protection of the gastroduodenal mucosa in humans: a critical review. J. Clin. Pharmacol., 25: 564–582.

Ciabattoni, G., Boss, A.H., Patrignani, P., Catella, F., Simonetti, B.M., Pierucci, A., Pugliese, F., Filabozzi, P. and Patrono, C. (1987) Effects of sulindac on renal and extrarenal eicosanoid synthesis. Clin. Pharmacol. Ther., 41: 380–383.

Davies-Caradoc, T.H. (1984) Nonsteroidal antiinflammatory drugs and gastrointestinal bleeding in elderly in-patients. Age Ageing, 13: 295–298.

Dawood, M.Y. (1983) Dysmenorrhea. Clin. Obstet. Gynecol., 26: 719–727.

Donaldson, R.M. (1975) Factors complicating observed associations between peptic ulcer and other diseases. Gastroenterology, 68: 1608–1614.

Dunn, M.J., Patrono, C. and Cinotti, G.A. (Eds.) (1983) Prostaglandins and the Kidney: Biochemistry, Physiology, Pharmacology and Clinical Applications, Plenum, New York.

Emmanuel, J.H. and Montgomery, R.D. (1971) Gastric ulcer and the anti-arthritic drugs. Postgrad. Med. J., 47: 227–232.

Ferriera, S.M. (1972) Prostaglandins, aspirin-like drugs and analgesia. Nature, 240: 200–203.

Graham, D.Y., Smith, J.L. and Dobbs, S.M. (1983) Gastric adaptation occurs with aspirin administration in man. Digest. Dis. Sci., 28: 1–6.

Halsey, J.P. and Cardoe, N. (1982) Benoxaprofen: side-effect profile in 300 patients. Br. Med. J., 284: 1365–1369.

Hanson, G., Bjork, T., Dahlen, S.E., Scott, J. and Cohen, Z. (1983) Specific allergen induces contraction of bronchi and formation of leukotrienes C_4, D_4, and E_4, in human asthmatic lung. Adv. Prostaglandin Thromboxane Leukotriene Res., 12: 153–157.

Higgs, G.A., Salmon, J.A., Henderson, B. and Vane, J. (1987) Pharmacokinetics of aspirin and salicylate in relation to inhibition of arachidonate cyclooxygenase and anti-inflammatory activity. Proc. Natl. Acad. Sci. USA, 84: 1417–1420.

Humes, J.L., Winter, C.A., Sadowski, S.J. and Kuehl, F.A. Jr.

(1981) Multiple sites on prostaglandin cyclooxygenase are determinants in the action of non-steroidal anti-inflammatory agents. Proc. Natl. Acad. Sci. USA, 78: 2053–2056.

Jick, H. and Porter, J. (1978) Drug-induced gastrointestinal bleeding. Lancet, ii: 87–89.

Johannson, C., Kollberg, B. and Nordemar, R. (1980) Protective effect of prostaglandin E_2 in the gastrointestinal tract during indomethacin treatment of rheumatic diseases. Gastroenterology, 78: 479–483.

Kantor, T.G. (1986) Ketoprofen: A review of its pharmacologic and clinical properties. Pharmacotherapy, 6: 93–103.

Kuehl, F.A. Jr., Humes, J.L. and Egan, R.W. (1977) Role of prostaglandin endoperoxide PGG_2 in anti-inflammatory processes. Nature, 265: 170–173.

Lanza, F.L., Royer, G.L. and Nelson, R.S. (1975) Endoscopic evaluation of the effects of nonsteroidal anti-inflammatory drugs on the gastric mucosa. Gastrointest. Endocrinol., 21: 103–105.

Levine, J.D., Lau, W., Kwiat, G. and Goetzl, E. (1984) Leukotriene B_4 produces hyperalgesia that is dependent on polymorphonuclear leukocytes. Science, 225: 225–243.

Levy, I.S. and DeLa Fuente, A.A. (1963) A post-mortem study of gastric and duodenal peptic lesions. Gut, 4: 349–359.

McGiff, J.C. (1980) Interaction of prostaglandins with the kallikrein-kinin and renin-angiotensin systems. Clin. Sci., 59: 105s–116s.

Orozco-Alcala, J.J. and Baum, J. (1979) Regular and enteric coated aspirin: a reevaluation. Arthritis Rheum., 22: 1034–1037.

Parry, D.J. and Wood, P.H.N. (1967) Relationship between aspirin taking and gastroduodenal hemorrhage. Gut, 8: 301–307.

Pemberton, R.E. and Strand, L.J. (1979) A review of upper gastrointestinal effects of the newer nonsteroidal anti-inflammatory agents. Digest. Dis. Sci., 24: 53–64.

Roth, S.H. and Boost, G. (1975) An open trial of naproxen in rheumatoid arthritis patients with significant esophageal, gastric and duodenal lesions. J. Clin. Pharmacol., 15: 378–381.

Roth, G.J., Stanford, N. and Majerus, P.W. (1975) Acetylation of prostaglandin synthetase by aspirin. Proc. Natl. Acad. Sci. USA, 72: 3073–3076.

Samter, M. (1973) Intolerance to aspirin. Hosp. Practice, 8: 85–100.

Sunshine, A., Eighelboim, I., Olson, N. and Laska, E. (1987) Flurbiprofen, flurbiprofen dextrorotatory component (BTS 24332) and placebo in post-episiotomy pain. Clin. Pharmacol. Ther., 41: 162 (Abstr.)

Vane, J.R. (1972) Prostaglandins and the aspirin-like drugs. Hosp. Practice, 7: 61–71.

Zurier, R.B. and Quagliata, F. (1971) Effect of prostaglandin E_1 on adjuvant arthritis, Nature, 234: 304–306.

Neuropathic Pain: Mechanisms and Treatment

R. Dubner, G.F. Gebhart & M.R. Bond (Eds.)
Proceedings of the Vth World Congress on Pain
© 1988 Elsevier Science Publishers BV (Biomedical Division)

CHAPTER 11

Pathophysiology of nerve following mechanical injury

Wilfrid Jänig

Physiologisches Institut, Christian-Albrechts-Universität zu Kiel, Olshausenstr. 40, 2300 Kiel, FRG

Summary

Mechanical injuries of peripheral nerves disturb the reciprocal fast and slow communication between periphery and CNS and may eventually lead to a variety of clinical pain syndromes. Several neurobiological processes which have been observed in afferent neurons after experimental lesions of nerves in animals may be important in the generation of these clinical syndromes.

(1) The axons start to sprout from the lesion distally and possibly proximally along the nerve trunk. Sprouts may reach their original target tissue or may innervate inappropriate tissue.

(2) If no connection to the periphery is established, sprouts, invading fibroblasts and proliferating Schwann cells form a neuroma. The cell bodies and axons of the neurons which project into the lesioned nerve shrink and (afferent and postganglionic) neurons with unmyelinated axons may finally die. As a result the conduction velocity of surviving axons decreases and cell death causes partial central deafferentation.

(3) The lesioned afferent neurons may generate activity due to changed membrane properties. This activity normally originates from the sprouts in the periphery, but it can possibly also be generated by the cell soma in the dorsal root ganglia. The percentage of unmyelinated fibers with ongoing activity increases with time after the lesion. The activity is mostly below 1 Hz and irregular, particularly in unmyelinated fibers. High rates of ongoing activity are rare, but can occur in myelinated fibers, occasionally with intermittent high-frequency bursts.

(4) Many sprouts are mechanosensitive and thresholds are often very low. Some afferents exhibit after-discharges lasting even for minutes following the mechanical stimulus. Mechanosensitivity is prominent in the neuroma, but was not found along the nerve trunk.

(5) Ephaptic transmission occurs between afferent fibers in the neuroma and also along the damaged nerve. This 'cross-talk' occurs between fibers of all sizes, yet it has not been shown to occur between postganglionic and afferent fibers. Ephaptic transmission is rare in the first weeks after nerve injury, but is regularly seen in chronic neuromas. The morphological correlates of this 'cross-talk' are probably close appositions between axon profiles without intervening Schwann cell cytoplasm.

(6) Axons which can be ephaptically activated may exhibit ongoing activity, mechanosensitivity and chemosensitivity. It is possible that excitation elicited in a neuroma or by natural stimulation of receptors of a partially reinnervated target tissue may spread via ephapses from axon to axon, thereby creating a strong barrage of impulses impinging on the CNS.

(7) Sprouts develop chemosensitivity and may respond to noradrenalin either when administered systemically or when released from postganglionic sympathetic axons. This excitatory effect is α-ad-

renergic. Experiments conducted recently demonstrate that unmyelinated afferents from a neuroma in a nerve can be excited by frequencies of activity in sympathetic neurons that occur physiologically.

All of these individual pathophysiological processes may contribute to the generation of the clinical phenomena following chronic nerve injuries, in particular neuropathic pains and reflex sympathetic dystrophy. Only a minority of patients with nerve injury develop pain and related clinical phenomena. Thus clinically relevant states may only appear after nerve damage when several or all pathophysiological processes quantitatively exceed a crucial level. Finally it must be kept in mind that (in the chronic state) the abnormal peripheral afferent messages impinge on a central neuronal machinery which is also changed as a consequence of the peripheral nerve injury.

Introduction

Mechanical injuries of peripheral nerves in humans may entail clinical syndromes consisting of pain, paresthesias, skeletomotor disturbances and autonomic disturbances. The clinical phenomena depend on the nerve(s) lesioned, the type of lesion (e.g. complete or partial lesion, with and without regeneration) and the time after the lesion. The pathobiological mechanisms which are associated with the clinical phenomena are the acute and chronic consequences of the lesion at the primary afferent neurons (Aldskogius et al., 1985; Lieberman, 1974; Sunderland, 1978; see also Culp and Ochoa, 1982; Pubols and Sessle, 1987) and the acute and chronic central changes, preferentially in the spinal cord (Wall, 1987 and Chapter 2 of this volume; see Pubols and Sessle, 1987). After a nerve lesion the messages from the periphery impinge on a central neuronal machinery which also changes as a consequence of the peripheral nerve injury and which may act back on the periphery via the efferent systems to skeletal muscle and autonomic effector organs (see Chapter 13 of this volume; and Blumberg and Jänig, 1983; Jänig, 1985b; Jänig and

Kollmann, 1984). Abnormal sensations and distorted regulations of skeletomotor and autonomic systems are therefore also the "consequence of disorder of the central control systems that establish the normal routing and amplification of sensory signals" (Wall, 1984, 1985). Because of the interacting peripheral and central pathobiological mechanisms it is mostly difficult to relate individual processes to individual clinical phenomena. Yet central disorders are triggered from the periphery when a nerve is lesioned. Therefore it is important to work out all possible peripheral pathobiological mechanisms which may contribute to the central disorders and their clinical consequences.

The present paper reviews peripheral pathobiological mechanisms which may contribute to pain and associated processes after mechanical injury to peripheral nerves. Most data were obtained in experiments on rat and cat in which a nerve of one hindlimb (sciatic, saphenal, superficial peroneal, sural, tibial nerve) was cut and ligated. Some data were obtained in experiments in which the central cut stump of one nerve was sutured to the peripheral stump of another nerve. Special emphasis will be laid on afferent neurons with unmyelinated axons.

The normal nerve, the lesioned nerve: some general considerations

Fig. 1 summarizes schematically the general functions of peripheral nerves supplying skin and deep somatic tissues (A) and the consequences of disrupting the communication between the periphery and the spinal cord (B). Under normal healthy conditions the nerve fibers serve centripetal and centrifugal impulse traffic via myelinated and unmyelinated axons. The axons are electrically well isolated by Schwann cell cytoplasm, guaranteeing in this way that the CNS can quickly communicate with the periphery by a large number of separate channels. Two points will be emphasized.

First, by far the most frequent nerve fibers in peripheral nerves are unmyelinated (afferent and postganglionic) (Carter and Lisney, 1987; McLachlan and Jänig, 1983; Peyronnard et al., 1986). Unmyelinated afferent axons may outnumber myelinated ones by a factor of 3 to 4 in skin nerves; in muscle nerves this factor is smaller. The fraction of postganglionic sympathetic axons amounts to 20–60% of all unmyelinated axons, depending on the tissue supplied by the nerve, the location of the tissue (e.g. proximal or distal skin), and possibly the species (e.g. rat or cat) (Baron et al., 1988; McLachlan and Jänig, 1983; Peyronnard et al., 1986a,b; Sittiracha and McLachlan, 1986). For example, muscle nerves seem to have relatively more postganglionic axons than unmyelinated afferent ones, skin nerves to distal parts of the extremities relatively more postganglionic axons than skin nerves to more proximal parts, and nerves to the rat hindlimb relatively fewer postganglionic axons than nerves to the cat hindlimb.

Second, periphery, afferent cell body and spinal cord communicate reciprocally via slow and fast axoplasmic transports of chemicals in the axons. These transport processes are probably of the utmost importance for the maintenance of the functionally specific central and peripheral connections of the primary afferent neurons. The primary afferent neurons with unmyelinated axons are in this respect of particular interest: many of them may primarily not be used for centripetal conduction of impulses but as transport channels ("trophic function of unmyelinated afferents", Wall and Fitzgerald, 1982).

Mechanical lesions of peripheral nerves lead to radical changes of the primary afferent neurons at all levels (Fig. 1B). The biochemical, morphological and functional changes that occur at the neurons

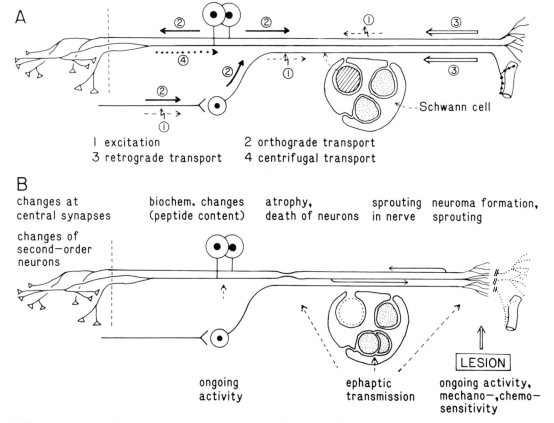

Fig. 1. The normal nerve with afferent and postganglionic fibers (A) and possible changes occurring as consequence of a peripheral nerve lesion (B).

may be interpreted as active regenerative processes in order to restore the connection between spinal cord and the appropriate target tissue and to repair the original function. If recovery of the original function does not occur, the neurons may revert to a reduced and changed functional state; they may finally disintegrate, resulting in a permanent cell loss and therefore irreversible damage. The latter applies particularly to neurons with unmyelinated axons (Aldskogius et al., 1985; Lieberman, 1974). In the following sections the functional changes and some morphological changes that occur at the primary afferent neurons as consequence of lesion to their peripheral axons will be reviewed. All changes may finally contribute to the clinical phenomena that are observed in patients with nerve lesions.

Morphological changes

Neurons which project in a peripheral nerve undergo considerable retrograde changes when their peripheral axons are cut and regeneration to the target tissue is prevented. The axons and cell bodies shrink (Fig. 2A–C) (Dyck et al., 1984a,b; Jänig and McLachlan, 1984; Peyronnard et al., 1986a). This shrinkage of the diameters leads to a decrease of the conduction velocity of myelinated and unmyelinated axons (Blumberg and Jänig, 1982a; Cragg and Thomas, 1961; Davis et al., 1978). This is illustrated in Fig. 2D,E for unmyelinated afferent and sympathetic postganglionic axons which project in nerves to the hairy skin of the cat hindlimb.

Many neurons may finally die. This has now been convincingly shown in rat and cat (Arvidson et al., 1986; Devor et al., 1985; Jänig and McLachlan, 1984; Risling et al., 1983; Ygge and Aldskogius, 1984). Up to 50% of the lesioned neurons may die 60 days or more after the peripheral nerve damage. Interestingly, neurons with myelinated axons do not die (at least up to about 22 weeks after the nerve lesion in cats (Jänig and McLachlan, 1984) and up to 80 weeks after the nerve lesion in rats (Peyronnard et al., 1986a)), but only (afferent and postganglionic) neurons with unmyelinated axons

(Jänig and McLachlan, 1984). The latter point is somewhat controversial: Peyronnard et al. (1986a) found that axotomy at the rat hindlimb does not affect postganglionic (sympathetic) neurons. The death of neurons leads to a partial central deaffe-

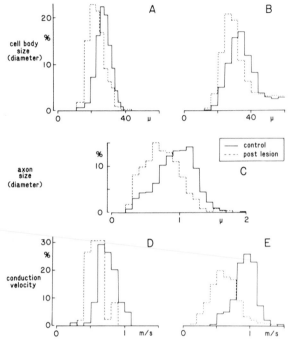

Fig. 2. Changes of size of small cells in dorsal root ganglia (B) and sympathetic ganglia (A), of unmyelinated fibers in peripheral nerve (C) and of conduction velocity in unmyelinated fibers (D,B) after ligating and cutting the superficial peroneal nerve in the cat. A,B. The cell bodies were labeled by horseradish peroxidase (HRP) which was applied to the central cut end of the experimentally lesioned nerve and of the contralateral control nerve. Each histogram is the mean of three nerves; ≧ 400 cells per nerve were measured. The nerve lesions were performed 144, 151 and 159 days before the application of HRP. Modified from Jänig and McLachlan (1984). C. Diameter of unmyelinated axons in control SP nerve (contralateral) and in SP nerve 30 mm proximal to the neuroma 245 days after the nerve lesion. The diameters were calculated from the areas of the axon profiles assuming spherical shape (n = 1081 fibers for control nerve and n = 604 fibers for lesioned nerve). From Christiane Vahle-Hinz and K. Gottschaldt, unpublished observation. D,E. Conduction velocity of unmyelinated axons. The control data were obtained in 4 experiments (D, 94 axons; E, 292 axons). The data on the lesioned axons were obtained in 13 experiments, 13–245 days after the nerve lesion (D: 46 axons, E: 915 axons). Modified from Blumberg and Jänig (1982a).

rentation and therefore also to central long-term changes which may be important for the understanding of the chronic consequences following peripheral nerve lesions (see Aldskogius et al., 1985). The death of neurons with unmyelinated axons may be reflected in a decrease of unmyelinated axons in the cut and ligated nerve proximal to the neuroma (Peyronnard et al., 1986a). The number of unmyelinated fibers increases from proximal to distal in the neuroma nerves, while their axon diameter decreases in the same direction (Vahle-Hinz et al., 1987). This may mean that unmyelinated axons in nerves with a stump neuroma sprout very far proximal to the neuroma.

Similar results were obtained in experiments on rats in which a saphenous nerve was transected and resutured (Carter and Lisney, 1987). Six months after the nerve lesion the number of myelinated fibers did not change proximal to the nerve lesion, but there was a 40% reduction in the number of unmyelinated ones. This result may appear somewhat surprising, since the events that occur in a neuron are probably quite different depending on whether its axon can regenerate or not.

Another change which is probably important for the understanding of ephaptic cross talk (see below) is the breakdown of the isolation between unmyelinated fibers by Schwann cell cytoplasm. In the neuroma as well as proximal to the neuroma close appositions of unmyelinated fiber profiles without intervening Schwann cell processes are present in preparations which have been lesioned a long time before (Fig. 3). The appositions are frequent in a neuroma which has developed after cutting and ligating a nerve (Bernstein and Pagnanelli, 1982; Devor and Bernstein, 1982; Vahle-Hinz et al., 1987), but less obvious proximal to the neuroma in the neuroma nerve. Close appositions between unmyelinated fibers in the neuroma nerve are difficult to detect in the electron microscope even if they are very common with respect to the number of unmyelinated fibers. These close appositions in the neuroma nerve may be brought about by the reorganization of the Schwann cell nerve fiber complexes induced by degeneration and sprouting of axons

and may be distributed along the whole neuroma nerve (see also Thomas, 1982).

Ongoing activity

Lesioned primary afferents which end in a neuroma may develop ongoing activity. This ongoing activity is generated in the neuroma by the sprouts: cutting the nerve proximal to the recording electrode (see Fig. 4A) does not affect the rate or pattern of ongoing activity (Fig. 4B; see Blumberg and Jänig, 1984; Govrin-Lippmann and Devor, 1978). Thus this ongoing activity is probably not related in any way to activity in postganglionic sympathetic neurons which project to the neuroma (see Blumberg and Jänig, 1985). Development of ongoing activity, percentage of fibers with ongoing activity, and rate and pattern of ongoing activity vary, depending on the species investigated, the type of nerve fiber (myelinated, unmyelinated) and the time after the nerve lesion (see Table I).

In *rodents* (mouse, rat) the percentage of fibers with ongoing activity may initially, in the first 2–3 weeks, reach values of 20–30%. On average 4–5% of the afferent units have ongoing activity 3–16 days after the nerve lesion in mice (Scadding, 1981) and Lewis rats (Devor et al., 1982) but about 18% in Wistar-derived Sabra rats (Govrin-Lippmann and Devor, 1978). Devor (1983; Devor et al., 1982) believes that the differences in frequency of ongoing activity between Sabra and Lewis rats are genetically determined. The ongoing activity occurs in myelinated fibers, reaches frequencies of up to 70 Hz and is mostly regular or regular bursting in its pattern (Burchiel, 1984a,b; Govrin-Lippmann and Devor, 1978; Scadding, 1981). Recently it has been shown by Matzner and Devor (1987) that unmyelinated fibers from rat neuromas also exhibit ongoing activity; most of this activity develops after 3 weeks or later, occurs in 6% or less of the unmyelinated units and is of low frequency of about 1 Hz or less. Burchiel and Russell (1987) conclude from their experiments on afferents from neuromas of the saphenous nerve of Sprague–Dawley rats 1–4 weeks postoperatively that unmyelinated fibers do not develop ongoing activity and that some ongoing activity in A fibers may be produced experimentally by gallamine (a potent potassium-channel blocking agent) which is used to immobilize the animals. They therefore believe that ongoing activity in experimental neuromas has been overestimated in previous studies. Govrin-Lippmann and Devor

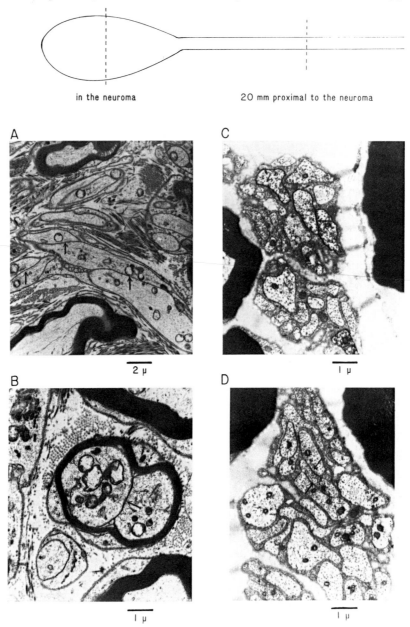

Fig. 3. Close appositions of unmyelinated axon profiles (arrows) without intervening Schwann cell cytoplasm in the neuroma (A,B) and in the neuroma nerve 20 mm proximal to the neuroma (C,D) 245 days (A,B) and 212 days (C,D) after cutting and ligating the superficial peroneal nerve. Note that the closely apposed axon profiles in B are surrounded by myelin. Both preparations have been investigated neurophysiologically and exhibited many ephaptically connected axons. From Christiane Vahle-Hinz and K. Gottschaldt, unpublished observations.

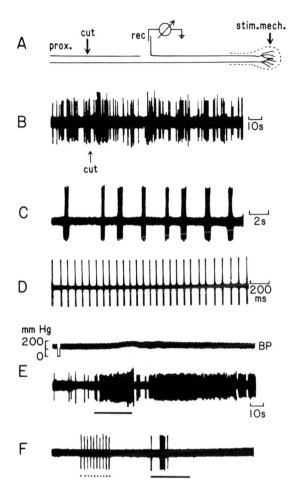

Fig. 4. Ongoing activity and mechanosensitivity in afferent units from neuromas of the superficial peroneal nerve. A. Experimental set-up. The arrow indicates the site at which the nerve was cut in B. B. Multi-unit bundle containing 2–3 unmyelinated fibers. C. Myelinated fiber (24 m/s) with bursting activity. D. Regularly discharging myelinated fiber (38 m/s). E,F. Unmyelinated afferent units (0.6 m/s, 0.9 m/s) responding to strong (E) and weak (F) mechanical stimulation of the neuroma with a blunt glass rod (tip diameter about 1 mm) (black bars). Note the ongoing activity and the afterdischarge in E. Upper trace in E arterial blood pressure. 108 (B), 6 (C,D) and 195 days (E,F) after the nerve lesion. Cat. Modified from Blumberg and Jänig (1984).

(1978) have already showed that the frequency of fibers with ongoing activity is somewhat higher under Flaxedil.

In *cat* and *monkey* the initial high rate of ongoing activity from neuromas of cutaneous nerves is practically absent; only very few myelinated fibers

exhibit ongoing activity, reaching rates of maximally 20 Hz; the discharge pattern in these fibers is normally regular or bursting (see Fig. 4C,D). Most of the fibers which display ongoing activity in the chronic state are unmyelinated; the discharge rates are around 1 Hz or less, the discharge pattern is irregular (Fig. 4B). The proportion of afferent units with ongoing activity is initially very low and may reach 15% or more 50 days or later after the nerve lesion.

Recently it has been shown in rats that dorsal root ganglion cells may generate ongoing activity after peripheral axotomy. This activity which probably occurred only in DRG ganglion cells with myelinated fibers had frequencies of about 0.2 to 15 Hz, and the discharges were irregular (Burchiel 1984a,b; Howe et al., 1977; Kirk, 1974; Wall and Devor, 1983). In the cat such generation of activity after peripheral axotomy has not been observed in our experiments (Blumberg and Jänig, 1984). This may be for several reasons.

First, in our experiments the vertebral canal was not opened and the dorsal root ganglia were left in situ. The activity of the afferent units was recorded from bundles which were isolated from the neuroma nerve and cut to the periphery. Using this approach, activity in (unmyelinated) postganglionic fibers could readily be recognized. It is therefore practically impossible to overlook antidromic activity in myelinated and unmyelinated afferent fibers which originates in the dorsal root ganglia (Blumberg and Jänig, 1984, 1985). In the studies mentioned above the vertebral canal was opened; in this way the dorsal root ganglia were also exposed. In the experiments on cats (Kirk, 1974) the nerve lesions were performed very close to the dorsal root ganglia with opened vertebral canal. This procedure may have produced a mechanical irritation of the dorsal root ganglia.

Second, in the cat the earliest experiments were done on days 6 and 13 after the nerve lesion and most experiments were done later (see Blumberg and Jänig, 1982b, 1984). Most experiments on rats were conducted in the first 10 days after the nerve lesion. The experiments on cats by Kirk (1974) were

TABLE I

Comparison of the functional properties of afferent units from experimentally produced stump neuromas of peripheral nerves in the mouse, rat, cat, and monkey

	Mouse	Rat[a]	Cat	Monkey
Type of neuroma	Sciatic nerve (mixed nerve)	Sciatic nerve, tibial nerve (mixed nerves)	Superficial peroneal nerve (skin nerve)	Superficial radial nerve (skin nerve)
Type of afferent fibers investigated	Myelinated	Myelinated (M), unmyelinated (U)	Myelinated (M), unmyelinated (U)	Myelinated (M) unmyelinated (U)
Ongoing activity: Peak	2–3 weeks	M: 1–2 weeks U: >3 weeks	M earlier than U, U: >7 weeks	
Percentage of units	$4.2 \pm 5.1\%$ (26) (3–16 d)[c], max ~20%; later 0–5% (higher after deducting motor fibers)	M: $17.9 \pm 7.8\%$ (11) (3–16 d)[b], max ~25%; later ≤5% (higher after deducting motor fibers); U: ≤6%	~4% (6–27 d; mostly M); $13\% \pm 10.7\%$ (9) (53–245 d), mostly U), max ~40%	8–18% (mostly U)
Average discharge rate	~23 (1–70) imp/s	M: 25 ± 11 (1–50) imp/s; U: close to 1 imp/s	M: 6.2 ± 7.2 imp/s (16) U: 0.5 ± 0.5 imp/s (42)	M: 0.2 ± 0.1 imp/s (10) U: 0.6 ± 0.2 imp/s (17)
Discharge pattern	Regular, irregular intermittent	M: regular, some bursting; U: irregular	M: regular, some bursting; U: irregular	Fairly regular, some bursting
Response to mechanical stimulation of neuroma	$19 \pm 11\%$ (26) (3–16 d)[c]; max ~50%; later ≤10%, (higher after deducting motor fibers)	Many	$19.4 \pm 9.6\%$ (6) (6–27 d) $32.8 \pm 14.9\%$ (8) (53–222 d) max ~50% some with longlasting afterdischarge	17–18% (1–4 months) 4% (7 months)
Ephaptic transmission		Yes (M)	Yes afferent→afferent (M,U) (not postganglionic → afferent) $2.5\% \pm 1.9\%$ (5) (6–27 d) $20\% \pm 6\%$ (5) (105–245 d)	yes (M,U) 0% (1–2 months) 4% (2–7 months)
Response to systemic adrenalin/noradrenalin	Total ~3%; 60% of units with ongoing activity, some silent units (α-adrenergic)	60–80% of units with ongoing activity, some silent units (M) (α-adrenergic)	Weak effects 40% of units with ongoing activity (M,U) (see Häbler et al. '87)	
Response to stimulation of the sympathetic trunk		~80% of units with ongoing activity (M), α-adrenergic, probably also unmyelinated units	Weak effects ~26% of units with ongoing activity (M,U) (see Häbler et al. '87)	

	Mouse	Rat[a]	Cat	Monkey
Literature	Scadding ('81)	Blumberg and Jänig ('81)	Blumberg and Jänig, ('81, '82, '84)	Meyer et al. ('85)
		Burchiel ('84a,b)	Lisney and Pover ('83)	
		Devor and Jänig, ('81)		
		Devor et al. ('82)		
		Govrin-Lippmann and Devor ('78)		
		Korenman and Devor ('81)		
		Seltzer and Devor ('79)		

[a]All numerical values obtained from Wistar-derived Sabra strain rats.
[b]Lewis rats: $4.5 \pm 4.2\%$ (10) (3–16 d), see Devor et al. (1982).
[c]Numerical values calculated from graphical data in Scadding (1981).
Numerical values: mean $\pm$ SD (n), mean $\pm$ standard deviation (number of measurements or animals); M, myelinated; U, unmyelinated; d, days.

conducted 1–21 days after the nerve lesion.

Third, the ectopic impulse generation by dorsal root ganglion cells may also be due to species differences.

Reactions to mechanical stimulation

All afferent units from a neuroma with ongoing activity can be activated by mechanical stimulation of the neuroma in the cat (Fig. 4E; see Blumberg and Jänig, 1984). This probably also applies to neuromas in rodents and monkeys (Meyer et al., 1985; Scadding, 1981). In both the cat and the mouse there are, however, many silent units which are mechanosensitive (Fig. 4F); thus the percentage of mechanosensitive afferent units is considerably higher than that of units with ongoing activity, amounting in both species to about 5–30% in the first 4 weeks and, in the cat, to 10–50% at later times after the axotomy (Table I). The latter percentages are on the average higher than those obtained in the mouse after 4 weeks (Scadding, 1981) and in the monkey (Meyer et al., 1985). Two reasons may account for these differences: first, the neuroma of the superficial peroneal nerve in the cat was always easily accessible during the experiments; second, a large proportion of the fibers which were isolated from the neuroma nerve in the cat were unmyelinated.

In the cat, no afferent units were found which could be activated by mechanical stimulation of the lesioned nerve more than 1 mm proximal to the neuroma. Many afferents have circumscribed spot-like receptive fields on the neuroma and the mechanical thresholds vary considerably (both probably because of the position of the mechanoreceptive endings in the neuroma).

The responses elicited by mechanical stimulation initially show a phasic component and adapt to a lower discharge rate throughout the stimulus. Some afferent units exhibit after-discharges when mechanically stimulated; these discharges appear particularly after strong stimuli and may last for 1–5 min after removing a 10–30 s stimulus (Fig. 4E). The discharges and after-discharges elicited by mechanical stimulation of the neuroma are very often accompanied by an increase of the arterial blood pressure (see upper trace in Fig. 4E).

In the cat, most mechanosensitive afferent units are unmyelinated (Fig. 4E,F). Preliminary experiments show that in rats unmyelinated afferents from neuromas may also develop mechanosensitivity (Jänig, unpublished observations).

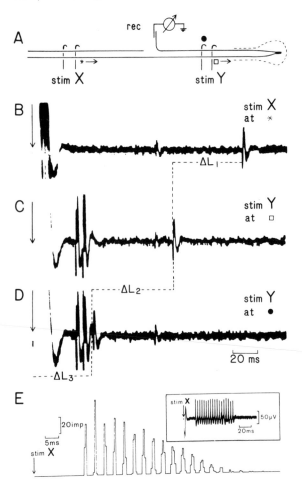

Fig. 5. Excitation of fibers from a neuroma by electrical stimulation of other fibers in the neuroma nerve. A. Arrangement of stimulation and recording electrodes. The sites at which the axons were stimulated are indicated by the symbols. B,C. Ephaptic excitation of an unmyelinated fiber by electrical stimulation of other unmyelinated fibers (signal connected by the interrupted lines). Both sites of the nerve (X,Y) were stimulated simultaneously with single pulses (B, 6 V at X, 5 V at Y; C, 6 V at X, 10 V at Y; D, 6 V at X, 11 V at Y; pulse duration 0.5 ms). ΔL1, latency difference between X* and Y□; ΔL2, latency difference between Y□ and Y● via the neuroma; ΔL3, latency to direct stimulation of the axon recorded from. Each trace 5 times superimposed. Note a second indirectly elicited response at 93 ms. E. Repetitive response of an afferent fiber to single shock stimulation of the nerve at X (1 V, 0.2 ms). The fiber responded with 2 to 19 impulses. The inset illustrates a specimen record with 18 impulses. The histogram was obtained from 100 superimposed trials (bin width 0.5 ms; repetition rate of stimuli 0.3 Hz). 108 days (B–D) and 6 days (E) after the nerve lesion. Modified from Blumberg and Jänig (1982b).

Ephaptic transmission

Fibers which are isolated from a neuroma nerve in the cat and cut centrally, thus leaving the connection to the neuroma intact, may be excited by stimulation of other fibers in the same nerve proximal or distal to the recording site (Fig. 5A). Fig. 5B,C illustrates such a type of activation for an unmyelinated afferent fiber (Fig. 5D). Blocking the conduction in the nerve just proximal to the neuroma by cooling normally abolishes this response, arguing that the transmission of impulses occurs in the neuroma. Normally the responses faithfully follow electrical stimulation at high frequencies (depending on the conduction velocity of the fibers) and have constant latencies and constant electrical thresholds. Most stimulated and recorded fibers are unmyelinated (63.5% and 83%, respectively), the rest are myelinated (36.5% and 17%, respectively). In the first 30 days after the nerve cut the event is rare, later it is more common, involving $20 \pm 6\%$ (mean $\pm$ SD) of all fibers (Blumberg and Jänig, 1982b). Similar results have been obtained on fibers ending in a neuroma of the sural nerve in the cat (Lisney and Pover, 1983), on myelinated fibers ending in a neuroma of the sciatic nerve in the rat (Seltzer and Devor, 1979) and on fibers ending in a neuroma of the superficial radial nerve in the monkey (Meyer et al., 1985). Also in these experiments the event was absent in the first 30–60 days after the nerve lesion. In the monkey it occurred between all types of fibers, but was generally rare.

The phenomenon may be explained either by ephaptic transmission ('cross-talk') between the fibers in the neuroma or by retrograde sprouting of fibers in the nerve from the neuroma over long distances. I favor the first possibility for the following reasons.

First, the phenomenon had already been observed in a few fibers 6 and 13 days after the nerve lesion (Blumberg and Jänig, 1982b). Retrograde sprouting appears unlikely in 6–13 days. At distances of 60–75 mm between neuroma and recording site it would require a sprouting at speeds of 6–12 mm/day.

Second, anterograde degeneration of retrogradely sprouted axons has not been found several centimeters proximal to the neuroma after cutting away the neuroma. Furthermore, the numbers of myelinated and unmyelinated fibers increase from proximal to distal in the neuroma nerves (Vahle-Hinz et al., 1987).

Third, Lisney and Pover (1983) and Seltzer and Devor (1979) recorded their activity from dorsal root fibers. Retrograde sprouting into dorsal roots is unlikely to occur (Risling et al., 1983).

Fourth, close appositions between profiles of fibers are very common in neuromas (see Fig. 3A,B; Bernstein and Pagnanelli, 1982; Devor and Bernstein, 1982; Vahle-Hinz et al., 1987). These appositions are presumably the morphological substrates of ephaptic transmission between fibers in the neuromas.

Several additional points concerning ephaptic transmission are worth mentioning and may emphasize its importance under pathophysiological conditions.

First, some afferents being excited ephaptically have ongoing activity and are excited by mechanical stimulation of the neuroma. This is either an intrinsic property of the afferent units or generated by other afferents via ephaptic transmission (Blumberg and Jänig, 1984).

Second, ephaptic transmission may also occur in the neuroma nerve several centimeters proximal to the neuroma. The putative morphological substrate does exist (see above and Fig. 3C,D). We have neurophysiological evidence for its existence (Blumberg and Jänig, 1984): some fibers isolated from the neuroma nerve and cut distally can be excited by mechanical stimulation of the neuroma and by electrical stimulation of the neuroma nerve distal to the recording site. Most of these fibers are unmyelinated. This phenomenon can also be explained by axon collaterals that have sprouted distally in the neuroma nerve over long distances (see Fig. 1).

Third, neuromas that appear as a consequence of a nerve suture (e.g. connection of the central stump of the superficial nerve to the peripheral stump of the tibial nerve in the cat) do not exhibit ephaptic transmission, though some fibers originating in the neuroma-in-continuity exhibit ongoing activity and mechanosensitivity (Häbler et al., 1987). This shows that ephaptic transmission between axons develops when sprouting over long distances of most fibers in a lesioned nerve is prevented, as is the case in a stump neuroma.

Fourth, ephaptic transmission from postganglionic sympathetic axons to afferent axons has not been observed (see Fig. 7B). This negative result does not exclude the possibility that it may occur in other types of nerve lesion.

Fifth, some afferent fibers in neuroma nerves exhibit repetitive discharges to electrical stimulation of other fibers with single pulses (Fig. 5E). These discharges were time-locked to the stimulus, but showed larger variation in their latency (see histogram in Fig. 5E). This type of activation was observed in the cat in early neuromas (Blumberg and Jänig, 1982b). Recently Lisney and Devor (1987) found that myelinated afferent fibers from a neuroma of the sciatic nerve in rats could be excited by repetitive electrical stimulation of other myelinated fibers with 2–10 s trains at 100 Hz. Most of their activated fibers were spontaneously active. As argued by the authors, this interaction of fibers probably results from the accumulation of potassium ions induced by excessive activation of the fibers within the extracellular space around active neuroma fibers.

Ephaptic transmission between afferent fibers in a neuroma and neuroma nerve could be very important in the generation of paresthesias, neuropathic pain and associated phenomena. It could amplify afferent activity in few afferents, so that trivial stimuli, which are normally not painful, lead to barrages of activity in many afferents. Activity in low-threshold afferents could lead in this way to activity in afferents which have high thresholds.

Response to catecholamines and to sympathetic stimulation

An important component in the generation of pain

syndromes which are generally subsumed under the generic term 'reflex sympathetic dystrophy' (RSD) and which may develop after peripheral nerve lesions is the coupling between noradrenergic postganglionic sympathetic fibers and afferent fibers at the lesion site or in the lesioned nerve. It is believed that by way of this coupling in the periphery a vicious circle builds up leading to a continuous or intermittent excitation of afferents and clinically to the typical symptoms of RSD, such as pain, trophic changes in the periphery and possibly also abnormal regulation of cutaneous blood flow and of sweating. Repeated temporary blockade of the sympathetic activity may abolish all symptoms and therefore RSD (Fig. 6; for extensive discussion see Blumberg and Jänig, 1983; Jänig, 1985b; Jänig and Kollmann, 1984; Schott, 1986).

Convincing experimental evidence is available for a chemical coupling between postganglionic noradrenergic axons and afferent myelinated and unmyelinated axons following peripheral nerve lesions (Fig. 7A). In rodents most myelinated afferent units from stump neuromas with ongoing activity are activated by adrenalin and noradrenalin applied i.v. or intraarterially (Fig. $8B_2$). The same activation is also elicited by repetitive electrical stimulation of the sympathetic chain (Fig. $8B_1$). Both effects are α-adrenergic and are blocked by α-adrenergic antagonists (Fig. $8B_3,B_4$) (Burchiel, 1984a,b; Devor and Jänig, 1981; Korenman and Devor, 1981; Scadding, 1981). In cats the effects of systemically applied adrenalin or noradrenalin and of electrical stimulation of the sympathetic supply

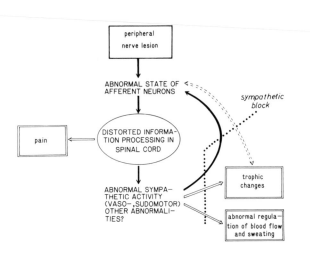

Fig. 6. Schematic and simplified expression of Livingston's hypothesis (Livingston 1976) about the neural mechanisms of generation of reflex sympathetic dystrophy following peripheral nerve lesions. Note the vicious circle (arrows in black). One important component of this circle is the excitatory influence of postganglionic sympathetic axons on primary afferent fibers in the periphery. This influence leads to orthodromic afferent impulse activity. But it may also induce antidromically conducted impulses in unmyelinated afferents to the periphery which may contribute to the trophic changes (i.e. by release of substances due to antidromic invasion of axon terminals which leads to vasodilation and plasma extravasation). These trophic changes may in turn influence the coupling between postganglionic axons and afferent axons (see interrupted double arrow). Modified from Blumberg and Jänig (1983), Jänig and Kollmann (1984).

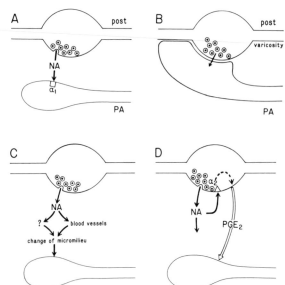

Fig. 7. Possible modes of coupling between postganglionic sympathetic axons (post) and primary afferent axons (PA) under pathophysiological conditions. A. Chemical coupling by release of noradrenalin (NA). The postsynaptic effect is α1-adrenergic. B. Ephaptic coupling by close appositions between postganglionic and afferent axons (see Fig. 3). C. Indirect coupling by change of the micromilieu of the primary afferent sensory terminals. D. Indirect coupling by release of prostaglandin (PGE) induced by presynaptic action of noradrenalin (see Levine et al., 1986). Note that other compounds (such as ATP, neuropeptide Y; see Burnstock, 1986, Lundberg and Hökfelt, 1986) may be released by the adrenergic terminals. For details see text.

on myelinated and unmyelinated afferent units ending in a neuroma are weak (Fig. 8A). About 20–40% of all units with ongoing activity respond to these adrenergic stimuli (Blumberg and Jänig, 1984). In both cats and rats, noticeable excitation of afferents ending in neuromas was observed at frequencies of 10 Hz or more. These discharge frequencies occur in post- or preganglionic sympathetic neurons only under extreme conditions, if at all (Jänig, 1985a, 1988), and sympathetic neurons projecting in chronically injured nerves do not seem to

increase their ongoing activity (Blumberg and Jänig, 1985). Preliminary work shows that unmyelinated fibers from rat neuromas can also be activated by sympathetic stimuli, and that this activation requires frequencies of 0.5 to 4 Hz; however, it could not be demonstrated that this activation is α-adrenergic (Blumberg and Jänig, 1981; Jänig, unpublished observations).

A very exciting experiment has been conducted recently in my laboratory, indicating that the efficiency of coupling between sympathetic postgang-

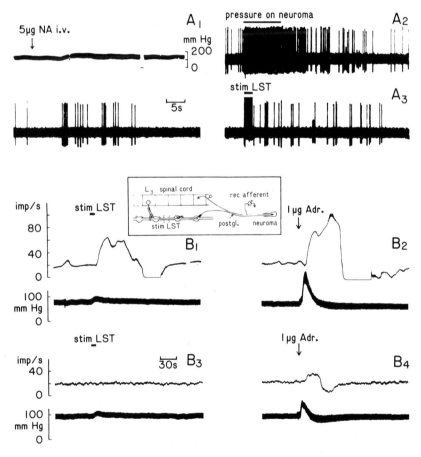

Fig. 8. Effects of noradrenalin (NA) and adrenalin (Adr) and stimulation of the sympathetic supply (stim LST, lumbar sympathetic trunk, see inset) on afferent activity from neuromas. A. Cat 13 days after ligating and cutting the superficial peroneal nerve. Myelinated mechanosensitive (A₂) unit (6.7 m/s). A₁, intravenous injection of 5 μg NA. A₃, repetitive electrical stimulation of the LST (10 V, 0.2 ms pulse duration, 50 stimuli at 25 Hz). Modified from Blumberg and Jänig (1984). B. Rat. Ten days after cutting and ligating the sciatic nerve. Myelinated unit with ongoing activity of about 20 Hz. B₁, B₃, repetitive maximal stimulation of the LST (pulse duration 0.2 ms, 200 stimuli at 20 Hz). B₂, B₄, intravenous injection of 1 μg adrenalin, B₃, B₄, after intravenous injection of 1 μg phentolamine. Modified from Devor and Jänig (1981).

lionic neurons and afferents probably depends on special conditions of the nerve lesion and that the stump neuroma may not be an appropriate model to study this coupling. In cats the central cut stump of either the sural or superficial peroneal nerve was anastomosed with the peripheral stump of the cut tibial nerve, leading to imperfect adaptation and regeneration of the injured central stump, a 'neuroma-in-continuity' and also regeneration of fibers into the peripheral stump. 330–640 days after this operation, unmyelinated afferent fibers in the lesioned nerve (experimental set-up, see Fig. 9A) could be activated by electrical low-frequency stimulation of the sympathetic supply at 1–5 Hz (Fig. 9B,C). The coupling was α-adrenergic and the afferent fibers could also be excited by reflex excitation

of the postganglionic neurons (Häbler et al., 1987). Whether the coupling occurred in the neuroma at the lesion site or more distally is unclear (see Fig. 9A). As mentioned in the last section, ephaptic connections between fibers in the lesioned nerve practically do not exist in this preparation.

Other modes of coupling between postganglionic sympathetic fibers and afferent fibers have been proposed (Fig. 7B-D), but are not supported directly by experimental evidence, nor are they refuted, taking into account the extreme variability of the pathophysiological conditions that may occur.

First, ephaptic transmission (Fig. 7B) has not been observed (see above). However, the possibility cannot be ruled out that it may develop after special nerve lesions, such as partial lesions of proximal

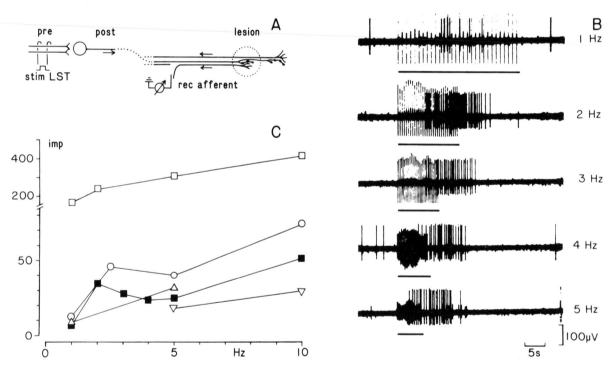

Fig. 9. Response of afferent units to electrical sympathetic stimulation in a preparation in which the central cut stump of the superficial peroneal nerve was sutured to the peripheral cut stump of the tibial nerve 330 to 640 days before the experiment in cats. A. Experimental set-up. Pre, preganglionic. Post, postganglionic. LST, lumbar sympathetic trunk. B. Record from a single afferent unit (1.3 m/s). Stimulation of the LST with 30 pulses of 10 V (pulse duration 0.2 ms) at 1 to 5 Hz. Note that the afferent unit had some low rate of ongoing activity and that a second unit was recruited at 5 Hz. C. Stimulus response curve for the single unit (■) and four multifilaments with 2–3 (○, ▽, △) and more than 5 units (□) in response to 30 pulses at graded frequencies delivered to the LST. Ordinate scale is the total number of impulses exceeding ongoing activity for each response. The ongoing activities as determined for 2–3 min before any series of trains of stimuli were 0.05 (■), 0.2 (○), 0.5 (▽), 0.6 (△) and 9.3 Hz (□). B and C from Häbler et al. (1987).

nerves induced by high-velocity bullets, which lead to classical causalgia. The development of causalgia is apparently not correlated with the degree of visible damage and appears far more common in lesions that ultimately recover spontaneously (see Sunderland, 1978). This clinical observation indicates that rapid and violent deformation of main nerve trunks (such as the sciatic nerve, median nerve or brachial plexus) entails interruptions of part of the nerve fibers which are distributed all over the nerve, leaving the nerve macroscopically intact. The disseminated damage of axons in the proximal nerve trunks may increase the likelihood of coupling between postganglionic and afferent axons and amongst afferent axons.

Second, noradrenalin may change the micromilieu of the primary afferent fibers by influencing the blood vessels or other unknown processes (Fig. 7C). This possibility is very complex and barely testable, but can also not be refuted. This is quite obvious from observations made by Wallin et al. (1976) on 4 patients with causalgia (two patients 11 days and 2 years after sympathectomy and 2 patients who had not been subjected to sympathectomy but were successfully treated by transcutaneous nerve stimulation). After iontophoretic application of noradrenalin to the previously causalgic skin area (in which light touch stimuli were perceived as normal after the treatment) allodynia developed; the size of the hyperalgesic zone increased considerably and finally spontaneous pain developed. The latter had the same character as the pain before the treatment. It is most interesting, in the present context, that the allodynia developed 30 min after application of the noradrenalin in two patients, though skin blood flow and skin temperature dropped immediately. This long latency may indicate that noradrenalin did not act directly on the afferent fiber terminals, but by some unknown mechanism via the change in the micromilieu (Fig. 7C).

Third, a further way of coupling has been proposed recently by Levine et al. (1986). The authors used rats in which the dorsum of one hindpaw was made hyperalgesic by daily application of chloroform to the skin surface. In these hyperalgesic ani-

mals the behavioral nociceptive threshold to pressure stimuli applied to the hyperalgesic skin was tested quantitatively under various pharmacological and other conditions (α-adrenergic agonists and antagonists, indomethacin, prostaglandin E, surgical and chemical sympathectomies). On the basis of the experiments the authors concluded that noradrenalin released by the postganglionic axon terminals acts presynaptically on α_2-adrenergic receptors and leads in this way to release of prostaglandin which in turn decreases the threshold of nociceptive afferents (Fig. 7D). This interesting hypothesis is entirely based on pharmacological arguments and is difficult to test directly.

Finally it remains to be mentioned that the influence of sympathetic activity on sensory receptors in normal skin and skeletal muscle appears to be weak and negligible or absent under normal physiological conditions. Some receptors in skin and skeletal muscle with myelinated fibers are continuously or transiently weakly activated by repetitive electrical stimulation of the sympathetic supply, some afferents with unmyelinated fibers decrease in their activity. Nociceptors with Group III fibers with high mechanical thresholds can be activated by sympathetic stimulation after sensitization by noxious heat (Roberts and Elardo, 1985b), yet nociceptors with Group IV fibers cannot (Barasi and Lynn, 1986; Roberts and Elardo, 1985a; Shea and Perl, 1986). Some mechano- and thermosensitive units with Group IV fibers may be activated by sympathetic stimulation (Barasi and Lynn, 1986; Roberts and Elardo, 1985a). It can generally be stated that the effect of sympathetic stimulation on some types of receptors in skin and skeletal muscle of cat and rabbit is weak and requires high rates of sympathetic efferent activity which occur either only under extreme conditions or not at all (for further discussion see Jänig, 1985a; Jänig and Kollmann, 1984; Roberts, 1985).

Roberts (1987) showed in anesthetized cats that many wide-dynamic-range (WDR) neurons in the lumbar spinal cord can be activated by electrical stimulation of the lumbar sympathetic trunk. This activation was blocked by local anesthesia or cooling of the receptive field of the WDR neurons or by α-adrenergic antagonists and was therefore elicited via the excitation of cutaneous receptors. The activation was common in WDR neurons with low mechanical thresholds, whereas WDR neurons with high mechanical thresholds were much less responsive. Whether sympathetically maintained pain (see Roberts, 1985) is to be mediated by activation of a subset of sensitized WDR neurons, as Roberts believes, remains to be sustantiated.

Comments and synopsis

The mechanisms by which complex peripheral and central changes following peripheral nerve lesions lead to various forms of paresthesias and pain and associated skeletomotor and autonomic abnormalities are only marginally understood. Consequently it is difficult to judge the importance of the individual pathobiological processes discussed above in the generation of clinically relevant symptoms. It must be kept in mind that only a minority of patients with nerve lesions suffer from neuropathic pain and develop, e.g., reflex sympathetic dystrophy. As already mentioned in the introduction, it appears unlikely that individual pathophysiological processes are related to individual clinical symptoms observed in patients. It may well be possible that clinically relevant states only appear after nerve damage when several pathophysiological processes quantitatively exceed a crucial level. All mechanisms described above (see Fig. 1B) are probably important and the quantitative predominance of a particular mechanism depends on the type of the nerve lesion. This is indicated when one compares the stump neuroma model, in which the nerve fibers are prevented from regenerating to their target organs, with the nerve suture model in which many fibers can regenerate to the periphery: in the first model the reactions of the afferents to adrenergic stimuli are usually weak and ephaptic transmission may be very prominent; in the second model adrenergic stimuli may have powerful effects on afferent fibers, but ephaptic transmission between fibers is

virtually absent (Häbler et al., 1987). It is also indicated by various behavioral animal models of chronic pain. The type of (abnormal) behavior displayed by the experimental animals depends on the type of nerve lesion: cutting and ligating whole nerves (Coderre et al., 1987), partial sciatic nerve lesion (Hylden et al., 1987), partial ligation of the sciatic nerve (Bennett and Xie, 1987), dorsal rhizotomy (Albe-Fessard et al., 1979; Albe-Fessard and Lombard, 1980).

It is commonly argued that the neuroma model, which is the most easily controllable nerve lesion, is not the appropriate animal model to study peripheral mechanisms of pain, paresthesias, reflex sympathetic dystrophy, etc., since patients with neuromas exhibit only very rarely these clinical phenomena. That is certainly true as far as the full development of the syndromes is concerned. Nevertheless, for the study of most pathophysiological neuronal processes occurring at the afferent side, the neuroma model seems to be particularly well-suited. Furthermore most animals with these types of controlled lesions do not seem to be disturbed at all, if the lesion is not too extensive, e.g. rats barely develop autotomy behavior when only the saphenous nerve or sural nerve is cut and ligated, but they may do so when the sciatic nerve or sciatic nerve and saphenous nerves are cut (Wall et al., 1979a,b; for review see Coderre et al., 1987).

One way to test which peripheral processes are relevant in humans is to perform systematic microneurographic investigations on afferent fibers in human neuroma nerves, and to correlate the microneurographically obtained data with the clinical symptoms. It is important to analyse afferent units from neuromata which are painful as well as from those which are not. Such an experimental approach on humans is of course limited: it is difficult to obtain enough quantitative data with this technique, and this applies particularly to unmyelinated afferents. In patients with chronic nerve injuries and in volunteers undergoing ischemia of nerve, stimuli and distorted sensations were correlated with the impulse activity in primary sensory units (Nordin et al., 1984; Nyström and Hagbarth, 1981; Ochoa,

1985; Ochoa et al., 1982, 1985, 1987; Ochoa and Torebjörk, 1980; Torebjörk et al., 1979).

Another way to test which peripheral pathobiological processes are relevant is the use of behavioral animal models of chronic pain. Such models are, for example, the abnormal behaviors of laboratory animals (rats, mice) that appear after peripheral neurectomy (Coderre et al., 1987), dorsal rhizotomy (Albe-Fessard et al., 1979; Albe-Fessard and Lombard, 1980), after partial nerve lesion (Hylden et al., 1987), and after partial ligation of nerves (Bennett and Xie, 1987). The displayed abnormal behavior can be quantified as an appropriate measure of the degree of pain or dysesthesia resulting from the nerve lesion (for details see the excellent review by Coderre et al., 1987). Thus, using these and other animal models, it should be possible to work out which peripheral (and central) pathobiological mechanisms are important for the generation of the abnormal behaviors.

Acknowledgement

Supported by the Deutsche Forschungsgemeinschaft.

References

Albe-Fessard, D.G. and Lombard, M.C. (1980) Animal models for chronic pain. In H.W. Kosterlitz and L.Y. Terenius (Eds.), Pain and Society, Dahlem Konferenzen, Verlag Chemie GmbH, Weinheim, pp. 299–310.

Albe-Fessard, D., Nashold, B.S., Lombard, M.C., Yamaguchi, Y. and Boureau, F. (1979) Rat after dorsal rhizotomy, a possible model for chronic pain. In J.J. Bonica, J.C. Liebeskind and D.G. Albe-Fessard (Eds.), Advances in Pain Research and Therapy, Vol. 3, Raven Press, New York, pp. 761–766.

Aldskogius, H., Arvidson, J. and Grant, G. (1985) The reaction of primary sensory neurons to peripheral nerve injury with particular emphasis on transganglionic changes. Brain Res. Rev., 10: 27–46.

Arvidson, J., Ygge, J. and Grant, G. (1986) Cell loss in lumbar dorsal root ganglia and transganglionic degeneration after sciatic nerve resection in the rat. Brain Res., 373: 15–21.

Barasi, S. and Lynn, B. (1986) Effects of sympathetic stimulation on mechanoreceptive and nociceptive afferent units from the rabbit pinna. Brain Res., 378: 21–27.

Baron, R., Jänig, W. and Kollmann, W. (1988) Sympathetic and afferent somata projecting in hindlimb nerves and the anatomical organization of the lumbar sympathetic nervous system of the rat. J. Comp. Neurol., in press.

Bennett, G.J. and Xie, Y. (1988) A peripheral mononeuropathy in rat that produces disorders of pain sensation like those seen in man. Pain, in press.

Bernstein, J.J. and Pagnanelli, D. (1982) Long-term axonal apposition in rat sciatic nerve neuroma. J. Neurosurg., 57: 682–684.

Blumberg, H. and Jänig, W. (1981) Neurophysiological analysis of efferent sympathetic and afferent fibers in skin nerves with experimentally produced neuromata. In J. Siegfried and M. Zimmermann (Eds.), Phantom and Stump Pain, Springer-Verlag, Berlin Heidelberg, pp. 15–31.

Blumberg, H. and Jänig, W. (1982a) Changes in unmyelinated fibers including sympathetic postganglionic fibers of a skin nerve after peripheral neuroma formation. J. Auton. Nerv. Syst., 6: 173–183.

Blumberg, H. and Jänig, W. (1982b) Activation of fibers via experimentally produced stump neuromas of skin nerves: ephaptic transmission or retrograde sprouting? Exp. Neurol., 76: 468–482.

Blumberg, H. and Jänig, W. (1983) Changes of reflexes in vasoconstrictor neurons supplying the cat hindlimb following chronic nerve lesions: a model for studying mechanisms of reflex sympathetic dystrophy? J. Auton. Nerv. Syst., 7: 399–411.

Blumberg, H. and Jänig, W. (1984) Discharge pattern of afferent fibers from a neuroma. Pain, 20: 335–353.

Blumberg, H. and Jänig, W. (1985) Reflex patterns in postganglionic vasoconstrictor neurons following chronic nerve lesions. J. Auton. Nerv. Syst., 14: 157–180.

Burchiel, K.J. (1984a) Spontaneous impulse generation in normal and denervated dorsal root ganglia: sensitivity to alpha-adrenergic stimulation and hypoxia. Exp. Neurol., 85: 257–272.

Burchiel, K.J. (1984b) Effects of electrical and mechanical stimulation on two foci of spontaneous activity which develop in primary afferent neurons after peripheral axotomy. Pain, 18: 249–265.

Burchiel, K.J. and Russell, L.C. (1987) Has the amount of spontaneous electrical activity in experimental neuromas been overestimated? In L.M. Pubols and B.J. Sessels (Eds.), Effects of Injury on Trigeminal and Spinal Somatosensory Systems, Alan Liss, New York, pp. 77–83.

Burnstock, G. (1986) The changing face of autonomic neurotransmission. Acta Physiol. Scand., 126: 67–91.

Carter, D.A. and Lisney, S.J.W. (1987) The numbers of unmyelinated and myelinated axons in normal and regenerated rat saphenous nerves. J. Neurol. Sci., 80: 163–171.

Coderre, T.J., Grimes, R.W. and Melzack, R. (1986) Deafferentation and chronic pain in animals: an evaluation of evidence suggesting autotomy is related to pain. Pain, 26: 61–84.

Cragg, G.B. and Thomas, P.K. (1961) Changes in conduction velocity and fibre size proximal to peripheral nerve lesions. J. Physiol. (Lond.), 157: 315–327.

Culp, W.J. and Ochoa, J. (Eds.) (1982) Abnormal Nerves and Muscles as Impulse Generators, Oxford University Press, London.

Davis, L.A., Gordon, T., Hoffer, J.A., Jhamandas, J. and Stein, R.B. (1979) Compound action potentials recorded from mammalian peripheral nerves following ligation and resuturing. J. Physiol. (Lond.), 285: 543–559.

Devor, M. (1983) Nerve pathophysiology and mechanisms of pain in causalgia. J. Auton. Nerv. Syst., 7: 371–384.

Devor, M. and Bernstein, J.J. (1982) Abnormal impulse generation in neuromas: electrophysiology and ultrastructure. In W.J. Culp and J. Ochoa (Eds.), Abnormal Nerves and Muscles as Impulse Generators, Oxford University Press, London, pp. 363–380.

Devor, M. and Govrin-Lippmann, R. (1985) Spontaneous neural discharge in neuroma C-fibers in rat sciatic nerve. Neurosci. Lett., Suppl., 22: S32.

Devor, M., Inbal, R. and Govrin-Lippmann, R. (1982) Genetic factors in the development of chronic pain. In I. Lieblich (Ed.), Genetics of the Brain, Elsevier, Amsterdam, pp. 273–296.

Devor, M. and Jänig, W. (1981) Activation of myelinated afferents ending in a neuroma by stimulation of the sympathetic supply in the rat. Neurosci. Lett., 24: 43–47.

Dyck, P.J., Karnes, J., Lais, A., Lofgren, E.P. and Stevens, J.C. (1984a) Pathologic alterations of the peripheral nervous system of humans. In P.J. Dyck, P.K. Thomas, E.H. Lambert and R. Bunge (Eds.), Peripheral Neuropathy, Vol. I, Saunders, Philadelphia, pp. 760–870.

Dyck, P.J., Nukada, H., Lais, A.C. and Karnes, J.L. (1984b) Permanent axotomy: a model of chronic neuronal degeneration preceded by axonal atrophy, myelin remodeling, and degeneration. In P.J. Dyck, P.K. Thomas, E.H. Lambert and R. Bunge (Eds.), Peripheral Neuropathy, Vol. I, Saunders, Philadelphia, pp. 666–706.

Govrin-Lippmann, R. and Devor, M. (1978) Ongoing activity in severed nerves: source and variation with time. Brain Res., 159: 406–410.

Häbler, H.-J., Jänig, W. and Koltzenburg, M. (1987) Activation of unmyelinated afferents in chronically lesioned nerves by adrenaline and excitation of sympathetic efferents in the cat. Neurosci. Lett., 82: 35–40.

Howe, J.F., Loeser, J.D. and Calvin, W.H. (1977) Mechanosensitivity of dorsal root ganglia and chronically injured axons: a physiological basis for radicular pain of nerve root compression. Pain, 3: 25–41.

Hylden, I.L.K., Nahin, R.L., Humphrey, E., Seltzer, Z. and Dubner, R. (1987) An animal model of hyperalgesia: partial sciatic nerve lesion. Pain, Suppl. 4: S274.

Jänig, W. (1985a) Organization of the lumbar sympathetic outflow to skeletal muscle and skin of the cat hindlimb and tail. Rev. Physiol. Biochem. Pharmacol., 102: 119–213.

Jänig, W. (1985b) Causalgia and reflex sympathetic dystrophy: in which way is the sympathetic nervous system involved? Trends Neurosci., 8: 471–477.

Jänig, W. (1988) Pre- and postganglionic vasoconstrictor neurons: differentiation, types and discharge properties. Annu. Rev. Physiol., 50: 525–539.

Jänig, W. and Kollmann, W. (1984) The involvement of the sympathetic nervous system in pain. Arzneim.-Forsch./Drug. Res., 34 (II): 1066–1073.

Jänig, W. and McLachlan, E.M. (1985) On the fate of sympathetic and sensory neurons projecting into a neuroma of the superficial peroneal nerve in the cat. J. Comp. Neurol., 225: 302–311.

Kirk, E.J. (1974) Impulses in dorsal spinal nerve rootlets in cats and rabbits arising from dorsal root ganglia isolated from the periphery. J. Comp. Neurol., 155: 165–176.

Korenman, E.M.D. and Devor, M. (1981) Ectopic adrenergic sensitivity in damaged peripheral nerve axons in the rat. Exp. Neurol., 72: 63–81.

Levine, J.D., Tairo, Y.O., Collins, S.D. and Tam, J.K. (1986) Noradrenaline hyperalgesia is mediated through interaction with sympathetic postganglionic neurone terminals rather than activation of primary afferent nociceptors. Nature, 323: 158–169.

Lieberman, A.R. (1974) Some factors affecting retrograde neuronal responses to axonal lesions. In R. Bellairs and E.G. Gray (Eds.), Essays on the Nervous System; A Festschrift for Prof. J.Z. Young, Clarendon Press, pp. 71–105.

Lisney, S.J.W. and Devor, M. (1987) Afterdischarge and interactions among fibers in damaged peripheral nerve in the rat. Brain Res., 415: 122–136.

Lisney, S.J.W. and Pover, C.M. (1983) Coupling between fibers involved in sensory neuromata in cats. J. Neurol. Sci., 59: 255–264.

Livingston, W.K. (1976) Pain Mechanisms. A Physiologic Interpretation of Causalgia and its Related States, Plenum Press, New York, London. Reprint of the 1943 edn. published by Macmillan, New York.

Lundberg, J.M. and Hökfelt, T. (1986) Multiple co-existence of peptides and classical transmitters in peripheral autonomic and sensory neurones – functional and pharmacological implications. Prog. Brain Res., 68: 241–262.

Matzner, O. and Devor, M. (1987) Contrasting thermal sensitivity of spontaneously active A- and C-fibers in experimental nerve-end neuromas. Pain, 30: 373–384.

McLachlan, E.M. and Jänig, W. (1983) The cell bodies of origin of sympathetic and sensory axons in some skin and muscle nerves of the cat hindlimb. J. Comp. Neurol., 214: 115–130.

Meyer, R.A., Raja, S.N., Campbell, J.N., Mackinnon, S.E. and Dellon, A.L. (1985) Neural activity originating from a neuroma in the baboon. Brain Res., 325: 255–260.

Nordin, M., Nyström, B., Wallin, U. and Hagbarth, K.-E. (1984) Ectopic sensory discharges and paresthesiae in patients with disorders of peripheral nerves, dorsal roots and dorsal columns. Pain, 20: 231–245.

Nyström, B. and Hagbarth, K.E. (1981) Microelectrode recordings from transected nerves in amputees with phantom limb pain. Neurosci. Lett., 27: 211–216.

Ochoa, J. (1982) Pain in local nerve lesions. In W.J. Culp and J. Ochoa (Eds.), Abnormal Nerves and Muscles as Impulse Generators, Oxford University Press, London, pp. 568–587.

Ochoa, J.L. and Tjorebjörk, H.E. (1980) Paresthesiae from impulse generation in human sensory nerves. Brain, 103: 835–853.

Ochoa, J.L., Tjorebjörk, H.E., Culp, W.J. and Schady, W. (1982) Abnormal spontaneous activity in single sensory nerve fibers in humans. Muscle Nerve, 5: S74–S77.

Ochoa, J.L., Tjorebjörk, H.E., Marchettini, P. and Sivak, M. (1985) Mechanisms of neuropathic pain: cumulative observations, new experiments, and further speculation. In H.L. Field, R. Dubner and F. Cervero (Eds.), Advances in Pain Research and Therapy, Vol. 9, Raven Press, New York, pp. 431–450.

Ochoa, J., Cline, M., Dotson, R. and Marchettini, P. (1987) Pain and paresthesias provoked mechanically in human cervical root entrapment (Sign of Spurling). Single sensory unit antidromic recording of ectopic, bursting, propagated nerve impulse activity. In L.M. Pubols and B.J. Sessle (Eds.), Effects of Injury on Trigeminal and Spinal Somatosensory Systems, Alan Liss, New York, pp. 389–397.

Peyronnard, J.M., Charron, L.F., Lavoie, J. and Messier, J.P. (1986a) Differences in horseradish peroxidase labeling of sensory, motor and sympathetic neurons following chronic axotomy of the rat sural nerve. Brain Res., 364: 137–150.

Peyronnard, J.M., Charron, L.F., Lavoie, J. and Messier, J.P. (1986b) Motor, sympathetic and sensory innervation of rat skeletal muscles. Brain Res., 373: 288–302.

Pubols, L.M. and Sessle, B.J. (Eds.) (1987) Effects of Injury on Trigeminal and Spinal Somatosensory Systems, Alan Liss, New York.

Risling, M., Aldskogius, H., Hildebrand, C. and Remahl, S. (1983) Effects of sciatic nerve resection on L7 spinal roots and dorsal root ganglia in adult cats. Exp. Neurol., 82: 568–580.

Roberts, W.J. (1986) A hypothesis on the physiological basis for causalgia and related pains. Pain, 24: 297–311.

Roberts, W.J. (1987) Which spinal nociceptive neurons are capable of mediating sympathetically maintained pain? Pain, Suppl., 4: S194.

Roberts, W.J. and Elardo, S.M. (1985a) Sympathetic activation of unmyelinated mechanoreceptors in cat skin. Brain Res., 339: 123–125.

Roberts, W.J. and Elardo, S.M. (1985b) Sympathetic activation of A-delta nociceptors. Somatosens. Res., 3: 33–44.

Scadding, J.W. (1981) Development of ongoing activity, mechanosensitivity, and adrenaline sensitivity in severed peripheral nerve axons. Exp. Neurol., 73: 345–364.

Schott, G.D. (1986) Mechanisms of causalgia and related clinical conditions. The role of the central and of the sympathetic nervous system. Brain, 109: 717–738.

Seltzer, Z. and Devor, M. (1979) Ephaptic transmission in chronically damaged peripheral nerves. Neurology (Mineap.), 29: 1061–1064.

Shea, V.K. and Perl, E.R. (1985) Failure of sympathetic stimulation to affect responsiveness of rabbit polymodal nociceptors. J. Neurophysiol., 54: 513–519.

Sittiracha, T. and McLachlan, E.M. (1986) Evaluation of the effects of various additives on retrograde labelling by horseradish peroxidase applied to intact and transected hindlimb nerves of rat and rabbit. Neuroscience, 18: 763–772.

Sunderland, S. (1978) Nerves and Nerve Injuries, 2nd edn., Churchill Livingstone, Edinburgh.

Thomas, P.K. (1982) Pain in peripheral neuropathy: clinical and morphological aspects. In W.J. Culp and J. Ochoa (Eds.), Abnormal Nerves and Muscles as Impulse Generators, Oxford University Press, London, pp. 553–567.

Torebjörk, H.E., Ochoa, J.L. and McCann, F.V. (1979) Paresthesiae: Abnormal impulse generation in sensory nerve fibers in man. Acta Physiol. Scand., 105: 518–520.

Vahle-Hinz, C., Gottschaldt, K.-M. and Kräft, H. (1987) Morphological basis for 'ephaptic' excitation in neuroma nerves. In L.M. Pubols and B.J. Sessle (Eds.), Effects of Injury on Trigeminal and Spinal Somatosensory Systems, Alan Liss, New York, pp. 487.

Wall, P.D. (1984) Mechanism of acute and chronic pain. In L. Kruger and J.C. Liebeskind (Eds.), Advances in Pain Research and Therapy, Vol. 6, Raven Press, New York, pp. 95–104.

Wall, P.D. (1985) Pain and no pain. In C.W. Coen (Ed.), Functions of the Brain, Clarendon Press, Oxford, pp. 44–66.

Wall, P.D. (1987) The control of neural connections by three physiological mechanisms. In F.J. Seil, E. Herbert and B.M. Carlson (Eds.), Neural Regeneration, Progress in Brain Research, Vol. 71, Elsevier, Amsterdam, pp. 239–247.

Wall, P.D. and Devor, M. (1983) Sensory afferent impulses originate from dorsal root ganglia as well as from the periphery in normal and nerve injured rats. Pain, 17: 321–339.

Wall, P.D. and Fitzgerald, M. (1982) If substance P fails to fulfill the criteria as a neurotransmitter in somatosensory afferents, what might be its function? In: Substance P in the Nervous System (Ciba Foundation Symposium 91), Pitman, London, pp. 249–266.

Wall, P.D., Devor, M., Inbal, R., Scadding, J.W., Schonfeld, D., Seltzer, Z. and Tomkiewicz, M.M. (1979) Autotomy following peripheral nerve lesions: experimental anaesthesia dolorosa. Pain, 7: 103–113.

Wall, P.D., Scadding, J.W. and Tomkiewicz, M.M. (1979) The production and prevention of experimental anaesthesia dolorosa. Pain, 6: 175–182.

Wallin, G., Torebjörk, E. and Hallin, R. (1976) Preliminary observations on the pathophysiology of hyperalgesia in the causalgic pain syndrome. In Y. Zottermann (Ed.), Sensory Functions of the Skin in Primates, Pergamon Press, Oxford, New York, pp. 489–499.

Ygge, J. and Aldskogius, H. (1984) Intercostal nerve transection and its effect on the dorsal root ganglion. A quantitative study on thoracic ganglion cell numbers and sizes in the rat. Exp. Brain Res., 55: 402–408.

R. Dubner, G.F. Gebhart & M.R. Bond (Eds.)
Proceedings of the Vth World Congress on Pain
© 1988 Elsevier Science Publishers BV (Biomedical Division)

CHAPTER 12

Changes in the content and release of substance P and calcitonin gene-related peptide in rat cutaneous nerve neuroma

D.M. White and M. Zimmermann

II Physiologisches Institut, Universität Heidelberg, Im Neuenheimer Feld 326, D-6900 Heidelberg, FRG

Summary

In this study, we investigated the changes in substance P-like immunoreactivity (SP-LI) and calcitonin gene-related peptide-like immunoreactivity (CGRP-LI) content and release from nerve fibre endings in rat saphenous nerve end neuromas. SP-LI and CGRP-LI contents are maximally depleted in 3-week-old neuromas. Similarly, bradykinin-induced release of SP-LI is also reduced in the 3-week-old neuroma as compared to the 5-week-old neuroma. Furthermore, unlike normal cutaneous nerve terminals, electrical stimulation of the saphenous nerve fails to induce a release of SP-LI from nerve fibre endings of the neuroma. We also find that veratridine and 40 mM K^+ fail to induce a release of SP-LI from neuroma nerve fibre endings. The bradykinin-induced release of SP-LI, therefore, is a chemically mediated release which is independent of electrophysiological excitation and may be indicative of a more general phenomenon in the nervous system.

Introduction

Substance P (SP) and calcitonin gene-related peptide (CGRP) are localized, and often co-localized, in small diameter, unmyelinated fibres of somatosensory primary afferent neurons (Hokfelt et al., 1975; Lee et al., 1985) where these peptides are synthesized in cell bodies of the dorsal root ganglia (Keen et al., 1982). Release of SP and CGRP from both the central and peripheral terminals of primary afferent nerve fibres has been demonstrated following electrical stimulation (Otsuka and Konishi, 1976; Yaksh et al., 1980; White and Helme, 1985; Wahlestedt et al., 1986) and potassium-induced depolarization (Moskowitz et al., 1983; Saria et al., 1986). The action of neuropeptides on the peripheral terminals of sensory nerve fibres has not been thoroughly studied, although there is evidence that superfusion of nerve fibre endings in the cat neuroma with SP inhibits C-fibre responses to noxious chemical and thermal stimulation (Zimmermann et al., 1987). It is well established that SP, released from peripheral nerve terminals, mediates, in part, the neurogenic inflammatory response (Lembeck and Gamse, 1982) and there is evidence that CGRP potentiates the actions of SP in this function (Gamse and Saria, 1985). It is also speculated that SP has trophic properties since it is released from cutaneous nerve terminals following thermal injury (Helme et al., 1986; Jonsson et al., 1986) and enhances the growth of connective tissue (Nilsson et al., 1985). CGRP has also been shown to act trophically by increasing the synthesis of acetylcholine receptors in neuromuscular junctions (New and

Mudge, 1986).

It is known that injury to a peripheral nerve leads to dramatic changes in the synthesis of peptides in primary sensory neurons (Shebab and Atkinson, 1986). The release, however, of peptides from injured and regenerating nerve fibre endings has not been examined. Considering the above, changes in the content and release of neuropeptides following nerve injury may have important consequences on both the sensory function and regrowth of damaged nerve fibres. This study examined the content and release of SP-like immunoreactivity (SP-LI) and CGRP-like immunoreactivity (CGRP-LI) in nerve fibre endings in rat cutaneous nerve neuroma.

Methods

Preparation of Neuromas

Neuromas were induced by ligating and cutting the saphenous nerve in male Sprague-Dawley rats anaesthetized with pentobarbitone sodium (50 mg/kg, i.p.) The behaviour of the rats, postoperatively, was indistinguishable from normal rats. The content and release of neuropeptides were then examined at one, 3 or 5 weeks after preparing the neuromas.

Content in neuropeptides

The SP-LI and CGRP-LI content of 1-, 3- and 5-week-old neuromas and normal saphenous nerve was quantified by radioimmunoassay. The rats were killed by an overdose of pentobarbitone sodium and 4 mm segments of nerve with neuromas were removed. A 4 mm segment of saphenous nerve was also removed from normal rats. The tissue samples were homogenized in ice cold 2 N acetic acid. The homogenates were centrifuged and the supernatants were lyophilized.

Release of SP-LI and CGRP-LI

To study the release of the neuropeptides following chemical and electrical stimulation, neuromas were dissected free from connective tissue, desheathed and placed in a perspex chamber, in situ, and superfused with Tyrode solution. An initial superfusion period of 15 min with 1 ml Tyrode solution served as the control. For the second 15 min interval the neuroma was superfused with 1 ml Tyrode solution containing 90 μM bradykinin, 50 μM veratridine or 40 mM K^+. In the Tyrode solution with 40 mM K^+, the NaCl concentration was reduced to 100 mM to maintain osmolarity. The calcium dependence of the bradykinin-induced release of SP was determined by using Tyrode solution without $CaCl_2$ and with an increased concentration of $MgCl_2$ (1.8 mM).

The release of SP-LI following electrical stimulation was also examined by placing platinum electrodes under the saphenous nerve proximal to the neuroma and stimulating the nerve for 30 min at 5 Hz with square pulses of 50 V, 0.5 ms. The neuroma was superfused for 30 min with 1 ml Tyrode solution before and during stimulation.

Superfusates to be assayed for SP-LI were passed through Sep-Pak cartridges. The cartridges were first washed with 10 ml 0.1% trifluoroacetic acid in 0.06 M NaCl. The samples were added to the column and SP was eluted with 2 ml 80% methanol and 0.1% trifluoroacetic acid in 0.06 M NaCl. The eluates were dried by evaporation using a Savant Speed Vac Concentrator. Superfusates to be assayed for CGRP-LI were lyophilized.

Radioimmunoassay

Dried superfusates and tissue extracts were reconstituted in assay buffer (Helme and White, 1981) immediately prior to being assayed. For the SP radioimmunoassay, a C-terminal-directed antibody (a gift from Dr S.E. Leeman) was used (Mroz and Leeman, 1979). The tracer, $[^{125}I]Tyr^8$-substance P was purchased from Amersham Buchler GmbH & Co. A dextran 10-coated charcoal separation method was used and assay sensitivity was 2 pg per tube (Helme and White, 1981). For the CGRP radioimmunoassay, the antibody, a rabbit anti-rat CGRP antibody, and the tracer, $[^{125}I]Tyr^0$-rat CGRP, were purchased from Peninsula Laboratories Europe, Ltd. A double antibody separation technique, using goat anti-rabbit IgG serum (Peninsula Laboratories Europe, Ltd.) was employed. Assay sensitivity was 125 pg per tube.

The crossreactivity of the bradykinin solution in the SP and CGRP radioimmunoassays was tested prior to the superfusion experiments and was found to be the same as the Tyrode controls.

The results are expressed as mean ± SEM. The statistical analysis was done using Student's *t*-test.

Results

SP-LI and CGRP-LI content
There is a significant decrease of SP-LI and CGRP-LI content in the 3-week-old neuroma as compared to normal saphenous nerve. In the 5-week-old neuroma the peptide content recovers to be equivalent to that measured in normal nerve (Fig. 1).

Release of SP-LI and CGRP-LI
Superfusion of 5-week-old neuromas with bradykinin results in a significant increase of SP-LI and CGRP-LI in the superfusate (Fig. 2). Further examination of the release of SP-LI, induced by bradykinin, shows that it is calcium-dependent (Table 1) and that the amount of SP-LI released varies with the age of the neuroma. Significantly less SP-LI is released from 3-week-old neuromas as compared to 5-week-old neuromas (Table 2).

Superfusion of the neuroma with 50 μM veratri-

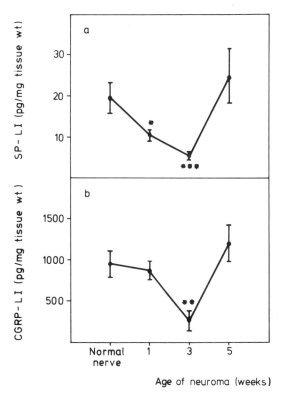

Fig. 1 (a) SP-LI content in normal saphenous nerve ($n=7$) and 1- ($n=8$), 3- ($n=8$) and 5- ($n=8$) week-old neuromas. SP-LI content in 1- and 3-week-old neuromas was significantly different from that in normal nerve (*$P<0.05$; ***$P<0.01$). (b) CGRP-LI content in normal saphenous nerve ($n=6$) and 1- ($n=4$), 3- ($n=4$) and 5- ($n=4$) week-old neuromas. CGRP-LI content in 3-week-old neuromas was significantly different from that in normal nerve (**$P<0.025$).

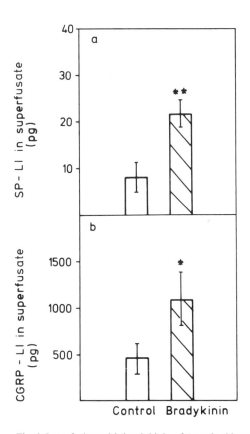

Fig. 2 Superfusion with bradykinin of 5-week-old neuromas results in a significant increase of (a) SP-LI ($n=15$) and (b) CGRP-LI ($n=9$) in the superfusate as compared to Tyrode solution controls (*$P<0.05$; **$P<0.01$).

TABLE I

The release of SP-LI from nerve fibre endings in rat saphenous nerve neuroma.

Stimulus	n	Change in SP-LI in super-fusate[a] (pg/15 min)
90 μM bradykinin	15	12.2 ± 2.6[b]
90 μM bradykinin without Ca^{2+}	10	1.2 ± 0.7
40 mM K^+	10	1.0 ± 0.9
50 μM veratridine	4	1.9 ± 2.5
Electrical stimulation	6	2.3 ± 1.6

[a]Calculated as: (pg SP-LI in test superfusate) − (pg SP-LI in control superfusate).
[b]Significantly different from control, $P < 0.01$.

TABLE II

Bradykinin-induced release of SP-LI from nerve fibre endings in rat saphenous nerve neuromas of various ages

Age of neuroma (weeks)	n	Increase of SP-LI in su-perfusate[a] (pg/15 min)
1	10	9.5 ± 2.8
3	8	4.5 ± 1.0[b]
5	14	8.8 ± 2.1

[a]Calculated as: (pg SP-LI in bradykinin superfusate) − (pg SP-LI in the control superfusate).
[b]Significantly different from 5-week-old neuromas, $P < 0.05$.

dine or 40 mM K^+ do not induce a release of SP-LI. Similarly, electrical stimulation of the saphenous nerve also fails to induce a release of SP-LI from nerve endings in the neuroma (Table 1).

Discussion

The results of this study show that both the content and release of peptides from nerve endings are altered during neuroma formation. The depletion of peptide content in the 3-week-old neuroma is most likely due to decreased synthesis and/or axonal transport of the peptides and not a result of increased rate of release of the peptides since bradykinin-induced release of SP-LI is also reduced in the 3-week-old neuroma.

The functional significance of the decrease in peptide content and release in 3-week-old neuromas is unclear. The local environment of the peripheral terminals is very important for determining the gene expression of peptidergic neurons (McMahon and Gibson, 1987). The decrease in synthesis of SP and CGRP may be a passive change in consequence of depriving the neurons of their normal environment. A recent discovery, however, has shown that SP inhibits the release of nerve growth factor from rat saphenous nerve neuromas (White et al., un-

published). It is more likely, therefore, that the decrease in SP-LI and CGRP-LI content and release is a genome-controlled reaction of the neuron to axotomy because these peptides are unnecessary or even impede regrowth.

The most surprising result of this study is that SP-LI is released by bradykinin but not released following electrical stimulation of the saphenous nerve. Stimulation of a peripheral nerve, using parameters similar to those used here, has been shown to induce a release of SP-LI from its central terminals in the spinal cord (Yaksh et al., 1980) and from the peripheral terminals in the skin (White and Helme, 1986). Furthermore, SP-LI was not released following superfusion of the neuroma with 40 mM K^+ or 50 μM veratridine. Veratridine- and potassium-induced depolarization of neurons are widely used methods for inducing the release of peptides throughout the nervous system. For example, high concentrations of K^+ induces a release of SP-LI from nerve terminals in the rat spinal cord (Otsuka and Konishi, 1976; Yaksh et al., 1980) and the cat pia arachnoid (Moskowitz et al., 1983) and veratridine induces a release of CGRP from cultured trigeminal ganglion cells (Peterfreund and Vale, 1986). It appears, therefore, that the mechanism whereby SP-LI is released from normal nerve terminals following cellular depolarization is absent in nerve fibre endings in rat saphenous nerve neuromas.

We conclude, first, that the bradykinin-induced release of SP-LI involves a neurochemical interaction which is not related to terminal depolarization. This raises the possibility that, for neuropeptides in general, there exist two separate release mechanisms at normal peripheral and central nerve terminals. Second, the changes in the content and release of SP-LI from neuroma nerve fibre endings, compared with normal nerve terminals, have important implications for future studies of the regulatory roles of neuropeptides in peripheral sensory nerve terminals.

Acknowledgements

This work is being supported by the Deutsche Forschungsgemeinschaft (Grant Zi 110). D. White was an Alexander von Humboldt Fellow.

References

Gamse, R. and Saria, A. (1985) Potentiation of tachykinin-induced plasma protein extravasation by calcitonin gene-related peptide. Eur. J. Pharmacol., 114:61–66.

Helme, R.D., Koschorke, G.M. and Zimmermann, M. (1986) Immunoreactive substance P release from skin nerves in the rat by noxious thermal stimulation. Neurosci. Lett., 63:295–299.

Helme, R.D. and White, D.M. (1981) Substance P in the central nervous system. Clin. Exp. Neurol., 18:156–160.

Hokfelt, T., Kellerth, J.O., Nilsson, G. and Pernow, B. (1975) Experimental immunohistochemical studies on the localization and distribution of substance P in cat primary sensory neurones. Brain Res., 100:235–252.

Jonsson, C-E., Brodin, E., Dalsgaard, C-J. and Haegerstrand, A. (1986) Release of substance P-like immunoreactivity in dog paw lymph after scalding injury. Acta Physiol. Scand., 126:21–24.

Keen, P., Harmar, A.J., Spears, F. and Winter, E. (1982) Biosynthesis, axonal transport and turnover of neuronal substance P. In R. Porter and M. O'Connor (Eds.), Substance P in the Nervous System, Ciba Foundation Symposium 91, Pitmman, London, pp. 145–160.

Lee, Y., Takami, K., Kawai, Y., Girgis, S., Hillyard, C.J., MacIntyre, I., Emson, P.C. and Tohyama, M. (1985) Distribution of calcitonin gene-related peptide in the rat peripheral nervous system with reference to its coexistence with substance P. Neuroscience, 15:1227-1237.

Lembeck, F. and Gamse, R. (1982) Substance P in peripheral sensory processes. In R. Porter and M. O'Connor (Eds.), Substance P in the Nervous System, Ciba Foundation Symposium 91, Pitman, London, pp. 35–49.

McMahon, S.B. and Gibson, S. (1987) Peptide expression is altered when afferent nerves reinnervate inappropriate tissue. Neurosci. Lett., 73:9–15.

Moskowitz, M.A., Brody, M. and Liu-Chen, L-Y. (1983) In vitro release of immunoreactive substance P from putative afferent nerve endings in bovine pia arachnoid. Neuroscience, 9:809–814.

Mroz, E.A. and Leeman, S.E. (1979) Substance P. in B.M. Jaffe and H.R. Behrman (Eds.), Methods of Hormone Radioimmunoassay. 2nd edn., Academic Press, New York, pp. 121–138.

New, H.V. and Mudge, A.W. (1986) Calcitonon gene-related peptide regulates muscle acetylcholine receptor synthesis. Nature, 323:809–811.

Nilsson, J., von Euler, A.M. and Dalsgaard, C-J. (1985) Stimulation of connective tissue cell growth by substance P and substance K. Nature, 315:61–63.

Otsuka, M. and Konishi, S. (1976) Release of substance P-like immunoreactivity from isolated spinal cord of newborn rat. Nature, 264:83–84.

Peterfreund, R.A. and Vale, W.W. (1986) Local anesthetics inhibit veratridine-induced secretion of calcitonin gene-related peptide (CGRP) from cultured rat trigeminal ganglion cells. Brain Res., 380:159–161.

Saria, A., Gamse, R., Peterfreund, J., Fischer, J.A., Theodorsson-Norheim, E. and Lundberg, J.M. (1986) Simultaneous release of several tachykinins and calcitonin gene-related peptide from rat spinal cord slices. Neurosci. Lett., 63:310–314.

Shebab, S.A.S. and Atkinson, E. (1986) Vasoactive Intestinal Polypeptide (VIP) increases in the spinal cord after peripheral axotomy of the sciatic nerve originate from afferent neurons. Brain Res., 37–44.

Wahlestedt, C., Beding, B., Ekman, R., Oksala, O., Stjernschantz, J. and Hakanson, R. (1986) Calcitonin gene-related peptide in the eye: release by sensory nerve stimulation and effects associated with neurogenic inflammation. Regulat. Pept., 16:107–115.

White, D.M. and Helme, R.D. (1986) Release of substance P from peripheral nerve terminals following electrical stimulation of the sciatic nerve. Brain Res., 336:27–31.

Yaksh, T.L., Jessell, T.M., Gamse, R., Mudge, A.W. and Leeman, S.E. (1980) Intrathecal morphine inhibits substance P release from mammalian spinal cord in vivo. Nature, 286:155–157.

Zimmermann, M., Koschorke, G.M. and Sanders, K. (1987) Response characteristics of fibres in regenerating and regenerated cutaneous nerves in cat and rat. In L.M. Pubols and B.J. Sessle (Eds.), Effects of Injury on Trigeminal and Spinal Somatosensory Systems, Neurology and Neurobiology, Vol. 30, Alan R. Liss, Inc., New York, pp. 93–103.

R. Dubner, G.F. Gebhart & M.R. Bond (Eds.)
Proceedings of the Vth World Congress on Pain
© 1988 Elsevier Science Publishers BV (Biomedical Division)

CHAPTER 13

Central changes mediating neuropathic pain

Marshall Devor

Department of Zoology, Life Sciences Institute, Hebrew University of Jerusalem, Jerusalem 91904, Israel

Summary

Peculiarities about certain chronic pains associated with peripheral nerve injury or disease suggest that the root cause may reside in the CNS rather than in the injured nerve or its dorsal root ganglia. The afferent imbalance feature of the 'Gate Control' theory does not provide a comprehensive explanation, particularly for conditions in which pain is evoked by weak, normally non-painful stimuli (allodynia). Is it possible that CNS changes triggered by peripheral injury might bring about the activation of central pain circuits by innocuous stimuli?

An animal model of this condition suitable for analysing the underlying mechanism has yet to be established. However, there are other examples of central connectivity altered by nerve injury which provide useful insights. One such example, somatotopic remapping, was used in this chapter to analyse the type of change that could result in central pain. By analogy to somatotopic remapping, it is suggested that disruption of the trophic relationship between peripheral tissue and the spinal cord could trigger the strengthening of pre-existing relatively ineffective synaptic contacts that were previously unexpressed. Imagine relatively weak, or even functionally latent, input from low-threshold afferent fibers converging onto central neurons whose strong activation normally signals pain to a conscious brain. The strengthening of these relatively ineffective synapses would yield allodynia and hyperalgesia.

Introduction

The clinical fact that injury or disease involving peripheral nerves can trigger chronic pain poses a real challenge to the biologist attempting to understand pain mechanisms. In principle, disruption of nerves ought to reduce the sensory signal arriving at the central nervous system (CNS) and ultimately its conscious appreciation. With a few possible exceptions, this is exactly what happens when special sensory nerves such as the optic or auditory nerves are injured. Why, then, does injury to a somatic sensory nerve frequently yield more, rather than less, sensation?

The 'Gate Control' theory
The afferent imbalance feature of Melzack and Wall's (1965) 'Gate Control' theory offers a possible explanation. If the injury/disease process preferentially attacked large-diameter, low-threshold afferent fibers, then the resulting disinhibition in the spinal gate circuit would, in effect, amplify the sensory consequences of nociceptor input. Such disinhibition, however, cannot give a full explanation of neuropathic pain for two reasons. First, both the clinical neuropathological data on patients with chronic pain, and the sensory status of patients who indeed have relatively selective large fiber loss, frequently do not jibe with the prediction of the theory (Wall and Devor, 1978). Second, one of the most common symptoms of neuropathic pain is in direct violation of the straightforward prediction of affe-

rent imbalance. Specifically, weak stimuli capable of activating normal low-threshold afferents but not nociceptors are expected to close the spinal gate and relieve pain. They should not produce pain, i.e. allodynia. (Allodynia is pain from stimuli which are normally nonpainful (Mersky, 1986).) Some other process(es) must be at play in addition to afferent imbalance.

Alternative theories
The fundamental paradox, then, is pain from weak stimuli. In recent years, preliminary outlines of three distinct classes of explanation have begun to emerge, or more correctly re-emerge. None of these is mutually contradictory, nor is any fundamentally incompatible with the afferent imbalance concept of 'Gate Control'. Indeed, I believe that all four processes may be at work, individually or in combinations, following nerve injury and/or disease.

(1) Sensitization and nerve pathophysiology It is possible that nociceptive afferents change their sensitivity (i.e. transduction properties) in the periphery so that they fire spontaneously (yielding ongoing pain) or so that weak stimuli are now adequate to cause them to generate action potentials (hence allodynia). This idea actually comes in two parts. First, the high-threshold receptor ending might become 'sensitized' (see Chapter 15). Second, nociceptors may develop 'pathophysiological' impulse-generating capabilities at ectopic sites (reviewed in Devor, 1988).

(2) Crosstalk It is possible that low-threshold fibers excited by weak stimuli secondarily activate nociceptors by pathophysiological crosstalk. In fact, several different forms of fiber-to-fiber crosstalk have recently been identified in experimental nerve injury preparations (reviewed in Devor, 1988), and the technology (peripheral neurography) is now available to determine whether one or another of these is at issue in any of the clinical pain syndromes (e.g. Torebjork et al., 1987).

(3) Changes in central processing It is possible

that following nerve injury, those cell assemblies whose activity normally yields a conscious appreciation of pain come to be activated by inputs which did not previously activate them. This type of process is the subject of the present chapter.

Central changes mediating neuropathic pain

Is there a need for a new CNS theory?
The 'Gate Control' theory arose primarily out of a need to explain a range of clinical pain phenomena that were not adequately explained within the framework of prior 'Specificity' theory. With only a few exceptions, 'Specificity' theory was, and remains, reasonably successful at accounting for the psychophysics of normal somatic sensation. However, it fails to account for spontaneous pain or pain upon weak stimulation. But if the new data on nerve pathophysiology can fill this void (and note that they do so within a framework that is fundamentally related to 'Specificity' theory), is there any real need to continue looking into the CNS?

The answer to this question is a tentative yes; yes on account of a number of clinical observations which continue to have a central flavor even in the light of nerve pathophysiology, but tentative because of the frequently anecdotal and weakly documented nature of the clinical data. Some examples:

(1) There are numerous descriptions of pains associated with peripheral nerve injury, particularly in phantom limbs, in which the sensations take highly idiosyncratic forms that could not reasonably be generated by abnormal discharge generated in the injured nerve or its dorsal root ganglia. Examples are rings worn, ulcers present, and peculiar orientations of the limb prior to amputation, which continue to be felt in the phantom (Riddoch, 1941; Henderson and Smyth, 1948; Haber, 1956).

(2) Phantoms may persist despite what is believed to be total conduction block of neuromas in the stump (Livingston, 1945). It is possible, of course, that abnormal discharges originate upstream of the block but still in the periphery (viz. in dorsal root ganglia (e.g. Wall and Devor, 1983)). However,

neuropathic pain is also said to occasionally survive segmental dorsal rhizotomy and even spinal cord block, again apparently with remarkable preservation of its sensory quality (Bors, 1951; Cook and Druckemiller, 1952; Appenzeller and Bicknell, 1969; Mackenzie, 1983).

(3) Sometimes neuropathic pain has peculiar abnormalities in the temporal and spatial domains (hyperpathia), including delay, slow cumulative build-up, and reference to locations too distant to be explained convincingly by collateral sprouting in the periphery (Noordenbos, 1959). Stimulation proximal to amputation stumps may evoke sensations in a phantom hand (Cronholm, 1951; Howe, 1983; Nurmikko and Pertovaara, 1984), and two-point discrimination on the stump is better than normal (Teuber et al., 1949; Haber, 1955).

(4) Campbell, LaMotte and collaborators have presented data indicating that cutaneous allodynia to mechanical stimuli is not accompanied by sensitization of nociceptive afferents and disappears when conduction in large-diameter afferents is blocked (see Chapter 15 in this volume, but see also Cline and Ochoa, 1986).

(5) Dorsal root avulsion, which produces notoriously severe and persistent pain (Wynn Parry, 1980), leaves no route for abnormal peripheral impulses to enter the CNS. It is not clear, however, whether this situation is rightfully classified along with dorsal rhizotomy as a peripheral injury, in the light of the substantial spinal cord trauma involved.

Together, observations such as these suggest that, in man, peripheral nerve injury might be capable of 'centralizing' pain, that is, of inducing changes in the CNS whereby afferent input along low-threshold fibers comes to activate central pain circuits.

Experimental evidence of functional rewiring in adult CNS following nerve injury

A great deal of evidence has accumulated over the past 20 years on plastic rearrangement of CNS circuitry in newborn animals following selective CNS injury, deafferentation, and even manipulation of sensory experience. In most systems, this develop-mental neuroplasticity freezes up within the first few days or weeks after birth, and cannot be demonstrated in the adult. There are several exceptions to this, however, the most striking being the central somatosensory system! Here, a most remarkable malleability is preserved into adulthood.

The first indication of this came with the work of Liu and Chambers (1958). They presented evidence that after dorsal rhizotomy in adult cats, and consequent degeneration of afferent synaptic terminals in the dorsal horn, some of the lost synapses are replaced by new growth from fibers in neighboring, intact dorsal roots. Although it is fairly clear today that the distance over which such reactive sprouting occurs was overestimated by Liu and Chambers (Brown, 1987), evidence for local, short-range synaptic replacement continues to accumulate (Goldberger and Murray, 1974; Murray et al., 1986).

A different and in many ways more interesting paradigm for examining post-traumatic changes in CNS connectivity was developed by Wall and Egger (1971). Their approach was to delineate the somatotopic (body surface) map in the somatosensory thalamus (VPL) in rats, and then to deafferent the hindlimb part of the map by destroying the nucleus gracilis. This, as expected, eliminated the response of former hindlimb neurons without affecting forelimb neurons. However, some days later, it was found that at least some of the neurons in the deafferented and unresponsive hindlimb region of the thalamus had become reconnected, and now responded to stimulation of forelimb skin. Rhoades et al. (1987) have recently performed a similar study in which VPM cells were shown to acquire a novel drive from the trigeminal nucleus interpolaris after destruction of the trigeminal nucleus principalis. Since the Wall and Egger (1971) study, corresponding somatotopic respecification has been demonstrated, using adult cats and primates as well as rodents, in all of the various CNS body-surface maps in which it has been sought. These include the spinal cord, the dorsal column nuclei, the trigeminal nucleus, the tectum, and the somatosensory cortex in addition to the thalamus (see references in Kaas et al., 1983; Devor et al., 1986). Indeed, in the majority of these studies, which now number well in excess of thirty, the initial functional deafferentation involved injury to a peripheral nerve. Only two studies involving nerve injury, to the best of my knowledge, have failed to obtain such somatotopic reordering (Brown et al., 1984; Pubols, 1984).

Because of the special relevance of this body of data to the problem of neuropathic pain, I will describe one of these studies in some more detail. In normal animals, the skin surface is mapped somatotopically in the upper layers of the spinal grey matter, the foot, and particularly the toes, occupying a particularly large proportion of the map (Brown and Fuchs, 1975). In this toe-foot region, which occupies the medial half–two-thirds of the lower lumbar spinal segments, cells respond to brushing, touching and/or pinching of the foot, and fail to respond to cutaneous stimulation elsewhere on the body. Their receptive field is restricted to the foot. Using barbiturate-anesthetized rats and decerebrate spinal cats, Wall and I (Devor and Wall, 1978, 1981a,b; also see Dostrovsky et al., 1976, 1982; Lisney, 1983; Markus et al., 1984; Snow and Wilson, 1985; Hylden et al., 1987; Wilson, 1987) cut and ligated the sciatic and the saphenous nerves, completely denervating the foot. The nerve injury, of course, also deafferented the spinal toe-foot cells, leaving them unresponsive to any cutaneous stimuli. However, after only a few days in rats, or a few weeks in cats, a substantial proportion of the cells in the former foot region began once again to respond to cutaneous stimulation, but now the responsive area was the upper leg, thigh and perineum. There had been a functional reconnection of neurons that lost their normal sensory input from the foot. Fig. 1 shows results of a typical experiment of this type in a cat, and Table I summarizes results from a series of cats.

In principle, such reconnection could reflect changes in the periphery, either anomalous growth of cut foot afferents into skin of the upper leg, or crosstalk between thigh and foot afferents. These peripheral explanations were specifically ruled out, however (Devor and Wall, 1981a,b; Devor, 1983). Acutely recutting the stumps of the sciatic and sa-

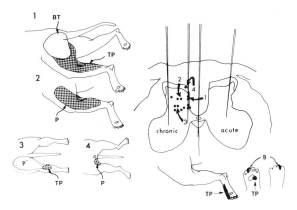

Fig. 1. This experiment, performed on an adult decerebrate spinal cat, illustrates somatotopic remodelling. Receptive fields in the medial part of the intact right dorsal horn were small, and limited to the toes and foot (black patches in figurines in lower right). Transection of the sciatic and saphenous nerves (acute) eliminated the receptive fields. On the left side, where the nerves had been cut 61 days earlier, numerous cells with novel proximal receptive fields were encountered. The location and response of four such cells are indicated, where BT indicates excitatory response to brushing hairs and light touch on the skin, TP indicates response to touch and pinch, P response to pinch only, and P⁻ inhibition to pinch. Maps of acute and chronic sides were always made at the same anteroposterior level. The mediolateral location of responsive cells was calculated with respect to marker electrodes left in the tissue after recording (see Devor and Wall, 1986). The four electrodes indicated are not reconstructions. They were traced from a projection of the original histological section which still contains the tips of the actual recording electrodes. Note that four responsive cells, each with a different receptive field, were observed along the electrode track of the cell labelled 1.

phenous nerves, for example, had no effect on the novel proximal receptive fields, but cutting the thigh nerves eliminated them. Similarly, electrophysiological recording from the thigh and foot nerves yielded no sign of aberrant crosstalk between the two (Devor et al., 1984). The functional rewiring had occurred in the spinal cord proper.

Shifts in receptive field submodality could explain allodynia

The foregoing example of spinal map respecification demonstrates the formation of new functional connections in the spatial domain, but not in the modality domain (i.e. the domain of sensory quali-

TABLE I

Emergence of neurons in the medial part of the dorsal horn with a cutaneous receptive field (RF) extending proximal to the ankle following permanent transection of the sciatic and saphenous nerves (data on decerebrate L1 spinal cats from Devor and Wall, 1978, 1981b).

Cat (L/R side)	Survival time (days p.o.)	No. medial penetrations	No. cells with a prox. RF	Cells with prox. RF per penetration
7R	intact	13	6	0.5
8R	intact	6	0	0
9R	intact	19	0	0
10L	intact	12	0	0
11R	intact	14	2	0.2
22L	intact	6	0	0
28L	intact	9	5	0.6
Mean ($n=7$)	intact	11.3	1.9	0.2
5L	0 (acute)	7	0	0
8R	0	7	0	0
9L	0	16	0	0
10L	0	10	0	0
12R	0	12	1	0.1
13R	0	16	0	0
14R	0	10	1	0.1
16R	0	4	1	0.3
18R	0	9	0	0
27R	0	3	1	0.3
31L	0	9	1	0.1
32L	0	8	3	0.4
Mean ($n=12$)	0	9.3	0.7[a]	0.1
7L	6	19	13	0.7
11L	6	13	4	0.3
30L	13	15	14	0.9
29L	15	8	11	1.4
8L	18	20	34	1.7
12L	19	12	19	1.6
Mean ($n=6$)	12.8	14.5	15.8	1.1
27L	28	7	18	2.6
18L	31	10	20	2.0
25L	34	12	23	1.9
14L	54	16	30	1.9
21L	61	6	7	1.2
13L	70	9	7	0.8
16L	105	9	32	3.6
Mean ($n=7$)	54.7	9.9	19.6[b]	2.0

[a] All of these cells required firm pressure or pinch.

[b] 68 % of these cells responded to hair movements or non-noxious touch over at least part of the receptive field.

ty). Do neurons that formerly responded primarily to noxious stimulation of the foot, and which are therefore good candidates for being involved in the forward transmission of a pain message, come to respond to brush or light touch of thigh skin? If so, this change would neatly account for allodynia.

The answer at this time is inconclusive. The receptive field submodality in samples of neurons encountered after rewiring does tend to be subtly different from normal. Many studies, for example, report a relative increase in the proportion of noxious input, especially early in the process (e.g. Devor and Wall, 1981a,b; Pubols and Brenowitz, 1981; Sedevic et al., 1981; Lisney, 1983; Wilson, 1987). Sometimes responses habituate, or require special manoeuvres such as flicking of hairs. These observations suggest a relatively tenuous synaptic drive which is aided by temporal summation of the afferent volley. The trouble is that observed changes in submodality convergence do not prove that cells have actually changed their submodality convergence. It is entirely possible that cell types that originally had little nociceptive drive are relatively unlikely to acquire a new receptive field. If so, these cells would be under-represented in any cell sample made after remodelling.

Unlike certain lower animal forms, it is not yet possible in the mammalian CNS to study a neuron, and then return to the same neuron days later to study the effects of a manipulation. We are forced to work with populations of neurons, which can be characterized in only limited ways. The whole beauty of Wall and Egger's (1971) paradigm is that at least one of the properties of a neuron, the original receptive field location, is known on the basis of the cell's physical location, even after obliteration of the receptive field by the nerve injury. What we need is some definite anatomical, electrophysiological or biochemical marker for spinal nociceptive neurons. We could then ask following transection of foot nerves whether such neurons in the foot region of the dorsal horn come to respond to low-threshold sensory stimulation of the thigh. A recent attempt at this design was carried out by Hylden et al. (1987). They defined a group of neurons in cat

lumbosacral spinal lamina I, many of which normally have exclusive nociceptive drive. Novel proximal receptive fields were observed, but the amount of low-threshold input did not increase noticeably.

My guess is that simple nerve section in rats and cats will continue to yield negative results of this sort. The reason is that substantially increased low-threshold drive of central nociceptive neurons ought to result in allodynia. Hylden et al.'s (1987) cats did not show any obvious allodynia on the thigh (personal communication), and this is in keeping with my experience with animals that have suffered hindlimb deafferentation (but see Markus et al., 1984). Note that when allodynia occurs clinically it is hard to miss! Nerve-injured animals do, however, frequently show a syndrome termed 'autotomy' which is reminiscent of anesthesia dolorosa (Wall et al., 1979). It will be most interesting to perform Hylden et al.'s (1987) experiment again once an appropriate animal model of allodynia emerges.

Other examples of functional remodelling
Although somatotopic remodelling stands out as an example of central rewiring induced by peripheral injury, it is not the only example. Long-term changes in several spinal reflexes have also been reported. These include alterations in the amplitude and time course of somatic mono- and polysynaptic motor reflexes (Eccles and MacIntyre, 1953; Woolf, 1983) and a frank reversal of sign in at least one visceral reflex (cutaneous postganglionic vasoconstrictor neurons, normally *inhibited* by arterial chemoreceptor stimulation and by noxious pinch, come to be *excited* by these stimuli (Blumberg and Jänig, 1985)).

One particularly interesting example from the point of view of mechanism is the reduced dorsal root potential and reflex evoked from injured nerves. This spinal reflex, which results from presynaptic depolarization of primary afferent terminals, normally plays an inhibitory role in spinal afferent transmission. Its decline, which is closely time-locked to the emergence of somatotopically inappropriate receptive fields, suggests that spinal disinhibition may be important for functional remodelling (Devor and Wall, 1981a; Wall and Devor, 1981; Horch and Lisney, 1981; Wall, 1982). Postsynaptic inhibition exerted by large-diameter fibers is also reduced by chronic nerve injury (Woolf and Wall, 1982).

Mechanisms of somatotopic remodelling

Despite the fact that there is, at present, no clear experimental evidence for the involvement of somatotopic remodelling or altered spinal reflexes in neuropathic pain, these phenomena are useful analogues of the predicted type of change. For lack of a really good model of peripherally evoked central pain itself, it is worthwhile examining such analogues. Virtually all of the available evidence relates to mechanisms of somatotopic remodelling.

Sprouting

The most obvious explanation for the creation of new functional connectivity is the growth of new axons across former somatotopic boundaries, that is, 'long-distance' sprouting. One of the advantages of examining somatotopic respecification at the spinal level as opposed, say, to the somatosensory cortex, is that one can be quite specific about the anticipated trajectory of such sprouting. For primary afferents, growth would have to be from the region surrounding the dorsal horn foot representation. Experiments using a range of different axon tracing techniques, however, have consistently failed to find evidence of 'long-distance' sprouting (e.g. Devor and Claman, 1980; Barbut et al., 1981; Seltzer and Devor, 1983). Primary afferent fibers also fail to undergo 'long-distance' intraspinal sprouting after transection of adjacent dorsal roots (Goldberger and Murray, 1974; Rodin et al., 1983) even though such surgery also induces shifts in somatotopic maps (e.g. Basbaum and Wall, 1976). Finally, it has also been impossible to demonstrate 'long-distance' dendritic sprouting over the predicted trajectory following either nerve or dorsal root injury

(e.g. Devor, 1983; Sedevic et al., 1985).

'Long-distance' sprouting cannot yet be ruled out entirely. Sprouting of interneurons, for example, has not been examined adequately. Nonetheless, the most immediate and likely options are excluded and this encourages exploration in other directions.

Increased effectiveness of a pre-existing synaptic channel

Indeed, from the very start an entirely different hypothesis was raised as an alternative to long-distance sprouting (Wall, 1977). According to this hypothesis, some neurons normally have wide-ranging synaptic inputs which are not normally expressed. These weak or 'silent' synapses are in addition to the strong ones which determine the expressed receptive field. New functional connections would appear in the absence of overt growth if these relatively ineffective synapses underwent an appropriate increase in their synaptic effectiveness. Indeed, such a process is demanded in the few instances in which cells have been reported to shift location instantly and reversibly (e.g. Dostrovsky et al., 1976). Rapid remapping, however, seems to be the exception.

When originally proposed, this hypothesis struck many as perversely unconventional, distressingly ad hoc. Ghost synapses were being invoked to create new connections out of thin air, by positing that they existed all along!

In the intervening years, however, largely as a result of research in invertebrates on the neural basis of learning, the idea that synaptic efficacy is subject to modulation has changed status from fantasy to dogma (e.g. Kandel and Schwartz, 1982; Black et al., 1987; Kaczmarek and Levitan, 1987). Indeed, the notion of 'strength' can be given a precise meaning in terms of membrane currents, and a large number of biophysical processes have been identified, both pre- and postsynaptic, that are capable of up- or down-regulating it. But what of the pre-existing synaptic channel that is supposed to be strengthened to reveal novel connectivity? Can unexpressed, somatotopically inappropriate connections be demonstrated to exist in the intact animal?

Evidence for somatotopically inappropriate connections

Progress has come mostly from the spinal cord preparation, once again due to the possibility of predicting with precision where such connections ought to be. There are basically two lines of evidence: neuronal tracing, and postsynaptic responses to synchronous electrical nerve stimulation.

Neuronal tracing Studies using antidromic electrical stimulation and anterograde axon tracing methods have shown that primary afferent axons may range for very long distances rostrocaudally in the spinal cord. In particular, they may reach well beyond the somatotopic boundaries of the expressed receptive fields of the immediately subjacent neurons (e.g. Wall and Werman, 1976; Meyers and Snow, 1982). Such axons are not numerous, and there is no proof that they actually form relatively ineffective synaptic contacts. They are, however, just what the hypothesis predicts as a basis for somatotopic remodelling after dorsal rhizotomy.

There are similar data for spinal somatotopic remapping following nerve injury. In normal, unoperated rats afferent fibers from thigh nerves can be traced along a trajectory that runs through the medial L4,5 dorsal horn (Seltzer and Devor, 1983; Devor et al., 1986), precisely the region where novel thigh receptive fields appear following transection of the foot nerves (Fig. 2a). What is more, electron microscopic images show that these afferents may make synaptic contacts on local dendrites on their way through (Fig. 2b).

Looking at intrinsic spinal cord circuitry, as opposed to primary afferent input, two additional candidate pathways can be found in normal animals. First, both Golgi and intracellular labelling studies reveal dorsal horn neurons whose ascending axon makes a plexus of mediolaterally directed branches at the segmental level of the cell soma. Laterally located neurons of this type are well placed to project relatively ineffective synaptic input into the medial dorsal horn. Higher-order spinal interneurons could also contribute to this channel. Finally, some medially located neurons, particularly

ones located in the deeper laminae of the dorsal horn, have dendritic arbors that extend laterally well into the thigh map region (e.g. Brown, 1981; Egger et al., 1981; Devor, 1983; Ritz and Greenspan, 1985; Woolf, 1987).

Postsynaptic responses to nerve stimulation Not only does a potential anatomical substrate exist for somatotopically inappropriate synaptic connections in intact animals, but it is relatively simple to demonstrate them using electrical nerve stimulation. The first such demonstration was by Merrill and Wall (1972). They recorded from neurons in the medial dorsal horn which had foot-receptive fields, and then cut the dorsal rootlets which provided the cutaneous receptive field. Despite the fact that the cells were now totally unresponsive to cutaneous stimulation, they still responded to electrical stimulation of neighboring rootlets. This experiment has the potential flaw that the residual responses could have been from normal proprioceptive or visceral input that had not been cut, although the cell type chosen for this study makes such an interpretation most unlikely. A modified experimental design resolved this problem. Here, cells with restricted foot-receptive fields were shown to respond to electrical stimulation of cutaneous nerves of the thigh (Devor and Wall, 1981b). Many other variations on this theme have also appeared (e.g. Devor et al., 1977; Markus et al., 1984; Pubols et al., 1986). Frequently, responses are so rapid that monosynaptic drive is a likelihood. Unfortunately, response latency to nerve stimulation is an uncertain diagnostic (Berry and Pentreath, 1976), and so polysynaptic links can by no means be ruled out.

If cells respond to electrical stimulation of somatotopically distant nerves, why don't they respond to natural stimulation of distant cutaneous receptors? That is, why is the distant skin not a part of the receptive field? Ghosts again? The hypothesis, of course, suggests that the synaptic contacts formed by the distant afferent fibers are relatively ineffective, that is, that they produce only a small postsynaptic potential at the neuron's spike initiation zone. Indeed, intracellular recordings from

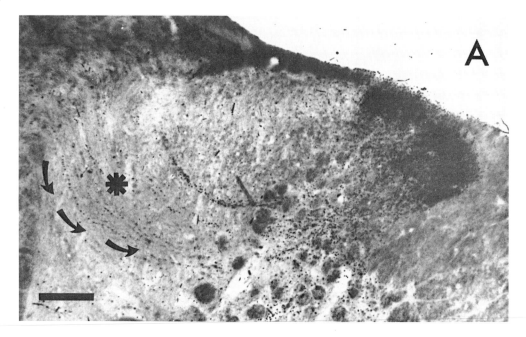

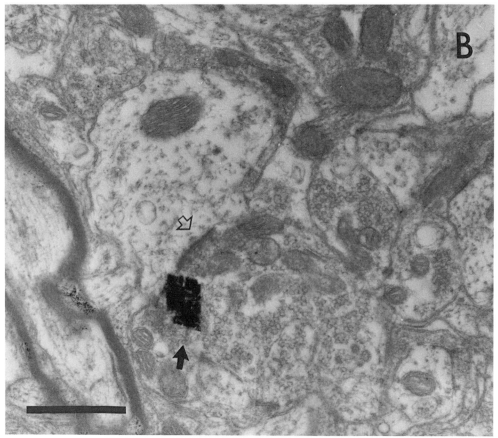

dorsal horn neurons always show at least a small subliminal fringe of subthreshold synaptic potentials (e.g. Mendell et al., 1978; Woolf, 1987). Electrical stimulation, by synchronizing the afferent volley, yields suprathreshold responses by temporal summation.

Precipitating events and the retrograde signal

Nerve injury precipitates a range of structural and neurophysiological changes in the spinal cord, one or more of which might be related to the types of functional remodelling implicated in chronic pain. Unfortunately, we only have the vaguest of hints which of these may be causally related, and which are merely coincidental.

Degeneration and atrophic changes
Nerve injury induces a complex of metabolic changes in axotomized sensory cell somata in the dorsal root ganglion, and some axotomized neurons subsequently die. Although the extent of this retrograde cell death is uncertain, some of the higher estimates quoted in the literature suggest that the *bulk* of sensory enurons may degenerate within a few weeks of injury. Obviously, massive cell death would much reduce the significance of abnormal discharge generated in the injured nerve, and would correspondingly emphasize the importance of changes in CNS processing. We have recently re-evaluated the extent of retrograde cell death, using the same population of rats used for the electrophysiological studies just described. Results of these experiments, which were done with special attention paid to the pitfalls inherent in quantitative morphometry, suggest that the significance of retrograde

cell death has heretofore been much overestimated (Devor et al., 1985).

A corollary of massive retrograde cell death is Wallerian degeneration of the synaptic terminals of primary afferents in the spinal cord. However, these synapses could degenerate even if the cell body remained viable. Again, the extent and significance of this effect is in dispute. The main difficulty here is defining criteria for synaptic degeneration. By all accounts, presynaptic terminals of afferents severed in the periphery can undergo a range of changes in their ultrastructural staining properties. Some authors are struck by the similarities between these changes and the ones that occur after dorsal rhizotomy, and therefore regard them as degenerative (e.g. Grant and Arvidsson, 1975; Westrum et al., 1976). Others, however, are struck by the differences, and regard the changes as a unique type of reversible 'atrophy' whose significance in terms of functional synaptic transmission needs to be determined (Sugimoto and Gobel, 1982; Csillik and Knyihar-Csillik, 1986).

The view that the transganglionic changes in primary afferent terminals are degenerative is consistent with the observaion of reactive gliosis (Gilmore and Skinner, 1979) and with the discovery of massive and rapid depletion of several of the neuroactive peptides contained in afferent terminals in the dorsal horn (including substance P (SP), somatostatin (SOM), fluoride-resistant acid phosphatase (FRAP) and cholecystokinin (CCK)). However, at least two others (vasoactive intestinal polypeptide (VIP) and the VIP-related peptide PHI) show substantial *increases*, a result clearly inconsistent with terminal degeneration (Shehab and Atkinson, 1984; McGregor et al., 1984). It is, of course, possible that both degenerative and non-degenerative pro-

---

←

Fig. 2. A. This negative print of a dark-field photomicrograph shows the spinal trajectory of axons labelled by the transganglionic transport of WGA-HRP injected into the posterior cutaneous nerve of the thigh (PCT) on the intact side of an adult rat. The PCT nerve innervates skin of the upper medial thigh. Note that some labelled axons pass through the medial part of the dorsal horn on the way to their somatotopically appropriate terminal field in the lateral dorsal horn (arrows). B. A thin section from the preparation shown in A illustrates a characteristic TMB reaction product crystal in a primary afferent terminal (solid arrow) located in the medial part of the dorsal horn at the position marked by an asterisk in A. An asymmetrical axodendritic contact formed by this synaptic terminal is marked with an open arrow (adapted from Seltzer and Devor, 1984; Devor et al., 1986). Scale bars: A 100 μm, B 1 μm.

cesses unfold simultaneously in different neuronal populations. Unfortunately, neither school has yet provided information on what types, and more important, what proportion of primary afferent terminals degenerate, or alternatively 'atrophy', following nerve section. Perhaps it is a negligible minority.

Because of the special importance of retrograde degeneration to any theory of neuropathic pain, Wall and Devor (1981) and Wall et al. (1981) sidestepped the problem of interpreting anatomical images, and used electrophysiological techniques to measure directly whether or not axons of proximal nerve stumps are capable of driving spinal neurons. During the initial period of ultrastructural degeneration/atrophy and peptide depletion, virtually no loss in synaptic transmission was observed for myelinated or unmyelinated afferent fiber types. Even after extended times, when a decline is expected by all accounts, the decline was not massive. The conclusion drawn was that whatever the significance of the anatomical and histochemical changes for spinal circuitry, axotomy does not cause functional destruction of most afferent synaptic terminals. In retrospect, this is clear from clinical observations. If retrograde cell degeneration, or even just terminal degeneration, were a massive process, there should be no Tinel sign, and palpation of amputation stump neuromas should not be felt.

The one major exception is during development. Nerve section before some critical age *does* result in rapid and irreversible loss of the large majority of axotomized sensory neurons (Yip et al., 1984; Devor et al., 1985). This could account, among other things, for the general absence of phantom limb sensation in early and congenital amputees (Simmel, 1962).

Transynaptic changes

Structural and biochemical changes extend well beyond the affected primary afferent terminal. SP, for example, depleted in the primary afferent neuron, is later partly restored by up-regulation in spinal cord interneurons (e.g. Tessler et al., 1981). Corresponding increases and decreases in various

other substances related to neurotransmission have also been reported (e.g. Sompa et al., 1985). There may even be degenerative changes in postsynaptic dendrites, and an eventual cascade of transsynaptic degeneration through the somatosensory pathway all the way to the cerebral cortex (Campbell, 1905; Johnson et al., 1983; Sugimoto and Gobel, 1984). Once again, however, it is not yet clear in what way these various changes relate to functional remodelling.

The retrograde signal

Assuming that one or more of the central changes mentioned above is indeed related to functional remodelling, an analysis of the precipitating event might suggest which one(s). For example, both the emergence of somatotopically inappropriate receptive fields in rat spinal cord and the collapse of the dorsal root reflex begin quite suddenly four days after sciatic and saphenous nerve injury, and both are induced by nerve transection but not by nerve crush (Devor and Wall, 1981a; Wall and Devor, 1981). These same peculiarities seem to hold for the depletion of dorsal horn SP (e.g. Barbut et al., 1981; McGregor et al., 1984). FRAP depletion, in contrast, is triggered equally by nerve crush and nerve section. This evidence tends to implicate SP, although the relationship could, of course, be purely coincidental.

Another potentially useful approach is consideration of the cellular mechanism responsible for provoking upstream change. One obvious possibility is an alteration in impulse activity. There is evidence, for example, that electrical activity in sympathetic ganglia can act at the level of gene transcription to up-regulate the synthesis of tyrosine hydroxylase and its mRNA, and down-regulate the synthesis of SP and its mRNA (Black et al., 1987). At least for somatotopic remapping, however, chronic afferent blockade by nerve crush and by pharmacological block is not sufficient to trigger the central change (Devor and Wall, 1981a; Wall et al., 1982). Rather, evidence has been slowly accumulating that the trigger event has to do with some trophic substance(s) transported along the nerve in the axoplasmic freight (Devor, 1983; Fitzgerald et al., 1985). But if so, we cannot be dealing with simple transport block, as nerve crush disrupts axoplasmic transport as completely as nerve cut. Here the trail fades. Why does one type of nerve injury reorder central synaptic effectiveness while another does not? Is there something special about the types of injury that are particularly likely to induce neuropathic pain?

Relatively ineffective synapses and neuropathic pain

Enough elements are now in place that the hypothesis of 'strengthening relatively ineffective synapses' is now widely quoted as a reasonable option to account for somatotopic remapping after nerve injury. By extension, this process is ideally suited as a central mechanism of neuropathic pain. How would this work (Fig. 3)?

Imagine a set of spinal neurons which, when activated at an appropriate level, evoke a conscious sensation of pain. These neurons are normally driven by noxious afferent input, although they may well have some low-threshold drive as well. That is, they are either nociceptive specific, or multireceptive neurons. Now imagine that in addition to this effective drive, they have relatively ineffective input from low-threshold afferents innervating skin or other tissue either within or outside their expressed receptive field. Some neuropathic process now attacks the nerves serving our cells, disrupts their normal trophic relations, and strengthens their previously ineffective synaptic input. Absolute sensory thresholds in the affected skin may well be elevated (a notable feature of hyperpathia) due to the destruction of some low-threshold afferents. The low-threshold afferents remaining, however, now drive a central pain circuit which they did not drive pre-

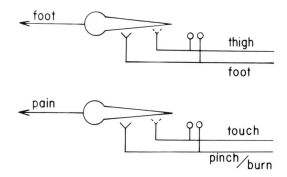

Fig. 3. Upper. A cell, or cell group, whose activity evokes sensation in the foot has 'relatively ineffective' input (dashed) from touch afferents. Strengthening of this input yields anomalous, somatotopically inappropriate receptive fields, and sensations referred from the thigh into the (phantom) foot (e.g. Cronholm, 1951). Lower. By analogy, a model of centrally mediated neuropathic pain is proposed. A cell (or cell group) whose activity evokes a sensation of pain has 'relatively ineffective' input (dashed) from touch afferents. Strengthening of such inputs would yield allodynia.

viously, or they drive it to a higher level of activity. The result: pain in response to normally non-painful stimuli (allodynia), and presumably also increased pain to stimuli which were previously painful (hyperalgesia).

Unfortunately, this scenario remains speculative. A test of the hypothesis will require the discovery of some mode of nerve injury or infection that consistently produces pain attributable to altered central processing. Without doubt, the most promising place to look for such a mode of injury is in the clinic.

Acknowledgements

The support of the United States – Israel Binational Science Foundation, the Israel Academy of Arts and Sciences, and the Leonard Wolinsky Memorial Fund is gratefully acknowledged.

References

Aldskogius, H., Arvidsson, J. and Grant, G. (1985) The reaction of primary sensory neurons to peripheral nerve injury with particular emphasis on transganglionic changes. Brain Res. Rev., 10: 27–46.

Appenzeller, O. and Bicknell, J.M. (1969) Effects of nervous system lesions on phantom experience in amputees. Neurology, 19: 141–146.

Arvidsson, J., Ygge, J. and Grant, G. (1986) Cell loss in lumbar dorsal root ganglia and transganglionic degeneration after sciatic nerve resection in the rat. Brain Res., 373: 15–21.

Barbut, D., Polak, J.M. and Wall, P.D. (1981) Substance P in spinal cord dorsal horn decreases following peripheral nerve injury. Brain Res., 205: 289–298.

Basbaum, A.I. and Wall, P.D. (1976) Chronic changes in the response of cells in adult cat dorsal horn following partial deafferentation: the appearance of responding cells in a previously non-responsive region. Brain Res., 116: 181–204.

Berry, M.S. and Pentreath, V.W. (1976) Criteria for distinguishing between monosynaptic and polysynaptic transmission. Brain Res., 105: 1–20.

Black, I.B., Adler, J.E., Dreyfus, C.F., Friedman, W.F., LaGamma, and E.F., Roach, A.H. (1987) Biochemistry of information storage in the nervous system. Science, 236: 1263–1268.

Blumberg, H. and Janig, W. (1985) Reflex patterns in postganglionic vasoconstrictor neurons following chronic nerve lesions. J. Auton. Nerv. Syst., 14: 157–180.

Bors, E. (1951) Phantom limbs of patients with spinal cord injury. Arch. Neurol. Psychiatry, 66: 610–631.

Brown, A.G. (1981) Organization in the Spinal Cord, Springer-Verlag, Berlin, pp. 130–134.

Brown, A.G., Fyffe, R.E.W., Noble, R. and Rowe, M. (1984) Effect of hindlimb nerve section on lumbosacral dorsal horn neurons in the cat. J. Physiol. (Lond.), 354: 375–394.

Brown, P.B. (1987) A reassessment of evidence for primary afferent sprouting in the dorsal horn. In L. Pubols and B. Sessle (Eds.), Effects of Injury on Spinal and Trigeminal Somatosensory Systems, Liss, New York, pp. 273–280.

Brown, P.B. and Fuchs, J.L. (1975) Somatotopic representation of hindlimb skin in cat dorsal horn. J. Neurophysiol., 38: 1–19.

Campbell, A.W. (1905) Histological Studies on the Localization of Cerebral Function. Cambridge University Press, Cambridge, pp. 47–60.

Cronholm, B. (1951) Phantom limbs in amputees. Acta Psychiat. Neurol. Scand., Suppl. 72: 1–310.

Cline, M. and Ochoa, J. (1986) Chronically sensitized C nociceptors in skin. Patient with hyperalgesia, hyperpathia and spontaneous pain. Soc. Neurosci. Abst. 12: 331.

Cook, A.W. and Druckemiller, W.H. (1952) Phantom limb in paraplegic patients. J. Neurosurg., 9: 508–516.

Csillik, B. and Knyihar-Csillik, E. (1986) The Protean Gate, Akademiai Kiado, Budapest.

Devor, M. (1983) Plasticity of spinal cord somatopy in adult mammals: involvement of relatively ineffective synapses. In B. Haber, J.R. Perez-Polo, G.A. Hashim, and A.-M. Giuffrida-Stella (Eds.), Nervous System Regeneration, Liss, New York, pp. 287–314.

Devor, M. (1988) The pathophysiology and anatomy of damaged nerve. In P.D. Wall and R. Melzack (Eds.), Textbook of Pain, Second edn., London, Churchill-Livingstone, in press.

Devor, M. and Wall, P.D. (1978) Reorganization of spinal cord sensory map after peripheral nerve injury. Nature, 275: 75–76.

Devor, M. and Claman, D. (1980) Mapping and plasticity of acid phosphatase afferents in the rat dorsal horn. Brain Res., 190: 17–28.

Devor, M. and Wall, P.D. (1981a) Plasticity in the spinal cord sensory map following peripheral nerve injury in rats. J. Neurosci., 1: 679–684.

Devor, M. and Wall, P.D. (1981b) The effect of peripheral nerve injury on receptive fields of cells in the cat spinal cord. J. Comp. Neurol., 199: 277–291.

Devor, M. and Wall, P.D. (1986) Spinal plasticity after nerve injury: Mediolateral localization of rewired cells. Exp. Brain Res., Suppl. 13: 142–149.

Devor, M., Merrill, E.G., Wall, P.D. (1977) Dorsal horn cells that respond to stimulation of distant dorsal roots. J. Physiol. (Lond.), 270: 519–531.

Devor, M., Wall, P.D. and McMahon, S.B. (1984) Dichotomizing somatic nerve fibers exist in rats but they are rare. Neurosci. Lett., 49: 187–192.

Devor, M., Govrin-Lippman, R., Frank, I. and Raber, P. (1985) Proliferation of primary sensory neurons in adult rat dorsal root ganglia and the kinetics of retrograde cell loss after sciatic nerve section. Somatosens Res., 3: 139–168.

Devor, M., Basbaum, A.I. and Seltzer, Z. (1986) Spinal somatotopic plasticity: possible anatomical basis for somatotopically inappropriate connections. In M.E. Goldberger, A. Gorio, M. Murray (Eds.), Development and Plasticity in the Mammalian Spinal Cord, Padova, Fidia Research Series Vol. 3, pp. 239–253.

Dostrovsky, J.O., Ball, G.J., Hu, J.W. and Sessle, B.J. (1982) Functional changes associated with partial tooth pulp removal in neurons of the trigeminal spinal tract nucleus, and their clinical implications. In R.G. Hill and B. Mathews (Eds.), Anatomical, Physiological and Pharmacological Aspects of Trigeminal Pain, Elsevier, Amsterdam.

Dostrovsky, J.O., Millar, J. and Wall, P.D. (1976) The immediate shift of afferent drive of dorsal column nucleus cells following deafferentation: a comparison of acute and chronic deafferentation in gracile nucleus and spinal cord. Exp. Neurol., 52: 480–495.

Eccles, J.C. and McIntyre, A.K. (1953) The effects of disuse and of activity on mammalian spinal reflexes. J. Physiol., 121: 492–516.

Egger, M.D., Freeman, N.C.G. and Proshansky, E. (1981) The significance of laminar arrangement. In A.G. Brown and M. Rethelyi (Eds.), Spinal Cord Sensation, Scottish Academic Press, Edinburgh, pp. 137–146.

Fitzgerald, M., Wall, P.D., Goedert, M. and Emson, P.C. (1985) Nerve growth factor counteracts the neurophysiological and neurochemical effects of chronic sciatic nerve section. Brain Res., 332: 131–141.

Gilmore, S.A. and Skinner, R.D. (1979) Intraspinal non-neuronal cellular responses to peripheral nerve injury. Anat. Rec., 194: 369–388.

Grant, G. and Arvidsson, J. (1975) Transganglionic degeneration in trigeminal primary sensory neurons. Brain Res., 95: 265–279.

Goldberger, M.E. and Murray, M. (1974) Restitution of function and collateral sprouting in the cat spinal cord: The deafferented animal. J. Comp. Neurol., 158: 37–54.

Haber, W.B. (1955) Effects of loss of limb on sensory functions. J. Psychol., 40: 115–123.

Haber, W.B. (1956) Observations on phantom-limb phenomena. Arch. Neurol. Psychiat., 75: 624–636.

Henderson, W.R. and Smyth, G.E. (1948) Phantom limbs. J. Neurol. Neurosurg. Psychiat., 11: 88–112.

Horch, K.W. and Lisney, S.J.W. (1981) Changes in primary afferent depolarization of sensory neurones during peripheral nerve regeneration in the cat. J. Physiol., 313: 287–299.

Hylden, J.L.K., Nahin, R.L. and Dubner, R. (1987) Altered responses of nociceptive cat lamina I spinal dorsal horn neurons after chronic sciatic neuroma formation. Brain Res., 411: 341–350.

Johnson, L.R., Westrum, L.E. and Canfield, R.C. (1983) Ultrastructural study of transganglionic degeneration following dental lesions. Exp. Brain Res., 52: 226–234.

Kaas, J.H., Merzenich, M.M., Killackey, H.P. (1983) The organization of somatosensory cortex following peripheral nerve damage in adult and developing mammals. Annu. Rev. Neurosci., 6: 325–356.

Kandel, E.R. and Schwartz, J.H. (1982) Molecular biology of learning: Modulation of transmitter release. Science, 218: 433–443.

Kaczmarek, L.K. and Levitan, I.B. (Eds.) (1987) Neuromodulation: the Biochemical Control of Neuronal Excitability, Oxford University Press, New York.

Li, C.-L. and Elvidge, A.R. (1951) Observations on phantom limb in a paraplegic patient. J. Neurosurg., 8: 524–527.

Lisney, S.J.W. (1983) Changes in the somatotopic organization of the cat lumbar spinal cord following peripheral nerve transection and regeneration. Brain Res., 259: 31–39.

Liu, C.N. and Chambers, W.W. (1958) Intraspinal sprouting of dorsal root axons. Arch. Neurol. Psychiat., 79: 46–61.

Livingston, K.E. (1945) The phantom limb syndrome: a discussion of the role of major peripheral nerve neuromas. J. Neurosurg., 2: 251–255.

Mackenzie, N. (1983) Phantom limb pain during spinal anaesthesia. Anaesthesia, 38: 886–887.

Markus, H., Pomeranz, B., Krushelnycky, D. (1984) Spread of saphenous projection map in spinal cord and hypersensitivity of the foot after chronic sciatic denervation in adult rat. Brain Res., 296: 27–39.

McGregor, G.P., Gibson, S.J., Sabate, I.M., Blank, M.A., Christofides, N.D., Wall, P.D., Polack, J.M. and Bloom, S.R. (1984) Effect of peripheral nerve section and nerve crush on spinal cord neuropeptides in the rat; increased VIP and PHI in the dorsal horn. Neuroscience, 13: 207–216.

Melzack, R. and Wall, P.D. (1965) Pain mechanisms: a new theory. Science, 150: 971–978.

Mendell, L.M., Sassoon, E.M. and Wall, P.D. (1978) Properties of synaptic linkage from long ranging afferents onto dorsal horn neurones in normal and deafferented cats. J. Physiol. (Lond.) 285: 299–310.

Merrill, E.G. and Wall, P.D. (1972) Factors forming the edge of a receptive field. The presence of relatively ineffective afferents. J. Physiol., 226: 825–846.

Merskey, H. (1986) Pain terms: a current list with definitions and notes on usage. Pain, suppl. 3: S215–S221.

Meyers, D.E.R. and Snow, P.J. (1982) Somatotopically inappropriate projections of single hair follicle afferent fibers to the cat spinal cord. J. Physiol. (Lond.), 347: 59–73.

Murray, M., Petry Battisti, M.E. and Goldberger, M.E. (1986) Quantitative electron microscopic correlates of sprouting in the adult cat spinal cord. In M. Goldberger, A. Gorio, M. Murray (Eds.), Development and Plasticity in the Mammalian Spinal Cord, Fidia Research Series, Vol. 3, Livinia Press, Padova, 163–178.

Noordenbos, W. (1959) Pain, Elsevier, Amsterdam.

Nurmikko, T. and Pertovaara, A. (1984) Painful hyperaesthesia following resection of the lateral cutaneous nerve of the thigh. J. Neurol. Neurosurg. Psychiat., 47: 320–321.

Pubols, L.M. (1984) The boundary of proximal hindlimb representation in the dorsal horn following peripheral nerve lesions in cats: a re-evaluation of plasticity in the somatotopic map. Somatosens. Res., 2: 19–32.

Pubols, L.M. and Brenowitz, G.L. (1981) Maintenance of dorsal horn somatotopic organization and increase in high threshold response after single root or spared root deafferentation in cats. J. Neurophysiol., 47: 103–112.

Pubols, L.M., Foglesong, M.E. and Vahle-Hinz, C. (1986) Electrical stimulation reveals relatively ineffective sural nerve projections to dorsal horn neurons in the cat. Brain Res., 371: 109–122.

Rhoades, R.W., Belford, G.R. and Killackey, H.P. (1987) Receptive-field properties of rat ventral posterior medial neurons before and after selective kainic acid lesions of the trigeminal brain stem complex. J. Neurophysiol., 5: 1577–1599.

Riddoch, G. (1941) Phantom limbs and body shape. Brain, 64: 197–222.

Ritz, L.A. and Greenspan, J.D. (1985) Morphological features of lamina V neurons receiving nociceptive input in cat sacrocaudal spinal cord. J. Comp. Neurol., 238: 440–452.

Rodin, B.E., Sampogna, S.L. and Kruger, L. (1983) An examination of intraspinal sprouting in dorsal root axons with the tracer horseradish peroxidase. J. Comp. Neurol., 215: 187–198.

Sedevic, M.J., Ovelmen-Levitt, J., Karp, R. and Mendell, L.M. (1983) Altered modality convergence after acute and chronic partial deafferentation of spinocervical tract cells in the cat spinal cord. J. Neurosci., 3: 1511–1519.

Sedevic, M.J., Capowski, J.J., and Mendell, L.M. (1986) Morphology of HRP-injected spinocervical tract neurons: effect of dorsal rhizotomy. J. Neurosci., 6: 661–672.

Seltzer, Z. and Devor, M. (1984) Effect of nerve section on the spinal distribution of neighboring nerves. Brain Res., 306: 31–37.

Shehab, S.A.S. and Atkinson, M.E. (1984) Vasoactive intestinal peptide increases in areas of the dorsal horn of the spinal cord from which other neuropeptides are depleted following peripheral axotomy. Exp. Brain Res., 62: 422–430.

Simmel, M.L. (1962) Phantom experiences following amputation in childhood. J. Neurol. Neurosurg. Psychiat., 25: 69–78.

Snow, P.J. and Wilson, P. (1985) Plasticity of somatosensory maps in the adult mammalian spinal cord. Soc. Neurosci. Abstr., 11: 965.

Sompa, C., Luttges, M.W. and Fisher, L.J. (1985) Plasticity in neurotransmitter systems of the spinal cord following sciatic nerve crush. Soc. Neurosci. Abstr., 11: 1104.

Sugimoto, T. and Gobel, S. (1982) Primary neurons maintain their axonal arbors in the spinal dorsal horn following peripheral nerve injury: an anatomical analysis using transganglionic transport of horseradish peroxidase. Brain Res., 248: 377–381.

Sugimoto, T. and Gobel, S. (1984) Dendritic changes in the spinal dorsal horn following transection of a peripheral nerve. Brain Res., 321: 199–208.

Tessler, A., Himes, B.T., Artymyshyn, R., Murray, M. and Goldberger, M.E. (1981) Spinal neurons mediate return of substance P following deafferentation of cat spinal cord. Brain Res., 230: 263–281.

Teuber, H.-L., Krieger, H.P. and Bendell, M.B. (1949) Reorganization of sensory function in amputation stumps: Two-point discrimination. Fed. Proc., 8: 156.

Torebjork, H.E., Ochoa, J.L. and Marchettini, P. (1987) Projections of pain from intraneural stimulation in normal subjects and in patients. Pain, Suppl. 4: S19.

Wall, P.D. (1977) The presence of ineffective synapses and circumstances which unmask them. Phil. Trans. R. Soc. London Ser. B., 278: 361–372.

Wall, P.D. (1982) The effect of peripheral nerve lesions and of neonatal capsaicin in the rat on primary afferent depolarization. J. Physiol., 329: 21–35.

Wall, P.D. and Devor, M. (1978) Physiology of sensation after peripheral nerve injury, regeneration and neuroma formation. In S.G. Waxman (Ed.), Physiology and Pathobiology of Axons, Raven Press, New York.

Wall, P.D. and Devor, M. (1981) The effect of peripheral nerve injury on dorsal root potentials and on transmission of afferent signals into the spinal cord. Brain Res., 209: 95–111.

Wall, P.D. and Devor, M. (1983) Sensory afferent impulses originate from dorsal root ganglia as well as from the periphery in normal and nerve injured rats. Pain, 17: 321–339.

Wall, P.D. and Egger, M.D. (1971) Formation of new connections in adult rat brains after partial deafferentation. Nature, 232: 542–545.

Wall, P.D. and Werman, R. (1976) The physiology and anatomy of long-ranging afferent fibers within the spinal cord. J. Physiol. (Lond.) 255: 321–334.

Wall, P.D., Devor, M., Inbal, R., Scadding, J.W., Schonfeld, D., Seltzer, Z. and Tomkiewicz, M.M. (1979) Autotomy following peripheral nerve lesions: Experimental anaesthesia dolorosa. Pain, 7: 103–113.

Wall, P.D., Fitzgerald, M. and Gibson, S.J. (1981) The response of rat spinal cord cells to unmyelinated afferents after peripheral nerve section and after changes in substance P levels. Neuroscience, 6: 2205–2215.

Wall, P.D., Mills, R., Fitzgerald, M. and Gibson, S.J. (1982) Chronic blockade of sciatic nerve transmission by tetrodotoxin does not produce central changes in the spinal cord of the rat. Neurosci. Lett., 30: 315–320.

Westrum, L.E., Canfield, R.C. and Black, R.G. (1976) Transganglionic degeneration in the spinal trigeminal nucleus following removal of tooth pulps in adult cats. Brain Res., 101: 137–140.

Wilson, P. (1987) Absence of mediolateral reorganization of dorsal horn somatotopy after peripheral deafferentation in the cat. Exp. Neurol., 95: 432–447.

Woolf, C.J. (1983) Evidence for a central component of post injury hypersensitivity. Nature, 332: 131–141.

Woolf, C.J. and King, A.E. (1987) Physiology and morphology of multireceptive neurons with C-fiber inputs in the deep dorsal horn of the rat lumbar spinal cord. J. Neurophysiol., 58: 460–479.

Woolf, C.J. and Wall, P.D. (1982) Chronic peripheral nerve section diminishes the primary A-fibre mediated inhibition of rat dorsal horn neurons. Brain Res., 242: 77–85.

Wynn Parry, C.B. (1980) Pain in avulsion lesions of the brachial plexus. Pain, 9: 41–53.

Yip, H.K., Rich, K.M., Lampe, P.A. and Johnson Jr., E.M. (1984) The effect of nerve growth factor and its antiserum on the postnatal development and survival after injury of sensory neurons in rat dorsal root ganglia. J. Neurosci., 12: 2986–2992.

R. Dubner, G.F. Gebhart & M.R. Bond (Eds.)
Proceedings of the Vth World Congress on Pain
© 1988 Elsevier Science Publishers BV (Biomedical Division)

CHAPTER 14

An experimental peripheral neuropathy in rat that produces abnormal pain sensation

Gary J. Bennett and Y.-K. Xie

*Neurobiology and Anesthesiology Branch, National Institute of Dental Research, National Institutes of Health, Bethesda,
MD 20892, USA*

Summary

The common sciatic nerve of adult rats was injured by tying loosely constrictive ligatures around the nerve. Postoperative behavior and pain tests indicated that this nerve injury produces the kinds of pain disorders that are seen in humans with peripheral neuropathies. Hyperalgesia was present to a marked degree for 2–3 months after the injury. The presence of allodynia was evident from the animals' responses to normally innocuous cold and mechanical stimulation. The possibility that spontaneous pain was present was suggested by the appearance of apparently spontaneous nocifensive reflexes and by a suppression of appetite. In addition, the experimental neuropathy produced abnormalities of cutaneous temperature regulation and claw growth. Investigation of this animal model may be of use for understanding the mechanisms that produce neuropathic pain in humans with peripheral nerve damage.

Introduction

We know very little about the neural mechanisms that underlie the distortions of pain perception that occur when peripheral nerves are damaged. Our ignorance has been due in no small part to our inability to reproduce these disorders in laboratory animals. However, we describe here an experimental injury of the rat's sciatic nerve that produces most of the signs of disordered pain perception that are seen in humans with painful peripheral neuropathies. A detailed account of this work is available elsewhere (Bennett and Xie, 1988).

Methods

The common sciatic nerve is exposed at mid-thigh level with sodium pentobarbital as the anesthetic. About 7 mm of nerve is freed of surrounding tissue and four ligatures (4–0 chromic gut) are tied loosely around the nerve with about 1 mm spacing. The desired degree of constriction reduces the diameter of the nerve by a just noticeable amount and retards, but does not occlude, the circulation through the superficial vasculature. The ligatures are left in place and the incision closed. An identical dissection is performed contralaterally but no ligatures are placed.

Results

We were first alerted to the existence of disordered pain perception in these animals when we noted that the animals limped. This was readily apparent by the first or second postoperative day and was pronounced for more than a month. Many of the animals were so reluctant to have the hindpaw touch the floor that they walked with it tucked up next to the flank. The hindpaw was also guarded from contact while the rats stood, sat, or slept (Fig. 1).

Pain thresholds were tested by measuring the latency of the withdrawal reflex evoked by radiant heat applied to the plantar hindpaw (for details see Hargreaves et al., 1988; Bennett and Xie, 1988). We express the results of this test as a difference score, computed by subtracting the withdrawal latency of the hindpaw on the control side from the withdrawal latency of the hindpaw on the nerve-damaged side. Negative difference scores thus indicate a lowered threshold (shorter latency) on the nerve-damaged side. Tests using normal (unoperated) rats showed that the distribution of difference scores averaged about zero, as one would expect, and had a standard deviation of about ±0.7 s. In these normal animals, the average latency of the withdrawal reflex (10.1 ± 1.8 s) occurred at a temperature of approximately 45°C.

The rats were obviously hyperalgesic after the

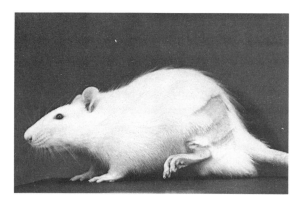

Fig. 1. The rat is standing quietly and holding its hindpaw in the typical guarded position. Note also that the nerve injury results in a deficit in the toe-spreading reflex, that the hindpaw is slightly everted, and that there is a slight degree of foot-drop, i.e., weakness of the hindpaw dorsiflexors (for further discussion see Bennett and Xie, 1988). The photograph was taken on the fifth postoperative day.

nerve injury. This was first apparent on the second postoperative day and persisted for about two months. After 2–3 months, the hyperalgesia was replaced by hypoalgesia, which appears to represent a permanent deficit (Bennett and Xie, 1988). The experiment shown in Figs. 2 and 3 illustrates the time course of the threshold changes produced by the nerve injury. The hyperalgesia was apparent not only from the changes in thresholds but also from the altered magnitude and duration of the withdrawal reflex. The normal response consisted of a brief (2–4 s) withdrawal of small amplitude (about 3 mm off the floor). The postoperative responses were often very much larger and longer. It was not uncommon to see the animal withdraw its hindpaw a centimeter or more above the floor and keep it there for more than 30 s, often while licking it continuously. These changes in the withdrawal reflex were confirmed with EMG recordings from the hamstring flexors (Bennett and Xie, 1988). Nocifensive responses from the control (sham operated) side were invariably normal in this and all the other pain tests.

We must consider whether the abnormal responses are dependent upon afferent volleys in the damaged sciatic afferents or in undamaged saphenous afferents. We examined this question by preparing two groups of rats, both with the usual sciatic injury but one with a complete transection of the ipsilateral saphenous nerve. As shown in Fig. 4, the presence or absence of an intact saphenous innervation had no bearing on the appearance of the hyperalgesic responses to noxious radiant heat (Bennett and Xie, 1988).

Allodynia is defined as the evocation of pain by stimuli that are normally innocuous. There is strong evidence that the nerve injury produces this symptom in the rats. We have already mentioned that the rats guard the affected hindpaw from incidental contact, suggesting that normally trivial mechanical stimulation produced pain. Patients with allodynia often report that innocuous cold stimulation evokes pain. To see whether the rats would respond similarly, we had them stand upon a metal plate that was chilled by an underlying cold water

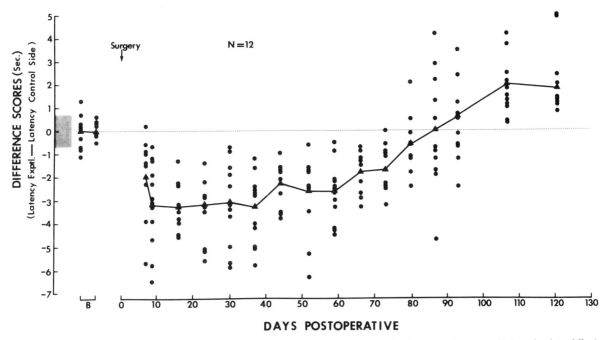

Fig. 2. Time course of hyperalgesia measured by the noxious heat-evoked withdrawal reflex. Negative scores (below the dotted line) indicate a lowered threshold on the side of the nerve damage. Individual scores ($n = 12$) are shown as filled circles and the group's mean score is given by the filled triangles and solid line. 'B' on the abscissa: the results of two preoperative baseline tests; note that these scores cluster around zero (i.e., the thresholds were the same for both hindpaws). The shaded region on the ordinate is equal to ± 0.7 s, which was one standard deviation for the distribution of a large sample ($n = 166$) of difference scores from unoperated rats (the mean of this distribution was 0.04 s). (From Bennett and Xie, 1988.)

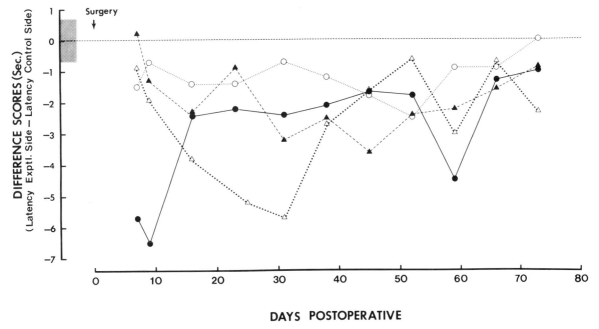

Fig. 3. Difference scores of 4 individual rats (from the experiment shown in Fig. 2) showing the typical variability encountered with sequential testing. (From Bennett and Xie, 1988.)

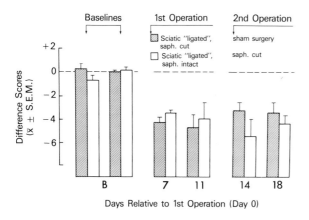

Fig. 4. The contribution of the saphenous innervation to the appearance of hyperalgesic responses to noxious heat. Two groups, each with 6 rats, were prepared. One group (cross-hatched bars) had the usual sciatic injury plus a complete transection of the saphenous nerve at the level of the knee. The other group (open bars) had the same sciatic injury; its saphenous nerve was exposed but not transected. Two postoperative test sessions showed that both groups were hyperalgesic. The rats were operated again immediately after the second test session. The group with the intact saphenous nerve had the nerve transected while the group with the already severed saphenous nerve had a sham surgery. Two postoperative tests again showed that both groups had the expected hyperalgesia. Thus afferent drive from the saphenous nerve is not necessary for the production or maintenance of heat-evoked hyperalgesia. The two preoperative baseline (B) tests were 3 and 8 days before the first surgery. The two groups degree of hyperalgesia does not differ significantly in any of the postoperative test sessions (Mann-Whitney U-test). (From Bennett and Xie, 1988.)

bath. The cold plate was not painful to ourselves (volar forearm skin) and it did not evoke any pain-related responses from control rats. Most of the rats with the neuropathy, however, clearly acted as if the cold evoked pain. The frequency of the cold-evoked hindpaw withdrawals and their cumulative duration were both significantly increased ($P < 0.01$ and $P < 0.05$, respectively) relative to the behavior seen on a thermally neutral surface (Bennett and Xie, 1988).

Spontaneous pain (or dysaesthesia) is a common complaint of people with peripheral neuropathy. It is thus most unfortunate that we have no sure way to establish the existence of this symptom in animals. Two observations, however, suggest that it

may be present. First, we commonly saw a rat that was standing quietly suddenly lift its affected hind-paw, lick it, and hold it in a guarded position. We think it likely that such responses are due to the onset of spontaneous pain but, of course, we cannot exclude the possibility that they are evoked by some undetected stimulus (e.g., the rat slightly shifting its weight towards the affected side). Second, we have shown that rats with the neuropathy gain weight more slowly than age-matched control (sham surgery) rats (Bennett and Xie, 1988). The suppression of biological drives is an expected outcome of chronic pain. It is possible that chronic, spontaneous pain accounts for the observed suppression of appetite.

Although the experimental nerve injury produces unmistakeable signs of disordered pain sensation, we have no reason to believe that the neuropathic condition produces debilitating pain or distress. For example, we saw no wounds or scars, indicating that the increased aggression expected of animals in severe pain was absent. Moreover, the animals groomed themselves normally, had normal levels of general activity, and could be handled without evoking squealing or biting. In addition, the severity of the hyperalgesia seen with the neuropathy was only about one-half that produced by a localized injection of carrageenan (an experimental model of tissue inflammation; Hargreaves et al., 1988).

There are several human neuropathies in which abnormal cutaneous temperature regulation and trophic changes of the skin and nails accompany the disorders of pain perception. The rat model presents two parallels (Bennett and Xie, 1988). The plantar surfaces of the hindpaws of a normal rat had, as expected, about the same temperature. Of 30 normal cases, only 1 had a temperature asymmetry larger than $\pm 1°C$. In contrast, 11 of 30 rats with the neuropathy had asymmetries exceeding $\pm 1°C$ and 4 of these had differences larger than $\pm 2°C$. Both abnormally warm and cold (relative to the control side) hindpaws were observed. The second parallel involved a change in the growth of the claws. About one-half of the cases showed a clearly abnormal thickening and curving elongation of the claws of the affected hindpaw. This was first detectable 1–2 months after the nerve injury.

About 70% of the cases displayed autotomy. It always began with damage to the tips of the claws, proceeded proximally until the root of the claw was bloodied, and usually proceeded no further. There was no relationship between the severity of autotomy and the degree of hyperalgesia or allodynia, and both of these latter symptoms were pronounced in the 30% of the cases that showed no autotomy.

We have not yet completed our examination of the microscopic anatomy of the nerve injury, but the gross anatomy of the nerve has been examined (dissecting microscope) with fixed specimens taken at postoperative intervals of 1–120 days. After 1 day, the nerves invariably have marked constrictions beneath each of the ligatures. We believe that the constrictions are due to intraneural edema opposing the unyielding ligatures so that the nerve self-strangulates (Sunderland, 1976). The constrictions reduce the nerve's diameter by 25–75% and at least partially occlude the nerve's vasculature. Within a few days the constrictions merge such that the nerve has a fairly uniform region of thinning. Backlighting desheathed nerves or examination of osmium-stained fascicles torn from this region show that there is very extensive demyelination. Preliminary electron microscopy (Y. Sahara and G.J. Bennett, unpublished data) shows that the demyelination is associated with very extensive degeneration that affects myelinated fibers to a much greater extent than unmyelinated fibers.

Conclusions

The experimental neuropathy described above produces disorders of pain perception like those seen in human cases. The cutaneous territory of the injured nerve is obviously hyperalgesic when tested with noxious heat. We have also shown that there are hyperalgesic responses to chemically-induced pain. We have not been able to document hyperalgesic responses to noxious mechanical stimulation, but we believe this to be a methodological problem (Bennett and Xie, 1988). The hyperalgesia is constant and lasts for about two months, a significantly long duration in a rat's life-span.

There is very strong evidence that allodynia is also present. The responses to cold are clearly abnormal and almost certainly pain-related. The frequent guarding behavior is analogous to that seen in humans and is reasonably assumed to be due to the evocation of pain by innocuous mechanical stimulation.

The presence of spontaneous pain is difficult to establish in one that does not speak, but the apparently spontaneous pain-related responses and the suppression of appetite are at least consistent with the idea that it is present.

The observed temperature asymmetries are comparable to those seen in the clinic (Shumacker et al., 1948; Tamoush et al., 1983) and the abnormal claw growth certainly calls to mind the overgrown nails of causalgia patients. Other trophic changes seen in human neuropathies (e.g., hair loss, shrinkage of the digital pads, and abnormal sudomotor function) are not seen in the rat model. We have noted elsewhere (Bennett and Xie, 1988) that such discrepancies might be due to species differences. For example, the rat's digital pads are heavily keratinized and adapted for locomotion rather than tactile discrimination.

Disorders of pain perception accompany many different kinds of peripheral neuropathies (Scadding, 1984). It seems improbable that any single experimental model will reproduce all of the neuropathic mechanisms involved in such a varied clinical picture. It seems equally improbable, however, that each of the many kinds of nerve damage might produce disordered pain perception by a unique neuropathic mechanism. Thus we hope that investigations of the neuropathic mechanisms arising from the experimental model that we have described will help us to understand at least some of the causes of human neuropathic pain.

References

Bennett, G.J. and Xie, Y.-K. (1988) A peripheral mononeuropathy in rat that produces disorders of pain sensation like those seen in man. Pain, in press.

Hargreaves, K., Dubner, R., Brown, F., Flores, C. and Joris, J. (1988) A new and sensitive method for measuring thermal nociception in cutaneous hyperalgesia. Pain, 32: 77–88.

Scadding, J.W. (1984) Peripheral neuropathies. In P.D. Wall and R. Melzack (Eds.), Textbook of Pain, Churchill Livingstone, Edinburgh, pp. 413–425.

Shumacker, H.B., Speigel, I.J., Upjohn, R.H. (1948) Causalgia II. The signs and symptoms, with particular reference to vasomotor disturbance, Surg. Gynecol. Obstet., 86: 452–460.

Sunderland, S. (1976) The nerve lesion in the carpal tunnel syndrome. J. Neurol. Neurosurg. Psychiat. 39: 615–626.

Tamoush, A.J., Malley, J. and Jennings, J.R. (1983) Skin conductance, temperature, and blood flow in causalgia. Neurology, 33: 1483–1486.

R. Dubner, G.F. Gebhart & M.R. Bond (Eds.)
Proceedings of the Vth World Congress on Pain
© 1988 Elsevier Science Publishers BV (Biomedical Division)

CHAPTER 15

Painful sequelae of nerve injury

James N. Campbell[1], Srinivasa N. Raja[2] and Richard A. Meyer[3]

[1]*Department of Neurosurgery,* [2]*Department of Anesthesiology and Critical Care Medicine, School of Medicine, Johns Hopkins University, and* [3]*Applied Physics Laboratory and Department of Neurosurgery, Johns Hopkins University, Baltimore, MD 21205, USA*

Some of the most dramatic, as well as challenging pain problems are those that emanate from injury to the peripheral nerve. In recent years, there has been increased interest in basic science and clinical spheres directed at understanding how pain develops from nerve injury. In this chapter, we will discuss the nature and mechanism of this pain, as well as techniques for establishing the different pathophysiological mechanisms. This discussion bears directly on treatment, and examples of this will be demonstrated through case studies.

An important manifestation of nerve-injury pain is hyperalgesia (Lindblom, 1985; Campbell et al., 1988; Frost et al., this volume) which is illustrated by the following case study.

A 40-year-old man had a laceration injury to the superficial peroneal nerve 5 years prior to evaluation. Subsequently the nerve was repaired, but hyperalgesia to mechanical stimuli developed weeks thereafter. Several nerve resection operations followed. Despite temporary relief (typically 6 weeks) with each operation, the pain returned each time. A lumbar sympathectomy led to no relief at all. The region of hyperalgesia was mapped by measuring the area over which pain was evoked by stroking a nylon probe across the skin. The region of hyperalgesia extended well beyond the region innervated by the superficial peroneal nerve, as is evident in Fig. 1. A resonating 256 Hz tuning fork placed on the patella outside the hyperalgesic region evoked pain, as did

small movements of hair follicles in the hyperalgesic region. On the dorsum of the foot, regions of reduced sensation were interspersed with regions of hyperalgesia. The common peroneal nerve was blocked by lidocaine injected just below the fibular head. The hyperalgesia disappeared for the duration of the block, not only in the region innervated by the peroneal nerve, but in the surrounding area also.

The hyperalgesia that follows cutaneous injury has been extensively investigated (Lewis, 1935; Hardy et al., 1952; LaMotte et al., 1982; LaMotte et al., 1983; Meyer and Campbell, 1981; Meyer et al., 1985a; Campbell and Meyer, 1986; Raja et al., 1984). An example of this is shown in Fig. 2, which illustrates the response to heat at the site of injury (primary hyperalgesia) before and after a burn. The leftward shift of the stimulus-response function identifies two essential elements of hyperalgesia: **(1)** a decrease in the threshold and **(2)** an increased pain to suprathreshold stimuli.

The International Association for the Study of Pain Committee on Taxonomy has suggested a new term, allodynia, to refer to the pain that results from low intensity (ordinarily innocuous) stimuli. Hyperalgesia was redefined to refer to the increased pain patients may have with noxious stimuli. With reference to Fig. 2, allodynia would refer to the left part of the upper curve, whereas hyperalgesia would refer to the right part of the upper curve. The purpose of developing a new term in order to distinguish changes in different parts of the stimulus

Correspondence: James N. Campbell, M.D., Department of Neurosurgery, School of Medicine, Johns Hopkins Hospital, Meyer 7-113, 600 N. Wolfe Street, Baltimore, MD 21205, U.S.A.

response function eludes the present authors. In particular the use of the root, 'allo' (meaning other), appears inappropriate since what we observe in patients seems not to be a change in the modality of stimulation that causes pain, but rather simply a leftward shift of the stimulus response function. We suggest that the term, allodynia, be put aside until results of future psychophysical studies provide a compelling rationale for use of such a term.

Foerster (1927) identified a different stimulus-evoked attribute of nerve-injury pain, termed hyperpathia. This is manifest by an increase in threshold for pain, but an increase in the slope of the stimulus-response function. Thus there is an explosive increase in pain as stimuli exceed threshold. Schematic illustrations in Fig. 3A and B contrast the phenomena of hyperalgesia and hyperpathia. Notably these phenomena may both occur in the same patient.

Other aspects of hyperpathic pain are shown in Fig. 3C. The time course for stimulus-induced pain is abnormal, as described by Foerster and later White and Sweet (1969). In contrast to what occurs with hyperalgesia, there is a marked delay between stimulus onset and onset of the pain. The pain is greater than normal, and the duration of pain far outlasts the stimulus duration. In addition to stimulus-induced pain and varying levels of ongoing pain, patients with nerve-injury pain may have sudden spontaneous jolts of pain, as is also shown in Fig. 3C.

Sensory testing was performed in 17 patients with mechanical hyperalgesia, to determine whether A or C fibers signalled the hyperalgesia (Campbell et al., 1988). An ischemic block of large fiber function was produced by a sphygmoma-

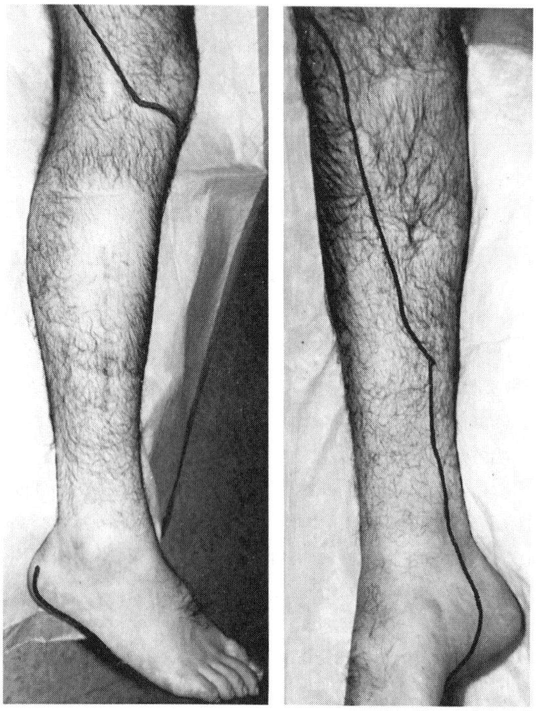

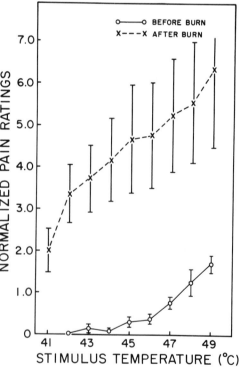

Fig. 1. The area of hyperalgesia in a patient who previously had injury to the superficial peroneal nerve near the lateral malleolus.

Fig. 2. Normalized subjective ratings of the painfulness of heat stimuli before and after a burn (53°C, 30 s) applied to the hand in human subjects. The leftward shift of the stimulus-response function induced by the injury stimulus indicates the presence of hyperalgesia (adapted from Raja et al., 1984).

nometer applied proximal to the site of nerve injury. The hyperalgesia was eliminated in 15 of 17 patients when A-fiber function was blocked, but when C-fiber function was still intact. In two patients tested, a selective block of C and A-delta fiber function with a local anesthetic block was associated with continued hyperalgesia. Finally, in corroboration of earlier studies of Lindblom and Verillo (1979), the latency for detection of pain produced by mechanical stimuli was short and required that the pain was signalled by A fibers. These three lines of evidence indicate that the hyperalgesia to mechanical stimuli following nerve injury is signalled by activity in large-diameter myelinated fibers.

One explanation that could account for this finding is that sensitized A-fiber nociceptors signal the pain. Nociceptors with conduction in the A-fiber range have been described in primates (Perl, 1968). Following a burn to their receptive field, these A-fiber nociceptors develop an enhanced response to heat, though there is no clear change in the response to mechanical stimuli (Campbell et al., 1979; Fitzgerald and Lynn, 1977). A-fiber nociceptors in rat have recently been shown to develop an enhanced response to mechanical stimuli after a mechanical injury (Reeh et al., 1987). Whether this sensitization is sufficient to account for the mechanical hyperalgesia observed in nerve-injury patients is not clear at the present time. Without invoking sensitization, it is unlikely that A-fiber nociceptors could explain hyperalgesia to mechanical stimuli, especially considering that small movements of hair follicles and vibratory stimuli may evoke pain.

Another possible explanation of the mechanical hyperalgesia is that crosstalk occurs between adjacent nerve fibers. Mechanical stimuli might activate low-threshold mechanoreceptors, which in turn crosstalk with nociceptive afferents at the site of nerve injury. Several laboratories have reported evidence that crosstalk between A and C fibers occurs following nerve injury (Seltzer and Devor, 1979; Blumberg and Janig, 1982; Lisney and Pover, 1983; Meyer et al., 1985b). However, it appears unlikely that crosstalk accounts for the hyperalgesia observed. Firstly, substantial crosstalk would likely

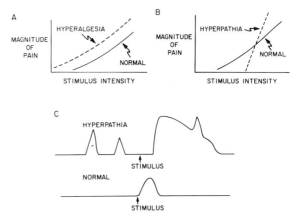

Fig. 3. Characteristics of nerve injury pain. A. Hyperalgesia is characterized by a decrease in pain threshold and increased pain to suprathreshold stimuli. B. Hyperpathia is characterized by an increase in the pain threshold, and an increase in the slope of the stimulus response function. C. Time course of pain in hyperpathic patients.

lead to prominent mislocalization. Yet, patients usually locate the site of painful mechanical stimulation quite precisely. Secondly, the fast latency for detection of pain from mechanical stimuli argues against A to C fiber crosstalk as being responsible for the hyperalgesia. Thirdly, as depicted in Fig. 1, the zone of hyperalgesia may extend outside the zone innervated by the injured nerve. Crosstalk provides no means to account for this.

A likely explanation is that mechanical hyperalgesia results from enhanced synaptic efficacy between low-threshold mechanoreceptors and central pain signalling neurons (CPSN). Collateral input of low threshold mechanoreceptors to CPSNs normally does not activate these neurons. As a result of peripheral nerve injury, central changes occur, such that primary afferents that normally signal touch sensation, now signal pain. Recent work in animal models supports the occurrence of central changes in hyperalgesia (Cook et al., 1987; Woolf, 1983). The implications of this are of considerable importance. It implies firstly that pain sensation does not always result solely from the activation of nociceptive afferents. Secondly, in contradistinction to such concepts as the gate control theory (Noordenbos, 1959; Melzack and Wall, 1965; Gybels et al., 1979;

Bini et al., 1984) large fibers signal pain in these patients, rather than inhibit pain. Thus, for hyperalgesia following nerve injury, the large fibers are the culprit, not the conveyor of pain relief.

Sympathetically maintained pain

An important factor in nerve injury pain is the influence of the sympathetic nervous system (Bonica, 1979; Nathan, 1947, 1983; Janig, 1985). It is useful to consider patients with chronic pain and hyperalgesia in two groups: those with sympathetically maintained pain (SMP, a phrase suggested by Roberts (1986)), and those whose pain is independent of sympathetic activity (SIP). The diagnosis of SMP is made when the pain, and specifically the hyperalgesia, is removed by blockade of the sympathetic efferents.

This criterion was applied to 30 patients who presented with chronic pain and hyperalgesia to mechanical stimuli (Frost et al., this volume). Nine of the patients had SMP, whereas 18 had SIP. Three other patients were considered indeterminate because of either incomplete or conflicting results from sympathetic blockade. Table I provides a breakdown of the relation between SMP, SIP and nerve injury. Of 18 patients with nerve injury, only four had SMP, whereas five of nine patients without nerve injury had SMP. This suggests that the emphasis on sympathetic mechanisms in nerve injury pain, what many might call causalgia, perhaps has been overstated (Schott, 1986). Indeed, many of the patients sent to us with nerve injury pain have

TABLE I

Incidence of nerve injury in patients with SMP and SIP

	Nerve injury	
	Yes	No
Sympathetically maintained pain (SMP)	4	5
Sympathetically independent pain (SIP)	14	4

already had a sympathectomy, in retrospect ill-advisedly. Another noteworthy point, particularly important when considering the mechanisms, is that nerve injury is not a prerequisite for SMP.

Lindblom and co-worker (Lindblom, 1985; Fruhstorfer and Lindblom, 1984) have pointed out that hyperalgesia is often not confined to mechanical stimuli. Patients may have in addition hyperalgesia to heat and/or cooling stimuli. Because many of our own patients had evidence of hyperalgesia to cooling stimuli, we investigated the relationship of this abnormality to the presence or absence of SMP. This work, presented elsewhere in this volume (Frost et al., Ch. 17) indicated that all patients with mechanical hyperalgesia and SMP had increased pain with mild cooling (1.5 to 2°C) of the skin. In contrast, only one third of the SIP patients had hyperalgesia to mild cooling stimuli. The skin can be cooled with several techniques, but the one we have found most convenient is to place gently a drop of acetone or ice water onto the area that is hyperalgesic to mechanical stimuli. A drop of water, warmed to 38°C, can be used as a control stimulus, to verify that the pressure of the droplet does not elicit pain. These data suggest that the demonstration of hyperalgesia to cooling stimuli may represent a simple and sensitive, but not specific test for SMP.

Roberts (1986) recently presented a model to explain the ongoing pain and hyperalgesia to mechanical stimuli which occurs in SMP. He postulated that injury produced enhanced responsiveness of wide-dynamic range (WDR) dorsal horn neurons to low-threshold mechanoreceptor activity. Since activity in sympathetic efferents evokes activity in mechanoreceptors normally (Calof et al., 1980; Loewenstein, 1956; Pierce and Roberts, 1981), this sympathetic activity can now evoke a response in WDR neurons resulting in pain.

Sympathetic efferent activity may also directly activate nociceptors to account for the ongoing pain in SMP. Afferent fibers ending in an experimental neuroma have been shown to develop alpha-adrenergic sensitivity (Wall and Gutnick, 1974; Korenman and Devor, 1981) and a response to sympathetic stimulation (Devor and Janig, 1981).

In addition, drugs that interfere with alpha-adrenergic function in SMP patients also relieve pain. Accordingly, drugs such as guanethidine (Hannington-Kiff, 1984; Hannington-Kiff, 1977), phenoxybenzamine (Ghostine et al., 1984) and prazosin (unpublished observations, Manning and Campbell) may significantly relieve pain in SMP patients. Finally, patients who have been relieved of SMP by surgical sympathectomy may have temporary rekindling of pain by injection of noradrenaline in the affected area (Wiesenfeld-Hallin and Hallin, 1984).

To account for these observations we propose a model somewhat different than that of Roberts. Ongoing nociceptive input leads to central changes such that CPSNs (the WDR cell is one possibility) can now be activated by low threshold mechanoreceptors and other low threshold receptor types. The ongoing nociceptive input might result from nerve injury (ectopic generators), and thus pain and hyperalgesia might be present without any sympathetic mechanism. We postulate that, in certain cases, as a result of soft tissue or nerve injury, alpha-adrenergic receptors become expressed on nociceptors. Thus sympathetic discharge through local release of norepinephrine now activates nociceptors. This in turn 'sensitizes' CPSN cells and they are then capable of being discharged by low threshold mechanoreceptors. Stimuli that evoke pain are well known to also stimulate sympathetic discharge. This increase in sympathetic discharge in turn activates further nociceptor activity through the release of norepinephrine, which in turn activates the alpha-adrenergic receptor which is expressed on the nociceptor. The elements for a vicious cycle are now all in place. Increases in sympathetic tone lead to nociceptor activation, which causes a further increase in sympathetic tone.

Hyperalgesia to cooling stimuli, a prominent feature of SMP as discussed above, might arise via sensitization of CPSN cells such that cold fiber input activates CPSN cells. Alternatively, hyperalgesia to cooling stimuli might be due to a reflex increase in sympathetic tone induced by CNS input of cold fibers. Once again the increase in sympathetic tone leads to activation of nociceptors through local release of norepinephrine and the presence of alpha-adrenergic receptors on the nociceptors.

The model proposed by Roberts does not explain the observation that, during sympathetic blockade, hyperalgesia is absent. Vigorous stimulation of the skin to activate mechanoreceptors does not result in pain when the patient is under the influence of a sympathetic block. In the model proposed here, the nociceptor input in SMP patients is maintained by the sympathetic discharge. The sympathetic block disrupts the vicious cycle by blocking the ongoing nociceptive input which results in desensitization of the CPSN cells and, thus, relief of hyperalgesia.

Diagnostic and therapeutic aspects of SMP

Patients may be improperly labelled as having SMP due to faulty performance or interpretation of sympathetic blocks. Errors in diagnosis of SMP are of two kinds, false positive and false negative. It deserves emphasis that the definitive diagnosis of SMP depends on the results of a selective sympathetic block. Selective blocks are not obtained by epidural blocks, or Bier blocks, as in each case there are other effects of the block which complicate interpretation of the block. Similar issues have been raised regarding the use of guanethidine blocks. To achieve specificity the sympathetic chain must be blocked by injecting a local anesthetic as close to the chain as possible. Only fluoroscopic visualization can assure this. A false negative may of course result from failure to block the sympathetic efferent fibers adequately. Demonstration of increased temperature in the region of interest or other objective signs of sympathetic blockade is useful to verify that a proper block has been done.

The nerve roots run in close proximity to the sympathetic chain, and thus another pitfall is a false positive block, where pain relief is due, not to the sympathetic blocks, but to a block of the somatic fiber for the adjoining nerve root. This is particularly an issue for knee pain because it is easy to block the L3 and L4 nerve roots with a lumbar sympathetic block. Sensory testing to verify that the affected area is not hypoesthetic should be performed. Placebo effects are always a worry, but if the patient has mechanical hyperalgesia and the skin can be rubbed without pain after the block (and there is no somatic block), placebo effects are unlikely.

Another more troublesome pitfall is that patients may have mixed SMP and SIP mechanisms. Thus pain from joint contracture that result from months or years of immobility will not likely improve from a simple sympathetic block.

Sympathetically independent pain

The majority of patients that present to us with nerve injury pain are not relieved of pain with sympathetic blockade. Since the mechanical hyperalgesia appears to be due to central changes, it might be concluded that therapeutic interventions directed to the peripheral neural lesion are destined to failure. Though this may be the situation with some patients, it certainly is not always the case. Invariably a block of the injured peripheral nerve proximal to the site of the lesion will provide temporary relief of pain. An example of this was provided earlier with the discussion of the patient whose area of hyperalgesia is illustrated in Fig. 1. With a block of the peroneal nerve, the hyperalgesia disappeared not only in the region innervated by the peroneal nerve, but also in the surrounding area.

Surgery of the peripheral nerve may be associated with dramatic pain relief, even in recalcitrant cases. Two examples are provided:

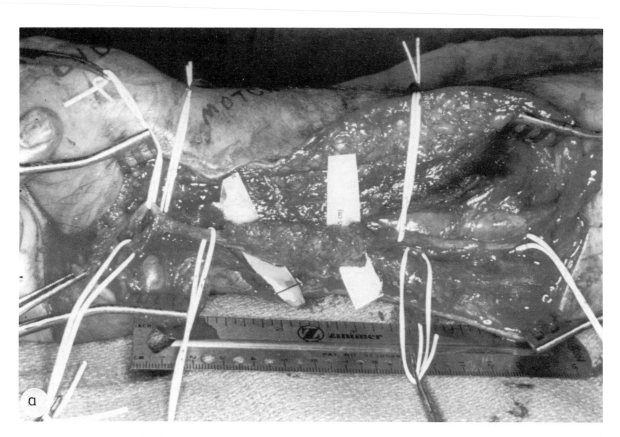

Fig. 4. Operative appearance of the ulnar nerve in a patient who had previously received a nerve graft for treatment of pain related to ulnar nerve injury. a. Before placement of new grafts. b. After placement of new grafts.

Four years prior to our evaluation, a 70-year-old man had a right shoulder manipulation for adhesive capsulitis complicated by shoulder dislocation. Post reduction he developed ulnar distribution pain. He clearly had a major injury to the brachial plexus but much of the weakness resolved to the point that he had intrinsic hand weakness, and ulnar distribution hyperalgesia and hyperpathia. He learned to wear a glove on the hand to help with the pain, which according to him helped because it kept the hand warm. The rumble of the bass notes from a church organ was among the many things that caused a marked increase in pain. Examination revealed that the ulnar nerve near the elbow was particularly tender to touch. A lidocaine block of the ulnar nerve above the elbow substantially relieved the pain. He underwent an intramuscular transposition of the ulnar nerve, and after this his pain was significantly (not completely) relieved. He now wears no glove, and can handle objects with the hand, a task which was impossible before the surgery.

This patient had what many would call a causalgic condition, yet a quite simple operative procedure aimed at relieving tension and compression of the *peripheral* nerve led to satisfactory relief of pain.

A 32-year-old man presented with pain in the lower medial forearm and ulnar side of the hand. Eight years earlier he had a laceration of the ulnar nerve in the lower forearm after an industrial accident. The nerve was repaired primarily, but the repair subsequently pulled apart and pain became a prominent problem. The nerve was subsequently grafted with sural nerve, but the pain persisted. A cervical sympathectomy was performed, which was complicated by injury to the intercosto brachial nerve. After this the hand no longer had sweating, but the pain was unaffected. On examination by us, he had a claw hand and marked tenderness over the trauma site where the ulnar nerve had been repaired. There was loss of touch and motor function in the distribution of the ulnar nerve. The appearance of the nerve at operation is shown in Fig. 4a. Obviously despite previous grafting there was an inadequate repair. The damaged segment of nerve was resected and grafted as shown in Fig. 4b. As of 2 years post-operatively, he continues to have excellent relief

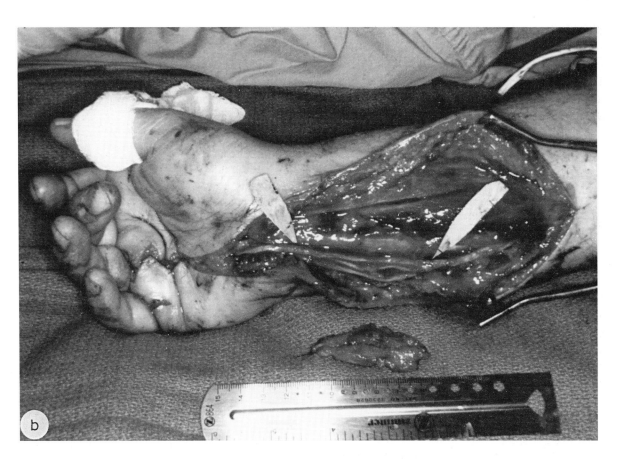

of pain. Though the claw hand deformity continues, he now handles utensils and performs other motor tasks, activities which were not possible prior to surgery.

The point here is that this patient had failed nerve surgery and persistent causalgia-like pain. The lesion in the nerve was still the offending problem, as reflected by the results of repeating the grafting procedure of the nerve.

The therapeutic nihilism that surrounds treatment of painful nerve lesions, sometimes expounded (Noordenbos and Wall, 1981), is to a considerable extent overstated. Another interpretation of failed surgery is that the surgery was inadequate for some reason. Many of the subtleties of certain nerve operations are only recently becoming apparent. For example, Mackinnon and Dellon (1987) noted that proximal resection of the superficial radial nerve frequently failed to relieve pain in patients with neuromas of the superficial radial nerve at the wrist. In cadaver dissections, they noted prominent overlap in the regions innervated by the superficial radial nerve and lateral cutaneous nerves of the forearm. The logical operation is therefore the proximal section of both the superficial radial nerve and lateral cutaneous nerves. When this was done the results of surgery improved substantially.

Conclusions

1. The pain and hyperalgesia following nerve injury is signalled not only by nociceptor input, but also by other receptor types. There exists therefore a central plasticity such that in pathologic circumstances the peripheral nervous system signal that triggers pain is in the domain of multiple receptor types.

2. Correction of the peripheral problem, even with central changes, may relieve the pain and correct the hyperalgesia.

3. The role of sympathetic efferents must be delineated by careful specific sympathetic blocks. If the pain is sympathetically maintained, treatment is best pursued through a series of sympathetic blocks, sympathectomy or medical techniques directed at interrupting the function of the alpha-adrenergic receptor in the tissue.

References

Bini, G., Crucci, G., Hagbarth, K.E., Schady, W. and Torebjork, E. (1984) Analgesic effect of vibration and cooling on pain induced by intraneural electrical stimulation. Pain, 18:239–248.

Blumberg, H. and Janig, W. (1982) Activation of fibers via experimentally produced stump neuromas of skin nerves: ephaptic transmission or retrograde sprouting. Exp. Neurol., 76:468–482.

Bonica, J.J. (1979) Causalgia and other reflex sympathetic dystrophies. In J.J. Bonica, J.C. Liebeskind, D.G. Albe-Fessard (Eds.), Advances in Pain Research and Therapy, Vol. 3, Raven Press, New York, pp. 141–166.

Calof, A.L., Jones, R.B. and Roberts, W.J. (1980) Sympathetic modulation of mechanoreceptor sensitivity in frog skin. J. Physiol., 310:481–499.

Campbell, J.N. and Meyer, R.A. (1986) Primary Afferents and Hyperalgesia. In T.L. Yaksh (Ed.), Spinal Afferent Processing, Plenum, New York, pp. 59–81.

Campbell, J.N., Raja, S.N., Meyer, R.A. and MacKinnon, S.E.

(1988) Myelinated afferents signal the hyperalgesia associated with nerve injury. Pain, 32:89–94.

Campbell, J.N., Meyer, R.A. and LaMotte, R.H. (1979) Sensitization of myelinated nociceptive afferents that innervate monkey hand. J. Neurophysiol., 42:1669–1679.

Cook, A.J., Woolf, C.J., Wall, P.D. and McMahon, S.B. (1987) Dynamic receptive field plasticity in rat spinal cord dorsal horn following C-primary afferent input. Nature, 325:151–153.

Devor, M. and Janig, W. (1981) Activation of myelinated afferents ending in a neuroma by stimulation of the sympathetic supply in the rat. Neurosci. Lett., 24:43–47.

Fitzgerald, M. and Lynn, B. (1977) The sensitization of high threshold mechanoreceptors with myelinated axons by repeated heating. J. Physiol,, 365:549–563.

Foerster, O. (1927) Die Leitungsbahnen des Schmerzgefuehls und die chirurgische Behandlung der Schmerzzustande, Urban and Schwarzenberg, Berlin.

Fruhstorfer, H. and Lindblom, U. (1984) Sensibility abnormalities in neuralgic patients studied by thermal and tactile pulse stimulation. In L.C. von Euler, O. Franzer, U. Lindblom, and

D. Ottoson (Eds.), Somatosensory Mechanisms, MacMillan, London, pp. 353–361.

Ghostine, S.Y., Comair, Y.G., Turner, D.M., Kassell, N.F. and Azar, C.G. (1984) Phenoxybenzamine in the treatment of causalgia. J. Neurosurg., 60:1263–1268.

Gybels, J., Handwerker, H.O. and Van Hees, J. (1979) A comparison between the discharges of human nociceptive nerve fibers and the subjects ratings of his sensations. J. Physiol. (London), 292:193–206.

Hannington-Kiff, J.G. (1977) Relief of Sudeck's atrophy by regional intravenous guanethidine. Lancet, i:1132–1133.

Hannington-Kiff, J.G. (1984) Pharmacologic target blocks in hand surgery and rehabilitation. J. Hand Surg., 9:29–36.

Hardy, J.D., Wolff, H.G. and Goodell, H. (1952) Experimental evidence on the nature of cutaneous hyperalgesia. J. Clin. Invest., 29:115–140.

Janig, W. (1985) Causalgia and reflex sympathetic dystrophy: In which way is the sympathetic nervous system involved? Trends Neurosci., 8:471–477.

Korenman, E.M.D. and Devor, M. (1981) Ectopic adrenergic sensitivity in damaged peripheral nerve axons in the rat. Exp. Neurol., 72:63–81.

LaMotte, R.H., Thalhammer, J.G., Torebjork, H.E. and Robinson, C.J. (1982) Peripheral neural mechanisms of cutaneous hyperalgesia following mild injury by heat. J. Neurosci., 2:765–781.

LaMotte, R.H., Thalhammer, J.G. and Robinson, C.J. (1983) Peripheral neural correlates of magnitude of cutaneous pain and hyperalgesia: a comparison of neural events in monkey with sensory judgements in human. J. Neurophysiol., 50:1–26.

Lewis, T. (1935) Experiments relating to cutaneous hyperalgesia and its spread through somatic fibres. Clin. Sci., 2:373–423.

Lindblom, U. (1985) Assessment of abnormal evoked pain in neurological pain patients and its relationship to spontaneous pain: A descriptive and conceptual model with some analytical results. In H.L. Fields, R. Dubner, and E. Cervero (Eds.) Advances in Pain Research and Therapy, Vol. 9, Raven Press, New York, pp. 409–424.

Lindblom, U. and Verrillo, R.T. (1979) Sensory functions in chronic neuralgia. J. Neurol. Neurosurg. Psychiatry, 42:422–435.

Lisney, S.J.W. and Pover, C.M. (1983) Coupling between fibers involved in sensory neuromata in cats. J. Neurol. Sci., 59:255–264.

Loewenstein, W.R. (1956) Modulation of cutaneous mechanoreceptors by sympathetic stimulation. J. Physiol., 132:40–60.

MacKinnon, S.E. and Dellon, A.L. (1987) Results of treatment of recurrent dorsoradial wrist neuromas. Ann. Plastic. Surg., 19:54–61.

Melzack, R. and Wall, P.D. (1965) Pain mechanisms: a new theory. Science, 150:971–979.

Meyer, R.A. and Campbell, J.N. (1981) Myelinated nociceptive afferents account for the hyperalgesia that follows a burn to the hand. Science, 213:1527–1529.

Meyer, R.A., Campbell, J.N. and Raja, S.N. (1985a) Peripheral neural mechanisms of cutaneous hyperalgesia. In H.L. Fields, R. Dubner and F. Cervero (Eds.) Advances in Pain Research and Therapy, Vol.9, Raven Press, New York, pp. 53–72.

Meyer, R.A., Raja, S.N., Campbell, J.N., MacKinnon, S.E. and Dellon, A.L. (1985b) Neural activity originating from a neuroma in the baboon. Brain Res., 325:255–260.

Nathan, P.W. (1947) On the pathogenesis of causalgia in peripheral nerve injuries. Brain, 70:145–171.

Nathan, P.W. (1983) Pain and the sympathetic system. J. Autonom. Nerv. Syst., 7:363–370.

Noordenbos, W. (1959) Pain. Elsevier, Amsterdam.

Noordenbos, W. and Wall, P.D. (1981) Implications of the failure of nerve resection and graft to cure chronic pain produced by nerve lesions. J. Neurol. Neurosurg. Psychiatry, 44:1068–1073.

Perl, E.R. (1968) Myelinated afferent fibres innervating the primate skin and their response to noxious stimuli. J. Physiol. (London), 197:593–615.

Pierce, J.P. and Roberts, W.J. (1981) Sympathetically induced changes in the responses of guard hair and type II receptors in the cat. J. Physiol., 314:411–428.

Raja, S.N., Campbell, J.N. and Meyer, R.A. (1984) Evidence for different mechanisms of primary and secondary hyperalgesia following heat injury to the glabrous skin. Brain, 107:1179–1188.

Reeh, P.W., Bayer, J., Kocher, L. and Handwerker, H.O. (1987) Sensitization of nociceptive cutaneous nerve fibers from the rat tail by noxious mechanical stimulation. Exp. Brain. Res., 65:505–512.

Roberts, W.J. (1986) A hypothesis on the physiological basis for causalgia and related pains. Pain, 24:297–311.

Schott, G.D. (1986) Mechanisms of causalgia and related clinical conditions. Brain, 109:717–738.

Seltzer, Z. and Devor, M. (1979) Ephaptic transmission in chronically damaged peripheral nerves. Neurology, 29:1061–1064.

Wall, P.D. and Gutnick, M. (1974) Ongoing activity in peripheral nerves: the physiology and pharmacology of impulses originating from a neuroma. Exp. Neurol., 43:580–593.

White, J.C. and Sweet, W.H. (1969) Pain and the Neurosurgeon: A forty year experience. Charles C. Thomas, Springfield, IL.

Wiesenfeld-Hallin, Z. and Hallin, R.G. (1984) The influence of the sympathetic system on mechanoreception and nociception. A review. Hum. Neurobiol., 3:41–46.

Woolf, C.J. (1983) Evidence for a central component of post-injury pain hypersensitivity. Nature, 306:686–688.

R. Dubner, G.F. Gebhart & M.R. Bond (Eds.)
Proceedings of the Vth World Congress on Pain
© 1988 Elsevier Science Publishers BV (Biomedical Division)

CHAPTER 16

Thoracic outlet syndrome: diagnostic value of sensibility testing, vibratory thresholds and somatosensory evoked potentials at rest and during perturbation with abduction and external rotation of the arm

Kristian Borg[1], Hans E. Persson[2] and Ulf Lindblom[1]

Departments of [1]Neurology and [2]Clinical Neurophysiology, Karolinska Hospital, S-104 01 Stockholm, Sweden

Summary

Patients with Thoracic Outlet Syndrome (TOS) were subjected to a detailed sensibility testing ($n = 18$), determinations of vibratory thresholds (VT), ($n = 18$) and somatosensory evoked potentials (SEP) ($n = 10$). The aim was to evaluate the diagnostic sensitivity of these procedures. VT and SEP were also recorded during perturbation with abduction and external rotation of the arm (AER) in an attempt to increase the diagnostic information.

Nine of the 18 TOS patients had abnormalities on sensibility testing. Eight patients had elevated VT on the finger pads of digit 3 and/or digit 5, 4 at rest and another 4 during AER. Five patients had reduced SEP over brachial plexus (N9 component), 4 at rest and another during AER. A significant average reduction of the N9 amplitude and a slight but significant average VT increase were also obtained in the controls during AER. The N9 amplitude reduction could be explained by the change in electrode position. The VT increase is discussed

and ischemia of the brachial plexus is suggested as the most probable cause.

It is concluded that sensibility testing, VT and SEP are almost equally sensitive as diagnostic tests for TOS. Sensibility testing is the first choice of the methods, since it is easy to perform and can be carried out as a routine along with the clinical examination. VT determination, at rest or during AER, adds diagnostic information in some patients. SEP may be abnormal in the resting position in cases with impaired sensibility, and may locate the level of the nerve lesion, but is technically difficult during AER.

Introduction

The diagnosis of Thoracic Outlet Syndrome (TOS) is difficult. Since the neurological symptoms dominate, neurophysiological techniques have been widely applied. Motor and sensory conduction velocities, sensory nerve action potentials in distal parts of the nerve as well as over the thoracic outlet, and F-wave latencies have been studied (Cherington, 1976; Daube, 1975; Dorfman, 1979; Eisen et al., 1977; Gilliat et al., 1978; Shahani et al., 1980;

Correspondence: Kristian Borg, MD, Department of Neurology, Karolinska Hospital, S-104 01 Stockholm, Sweden.

Urschel and Razzuk, 1972; Urschel et al., 1968, 1971; Wilbourn and Lederman, 1984; Wulff and Gilliatt, 1979), but all methods have shown limited diagnostic value.

In recent years, there has been increasing interest in somatosensory evoked potentials (SEP). Glover et al. (1981) and Jerrett et al. (1984) reported abnormal SEP in more than 2/3 of the TOS patients examined. However, these observations could not be verified in other studies (Moralez-Blanquez and Delwaide, 1982; Newmark et al., 1985). Abnormal SEP have been demonstrated only in patients with objective signs of neurological impairment (Yianik-kas and Walsh, 1983) and in patients with associated cervical ribs (Inouye and Buchtal, 1977) or muscle atrophy (Siivola et al., 1979).

Sensory testing with perception thresholds for warmth and cold has been evaluated and differences have been described between the symptomatic and nonsymptomatic side (Ryding et al., 1985). No study has reported vibratory threshold (VT) determinations in TOS patients.

In order to increase diagnostic sensitivity, neurophysiological techniques have been applied with the arm abducted and externally rotated in order to stress the nerve structures in the thoracic outlet. Chodoroff et al. (1985) found abnormal SEP and Glassenberg (1981) found reduced conduction velocity across the brachial plexus. On the other hand, Shahani et al. (1980) did not record any alterations in proximal nerve conduction during hyperabduction of the arm.

The aim of the present study was to evaluate the diagnostic properties of sensibility testing, VT and SEP at rest in TOS patients and to determine whether VT and SEP during perturbation with abduction and external rotation of the arm (AER) might add diagnostic information.

Patients and methods

Sensibility testing and VT determinations were performed in 18 patients (13 women, 5 men, median age 38 years, range 21–58 years) who were referred with tentative diagnosis of TOS. SEP was examined in 10 of these patients (Nos. 8–13, 15–18). For a detailed description of the patient group see Table I. All patients had pain in the shoulder region radiating down in the C8 dermatome and a positive 'elevated arm stress test' according to Roos (1976). The symptoms (median duration 2.5 years, range 7 months – 22 years) were aggravated by elevation of the arm. Routine neurological, neurophysiological and radiographical examinations were carried out before referral (Table I). Eighteen age-matched healthy volunteers (median age 37 years, range 21–58 years) were examined as controls.

Sensibility testing
The sensibility testing was carried out with cotton wool, pin-prick and warm and cold rollers according to Lindblom and Tegnér (1987).

Vibratory thresholds (VT)
A 100 Hz sine-wave vibration was produced by an electromagnetic vibrator according to Goldberg and Lindblom (1979). The vertical movement of the 13-mm-diameter probe was continuously recorded by means of an accelerometer and digitally displayed in micrometers. VT was defined as the average of (a) the perception appearance threshold, i.e., the amplitude at which vibration was first percieved when the stimulus was gradually increased from zero, and (b) the perception disappearance threshold, i.e., the amplitude at which the sensation disappeared on subsequent stimulus reduction. VT was determined on the finger pads of the little finger (digit 5, ulnar nerve region) and the middle finger (digit 3, median nerve region) in resting position and during perturbation produced by placing the arm in the abduction external rotation position (AER).

Somatosensory evoked potentials (SEP)
Stimulation of the ulnar or median nerves at the wrist was carried out with square-wave constant-current pulses (duration 0.3 ms, frequency 3 Hz) in resting position and with the arm in AER position. 512 or 1024 responses were averaged during 50 ms

TABLE I

Age, sex, symptom duration and results from the neurological, radiographical and neurophysiological examinations and findings on sensibility testing and VT determination at rest and during AER in the 18 TOS patients. + is an abnormal and − a normal finding. Ulnar nerve is abbreviated ULN, median nerve MED, sensory nerve conduction velocity SNCV, sensory nerve action potential SNAP and electromyography EMG.

Patient No.	Age (yr)	Sex	Symptom duration (months)	Neurological examination				Radiographical examination: cervical spondylosis	Neurophysiological examination				Sensibility on screening		Vibratory thresholds			
				Paresis		Atrophy			SNCV/SNAP		EMG				At rest		With AER	
				ULN	MED	ULN	MED		ULN	MED	ULN	MED	ULN	MED	ULN	MED	ULN	MED
1	34	m	9	−	−	−	−	Triangular shape C 6	−	−	−	−	−	−	−	−	−	−
2	34	m	12	−	−	−	−	−	−	−	−	−	−	−	−	−	−	−
3	42	m	70	−	−	−	−	+	−	−	−	−	−	−	−	−	−	−
4	41	f	24	−	−	−	−	+	−	−	−	−	−	−	−	−	−	−
5	49	f	8	+	−	−	−	−	−	−	−	−	−	−	−	−	−	+
6	25	f	24	−	+	−	−	+	−	−	−	−	+	−	−	+	+	−
7	39	f	60	−	−	−	−	−	−	−	−	−	+	−	−	−	+	+
8	26	f	48	−	−	−	−	−	−	−	+	−	+	+	−	−	−	−
9	35	f	264	−	−	−	−	−	−	−	−	+	+	+	+	+	+	−
10	52	m	36	+	−	+	−	−	+	−	+	+	+	+	+	+	+	+
11	38	m	14	+	−	+	−	+	+	−	+	+	+	−	−	−	−	−
12	41	f	36	+	−	−	−	+	−	−	−	+	+	−	−	−	−	+
13	40	f	60	+	+	−	−	+	−	−	+	+	+	−	−	−	−	−
14	21	f	12	−	−	−	−	Prolonged transverse process C7	−	−	−	+	+	−	−	−	−	−
15	31	f	72	−	−	−	−	Cervical rib	−	−	−	−	−	−	−	−	+	−
16	58	f	84	−	−	−	−	−	−	−	+	+	−	−	+	+	−	+
17	31	f	9	−	−	−	−	−	−	−	−	+	−	−	−	+	−	−
18	37	f	36	−	−	−	−	Fusion C₂ – C₃	−	−	+	−	+	−	+	+	−	−

following stimulation and recorded with silver/ silver cup electrodes attached to the skin of the ipsilateral supraclavicular fossa, over the 7th cervical spinous process and the 2nd cervical vertebrae at the dorsum of the neck, and on the scalp over the hand area of the contralateral somatosensory cortex (7 cm lateral and 2 cm posterior to the vertex). Peak latencies and peak-to-peak amplitudes of the N9 (supraclav), N13 (C7 or C2) and N20 (contralateral scalp) components were determined as well as plexus conduction time (PCT, N13–N9) and central conduction time (CCT, N20–N13). The latencies and the amplitudes were measured with the cursor system on the recording unit (Medelec 8 channel Sensor) and allowed measurements in steps of 0.1 ms and 0.2 μV.

The VT and SEP values obtained during AER were divided into 4 time classes (0–4 min, 5–9 min, 10–14 min and more than 15 min) and mean values were calculated for the whole AER period. The mean values for the four intervals did not indicate any trend or differences and are therefore not presented in the results. VT and SEP values were considered abnormal if they deviated by more than $\pm$ 2 SD from the mean values in the control group. Differences of VT and SEP values between AER and at rest, as well as between digits 5 and 3, were evaluated by means of the Wilcoxon matched-pairs signed-rank test. VT and SEP differences between patients and controls were analysed by means of the Mann-Whitney U-test. $P < 0.05$ was considered significant.

Results

Sensibility testing

Table I displays the patient data and distribution of abnormal findings (+). Nine patients (50%) had impaired sensibility on screening. Three of the patients (Nos. 7, 11, 13) were abnormal for all tested modalities in the ulnar nerve region and one patient (No. 10) in both ulnar and median nerve distributions. Two patients (Nos. 12, 18) had impairment for touch and pin-prick and one (No. 14) only for

temperature in the ulnar nerve region. Patient No. 8 had hyperesthesia for pin-prick in the ulnar nerve region and patient No. 9 had impairment for pin-prick in the median nerve region.

Among the 9 patients with sensibility impairment there were 7 who also exhibited other abnormalities (paresis, atrophy and/or positive neurophysiological examination and/or radiographical findings; see Table I). Among the 9 patients with normal sensibility (– in Table I) there were also 7 patients who had other abnormalities.

Vibratory thresholds

Eight of the 18 TOS patients (44%) exhibited abnormal VT, 4 at rest and another 4 during AER (Table I). The VT increase was located in digit 3 in 2 patients, in digit 5 in 2 and in both digits 3 and 5 in the other 4 patients. For unknown reasons one patient (No. 18) had abnormal VT at rest but normal VT during AER.

When the mean VT value during AER was compared with the value at rest (Table II), it was about

TABLE II

Numerical mean VT values (μm) in the little (digit 5) and the middle finger (digit 3) and mean SEP N9 latencies (lat, ms) and amplitudes (ampl, μV) on ulnar (ULN) and median (MED) nerve electrical stimulations in the TOS patients and normal controls at rest and during AER (SD within brackets).

			TOS		CONTROL	
VT		REST	AER		REST	AER
	Dig 5	1.1	2.2		0.5	0.6
		(2.4)	(5.7)		(0.3)	(0.4)
	Dig 3	1.3	2.2		0.5	0.7
		(2.7)	(4.8)		(0.3)	(0.5)
SEP	(N9)					
ULN	lat	10.7	10.9		11.1	11.4
		(1.2)	(1.0)		(1.2)	(1.3)
	ampl	4.4	2.8		4.8	3.3
		(2.9)	(2.5)		(1.3)	(1.3)
MED	lat	9.9	10.2		10.2	10.2
		(0.9)	(0.7)		(1.2)	(1.0)
	ampl	9.3	5.7		10.1	7.5
		(3.4)	(2.2)		(2.0)	(2.4)

doubled in the TOS patients and the change was statistically significant ($P < 0.0025$ in digit 5 and $P < 0.005$ in digit 3). A smaller (0.1–0.2 μm) but statistically significant VT increase ($P < 0.025$ in digit 5 and $P < 0.005$ in digit 3) was found in the controls. VT differences were obtained between the patients and the controls but were not statistically significant due to a great variation in the patient group.

Only 4 of the 8 TOS patients (Nos. 7, 10, 12, 18) with VT abnormalities had impairment on sensibility testing and 5 of the 10 patients (Nos. 8, 9, 11, 13, 14) with normal VT had sensibility impairment.

Somatosensory evoked potentials

Five of the 10 patients examined (50%) had abnormal SEP, 4 at rest and another during AER. Three of the patients exhibited abnormalities on both ulnar and median nerve stimulation and 2 patients on ulnar nerve stimulation only. All 5 had a reduced N9 amplitude and one had a reduced N13 amplitude as well.

During AER, a statistically significant mean N9 amplitude reduction was observed in the ulnar and median nerves in both TOS patients and controls (Table II). There were no significant differences between patients and controls at rest or during AER for the SEP components.

All 5 patients with abnormal SEP had impairment on sensibility testing, 2 (Nos. 10, 12) had VT abnormalities and 4 (Nos. 8, 10, 11, 13) had other neurophysiological (EMG, SNCV, SNAP) abnormalities.

Two (Nos. 9, 18) of the 5 patients with normal SEP had impairment on sensibility testing, 3 (Nos. 15, 16, 18) had VT abnormalities and 3 (Nos. 16, 17, 18) had positive findings in the other neurophysiological parameters.

In control experiments in two healthy subjects, the position of the recording electrode relative to the brachial plexus was checked radiographically at rest and during AER. Placing the arm in the AER position produced a significant change in the position of the recording electrode. With the arm in the resting position the electrode was moved approxi-

mately the same distance on the skin and another SEP recording was made. A significant N9 amplitude reduction was observed, which was of the same order as that during AER.

Discussion

Sensibility testing, VT, SEP and conventional electrophysiological examination were abnormal in half of the TOS patients examined and thus about equally sensitive. We cannot make a comparison with Ryding et al.'s finding (1985) of 27% (in 10 of 37 patients) with decreased temperature perception, since this test was not included in our study. The percentage difference may simply be due to patient selection.

The result that SEP was abnormal only in patients with objective signs on clinical examination corroborates the findings by Yiannikas and Walsh (1983), and the rate of abnormality (4 of 10 patients) is in accord with the studies of Moralez-Blanquez and Delwaide (1982) and Newmark et al. (1985). A higher incidence of SEP abnormality was reported by Glover et al. (1981) (13 of 19 patients) and Jerrett et al. (1984) (17 of 18 patients). These percentage differences may also be explained on the basis of patient selection. The symptoms of the patients in this study and in those of Moralez-Blanquez and Delwaide (1982) and Newmark et al. (1985) were relatively mild. It is conceivable, although not evident from the descriptions, that the patients of Glover et al. (1981) and Jerrett et al. (1984) were more advanced cases.

SEP recording with the arm in the AER position was performed by Chodoroff et al. (1985). SEP became abnormal during AER in 6 of 14 patients. In our study this occurred only in one additional patient. This discrepancy may be explained by differences in technique and interpretation. One has to consider that SEP can be reduced in amplitude in the AER position also in normals, as was demonstrated in our control experiment. The change in position of the arm during AER is obviously of great importance. Suboptimal stimulation and recording during a long period of AER may produce false-positive SEP findings.

Statistically, VT increased not only in the patients but also in the controls. It has been suggested that transitory nerve dysfunction during compression in carpal tunnel syndrome is due to ischemia (Borg and Lindblom, 1986; Marin et al., 1983; Ochoa and Nordenboos, 1979) rather than direct neuronal compression. It is conceivable that the same explanation applies to the VT changes during AER in our TOS patients, as well as the small increase in the controls. It is in keeping with such a pathophysiological mechanism that the dominating symptoms of TOS, pain and paresthesiae, are of a positive nature. It has been reported that transitory ischemia produces ectopic nerve impulses and paraesthesia (Ochoa and Torebjörk, 1980). An abnormal impulse discharge was indeed demonstrated in a TOS patient by Nordin et al. (1984) in a microneurographic study. The discharge was recorded concomantly with the occurrence of paraesthesia during elevation of the arm. The dominance of positive symptoms in TOS is compatible with the relatively low frequency of pathology found by SEP and by routine neurophysiological examinations, which only record loss of function.

Acknowledgements

This study was supported by grants from the Folksam Research Foundation, the Vivian L. Smith Foundation for Restorative Neurology and the Karolinska Institute. We are indebted to Mrs. Berit Lindblom for excellent technical assistance.

References

Borg, K. and Lindblom, U. (1986) Increase of vibration threshold during wrist flexion in patients with carpal tunnel syndrome. Pain, 26: 211–219.

Cherington, M. (1976) Ulnar conduction velocity in thoracic outlet syndrome. N. Engl. J. Med., 294: 1185.

Chodoroff, G., Lee, D.W. and Honet, J.C. (1985) Dynamic approach in the diagnosis of thoracic outlet syndrome using somatosensory evoked responses. Arch. Phys. Med. Rehab., 66: 3–6.

Daube, J.R. (1975) Nerve conduction studies in the thoracic outlet syndrome. Neurology, 25: 374.

Dorfman, L.J. (1979) F-wave latency in the cervical-rib-and-band syndrome. Muscle Nerve, 2: 158–159.

Eisen, A., Schomer, D. and Melmed, C. (1977) The application of F-wave measurements in the differentiation of proximal and distal upper limb entrapments. Neurology, 27: 662–668.

Gilliat, R.W., Willison, R.G., Dietz, V. and Williams, J.R. (1978) Peripheral nerve conduction in patients with a cervical rib and band. Ann. Neurol., 4: 124–129.

Glassenberg, M. (1981) The thoracic outlet syndrome: An assessment of 20 cases with regard to new clinical and electromyographic findings. Angiology, 32: 180–186.

Glover, J.L., Worth R.M., Bendick, P.J., Hall, P.V. and Markand, O.M. (1981) Evoked responses in the diagnosis of thoracic outlet syndrome. Surgery, 89: 86–93.

Goldberg, J.M. and Lindblom, U. (1979) Standardized method of determining vibratory perception thresholds for diagnosis and screening in neurological investigation. J. Neurol. Neurosurg. Psych., 42: 793–803.

Inouye, Y. and Buchtal, F. (1977) Segmental sensory innervation determined by potentials recorded from cervical spinal nerves. Brain, 100: 731–748.

Jerrett, S.A., Cuzzone, L.J. and Pasternak, B.M. (1984) Thoracic outlet syndrome, electrophysiological reappraisal. Arch. Neurol., 41: 960–963.

Lindblom, U. and Tegnér, R. (1988) Quantification of sensibility in mononeuropathy, polyneuropathy and central lesions. In: T. Munsat (Ed.) Quantification of Neurological deficit, in press.

Marin, E.L., Vernick, S. and Friedmann, L.W. (1983) Carpal tunnel syndrome: Median nerve stress test. Arch. Phys. Med. Rehab., 64: 206–208.

Moralez-Blanquez,G. and Delwaide, P.J. (1982) The thoracic outlet syndrome: an electrophysiological study. Electromyogr. Clin. Neurophysiol., 22: 255–263.

Newmark, J., Levy, S.R. and Hochberg, F.H. (1985) Somatosensory evoked potentials in thoracic outlet syndrome. Arch. Neurol., 42: 1036.

Nordin, M., Nyström, B., Wallin, U. and Hagbarth, K.E. (1984) Ectopic sensory discharges and paraesthesiae in patients with disorders of peripheral nerves, dorsal roots and dorsal columns. Pain, 20: 231–245.

Ochoa, J. and Nordenboos, W. (1979) Pathology and disordered sensation in local nerve lesions: An attempt at correlation. In J J Bonica et al. (Eds.), Advances in Pain Research and Therapy, Vol. 3, pp. 67–90. Raven Press, New York.

Ochoa, J. and Torebjörk, H.E. (1980) Paraesthesiae from ectopic impulse generation in human sensory nerves. Brain, 103: 835–853.

Roos, D.B. (1976) Congenital anomalies associated with thoracic outlet syndrome: Anatomy, symptoms, diagnosis and treatment. Am. J. Surg., 132: 771–778.

Ryding, E., Ribbe, E., Rosén, I. and Norgren, L. (1985) A neurophysiologic investigation of thoracic outlet syndrome. Acta Chir. Scand., 151: 327–331.

Shahani, B.T., Potts, F., Juguilon, A. and Young, R.R. (1980) Electrophysiological studies in 'thoracic outlet syndrome'. Muscle Nerve, 3: 182–183.

Siivola, I., Myllylä, V.V., Sulg, I. and Hokkanen, E. (1979) Brachial plexus and radicular neurography in relation to cortical evoked reponses. J. Neurol. Neurosurg. Psych., 42: 1151–1158.

Urschel, H.C., Paulson, D.L. and McNamara, J.J. (1968) Thoracic outlet syndrome. Ann. Thoracic Surg., 6: 1–10.

Urschel, H.C. and Razzuk, M.A. (1972) Management of the thoracic outlet syndrome. N. Engl. J. Med., 286: 1140–1143.

Urschel, H.C., Razzuk, M.A., Wood, R.E., Parekh, M. and Paulson, D.L. (1971) Objective diagnosis (ulnar nerve conduction velocity) and current therapy of the thoracic outlet syndrome. Ann. Thoracic Surg., 12: 608–620.

Wilbourn, A.J. and Lederman, R.J. (1984) Evidence for conduction delay in thoracic outlet syndrome is challenged. N. Engl. J. Med., 310: 1052–1053.

Wulff, C.H. and Gilliatt, R.W. (1979) F-waves in patients with hand wasting caused by a cervical rib and band. Muscle Nerve, 2: 452–457.

Yianikkas, C. and Walsh, J.C. (1983) Somatosensory evoked responses in the diagnosis of thoracic outlet syndrome. J. Neurol. Neurosurg. Psych., 46: 234–240.

R. Dubner, G.F. Gebhart & M.R. Bond (Eds.)
Proceedings of the Vth World Congress on Pain
© 1988 Elsevier Science Publishers BV (Biomedical Division)

CHAPTER 17

Does hyperalgesia to cooling stimuli characterize patients with sympathetically maintained pain (reflex sympathetic dystrophy)?

Sheila A. Frost[1], Srinivasa N. Raja[2], James N. Campbell[1], Richard A. Meyer[1,3] and Adil A. Khan[1]

[1]*Department of Neurosurgery, Johns Hopkins University,* [2]*Department of Anesthesiology and Critical Care Medicine, Johns Hopkins University, and* [3]*Applied Physics Laboratory, Johns Hopkins University, Baltimore, MD, USA*

Introduction

Trauma, with or without associated nerve injury, is sometimes complicated by the development of chronic pain (Livingston, 1943; Nathan, 1947; Bonica, 1979). In certain cases, the ongoing pain is accompanied by cutaneous hyperalgesia to mechanical stimuli. This altered state of cutaneous sensibility is characterized by a decrease in pain threshold and an increase in pain from suprathreshold stimuli. In some of these patients, the pain may be relieved by sympathetic blockade, in which case they are said to have sympathetically maintained pain (SMP) (Wallin et al., 1976; Nathan, 1983; Janig, 1985; Roberts, 1986). In other patients, however, their pain is clearly independent of the sympathetic nervous system, as evidenced by lack of signs of increased sympathetic tone or lack of relief by sympathetic blockade (Nathan, 1983; Schott, 1986). These patients are designated as having sympathetically independent pain (SIP).

Correspondence: Srinivasa N. Raja, M.D., Department of Anesthesiology and Critical Care Medicine, Meyer 8-134, Johns Hopkins Hospital, 600 N. Wolfe Street, Baltimore, MD 21205, U.S.A.

The aim of the present investigation was to characterize the sensations elicited by mechanical, vibratory and cooling stimuli in patients with cutaneous hyperalgesia. We sought to determine whether sensory testing could be used to distinguish between SMP and SIP, because sympathetic blockade can be therapeutic for SMP patients but has no beneficial effects for SIP patients. We demonstrate that a simple test can be performed during a routine neurological examination which may indicate the presence of a sympathetically maintained component of the pain.

Methods

Thirty patients who presented with chronic pain and cutaneous hyperalgesia to mechanical stimuli were tested with mechanical and cooling stimuli to characterize their sensory abnormalities. These patients were divided into two groups (SMP or SIP) based on whether their pain was dependent upon sympathetic activity in the involved area. Patients classified as SMP ($n=9$) had at least 1°C cooler skin in the painful area compared to the corresponding contralateral body part (Hendler et al., 1982), and obtained complete or nearly complete pain relief following sympathetic blockade. Patients with SIP ($n = 18$) either had no pain relief following sympathetic blockade, or had no clinical signs of increased sympathetic tone and their pain was eliminated by peripheral nerve surgeries. There were three other patients who could not be classified because of equivocal results of sympathetic blockade, and will not be discussed in this paper.

Patients were asked to keep their eyes closed so that they were blinded during the testing procedure. The zone of hyperalgesia was mapped by dragging a nylon probe across the skin until the patient reported that it was painful. Sensory testing was done in this hyperalgesic area, and at homologous sites on the contralateral normal side.

Detection (touch) and pain thresholds to mechanical stimuli were determined on both the normal and affected sides using von Frey probes. The detection threshold was considered to be that pressure which the patient reliably detected in the area being tested. The pain threshold was that which the patient felt confidently to be painful in the area being tested. Vibrating tuning forks (128 and 256 Hz) were applied outside the zone of hyperalgesia, usually at the closest bony prominence. A single hair follicle within the zone of hyperalgesia was moved with forceps, without touching the skin.

The presence of hyperalgesia to cold was tested by applying a drop of acetone to both the affected side and the contralateral normal side. In normal subjects, the acetone drop produced a temperature decrease of 1–2°C, and was perceived as cooling, never as painful. In addition, a drop of ice water and/or alcohol was applied in most of the patients tested. Because a drop of fluid also presents a mechanical stimulus, which could cause pain by itself, a drop of 38°C water was applied to the skin as a control stimulus. Testing was performed in a single blinded fashion.

Results

Pronounced cutaneous hyperalgesia to mechanical stimuli was observed in all 30 patients tested. Pa-

tients with SMP ranged in age from 11 to 56 years and included 7 female and 2 male subjects. Only 4 of the SMP patients had evidence of nerve injury. The others had either soft tissue or bony injuries without nerve injury ($n = 4$), or had no clear precipitating cause ($n = 1$). The region of hyperalgesia in most SMP patients (6/9) was not restricted to the cutaneous innervation of a given nerve, but was of a stocking-glove distribution.

Patients with SIP ranged in age from 18 to 68 years and included 10 female and 8 male subjects. In contrast to the SMP group, the majority of the SIP patients had evidence of nerve injury (14/18). The patients with nerve injury typically had hyperalgesia in the cutaneous innervation of the injured nerve, but the hyperalgesia was not necessarily restricted to this area.

Testing with mechanical stimuli

Threshold testing. The detection and pain thresholds in the SMP and SIP groups were similar (Fig. 1, t-test, $P > 0.6$) and thus the analysis for the two

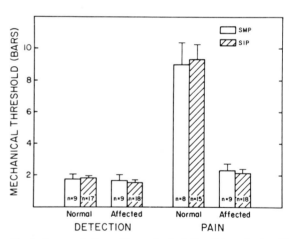

Fig. 1. Sensory testing with mechanical stimuli in patients with sympathetically maintained pain (SMP) and sympathetically independent pain (SIP) Mean mechanical thresholds in bars (1 bar = 10^6 dynes/cm²) for detection and pain on the normal and affected sides are shown for SMP and SIP patients. The pain threshold for mechanical stimuli on the affected side is significantly lower than for the contralateral normal side in both groups ($P < 0.001$). Notably, the pain threshold corresponded to the detection threshold in 16 of the 27 patients.

groups was combined. On the normal side, the touch threshold always corresponded to the detection threshold and was 1.8 ± 0.1 bars ($n = 26$, mean $\pm$ SEM, 1 bar $= 10^6$ dynes/cm^2). The pain threshold was 9.2 ± 0.8 bars ($n = 23$) on the normal side, which was significantly greater than the touch threshold (t-test, $P < 0.001$). The mean pain threshold on the affected side was 2.2 ± 0.2 bars ($n = 27$), which was significantly lower than the pain threshold on the normal side (t-test, $P < 0.001$). Notably, in the region of hyperalgesia, the pain threshold corresponded to the detection threshold in 16 of the 27 patients. Moreover, the pain threshold on the abnormal side did not differ significantly from the detection threshold on the normal side (t-test, $P > 0.1$).

Vibratory stimuli and hair follicle movement. The incidence of pain resulting from vibratory stimuli applied to a bony prominence near the hyperalgesic area was not significantly different between the SMP (4/5) and SIP (8/12) patients ($\chi^2 = 0.3$, df $= 1$, $P > 0.5$). Movement of a single hair follicle within the zone of hyperalgesia caused pain in 50% of the patients tested (3/6 SMP and 6/12 SIP).

Testing with cold stimuli

The SMP and SIP groups differed significantly with regard to responses to the cooling stimulus. The drop of 38°C water did not elicit pain in any of the patients. Pain in response to the drop of acetone in the affected area was present in all of the 7 SMP patients tested. A drop of ice water and a drop of isopropyl alcohol also evoked pain in all 7. In contrast, only 5 of 14 SIP patients tested reported pain response to cold ($\chi^2 = 7.88$, df $= 1$, $P < 0.01$). All 5 SIP patients with hyperalgesia to cold stimuli failed to obtain pain relief during sympathetic blockade. In 3 patients with SMP, sensory testing was done before and during sympathetic blockade. During the sympathetic blockade, the hyperalgesia to cooling as well as to mechanical stimuli was abolished.

In 11 of 11 patients (7 SMP and 4 SIP) with hyperalgesia to cooling stimuli, the skin was cooler in the affected area (1.0–3.5°C colder than the cor-

responding contralateral body part). Thermographic data were not available in the fifth SIP patient with cold hyperalgesia. Five SIP patients had cooler skin (1.0–1.3°C) but had no hyperalgesia to cooling stimuli. Four other SIP patients had no temperature difference (1 patient actually had a warmer extremity due to a previous sympathectomy), and no cold hyperalgesia was observed. Thus, there was a significantly greater incidence of hyperalgesia to cooling stimuli in patients whose affected area was cooler (≥ 1°C) than the corresponding contralateral normal body part ($\chi^2 = 6.11$, df $= 1$, $P < 0.02$).

Discussion

Patients with chronic hyperalgesia to mechanical stimuli after soft tissue or nerve injury may be classified into two groups, sympathetically maintained pain (SMP) and sympathetically independent pain (SIP). Patients with SMP have signs of increased sympathetic tone and achieve pain relief with sympathetic blockade. Sensory testing with mechanical and vibratory stimuli failed to reveal any significant differences between the SMP and SIP patients. Preliminary sensory testing with heat stimuli also has not suggested any significant differences between the two groups.

All SMP patients tested found cooling stimuli painful. In contrast, only about one-third of the SIP patients tested had a similar response to cooling stimuli. Each of the patients who had cold hyperalgesia also had signs of increased sympathetic tone, as reflected by a decrease in skin temperature compared to the corresponding normal body part [5]. It is possible that the SIP patients with hyperalgesia to cooling stimuli could have a mixed mechanism for their pain – a sympathetically dependent and an independent component. Thus, sympathetic blockade may not afford satisfactory relief of symptoms. It is suggested, therefore, that hyperalgesia to cold stimuli is a sensitive, but not specific, sign of SMP. Whether more intense cooling stimuli (> 2°C) also reveal differences between SIP and

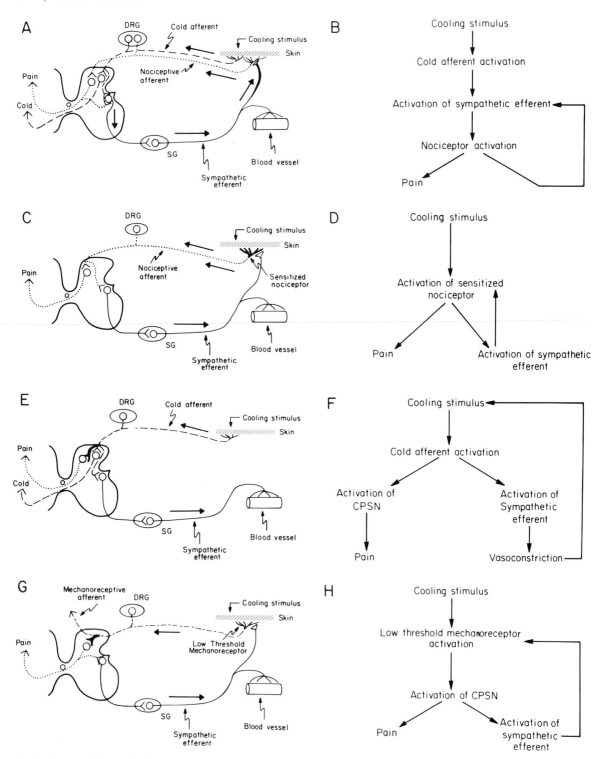

Fig. 2. Four possible mechanisms to account for the hyperalgesia to cooling stimuli in SMP patients are shown. The left half of the figure (A, C, E and G) shows a schematic diagram and the corresponding right half of the figure (B, D, F and H) shows a flow-chart of the pathways involved (see text for details). DRG = dorsal root ganglion, SG = sympathetic ganglion, CPSN = central pain-signalling neurons.

SMP patients will be of interest.

It might be argued that hyperalgesia to cooling stimuli is a non-specific finding associated with the relative temperature of the area. Accordingly, all patients with hyperalgesia to cooling stimuli had relatively cooler skin in the painful area. However, there were five SIP patients who had relatively cooler skin, but did not have hyperalgesia to cooling stimuli. Thus having relatively cooler skin in the painful area does not in itself predict the presence of cold hyperalgesia.

Lindblom and coworkers (1979, 1984) and Fruhstorfer and Lindblom (1984) have performed quantitative sensory testing in patients with neuralgia using mechanical and thermal stimuli. Their patients differed from ours in that they were hypoesthetic, with higher detection thresholds on the affected side. Similar to our observations, however, there were two groups of patients in their population. One group was characterized by hyperalgesia to thermal stimuli, while the other group of patients was hypoesthetic. In 4 of 6 patients, presumably with sympathetically independent pain, a lower threshold to pain from cold stimuli was observed (Fruhstorfer and Lindblom, 1984).

Four mechanisms may account for the hyperalgesia to cooling stimuli in SMP patients. The normal vasoconstriction reflex to cutaneous cooling is mediated by increased sympathetic discharge. The pain to cooling stimuli in SMP patients is due to this reflex increase in sympathetic tone in the hyperalgesic area (Fig. 2A). The release of catecholamines at the peripheral sympathetic nerve terminals results in vasoconstriction as well as a response in the nociceptors (Fig. 2B). In support of this hypothesis, there are reports on the development of adrenergic sensitivity in nociceptors after nerve injury (Wall and Gutnick, 1974; Devor and Janig, 1981; Korenman and Devor, 1981; Janig, 1985) and after cutaneous injury (Roberts and Elardo, 1985). In addition, hyperalgesia to cooling stimuli was abolished in the SMP patients in this study during the sympathetic block.

A second possible mechanism is that primary afferent nociceptors develop an enhanced response to cooling stimuli (Fig. 2C). Thus, the cooling stimuli activate the nociceptive afferents which lead to pain and an efferent discharge in the sympathetics (Fig. 2D). Again, the positive-feedback loop involves the development of an adrenergic sensitivity by the nociceptors.

Another possibility is that central changes may occur resulting in increased synaptic efficacy between cold fiber primary afferents and central pain-signalling neurons (Fig. 2E). Thus, the cooling stimulus activates normal cold afferents, which leads to pain and an increase in sympathetic discharge. The resulting vasoconstriction further cools the skin, which activates the cold receptor and thus completes the positive-feedback loop (Fig. 2F). A fourth possible explanation is that low-threshold mechanoreceptors could develop an increased synaptic efficacy with central pain-signalling neurons (Fig. 2G). It has been shown that slowly adapting mechanoreceptors normally respond to cooling of the skin (Janig, 1985). The cooling stimulus activates the low-threshold afferents, which leads to a response in the central pain signal neuron which results in pain as well as activation of the sympathetic efferents (Fig. 2H).

These results suggest that patients with hyperalgesia to mechanical stimuli should be tested for hyperalgesia to cooling stimuli. Patients with pain from mild cooling stimuli are likely to have SMP, and may therefore benefit from procedures directed at reducing sympathetic input to the involved area. As indicated by this study, psychophysical testing in patients with chronic pain may be of importance in deciphering the pathophysiological mechanisms of their pain.

Acknowledgements

We greatly appreciate the technical assistance of T.V. Hartke. This research was supported by NIH grant NS-14447, the Blaustein Fund, and a New Investigator Research Award (GM33451) to S.N.R.

References

Bonica, J.J. (1979) Causalgia and other reflex sympathetic dystrophies. In J.J. Bonica et al. (Eds.), Advances in Pain Research and Therapy, Vol. 3, Raven Press, New York, pp. 141–166.

Cook, A.J., Woolf, C.J., Wall, P.D. and McMahon, S.B. (1987) Dynamic receptive field spasticity in rat spinal cord dorsal horn following C-primary afferent input. Nature, 325: 151–153.

Devor, M. and Janig, W. (1981) Activation of myelinated afferents ending in neurons by stimulation of the sympathetic supply in the rat. Neurosci. Lett., 24: 43–47.

Fruhstorfer, H. and Lindblom, U. (1984) Sensibility abnormalities in neuralgic patients studied by thermal and tactile pulse stimulation. In C. von Euler et al. (Eds.), Somatosensory Mechanisms, Macmillan, London, pp. 353–361.

Hendler, N., Uematesu, S. and Long, D. (1982) Thermographic validation of physical complaints in 'psychogenic pain' patients. Psychomatics, 23: 283–287.

Janig, W. (1985) Causalgia and reflex sympathetic dystrophy: in which way is the sympathetic nervous system involved? Trends Neurosci., 8: 471–477.

Johnson, K.O., Darian-Smith, I. and LaMotte, C. (1973) Peripheral Neural Determinants of Temperature Discrimination in Man: A correlative study of responses to cooling skin. J. Neurophys., 36: 347–371.

Korenman, E.M.D. and Devor, M. (1981) Ectepic adrenergic sensitivity in damaged peripheral nerve axons in the rat. Exp. Neurol., 72: 63–81.

Lindblom, U. and Verillo, R. (1979) Sensory functions in chronic neuralgia. J. Neurol. Neurosurg. Psychiatry, 42: 422–435.

Lindblom, U. (1984) Neuralgia: Mechanisms and Therapeutic Prospects. In C. Benedetti (Ed.), Advances in Pain Research and Therapy, Vol. 7, Raven Press, New York, pp. 427–438.

Livingston, W.K. (1943) Pain Mechanisms. A physiologic interpretation of causalgia and its related states, Macmillan, New York.

Nathan, P.W. (1947) On the pathogenesis of causalgia in peripheral nerve injuries. Brain, 70: 145–171.

Nathan, P.W. (1983) Pain and the sympathetic system. J. Auton. Nerv. Sys., 7: 363–370.

Roberts, W.J. and Elardo, S.M. (1985) Sympathetic activation of a delta nociceptor. Somatosens. Res., 3: 33–44.

Roberts, W.J. (1986) A hypothesis on the physiological basis for causalgia and related pains. Pain, 24: 297–311.

Scadding, J.W. (1981) Development of ongoing activity, mechanosensitivity, and adrenaline sensitivity in severed peripheral nerve axons. Exp. Neurol., 73: 345–364.

Schott, G.D. (1986) Mechanisms of causalgia and related clinical conditions. Brain, 109: 717–738.

Wall, P.D. and Gutnick, M. (1974) Ongoing activity in peripheral nerves. The physiology and pharmacology of impulse originating from a neuroma. Exp. Neurol., 43: 580–593.

Wallin, G., Torebjork, E. and Hallin, R. (1976) Preliminary observations on the pathophysiology of hyperalgesia in the causalgic pain syndrome. In Y. Zotterman (Ed.), Sensory Functions of the Skin in Primates, Pergamon Press, New York, pp. 489–502.

R. Dubner, G.F. Gebhart & M.R. Bond (Eds.)
Proceedings of the Vth World Congress on Pain
© 1988 Elsevier Science Publishers BV (Biomedical Division)

CHAPTER 18

Abnormal single-unit activity and responses to stimulation in the presumed ventrocaudal nucleus of patients with central pain

Frederick A. Lenz[1], Ronald R. Tasker[1], Jonathan O. Dostrovsky[4], Hon C. Kwan[4,5], John Gorecki[1], Teruyasu Hirayama[1] and John T. Murphy[2,3,4]

Divisions of [1]Neurosurgery, [2]Neurology and [3]Clinical Neurophysiology, Toronto General Hospital, and Departments of [1]Surgery, [4]Physiology and [5]Engineering, University of Toronto, Toronto, Ontario, Canada

Summary

We have performed stimulation and single-unit analysis of the activity of cells in the presumed ventrocaudal nucleus of the thalamus in patients with central pain. Results in some patients with spinal cord injury indicated an increase in the size of the thalamic region representing the area of the body adjacent to that supplied by the spinal cord below the level of the injury. The spontaneous activity of cells in this region of the thalamus was increased and characterized by bursts of action potentials. Electrical stimulation in this region sometimes produced the sensation of pain.

Introduction

The results of electrical stimulation and recording in the central nervous system of patients with central pain have suggested the presence of significantly disordered function. Recordings from ten spinal

Correspondence: Dr. Frederick A. Lenz, c/o Division of Neurosurgery, 14-216 Eaton North Wing, Toronto General Hospital, 200 Elizabeth Street, Toronto, Ontario, Canada M5G 2C4.

neurons located above the level of a complete transection demonstrated abnormal activity with 'a tendency toward burst firing' (Loeser et al., 1968). Abnormal slow-wave activity was recorded in the midbrain tegmentum of a patient with central pain following a lesion of 'the left side of the brain extending from cerebral cortex through thalamus, internal capsule and the midbrain' (Nashold and Wilson, 1966). Abnormal low-frequency (1–3 Hz) slow-wave activity was recorded in the 6–8 mm lateral plane of the thalamus in three patients with pain secondary to spinal arachnoiditis, facial anesthesia dolorosa and the Déjèrine-Roussy syndrome (Gücer et al., 1978).

Somatosensory responses elicited by electrical stimulation of the human central nervous system include the sensations of paresthesias, heat, cold, muscle squeezing and movement of a body part. However, the sensation of pain is rarely evoked, except in patients suffering from chronic pain (Obrador and Dierssen, 1966; Tasker et al., 1982; cf. Sano, 1977). In these patients, the sensation of burning and pain was most frequently induced by stimulation of the mesencephalon caudal to the thalamus, less than 10 mm lateral to the midline (Tasker et al., 1982). Other sites in the thalamus and midbrain where pain can be evoked are the presumed centre médian, parafascicular, intralaminar nuclei (Levin, 1966; Hosobuchi et al., 1974) and midbrain tegmentum (Nashold and Wilson, 1966). The ventrocaudal nucleus (Vc) has rarely been studied (cf. Tasker et al., 1982, 1987), although studies in animals with lesions of ascending somatosensory pathways relaying in Vc indicate significant abnormalities of the somatosensory system proximal to the lesion. We now report results of studies of stimulation and single-unit analysis of cellular activity in presumed Vc of patients with central pain secondary to spinal cord injuries.

Methods

The studies reported here were carried out as part of the thalamic procedures for the treatment of patients suffering from a number of disorders, including parkinsonian tremor and pain secondary to spinal cord injury and supratentorial stroke. The protocol of these studies conforms to the principles of the International Association for the Study of Pain regarding use of human subjects and was reviewed and approved by the local human experimentation committee.

Thalamic exploration was performed as a two-stage procedure (Lenz et al., 1988a; Tasker et al., 1982). The first stage comprised radiological determination of the stereotactic coordinates of the anterior (AC) and posterior commissures (PC). During the second stage, the site of Vc, estimated from these coordinates, was explored with a high-impedance microelectrode (Lenz et al., 1988a). When a single unit was isolated, a sensory examination was performed in order to determine the optimum stimulus (light touch or non-nociceptive pressure), the receptive field and the response to a maintained stimulus (rapidly adapting (RA) or slowly adapting (SA)). For each cell, a 10–30 s period of spontaneous firing was observed. The microelectrode signal and a descriptive voice channel were recorded on tape throughout the recording session. After microelectrode exploration, a concentric bipolar stimulating electrode (1.1 mm diameter tip) was intro-

duced along the same trajectory, and sensations to threshold stimulation (60 Hz, pulse width 3 ms) were determined at 2-mm intervals (Tasker et al., 1982). In some patients, threshold microstimulation was carried out during the recording session by connecting the microelectrode to a constant-current stimulator at sites in presumed Vc, where single units with receptive fields could be recorded. Sensations were often evoked by microstimulation with a 0.5–2.0 s stimulus train consisting of 0.1–0.3 ms negative pulses at a frequency of 300 Hz.

The tapes of the microelectrode recordings were examined postoperatively. Single units were discriminated by standard techniques (Lenz et al., 1988a). The times of occurrence of action potentials were digitized and the resulting spike train was converted to an equivalent analog signal (French and Holden, 1971). Fast Fourier transforms were performed and the magnitudes of the resulting spectral estimates were averaged in consecutive groups of 16 to produce an autopower spectrum of the type illustrated in Fig. 2B (Lenz et al., 1984).

Results

All patients in the present report ($n = 9$, see Fig. 4) were studied by intraoperative analysis of neuronal activity and responses to stimulation. Postoperative single-unit analysis of the type described above has been completed in only one spinal cord injury patient (b7). We now report results of postoperative analysis in that patient and preliminary results in one further spinal cord injury patient (d2).

The first patient (b7) was involved in a motor vehicle accident and suffered a fracture dislocation at C4–5 with an immediate, clinically complete spinal cord transection at C5 (Lenz et al., 1987). One and one-half years later he developed a burning dysesthetic pain in the abdomen, thigh and perineum. Since his pain persisted despite a three-year course of conservative therapy, it was elected to attempt deep-brain stimulation for pain relief. Therefore, he underwent a thalamic exploration to determine the optimal location for the deep-brain electrode.

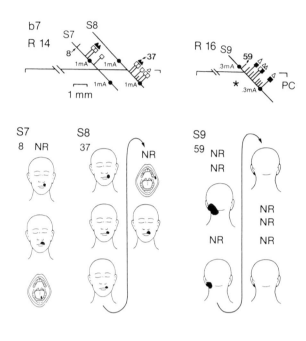

Fig. 1. Receptive field mapping along three trajectories, two (S7 and S8) in the parasagittal plane 14 mm to the right of the midline (R14), and one (S9) in the plane 16 mm to the right of the midline (R16) in a patient (b7) with a clinically complete spinal cord transection. In the upper portion of the figure, the three trajectories are shown relative to the intercommissural line (AC–PC distance 26.1 mm) and the posterior commissure (PC), labelled in the right hand panel. Lines at right-angles to the trajectories indicate the positions at which single units were recorded. The optimal responses of cells correspond to the following symbols: open squares = cutaneous responses to light touch, filled squares = cutaneous responses to non-nociceptive pressure. Filled triangles = SA cell, open triangles = RA cell. Short lines with no symbols indicate the location of single units having no identifiable receptive field. The figurines in the lower panels indicate the size and location of the RFs for each neuron identified in the upper panel. NR indicates a single unit having no identifiable receptive field. The number of the most anterior single unit along each trajectory and its corresponding figurine are labelled in the upper and lower panels, respectively. Single units located more posteriorly along each trajectory correspond to figurines arranged in vertical columns and numbered sequentially, as indicated. Dots along the trajectory indicate sites where stimulation was carried out. Stimulation (0.3 mA) along trajectory S9 produced pain (see text). Stimulation along trajectories S7 and S8 produced no sensation. The calibration bar indicates 1 mm in the brain. (From Lenz et al., 1987, with permission.)

During exploration of the 14 mm lateral sagittal plane, cells were found which responded to facial and intraoral tactile stimulation. These cells, located less than 5 mm anterior to the posterior commissure, were within presumed Vc (Lenz et al., 1988b). In patients with dyskinesia but no demonstrated sensory abnormality (controls), cells with similar receptive fields were characteristically found in the thalamic area representing facial and intraoral structures (Lenz et al., 1988b). Planes located 2 mm lateral to those containing the representation of intraoral and facial structures characteristically contain cells with receptive fields on the upper extremity (Lenz et al., 1988b). However, in this patient the plane 2 mm lateral to that containing the facial and intraoral representation contained cells with receptive fields on the occiput and ear (Fig. 1, trajectory S9). The representation of the occiput and ear is significantly larger in this case than in controls (Lenz et al., 1988b). Increased representation of areas adjacent to the deafferented area is characteristic of central nervous system structures which have lost their normal somatosensory input (reviewed in Lenz et al., 1987). Therefore we propose that cells in the 16 mm lateral plane have lost their normal sensory input because they are located in a region where (1) there is increased representation of body parts adjacent to the deafferented area and (2) cells with receptive fields on the hand area normally found.

Bipolar stimulation along trajectory S9 at currents of 0.3 mA produced a burning sensation in the left cheek, occiput, neck and throughout the left upper extremity. This sensation was similar to the patient's pain in quality, although its location was different. Stimulation along trajectories (S7 and S8) which contained cells having facial and intraoral receptive fields produced no sensation at currents of 1.0 mA.

Subjective assessment of cellular activity suggested that cells located in the 16 mm lateral plane had a tendency to fire spontaneously in bursts of action potentials. Spectral analysis was used to assess the firing patterns of these cells quantitatively. The bursts of high-frequency activity seen in the

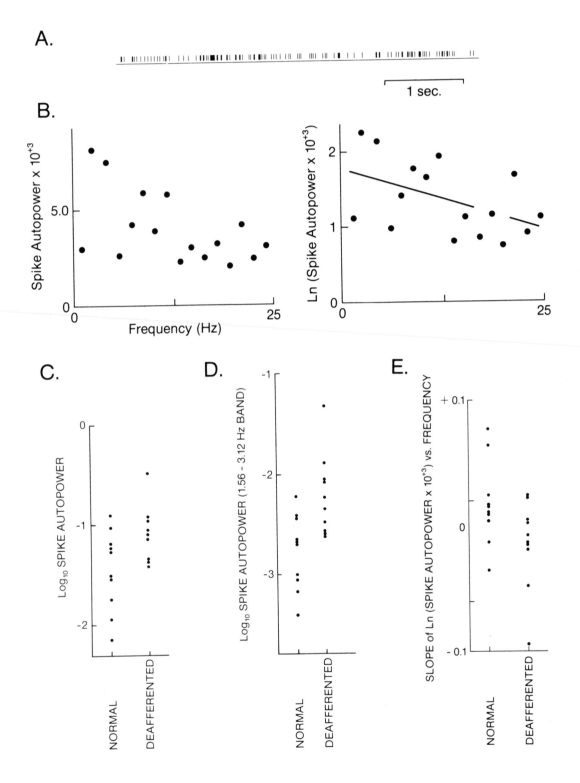

spike train (Fig. 2A) are reflected by an increase in low-frequency spectral power (Fig. 2B) because of the low-pass filtering which is essential in order to prevent errors due to aliasing (French and Holden, 1971). By comparison with cells in the 14 mm lateral plane, cells in the 16 mm lateral plane were found to have: (1) a higher mean firing rate, demonstrated in the higher spike autopower ($P<0.0001$, Fig. 2C), (2) a greater tendency to fire in bursts reflected by the higher power at low frequencies ($P<0.005$, Fig. 2D) and by the more negative slope of the graph of *ln* spike autopower vs. frequency ($P<0.05$, Fig. 2E). Since stimulation produced a pain in the area exhibiting abnormal spontaneous (Fig. 2) and evoked (Fig. 1) neuronal activity, these results suggested that stimulation-evoked pain might be a marker for abnormal neuronal activity involved in the generation of pain.

Preliminary results in other patients with pain secondary to spinal cord injury demonstrate some, but not all, of the abnormalities found in this patient. The region of the thalamus representing parts of the body adjacent to the deafferented area was explored in one further patient (d2) with a clinically complete spinal cord transection at T4. Preliminary results in this patient did demonstrate increased spontaneous and bursting activity in thalamic regions containing cells with receptive fields adjacent to the deafferented part of the body but did not demonstrate increased representation of those parts of the body.

The sensation of pain produced by electrical stimulation in Vc of patient b7 (Fig. 1) was not evoked by microstimulation in two other patients (d2 and d3) with pain secondary to spinal cord injury. Fig. 3 shows an example of the effect of thalamic microstimulation in a chronic pain patient. These results were obtained in the 17 mm right lateral parasagittal plane of a patient in whom a supratentorial stroke had given rise to the Déjèrine-Roussy syndrome. Areas along these trajectories where multiple cells had small receptive fields and well-defined sensory modalities were presumed to be located in Vc. Pain was evoked by microstimulation at many of these sites, demonstrating that pain can be evoked in chronic pain patients by microstimulation, which has rarely been applied in the human Vc.

The results of both bipolar stimulation and microstimulation in presumed Vc are summarized in Fig. 4 for patients with thalamic pain (2 patients), pain following spinal cord injuries (3 patients – b7, d2, d3) and parkinsonian tremor without pain (4 patients). Note that pain responses were not observed in any of the control (parkinsonian) patients. Numerous pain responses were evoked by stimulation in the ventrocaudal nucleus of patients with thalamic pain, as demonstrated in Fig. 3. However, in patients with pain secondary to spinal cord injury, only patient b7 (Fig. 1) reported the sensation of pain in response to electrical stimulation.

Conclusions

The present results in patients with pain secondary to spinal cord injury demonstrate several abnormalities, including (1) a reorganization of somatosensory representation characterized by an increase in the number of cells with receptive fields adjacent to the area of the body which has been deaffe-

---

Fig. 2. Spike train (A) and autopower (B) spectrum of the spontaneous activity for thalamic cell No. 62 located in the 16 mm lateral plane. In A, time is represented along the horizontal axis. B illustrates the autopower spectrum (left) and ln autopower spectrum (right) for the spike train illustrated in A. C gives the $\log_{10}$ of the sum of all components in the autopower spectrum (B, left) for cells in the deafferented and normal thalamus. Each dot represents the value for one cell. D shows the low-frequency spectral component in the autopower spectrum in normal and deafferented thalamus. The slope of the spectrum was estimated by linear regression after taking the $\log_e$ as illustrated in B, right. Slopes of spectra for deafferented and normal cells are given in E. (Adapted from Lenz et al., 1987, with permission.)

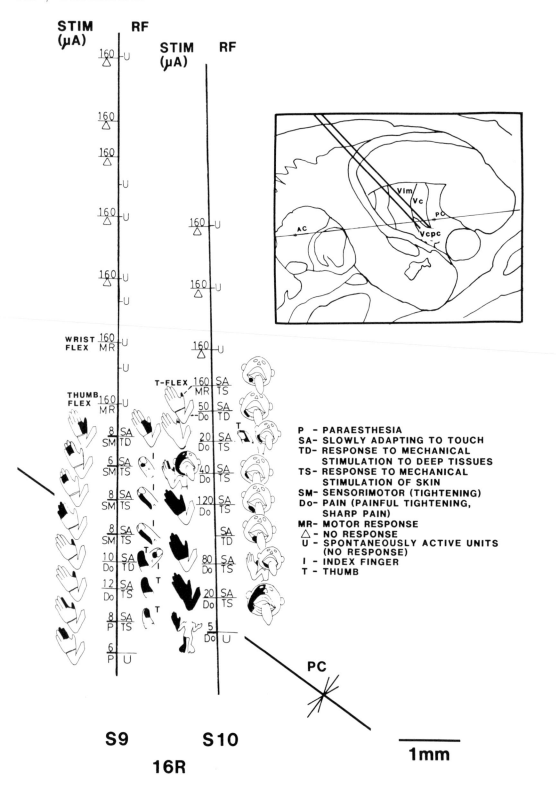

P - PARAESTHESIA
SA- SLOWLY ADAPTING TO TOUCH
TD- RESPONSE TO MECHANICAL
    STIMULATION TO DEEP TISSUES
TS- RESPONSE TO MECHANICAL
    STIMULATION OF SKIN
SM- SENSORIMOTOR (TIGHTENING)
Do- PAIN (PAINFUL TIGHTENING,
    SHARP PAIN)
MR- MOTOR RESPONSE
△ - NO RESPONSE
U - SPONTANEOUSLY ACTIVE UNITS
    (NO RESPONSE)
I - INDEX FINGER
T - THUMB

1mm

S9   S10

16R

rented, (2) abnormal spontaneous neuronal activity characterized by a tendency to fire in bursts of action potentials, (3) induction of pain by electrical stimulation. The reorganization of somatosensory representation and spontaneous bursting activity is similar to that identified in animal models of central and deafferentation pain (reviewed in Lenz et al., 1987). Preliminary evidence of reorganization of the presumed Vc was only found in one patient with spinal cord injury (Fig. 1). However, reorganized areas might not have been sampled in the limited exploration of the thalamus which is possible during these operative procedures. The finding of increased spontaneous firing characterized by bursts of action potentials appears to be consistent in both patients with spinal cord injuries studied thus far. Thus the activity of single units recorded in the thalamus of some patients with central pain secondary to spinal cord injury shows abnormalities similar to those recorded in animals with injuries to the somatosensory system.

We originally anticipated that clinical pain, stimulation-induced pain and abnormal neuronal activity could be related. However, stimulation-evoked pain was not observed in all patients with both central pain and abnormal spontaneous neuronal activity. These results suggest that abnormal neuronal activity is not consistently related to stimulation-evoked pain in patients with spinal cord injury.

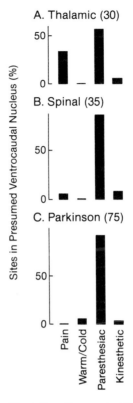

Fig. 4. Sensations evoked by stimulation at multiple sites in the presumed ventrocaudal nucleus of patients with parkinsonian tremor (C) and with pain secondary to supratentorial stroke (A) and spinal cord injury (B). Total numbers of stimulation sites for each type of patient are indicated in brackets.

Acknowledgements

We wish to thank Hoi Nguyen-Huu for writing the computer programs used in this study, Mary Teofilo and Allan Suran for technical assistance, and Sharon Norman and Prof. David Andrews of the Statistical Consulting Service for advice concerning the statistical analysis of the results.

←

Fig. 3. Results of microstimulation and microrecording along two trajectories (S9 and S10) in a patient with pain secondary to supratentorial stroke. Unlike the results shown in Fig. 1, these results are taken from the operative records and are not based on postoperative single-unit analysis of the tapes made during the operation. The two vertical lines are the trajectories, shown relative to the anterior commissure–posterior commissure line, with the posterior commissure (PC) as indicated. Figurines and letters to the right of each trajectory indicate the modality (TS or TD), response pattern (SA) and receptive field of cells recorded at the sites indicated along the trajectory. Letters, numbers and figurines to the left of each trajectory respectively indicate the stimulation-evoked sensation (Do, P or SM), stimulation threshold (in μA) and area to which the sensation was referred in response to stimulation at the site indicated along the trajectory. The estimated location of nuclear boundaries in relation to these trajectories is indicated on the parasagittal map of the thalamus shown in the inset. Scale is as indicated. Abbreviations are as listed in the figure plus: Vc, ventrocaudal; Vcpc, ventrocaudal, pars parvocellularis; Vim, ventralis intermedius.

This research was supported by the PSI Foundation, Toronto, Canada, The Parkinson's Foundation of Canada, and MRC (Canada). F.A.L. was a Fellow of the MRC (Canada) and a Schering Scholar of the American College of Surgeons.

References

French, A.S. and Holden, A.V. (1971) Alias-free sampling of neuronal spike trains. Kybernetic, 8: 165–171.

Gücer, G., Niedermeyer, E. and Long, D.M. (1978) Thalamic recordings in patients with chronic pain. J. Neurol., 219: 47–61.

Hosobuchi, Y., Adams, J.E. and Fields, H.L. (1974) Chronic thalamic and internal capsule stimulation for the control of facial anesthesia doloroasa and dysesthetia of thalamic syndrome. Adv. Neurol., 4: 783–787.

Lenz, F.A., Dostrovsky, J.O., Tasker, R.R., Yamashiro, K., Kwan, H.C. and Murphy, J.T. (1988b) Single unit analysis of the human ventral thalamic nuclear group: somatosensory responses. J. Neurophysiol., 59(2): in press.

Lenz, F.A., Dostrovsky, J.O., Tasker, R.R., Yamashiro, K., Kwan, H.C. and Murphy, I.T. (1988b) Single unit analysis of the human ventral thalamic nuclear group: somatosensory responses. J. Neurophysiol., 59(2): in press.

Lenz, F.A., Tasker, R.R., Dostrovsky, J.O., Kwan, H.C., Gorecki, J., Hirayama, T. and Murphy, J.T. (1987) Abnormal neuronal activity in the thalamus of a quadriplegic patient with central pain. Pain, 31: 225–236.

Lenz, F.A., Tasker, R.R., Kwan, H.C., Murphy, J.T. and Nguyen-Huu, H.H. (1984) Techniques for the study of spike trains in the human central nervous system. Acta Neurochir. Suppl., 33: 57–61.

Levin, G. (1966) Electrical stimulation of the globus pallidus and thalamus. J. Neurosurg., 24: 415.

Loeser, J.D., Ward, A.A. and White, L.E. (1968) Chronic deafferentation of human spinal cord neurons, J. Neurosurg., 29: 48–50.

Nashold, B.S. Jr. and Wilson, W.P. (1966) Central pain. Observations in man with chronic implanted electrodes in the midbrain tegmentum. Confin. Neurol. 27: 30–34.

Obrador, S. and Dierssen G. (1966) Sensory responses to subcortical stimulation and management of pain disorders by stereotactic methods. Confin. Neurol. 27: 45–52.

Sano, K. (1977) Intralaminar thalamotomy (thalamolaminotomy) and postero-medial hypothalamotomy in the treatment of intractable pain. In H. Krayenbuhl, P. Maspes, and W. Sweet (Eds.), Progress in Neurological Surgery, Vol. 8, Karger, Basel, pp. 50–103.

Tasker, R.R., Lenz, F.A., Yamashiro, K., Gorecki, J., Hirayama, T. and Dostrovsky, J.O. (1987) Microelectrode techniques in the localization of stereotactic targets. Neurol. Res., 9: 105–112.

Tasker, R.R., Organ, L.W. and Hawrylyshyn, P. (1982) The Thalamus and Midbrain in Man: A Physiologic Atlas Using Electrical Stimulation, Springfield, IL, Charles C. Thomas, 505 pp.

R. Dubner, G.F. Gebhart & M.R. Bond (Eds.)
Proceedings of the Vth World Congress on Pain
© 1988 Elsevier Science Publishers BV (Biomedical Division)

CHAPTER 19

Toward a rationale for the treatment of painful neuropathies

Kenneth L. Casey

VA Medical Center, 2215 Fuller Road, Ann Arbor, MI 48105, USA

Introduction

Although serendipity has played a major role in developing effective therapies for a variety of medical conditions, it is preferable to have a therapeutic rationale based on a knowledge of the pathophysiology of the disease. The pathophysiology of painful neuropathy is not known but, as the other contributors to this topic elsewhere (Lindblom, 1984; Maciewicz et al., 1985) and in this volume have shown, substantial progress is being made.

My purpose is to review very briefly some of the information relevant to the pathophysiology of painful neuropathies and to indicate how various treatments may be appropriate depending upon which pathophysiological process is affected. This approach may suggest new therapies or new insights into the physiological processes underlying the pain of certain neuropathies.

A few caveats are in order. First, most neuropathies are not associated with pain severe enough to become the patient's chief complaint. Second, there is no single pathophysiology of painful neuropathy because there are multiple etiologies and thus multiple ways in which pain may be produced. Therefore, there is no single treatment for

painful neuropathy. Finally, this paper is not a complete review of the pathophysiology of neuropathy or of its treatment; rather, it is intended to outline an approach to therapeutic strategy that may have some clinical utility.

I will consider pathophysiological processes that may affect the nervous system at various stages of information transfer from the receptor through the axon–ganglion complex to the primary afferent terminals in the central nervous system and the first central cells receiving nociceptive information. At each point, I will consider how various treatments may modify the pathological process that may be responsible for the pain. The argument is summarized in Fig. 1.

Receptors

Pathology
Painful conditions with many of the clinical characteristics of a neuropathy may develop without the peripheral fibers themselves being damaged. Thus, tissue damage and pain may lead to a painful condition even without neurological damage. The tissue trauma may be minimal, but pain appears to be a necessary condition. Persistent pain, local changes in cutaneous blood flow and temperature, swelling, osteoporosis and muscle atrophy may all appear in the absence of any evidence for central or peripheral neurologic disease. Homans (1940)

Correspondence: Kenneth L. Casey, M.D., Chief, Neurology Service (127), VA Medical Center, 2215 Fuller Road, Ann Arbor, MI 48105, USA.

called attention to a syndrome he referred to as minor causalgia. In these cases, local tissue injury was followed by persistent hyperesthesia. There was clinical evidence of increased sympathetic outflow, so the author suggested that a hyperactive neurovascular reflex was responsible and found that sympathectomy or sympathetic block was effective therapy. In these cases, it was not necessary that nervous tissue be damaged – only that local tissue injury had taken place. Steinbrocker (1947) later described the shoulder-hand syndrome, characterized by a painful shoulder with homolateral painful swelling and vasomotor changes in the hand.

Usually, but not always, there was an antecedent history of disease or trauma, but neurologic disease was not a necessary condition. In the same year, Evans (1947) used the term reflex sympathetic dystrophy to describe 57 cases with severe pain and evidence of sympathetic overactivity associated with tissue trauma, but without neurologic disease. Kozin et al. (1976) elaborated on what they termed the reflex sympathetic dystrophy syndrome (for review, see Schwartzman and McLellan, 1987). The clinical components include pain, signs of vasomotor instability, swelling and dystrophic skin changes. Again, no evidence for neurologic disease was necessary al-

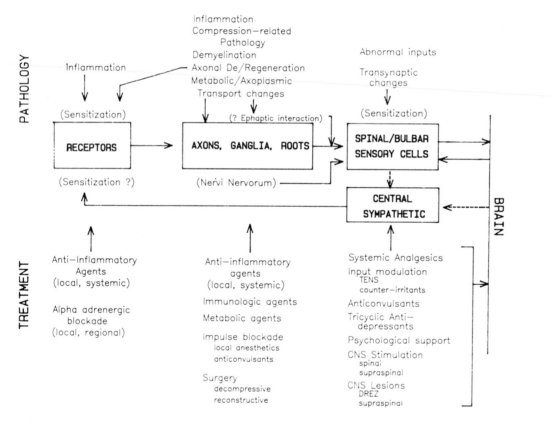

Fig. 1. Summary diagram of pathological processes (top) affecting neurologic function at three levels of the sensory transmission system and the treatments (below) that may counteract those processes to relieve pain. Receptors may be abnormally sensitized by the combined action of substances produced or released locally by sympathetic nerves and the inflammatory process. Degenerating and regenerating receptors may also have abnormal sensitivity. The various pathological processes that may affect axons, ganglia and roots lead to the generation of excessive and abnormal impulses. Central sensory and, possibly, sympathetic neurons may become pathologically hypersensitive because of the lack of neural impulse input controls and impaired biochemical communication from the periphery. Therapeutic measures at this level may affect spinal or bulbar sensory and sympathetic functions directly or they may act indirectly by enhancing sensory control systems in the brain.

though this was present in many cases. Steroids were advocated as effective therapy.

The existence of the syndromes mentioned above suggest that there are as yet unknown processes that occur in damaged tissue, leading to a sensitization of receptors and that this sensitization in some way leads to the continued presence of pain. Thus, the receptors, not the peripheral nerve fibers, may be the target of a pathological process.

The inflammatory process probably plays a critical role in establishing pathological receptor sensitization. The critical chemical or chemicals involved are not known. Chal (1979) concludes that there may be no single agent but that several compounds involved in the inflammatory response may be working in concert to produce the sensitization phenomenon. Perl et al. (1976) found that the heat-induced sensitization of nociceptors was not modified by antihistamines, antiprostaglandins, serotonin or epinephrine. However, as further details of the inflammatory process are known and as more is learned about the chemosensitivity of nociceptors, we may be able to identify the sensitizing mechanism that is produced by the inflammatory process.

There may be no necessary association between clinically evident sympathetic activity and the presence of persistent pain. Painful conditions may be associated with increased or decreased sympathetic activity. However, sympathetic blocks distal to the site of injury may significantly reduce or eliminate the pain (Hannington-Kiff, 1974) even when a sympathetic abnormality is not evident (Loh and Nathan, 1978). It may be, therefore, that some process in the inflammatory reaction exaggerates an additional sensitizing effect of sympathetic efferent activity. This may lead to sensitization of nociceptors and thus to increased pain, allodynia and hyperpathia. There is little doubt that sympathetic discharge has a potentially marked effect on receptor sensitivity even in the absence of the inflammatory response. Chernetski (1964) and Loewenstein (1956) demonstrated that stimulation of sympathetic efferents can elicit somatic afferent discharges in mechanoreceptors in amphibians and mammals. In

their review of this topic, Loh and Nathan (1978) refer to the Russian literature, which confirms these observations. Long (1977) found that afferent cold fibers show increased paradoxical response to noxious heat when cutaneous adrenergic efferent discharge is blocked or reduced. Roberts et al. (1985) and Roberts and Elardo (1985) have shown that sympathetic stimulation can change the responses of tactile receptors and activate A-delta nociceptors that have been sensitized by noxious heat. Wall and Gutnick (1974) showed that impulses originating in a neuroma of the rat sciatic nerve were increased by norepinephrine. Roberts (1986) has summarized the evidence and suggests that sympathetic outflow may sensitize low threshold mechanoreceptors, increasing the convergent input on to sensitized multireceptive spinal cord neurons to produce pain.

Whatever the mechanism, there is evidence that receptors alone may be pathologically sensitized by the combined actions of the inflammatory process and sympathetic efferent activity. Treatments directed at these processes should be useful.

Treatments

Anti-inflammatory agents, in particular corticosteroids, have been advocated in the treatment of these conditions (Kozin et al., 1976; Schwartzman and McLellan, 1987). However, early in the course of the problem, when the inflammatory response is still evident, the use of nonsteroidal anti-inflammatory agents may provide significant relief and may even serve to prevent further receptor sensitization (Huskisson, 1984). Other anti-inflammatory physical procedures such as the use of ice may also be beneficial.

Sympathetic blockade may be particularly useful, especially if hyperpathia is present, even in those conditions in which there is no evidence of sympathetic abnormality (Hannington-Kiff), 1974; Loh and Nathan, 1978; Bonica, 1979; Sweet, in press,b). Sympathetic blockade or sympathectomy is clearly indicated with causalgic syndromes (Schumacker, 1948; Bonica, 1979; Sweet in press,b). Recently, Ghostine et al. (1984) have reported remarkable success in causalgic syndromes using phenoxybenzamine (40–120 mg/day). When this drug was given within 2 weeks of the onset of the syndrome, 6–8 weeks of treatment resulted in a total resolution of pain in all of their 40 cases.

In summary, there is evidence that non-neurologic tissue damage leads to receptor sensitization due presumably to the interaction of inflammatory processes and the activity of sympathetic efferents. Treatment directed at these factors, especially when applied early, may cure or prevent the persistence of these painful states.

Axons, ganglia and roots

Pathology

There is substantial agreement that nociceptive afferent fibers are involved in virtually all cases of painful neuropathy. Dyck et al. (1976) and Thomas (1982) have reviewed the clinical evidence that, although large afferent fibers may also be affected in the pathological process, small fibers are invariably damaged. Dyck et al. (1976) have suggested that the degree of pain in these painful neuropathies may be related to the rate of degeneration of the small diameter afferent fibers (A delta and C).

The compression of a nerve or root produces a complex series of pathologic changes which have been reviewed recently by Gilliat and Harrison (1984). A primary effect of a nerve compression syndrome may be to produce nociceptive afferent input via the nervi nervorum as suggested by Asbury and Fields (1984). This will produce a familiar aching nerve trunk pain as distinguished from the dysesthetic pain due to abnormal discharges generated within the affected nerve. Another consequence of nerve compression may be the creation of ephaptic interactions as has been shown experimentally to occur in damaged nerve (Seltzer and Devor, 1979). In severely damaged nerve with neuroma formation, spontaneous afferent discharge, heightened mechanical and adrenergic sensitivity, and ephaptic interactions may all develop (Govrin-Lippmann and Devor, 1978; Blumberg and Janig, 1984). Secondarily, the compression may lead to

vascular compromise, demyelination and axonal degeneration and subsequent regeneration.

The polyneuropathies caused by metabolic, toxic or immunologic disease are also associated with demyelination and axonal degeneration. Pain is not always associated with these conditions, but among the more common painful neuropathies are those produced by diabetes mellitus (Brown et al., 1976; Archer et al., 1983), amyloid, alcoholic and nutritional disorders, heavy metals (especially arsenic and thallium), carcinoma (remote or direct effects), paraproteinemias, severe and rapidly progressive parainfectious idiopathic polyneuropathy (Guillain-Barre Syndrome) and the type I hereditary sensory neuropathies. A particularly painful condition associated with degeneration of large and small fibers is the inherited metabolic disorder of Fabry's disease.

Both the surgical and nonsurgical neuropathic conditions may lead to changes in axoplasmic transport and metabolism which ultimately affect the cell bodies in the dorsal root ganglion and even in the central nervous system (Aldskogius et al., 1985). These peripherally induced changes in proximally located structures may be associated with increased pathological firing (Burchiel, 1984) and with increased nociceptive nerve impulse generation via the nerve or nervi nervorum. The extent to which ephaptic interaction occurs in human pathologic conditions is debatable, but it has been shown experimentally and may lead to a significant amplification of afferent barrage from nociceptive afferents (Blumberg and Janig, 1984). Firing in bursts may be a prominent feature of afferents in these pathologic conditions (Devor and Bernstein, 1982). The spontaneous generation of impulses seen in these experimental conditions may not involve the discharge of nociceptors. However, as Roberts (1986) suggests, input from nociceptive afferents may not be necessary to produce pain if there are sensitized multireceptive central neurons.

Regenerating axons of damaged nerves and collateral spouts from intact fibers growing into the denervated area of a damaged nerve may also contribute to an increase in the generation of nociceptive impulses. This has been demonstrated by Nixon et al. (1984), Brenan (1986) and Zimmerman and Sanders (1982).

Treatment

The prompt initiation of anti-inflammatory therapy is appropriate in both surgical and nonsurgical diseases of nerve because the inflammatory process may easily lead to vascular compromise, demyelination and axonal degeneration. Thus, the use of nonsteroidal anti-inflammatory agents, as well as steroids in some instances, should be beneficial. My own experience has been that steroids are not usually necessary in the treatment of compressive radicular pain; treatment with non-steroidal anti-inflammatory agents and systemic analgesics has usually been sufficient.

It is of course necessary to use immunologic treatments such as plasma exchange or immunosuppressive agents to treat primary immunology neuropathies because these pathologic processes also produce demyelination and axonal degeneration, possibly leading to the generation of pathologic impulses. A particularly striking example of the effectiveness of metabolic treatment has been cited by Archer et al. (1983) in which the acute painful neuropathy of diabetes mellitus was greatly improved by prompt and careful control of the blood glucose.

Because most of the conditions cited above lead to the generation of abnormal impulses, measures designed to provide impulse blockade are appropriate. Local anesthetics are advocated in some cases of acute herpetic neuralgia (Portnoy et al., 1986). However, a partial, rather than complete blockade of impulse generation may be sufficient. Kastrup et al. (1987) have indicated that systemic lidocaine may be effective in cases of painful diabetic neuropathy. These authors suggest that the effect of systemic lidocaine may not be due to its local anesthetic effect on peripheral nerve, but to actions within the central nervous system. Anticonvulsants such as phenytoin and carbamazepine have been shown to be effective in a variety of painful conditions including amyloid neuropathy (Bada, 1977),

the lightning pains of tabes dorsalis (Ekbom, 1972), the lancinating pains of postherpetic neuralgia (Portnoy et al., 1986) and in trigeminal neuralgia (Fromm, 1984). Swerdlow and Cundill (1981) have shown that clonazepam may be especially effective in lancinating pain. The mechanism of action of certain anticonvulsants and of the local anesthetics may be very similar. Phenytoin and carbamazepine are known to prolong the inactivation of sodium channels and thus to be particularly effective in attenuating or preventing high frequency firing of neural impulses (Maclean and Macdonald, 1983, 1986).

In cases where surgery is appropriate, it is obvious that decompressive procedures will be necessary to prevent the secondary changes mentioned above. In some instances, reconstructive procedures, such as nerve grafts, may be indicated if the trauma is local. Reconstructive surgery may lead to more effective regeneration to appropriate targets and prevent further retrograde or anterograde degeneration which, in turn, may lead to further pathological peripheral and central changes (Gilliatt and Harrison, 1984).

There is little doubt, then, that various pathological etiologies may lead to abnormal impulse generation in axons, dorsal root ganglion cells, and perhaps dorsal roots. Many of the phenomena seen in experimental models may not be the cause of pain in humans, but they strongly suggest that the prevention of impulse generation is the main goal of treatment of disorders affecting these structures. Nociceptive impulses may also be generated in the nervi nervorum, resulting in nerve trunk pain. Treatments are therefore most effectively directed at the inflammatory process, impulse blockade, the treatment of the primary immunologic or metabolic disease and decompressive or reconstructive surgery.

Central nervous system

Pathology

There is no doubt that peripheral tissue damage

that produces increased nociceptive input may in turn produce significant anatomical and physiological changes in the central nervous system of animals (Woolf, 1984; Guilbaud et al., 1986a, b; Coderre and Melzack, 1985, 1987; Cook et al., 1987). There is also evidence that nerve damage of various kinds may lead to morphological and biochemical changes within peripheral sensory ganglia, the central processes of primary afferents and perhaps even central cells of the first synaptic relay (Aldskogius, 1985). These structural, physiological and biochemical changes do not appear permanently to affect the human central nervous system because it is common clinical experience that the effective treatment of pain, even chronic pain as in long-standing arthritis, leaves behind a central sensory apparatus that is capable of normally processing somatic sensory information. Mallow and Olson (1981), for example, have shown that the sensory responsiveness of chronic pain patients without neurologic damage returns to normal following effective treatment of the pain. However, the central changes that have been reported in experimental animals may reflect the presence of a pathophysiological process that may be responsible for sustaining pain at a pathological level so long as the responsible central or peripheral abnormality remains.

Whether denervation itself can produce a hyperexcitable state in central neurons and pain in humans remains a controversial issue. Tasker (1984) has extensively reviewed the evidence in favor of this concept. Wynn Parry (1980) has presented evidence that an anatomically confirmed avulsion of the brachial plexus is associated with a very high incidence of a painful syndrome; in contrast, severe plexus injuries that do not produce avulsion have a relatively low incidence of persistent pain. These clinical observations find support in evidence from experimental animals and humans (Loeser and Ward, 1967; Loeser et al., 1968) that deafferentation may produce abnormal spontaneous or evoked discharges in spinal cord cells, possibly due to a loss of afferent inhibition (Wall and Devor, 1981). In reviewing this issue, however, Kerr (1983) and Sweet (1984, in press, a) marshal experimental and clinical

evidence that fails to support the concept that denervation alone is the cause of pain. Pubols (1984) and Brown et al. (1984) have failed to confirm the induction of certain plastic changes on spinal cord neurons by peripheral nerve damage. Other studies of partial deafferentation by dorsal rhizotomy have found no evidence for a denervation hyperactivity or hyperresponsiveness that might provide a basis for deafferentation pain (Pubols and Goldberger, 1980; Brinkhus and Zimmermann, 1983). In reviewing the topic, Mendell (1984) points out that several technical and interpretive problems must be addressed before these different experimental results can be understood.

There is general agreement, however, that pain and itching may be remarkably alleviated by natural or electrical stimuli that activate the larger diameter tactile afferents (Wall and Sweet, 1967; Meyer and Fields, 1972) and that this effect may have a basis in the afferent-induced inhibition of dorsal horn cells (Hentall and Fields, 1979; Fitzgerald and Woolf, 1981; LeBars et al., 1979). Peripheral nerve lesions have been shown to reduce the inhibitory depolarization of primary afferent fibers (Horch and Lisney, 1981; Woolf and Wall, 1982) and section of a single dorsal root increased the number of dorsal horn cells responsive to high threshold stimuli (Pubols and Brenowitz, 1982). Thus, it is possible that a loss of large diameter tactile afferents may contribute, along with other pathological changes, to an enhanced nociceptive excitability of central cells.

Treatment

Systemically administered analgesics are appropriate for painful disease at any site in the nervous system. They are mentioned here because of the site of action: either directly on the dorsal horn or on descending mechanisms that attenuate the responses of dorsal horn neurons to noxious input (Basbaum and Fields, 1978, 1984).

Because of the experimental and clinical evidence that peripheral input can significantly attenuate the perception of nociceptive impulses, input modulation, either by transcutaneous electrical nerve stimulation (TENS) or by counter-irritant measures (which probably activate the lower threshold nociceptive afferents), is an appropriate therapeutic approach (Wall and Sweet, 1967; Meyer and Fields, 1972; Nathan and Wall, 1974; Lundeburg, 1984).

Anticonvulsants, including the sodium channel inactivators such as phenytoin and carbamazepine, may attenuate abnormal spontaneous and evoked activity at early levels of sensory transmission. In addition, compounds such as clonazepam and baclofen, which are presumed to act through GABAergic mechanisms (see also Sawynok, 1987), may contribute significantly to the suppression of abnormal discharges in the dorsal horn or more centrally (Swerdlow and Cundill, 1981; Fromm, 1984). Tricyclic antidepressants such as amitriptyline have been shown to be effective in painful diabetic neuropathy (Max et al., 1987) and postherpetic neuralgia (Watson et al., 1982). These compounds, which block the reuptake degradation of biogenic amines (Ross and Renyi, 1967), are thought to potentiate or activate central analgesic mechanisms (Fromm and Glass, 1977; Botney and Fields, 1983; Spiegel et al., 1983; Basbaum and Fields, 1984). There is, therefore, a good neuropharmacological basis for using such drugs to potentiate the analgesic effect of opiate narcotics. The sympathomimetic agent dextroamphetamine, for example, has been shown to both enhance analgesia and counteract the sedative effects of morphine given for post-operative pain (Forrest et al., 1977).

It is common clinical experience that strong psychological support by the physician and others involved in the patient's care is a highly important primary and adjunctive treatment of any painful condition. There is ample physiological, anatomical and behavioral support for the concept that higher cognitive processes generated within the brain may activate descending inhibitory systems and significantly attenuate both pain perception and the affective dimension of pain (Melzack and Casey, 1967).

When all reasonable non-invasive measures for pain relief have been tried and found unsatisfactory, it is appropriate to consider surgical procedures that modify central nervous system function. Stim-

ulation epidurally of spinal structures, presumably the larger diameter fibers, may be advocated for certain disorders (Long and Erickson, 1975), but patient selection is a critical determinant of the success of this procedure (Long et al., 1981). Among other neurosurgeons, there seems to be a greater enthusiasm for the effectiveness of electrical stimulation within the thalamus or internal capsule for the relief of intractable pain (Adams et al., 1974; Boivie and Meyerson, 1982; Hosobuchi, 1983).

If these 'neuroaugmentive procedures' are not effective or appropriate, dorsal root entry zone (DREZ) lesions may be recommended where the pain is localized within a segmental distribution (Nashold, 1979). Lesions within the primary thalamic or cortical somatosensory pathways produce a contralateral hypesthesia which is unacceptable for many patients. Sweet (1980) and Bouckoms (1984) have reviewed the evidence regarding the use of lesions within non-sensory subcortical and cortical structures that are functionally and anatomically related to the limbic system. Such lesions may relieve the patient of the affective component of chronic pain while preserving somatosensory discriminative functions, including the ability to recognize acute pain. Suprabulbar lesions for pain, however, are often reserved for patients with terminal disease.

In summary, it is apparent that increased nociceptive or other abnormal inputs may lead to changes in the excitability of central cells. These changes are not permanent, so near as can be determined by clinical examination, but they may sustain the painful condition beyond the period of acute disease and contribute significantly to the continuation of painful neuropathy. Whether denervation itself contributes significantly to increased central excitability and pain is not entirely clear, but there is little doubt that removal of some inputs to the dorsal horn will deprive the nervous system of another mechanism for inhibitory control over nociceptive input. The goal of therapy is to reduce the abnormal excitability of central nervous system cells by pharmacological, psychological or, if necessary, surgical intervention.

Concluding comments

Independent and interacting pathological processes may affect the peripheral nervous system at various points along the information transmission system, leading to persistent pain. At each level, different therapies can be directed at the pathological processes contributing to the pain. Receptors may be pathologically sensitized by the combined actions of the inflammatory process and sympathetic efferents, suggesting the use of anti-inflammatory agents and alpha adrenergic blockade. Axons, ganglion cells, nerve roots and the nervi nervorum may generate increased nociceptive or other abnormal inputs as a result of structural and biochemical changes induced by local or systemic pathology. In addition to medical or surgical therapies directed at the primary pathologic etiology, impulse blockade by local anesthesia or by sodium channel-inactivating anticonvulsants may be beneficial. Because persistent painful pathology may lead to central changes that tend to sustain the pain, it is appropriate to employ a variety of pharmacologic, physical and psychological measures to reduce the nociceptive excitability of central cells. If all other measures have failed to yield adequate relief, it may be necessary to resort to surgical intervention in the form of selectively stimulating or destroying portions of the central nervous system. In all cases, the therapeutic approach to the difficult problem of painful neuropathy may be improved by considering all the pathophysiologic processes involved in each case and directing therapy accordingly.

References

Adams, J.E., Hosobuchi, Y. and Fields, H.L. (1974) Stimulation of internal capsule for relief of chronic pain. J. Neurosurg., 41:740–744.

Aldskogius, H., Arvidsson, J. and Grant, G. (1985) The reaction of primary sensory neurons to peripheral nerve injury with particular emphasis on transganglionic changes. Brain Res. Rev., 10:27–46.

Archer, A.G., Watkins, P.J., Thomas, P.K., Sharma, A.K. and Payan, J (1983) The natural history of acute painful neuropathy in diabetes mellitus. J. Neurol. Neurosurg. Psychiatr., 46:491–499.

Asbury, A.K. and Fields, H.L. (1984) Pain due to peripheral nerve damage: An hypothesis. Neurology, 34:1587–1590.

Bada, J.L., Cervera, C. and Padro, L. (1977) Carbamazepine for amyloid neuropathy. New Engl. J. Med., 296:396.

Basbaum, A.I. and Fields, H.L. (1978) Endogenous pain control mechanisms: review and hypothesis. Ann. Neurol., 4:451–462.

Basbaum, A.I. and Fields, H.L. (1984) Endogenous pain control systems: Brainstem spinal pathways and endorphin circuitry. Annu. Rev. Neurosci. 7:309–338.

Blumber, H. and Janig, W. (1984) Discharge pattern of afferent fibers from a neuroma. Pain, 20:335–353.

Boivie, J. and Meyerson, B.A. (1982) A correlative anatomical and clinical study of pain suppression by deep brain stimulation. Pain, 13:113–126.

Bonica, J.J. (1979) Causalgia and other reflex sympathetic dystrophies. In J.J. Bonica, J.C. Liebeskind and D.G. Albe-Fessard (Eds.), Adv. Pain Res. Ther., Vol. 3, Raven Press, NY, pp. 141–166.

Botney, M. and Fields, H.L. (1983) Amitriptyline potentiates morphine analgesia by a direct action on the central nervous system. Ann. Neurol., 13:160–164.

Bouckoms, A.J. (1984) Psychosurgery. In P.D. Wall and R. Melzack (Eds.), Textbook of Pain, Churchill-Livingstone, Edinburgh, pp. 666–676.

Brenan, A. (1986) Collateral reinnervation of skin by C-fibres following nerve injury in the rat. Brain Res., 385:152–155.

Brinkhus, H.B. and Zimmerman, M. (1983) Characteristics of spinal dorsal horn neurons after partial chronic deafferentation by dorsal root transection. Pain, 15:221–236.

Brown, A.G., Fyffer, E.W., Noble, R. and Row, M.J. (1984) Effects of hindlimb nerve section on lumbosacral dorsal horn neurones in the cat. J. Physiol. (London), 354:375–394.

Brown, M.J., Martin, J. and Asbury, A.K. (1976) Painful diabetic neuropathy: a morphometric study. Arch. Neurol., 33:164–171.

Burchiel, K.J. (1984) Effects of electrical and mechanical stimulation on two foci of spontaneous activity which develop in primary afferent neurons after peripheral axotomy. Pain, 18:249–265.

Chernetski, K.E. (1964) Sympathetic enhancement of peripheral sensory input in the frog. J. Neurophysiol., 27:493–515.

Coderre, T.J. and Melzack, R. (1985) Increased pain sensitivity following heat injury involves a central mechanism. Behav. Brain Res., 15:259–262.

Coderre, T.J. and Melzack, R. (1987) Cutaneous hyperalgesia: contributions of the peripheral and central nervous systems to the increase in pain sensitivity after injury. Brain Res., 404:95–106.

Cook, A.J., Woolf, C.J., Wall, P.D. and McMahon, S.B. (1987) Dynamic receptive field plasticity in rat spinal cord dorsal horn following C-primary afferent input. Nature, 325:151–153.

Devor, M. and Bernstein, J.J. (1982) Abnormal impulse generation in neuromas: Electrophysiology and ultrastructure. In W.J. Culp and J. Ochoa (Eds), Abnormal Nerves and Muscles as Impulse Generators, Oxford, NY, pp. 363–380.

Dyck, P.J., Lambert, E.H. and O'Brien, P.C. (1976) Pain in peripheral neuropathy related to rate and kind of fiber degeneration. Neurology, 26:466–471.

Ekbom, K. (1972) Carbamazepine in the treatment of tabetic lightning pains. Arch. Neurol., 26:374–378.

Evans, J.A. (1947) Reflex sympathetic dystrophy: report of 57 cases. Ann. Int. Med., 26:417:426.

Fitzgerald, M. and Woolf, C.J. (1981) Effects of cutaneous nerve and intraspinal conditioning on C-fibre afferent terminal excitability in decerebrate spinal rats. J. Physiol. (London), 318:25–39.

Forrest, W.H., Jr., Brown, B.W., Jr., Brown, C.R., Defalque, R., Gold, M., Gordon, H.E., James, K.E., Katz, J., Mahler, D.L., Schroff, P. and Teutsch, G. (1977) Dextroamphetamine with morphine for the treatment of post-operative pain. N. Engl. J. Med., 296:712–715.

Fromm, G.H. and Glass, J.D. (1977) The effect of tricyclic antidepressants on corticofugal inhibition of the spinal trigeminal nucleus. Electroencephalogr. Clin. Neurophysiol., 43:637–645.

Fromm, G.H., Terrence, C.F. and Maroon, J.C. (1984) Trigeminal neuralgia: current concepts regarding etiology and pathogenesis. Arch. Neurol., 41:1204–1207.

Ghostine, S.Y., Comair, Y.G., Turner, D.M., Kassell, N.F. and Azar, C.G. (1984) Phenoxybenzamine in the treatment of causalgia. J. Neurosurg., 60:1263–1268.

Gilliatt, R.W. and Harrison, M.J.G. (1984) Nerve compression and entrapment. In A.K. Asbury and R.W. Gilliatt (Eds), Peripheral Nerve Disorders, Butterworth's, London, pp. 243–286.

Govrin-Lippmann, R. and Devor, M. (1978) Ongoing activity in severed nerves: source and variation with time. Brain Res., 159:406–410.

Guilbaud, G., Kayser, V., Benoist, J.M. and Gautron, M. (1986) Modifications in the responsiveness of rat ventrobasal thalamic neurons at different stages of carrageenin-produced inflammation. Brain Res., 385:86–98.

Guilbaud, G., Peschanski, M., Briand, A. and Gautron, M. (1986) The organization of spinal pathways to vetrobasal thalamus in an experimental model of pain (the arthritic rat). An electrophysiological study Pain, 26:301–312.

Hannington-Kiff, J.G. (974) Pain Relief, Lippincott, Philadelphia, pp. 68–79.

Hentall, I.D. and Fields, H.L. (1979) Segmental and descending influences on intraspinal thresholds of single C-fibers. J. Neurophysiol., 42:1527–1537.

Homans, J. (1940) Minor causalgia: a hyperesthetic neurovascular syndrome. New Engl. J. Med., 222:870–874.

Horch, K.W. and Lisney, S.J.W. (1981) Changes in primary afferent depolarization of sensory neurones during peripheral nerve regeneration in the cat. J. Physiol. (London), 313:287–299.

Hosobuchi, Y. (1983) Combined electrical stimulation of the periaqueductal gray matter and sensory thalamus. Appl. Neurophysiol., 46:112–115.

Huskisson, E.C. (1984) Non-narcotic analgesics. In P.D. Wall and R. Melzack (Eds), Textbook of Pain, Churchill-Livingstone, Edinburgh, pp. 505–513.

Kastrup, J., Petersen, P., Dejgard, A., Angelo, H.R. and Hilsted, J. (1987) Intravenous lidocaine infusion – a new treatment of chronic painful diabetic neuropathy? Pain, 28:69–75.

Kerr, F.W.L. (1983) Central nervous system changes and deafferentation pain: the role of reorganization and gliosis. In J.J. Bonica, U. Lindblom and A. Iggo (Eds), Adv. Pain Res. Ther., Vol. 5, Raven Press, NY, pp. 663–675.

Kozin, F., McCarthy, D.J., Sims, J. and Genant, H. (1976) The reflex sympathetic dystrophy syndrome. I. Clinical and histologic studies: evidence for bilaterality, response to corticosteroids and articular involvement. Am. J. Med., 60:321–331.

LeBars, D., Dickenson, A.H. and Besson, J.-M. (1979) Diffuse noxious inhibitory controls (DNIC). I. Effects on dorsal horn convergent neurones in the rat. Pain, 6:283–304.

Lindblom, U. (1984) Neuralgia: mechanisms and therapeutic prospects. In C. Bennedetti, C.R. Chapman and G. Monnica (Eds.), Adv. Pain Res. Ther., Vol. 7, Raven Press, NY, pp. 427–438.

Loeser, J.D. and Ward, A.A. (1967) Some effects of deafferentation on neurons of the cat spinal cord. Arch. Neurol., 17:629–636.

Loeser, J.D., Ward, A.A. and White, L.E. (1968) Chronic deafferentation of human spinal cord neurons. J. Neurosurg., 29:48–50.

Loewenstein, W.R. (1956) Modulation of cutaneous mechanoreceptors by sympathetic stimulation. J. Physiol. (London), 136:40–60.

Loh, L. and Nathan, P.W. (1978) Painful peripheral states and sympathetic blocks. J. Neurol. Neurosurg. Psychiatr., 41:664–671.

Long, D.M. and Erickson, D. (1975) Stimulation of the posterior columns of the spinal cord for relief of intractable pain. Surg. Neurol., 4:134–141.

Long, D.M., Erickson, D. Campbell, J. and North, R. (1981) Electrical stimulation of the spinal cord and peripheral nerves for pain control: 10 years experience. Appl. Neurophysiol., 44:207–217.

Long, R.R. (1977) Sensitivity of cutaneous cold fibers to noxious heat: paradoxical cold discharge. J. Neurophysiol., 40:489–502.

Lundeberg, T. (1984) The pain suppressive effect of vibratory stimulation and transcutaneous electrical nerve stimulation (TENS) as compared to aspirin. Brain Res., 294:201–210.

Maceiwicz, R., Bouckoms, A. and Martin, J.B. (1985) Drug therapy of neuropathic pain. Clin. J. Pain, 1:39–49.

Malow, R.M. and Olson, R.E. (1981) Changes in pain perception after treatment for chronic pain. Pain, 11:65–72.

Max, M.B., Culnane, M., Schafer, S.C., Gracely, R.H., Walther, D.J., Smoller, B. and Dubner, R. (1987) Amitriptyline relieves diabetic neuropathy pain in patients with normal or depressed mood. Neurology, 37:589–596.

McLean, M.J. and Macdonald, R.L. (1983) Multiple actions of phenytoin on mouse spinal cord neurons in cell culture. J. Pharmacol. Exp. Ther., 227:779–789.

McLean, M.J. and Macdonald, R.L. (1986) Carbamazepine and 10,11-epoxycarbamazepine produce use- and voltage-dependent limitation of rapidly firing action potentials of mouse central neurons in cell culture. J. Pharmacol. Exp. Ther., 238:727–738.

Melzack, R. and Casey, K.L. (1968) Sensory, motivational and central control determinants of pain. In D.R. Kenshalo (Ed.), The Skin Senses, C.C. Thomas, Springfield, pp. 423–439.

Mendell, L.M. (1984) Modifiability of spinal synapses. Physiol. Rev., 64:260–324.

Meyer, G.A. and Fields, H.L. (1972) Causalgia treated by selective large fiber stimulation of peripheral nerve. Brain, 95:163–168.

Nashold, B.S., Jr. and Ostdahl, R.H. (1979) Dorsal root entry zone lesions for pain relief. J. Neurosurg., 51:59–69.

Nathan, P.W. and Wall, P.D. (1974) Treatment of post-herpetic neuralgia by prolonged electric stimulation. Br. Med. J., 3:645–647.

Nixon, B.J., Doucette, R., Jackson, P.C. and Diamond, J. (1984) Impulse activity evokes precocious sprouting of nociceptive nerves into denervated skin. Somatosens. Res., 2:97–126.

Perl, E.R., Kumazawa, T., Lynn, B. and Kenins, P. (1976) Sensitization of high threshold receptors with unmyelinated (C) afferent fibers. In A. Iggo and O.B. Ilyinsky (Eds.), Somatosensory and Visceral Receptor Mechanisms, Progress in Brain Research, Vol. 43, Elsevier, Amsterdam, pp. 263–276.

Portenoy, R.K., Duma, C. and Foley, K.M. (1986) Acute herpetic and postherpetic neuralgia: Clinical review and current management. Ann. Neurol. 20:651–664.

Pubols, L.M. (1984) The boundary of proximal hindlimb representation in the dorsal horn following peripheral nerve lesions in cats: A reevaluation of plasticity in the somatotopic map. Somatosens. Res. 2:19–32.

Pubols, L.M. and Brenowitz, G.L. (1982) Maintenance of dorsal horn somatotopic organization and increased high-threshold response after single-root or spared-root deafferentation in cats. J. Neurophysiol., 47:103–112.

Pubols, L.M. and Golberger, M.E. (1980) Recovery of function in dorsal horn following partial deafferentation. J. Neurophysiol., 43:102–117.

Roberts, W.J. (1986) A hypothesis on the physiological basis for causalgia and related pains. Pain, 24:297–311.

Roberts, W.J. and Elardo, S.M. (1985) Sympathetic activation of A-delta nociceptors. Somatosens. Res., 3:33–44.

Roberts, W.J., Elardo, S.M. and King, K.A. (1985) Sympathetically induced changes in the responses of slowly adapting type I receptors in cat skin. Somatosens. Res., 2:223–236.

Ross, S.B. and Renyi, A.L. (1967) Inhibition of uptake of tritiated catecholamines by antidepressants and related drugs. Eur. J. Pharmacol., 2:181–186.

Sawynok, J. (1987) GABAergic mechanisms of analgesia: an update. Pharmacol. Biochem. Behav., 26:463–474.

Schumacker, H.B. (1948) Causalgia III. A general discussion. Surgery, 24:485–504.

Schwartzman, R.J. and McLellan, T.L. (1987) Reflex sympathetic dystrophy. A review, Arch. Neurol., 44:555–561.

Seltzer, Z. and Devor, M. (1979) Ephaptic transmission in chronically damaged peripheral nerves. Neurology, 29:1061–1064.

Spiegel, K., Kalb, R. and Pasternak, G.W. (1983) Analgesic activity of tricyclic antidepressants. Ann. Neurol., 13:462–465.

Steinbrocker, O. (1947) Shoulder-hand syndrome. Am. J. Med., 3:402–407.

Sweet, W.H. (1980) Central mechanisms of chronic pain (neuralgias and certain other neurogenic pain). In J. J. Bonica (Ed.), Pain. Assoc. Res. Nerv. Ment. Dis., Vol. 58, Raven Press, NY, pp. 287–303.

Sweet, W.H. (1984) Deafferentation pain after posterior rhizotomy, trauma to a limb, and herpes zoster. Neurosurgery 15:928–932.

Sweet, W.H. (1987a) Deafferentation pain in man. Applied Neurophysiol., (in press).

Sweet, W.H. (1987b) Sympathectomy for pain. In J.R. Youmans (Ed.), Neurological Surgery, 3rd edn., W.B. Saunders, PA, (in press).

Swerdlow, M. and Cundill, J.G. (1981) Anticonvulsant drugs used in the treatment of lancinating pain. A comparison. Anesthesia, 36:1129–1132.

Tasker, R.R. (1984) Deafferentation. In P.D. Wall and R. Melzack (Eds.), Textbook of Pain, Churchill-Livingstone, Edinburgh, pp. 119–132.

Thomas, P.K. (1982) Pain in peripheral neuropathy: clinical and morphological aspects. In W. Culp and J. Ochoa (Eds.), Abnormal Nerves and Muscles as Impulse Generators, Oxford Univ. Press, NY, pp. 553–567.

Wall, P.D. and Gutnick, M. (1974) Ongoing activity in peripheral nerves: The physiology and pharmacology of impulses originating from a neuroma. Exp. Neurol., 43:580–593.

Wall, P.D. and Sweet, W.H. (1967) Temporary abolition of pain in man. Science, 155:108–109.

Wall, P.D. and Devor, M. (1981) The effect of peripheral nerve injury on dorsal root potentials and on transmission of afferent signals into the spinal cord. Brain Res., 209:95–111.

Watson, C.P., Evans, R.J., Reed, K., Merskey, H., Goldsmith, L. and Warsh, J. (1982) Amitriptyline vs. placebo in postherpetic neuralgia. Neurology, 32:671–673.

Woolf, C.J. and Wall, P.D. (1982) Chronic peripheral nerve section diminishes the primary afferent A-fibre mediated inhibition of rat dorsal horn neurones. Brain Res., 242:77–86.

Woolf, C.J. (1984) Long term alterations in the excitability of the flexion reflex produced by peripheral tissue injury in the chronic decerebrate rat. Pain, 18:325–343.

Wynn Parry, C.B. (1980) Pain in avulsion lesions of the brachial plexus. Pain, 9:41–53.

Zimmerman, M. and Sanders, K. (1982) Responses of nerve axons and receptor endings to heat, ischemia, and algesic substances. Abnormal excitability of regenerating nerve endings. In W.J. Culp and J. Ochoa (Eds.), Abnormal Nerves and Muscles as Impulse Generators, Oxford, NY, pp. 513–532.

Musculoskeletal, Vascular and Visceral Pains

R. Dubner, G.F. Gebhart & M.R. Bond (Eds.)
Proceedings of the Vth World Congress on Pain
© 1988 Elsevier Science Publishers BV (Biomedical Division)

CHAPTER 20

The trigeminovascular system and pain mechanisms from cephalic blood vessels

Michael A. Moskowitz, Kiyoshi Saito, Damianos E. Sakas and Stephen Markowitz

Stroke Research Laboratory, Neurosurgery and Neurology Services, Massachusetts General Hospital, Harvard Medical School, Boston, MA 02114, USA

Introduction

Few topics in neurology are as controversial as the pathophysiology of migraine headaches. Wolff and his colleagues proposed that dilation of cephalic vessels caused the headaches of migraine (Graham and Wolff, 1938; Wolff, 1948). Wolff based his notions about pain upon pulse amplitude measurements of extracranial cephalic vessels. During the painful phase, increases in arterial pulsations were recorded. After headache relief by ergotamine tartrate administration, the pulse amplitude decreased. Wolff reasoned that pain was caused by stretching and distension of the arteries, and that ergotamine tartrate, a well-known smooth muscle contractor, relieved headaches by causing vasoconstriction. This explanation for both the cause of pain and the mechanism of ergot action became widely accepted and, in fact, continues to be embraced by both patients and doctors alike – despite (a) the reported failure of others to reproduce the characteristic amplitude tracings during pain (Heyck, 1956), (b) the publication of alternative interpretations of Wolff's own data (Blau, 1987), (c) the failure of more recent studies to identify characteristic blood flow increases with headache or to find a temporal correlation with pain when increases occurred (Lauritzen et al., 1983), and (d) the development of ergot preparations with minimal vasoconstrictor properties which relieve migraine headaches. This controversy

notwithstanding, Wolff's contributions to the study of headache remain monumental!

Very little is known about initiating stimuli. Numerous studies implicating circulating vasoactive molecules such as histamine, serotonin and small, biologically active peptides have not been validated. Sex hormones have been implicated in some forms of headache, particularly those that occur just before and during the menstrual periods. Severe mechanical stretch can depolarize sensory fibers and cause pain, but probably not to the degree required during most migraine headaches. One of the most reliable initiators is the migraine aura. In this instance, the pain characteristically follows 15–30 min after the onset of the focal neurological deficit, and is most often felt over the hemisphere causing the symptoms. The mechanism remains obscure. Despite incompleteness in our knowledge concerning the exact pathophysiology, vascular head pain specifies activation of a final common pain pathway involving depolarization of perivascular sensory axons. It follows, therefore, that a better understanding of migraine headaches can be achieved by paying particular attention to the anatomy, chemistry, physiology and pharmacology of sensory connections to cephalic blood vessels.

Some important background issues concerning the source of pain and initiating stimuli deserve comment. Most throbbing headaches are presumed to arise from a disturbance in cephalic blood vessels. This notion is inferred from the observations that similar headaches are associated with strokes, aneurysms and arteriovenous malformations, and from the demonstrations by Ray and Wolff, Penfield and others that blood vessels (dural and pial) are the only structures within the cranium which cause pain when stimulated, and that the symptoms elicited resemble those described by patients with vascular head pain (Penfield and McNaughton, 1940; Penfield, 1935; Ray and Wolff, 1940).

In the first part of this chapter, we review recent information concerning the source, distribution and neurotransmitter content of afferent projections to cephalic blood vessels, and describe how the established innervation in animals may relate to the localization and referral of vascular headaches in man. Next we will consider recent neurophysiological evidence establishing that electrical or chemical stimulation of these afferents activates units within the trigeminal nucleus caudalis. Some of these responding units exhibit properties of wide-dynamic-range neurons and receive a convergent input from cutaneous receptive fields within the first trigeminal division. Finally, we will examine evidence that depolarization of sensory fibers within the dura provokes neurogenic plasma extravasation in this tissue, and that ergot alkaloids useful in treating headaches block this response.

Anatomy

Retrograde and orthograde axonal tracing studies using horseradish peroxidase, wheat germ agglutinin or fluorescent dyes, or immunohistochemistry determined that the feline (Keller et al., 1985; Liu-Chen et al., 1984; Mayberg et al., 1981, 1984) guinea pig (Yamamoto et al., 1983), rat (Arbab et al., 1986) and gerbil (Matsuyama et al., 1985) pial vessels of Willis's circle and dural vessels receive a rich sensory innervation from the trigeminal ganglia. The innervation pattern (Fig. 1) is remarkably similar for the four species and resembles the findings expected in man if similar experiments were possible. These findings are summarized by the follow-

ing. For vessels which course away from the midline (e.g., the middle meningeal and middle cerebral arteries), projecting neurons are located in the ipsilateral ganglia, most often in the medial aspect corresponding to the first division. For vessels which course close to the midline (especially the anterior cerebral artery and sagittal sinus) projecting neurons are located in the same region but are represented bilaterally. On average, less than 100 cells are labelled per ganglia, although somewhat larger numbers are found for dural vessels. Projecting neurons tend not to cluster; rather, individual labelled cells lie in close approximation to those unlabelled neurons projecting to the forehead. Divergent axon collaterals supplying the intra- and extracranial arteries are rarely found, although widely branching axons supplying more than a single major pial artery are the rule rather than the exception (Borges and Moskowitz, 1983; McMahon et al., 1985). Some branching axons reportedly supply both pial and dural blood vessels (O'Connor and Van der Kooy, 1986). When one considers that the external carotid artery supplies the dura mater (in large part) whereas the internal carotid system supplies the circle of Willis, this arrangement suggests several intriguing possibilities for coupling sensory and motor functions in the two circulations.

It seems likely that sensory fibers course from the proximal to the distal portion of the vessel, and probably join the carotid system at the level of the cavernous sinus. Compatible with this notion are the findings that fewer labelled cells were present in the trigeminal ganglia following tracer application to the distal segments of the middle cerebral artery over the convexities, and retrograde labelling was abolished by placing a ligature around the middle cerebral artery proximal to the site of application.

The origin and distribution of perivascular afferents suggest several of the following unique explanations for vascular headache patterns experienced by man.

(a) The finding that the vertebral and basilar arteries are innervated by upper cervical dorsal root segments and that the rostral circulation is innervated by the trigeminal nerve explains the occipital and frontal locations of pain for diseases involving these two circulations, respectively.

(b) The predominantly ipsilateral distribution of trigeminal fibers explains the strictly ipsilateral location of many vascular headaches. (A strictly unilateral headache seems difficult to reconcile with headache theories which promote the importance of circulating substances. If substances in the vessel lumen are important, an additional factor(s) must also be present which independently modulates the two trigeminal systems.)

(c) The bilateral innervation of certain vessels suggests the possibility that disturbances within individual vessels can cause bilateral headaches, and may even give rise to headache on the 'wrong side'.

(d) The trigeminal innervation of the superior cerebellar artery provides an explanation for the frontal headache experienced by patients with cerebellar tumors.

(e) The dual innervation of the superior cerebellar, as well as of rostral basilar arteries (i.e., from upper cervical dorsal roots and trigeminal fibers), provides an anatomical basis for the co-existence of occipital and frontal headaches, a second alternative to the convergence of descending trigeminal impulses with inputs from upper cervical cord segments.

(f) The observation that some dural and pial arteries receive divergent axon collaterals from single trigeminal neurons may account for the difficulties

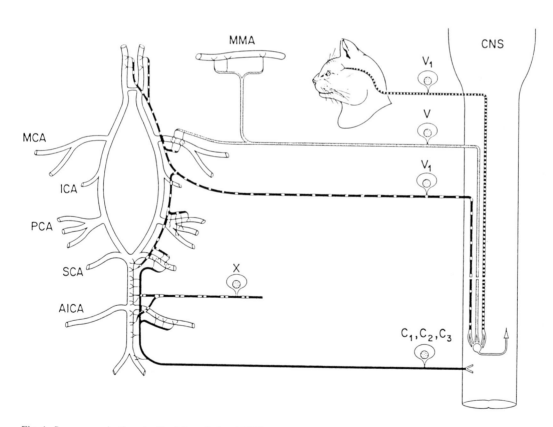

Fig. 1. Sensory projections to the feline circle of Willis. The trigeminal neurons (V_1) send axonal projections to the circle of Willis as shown. Some ganglion cells which innervate the circle of Willis also project to dural vessels (MMA). A separate population of ganglion cells innervate extracranial cephalic vessels (top ganglion cell). Ganglia cells in upper cervical DRG and superior vagal ganglia innervate the most caudal vessels (bottom ganglion cells).

in distinguishing between pain of dural or pial origin (i.e., the same neuron depolarizes with appropriate stimulation in both circulations).

Recent unpublished studies examining the transganglionic transport of wheat germ agglutinin-labelled horseradish peroxidase documented reaction product predominantly (but not exclusively) within the most caudal aspect of trigeminal nucleus caudalis after label had been placed around the superior sagittal sinus. Transported protein was particularly concentrated within laminae I and II, just above the level of C_1. Significant overlap existed between these sites and axon terminations from fibers within the supraorbital nerve. Such an arrangement suggests the possibility that visceral and somatic afferents converge onto individual sensory neurons to underlie the phenomenon of cutaneous referral of visceral pain. Recent electrophysiological data appear to support this possibility (see below).

Trigeminovascular chemistry

Results of trigeminal lesioning studies recently confirmed the existence of sensory projections to cephalic arteries, and have identified substance P and other sensory peptides within these perivascular fibers (Edvinsson et al., 1981; Edvinsson and Uddman, 1987; Liu-Chen et al., 1983; Norregaard and Moskowitz, 1985; Saito et al., 1987b). The list of contained peptides now includes neurokinin A (a tachykinin made from the same gene precursor as substance P) (Saito et al., 1987a), calcitonin gene-related peptide (CGRP, a 37-amino-acid-containing peptide formed by alternative processing of the calcitonin gene) (McCulloch et al., 1986), and perhaps cholecystokinin-8 (Liu-Chen et al., 1986b). Substance P and CGRP coexist within trigeminovascular fibers as they do in other neuropeptide-containing pathways. But unlike CGRP, only half the substance P is contained within sensory axons. The source of the remaining 50% is unknown, but most likely it is of parasympathetic origin. All three peptides are potent vasodilators (McCulloch et al., 1986; Moskowitz et al., 1987a); the tachykinins

promote leakage of plasma proteins from post-capillary venules as well (Markowitz et al., 1988; Saria et al., 1983).

Based on a recently published immunoelectron micrographic study, substance P is contained within finely varicosed small-diameter (200 nm), widely branching, unmyelinated axons which lie both perpendicular and parallel to the long axis of pial blood vessels (Liu-Chen et al., 1986a). These fibers traverse the adventitial lamina to reach the smooth muscle junction. At this location, immunopositive axons and axon terminations lie adjacent to those of adrenergic and cholinergic origin, but exhibit no unusual membrane specializations or apparent connections to autonomic fibers, and contain a relative abundance of mitochondria and vesicles (Matsuyama et al., 1985). Surrounding small blood vessels (especially venules) of the dura mater, unspecialized axon terminations lie close to both fenestrated and non-fenestrated endothelial cells (Andres et al., 1987).

The presence of neuropeptides within perivascular sensory fibers suggests the possibility that peptide release may occur upon depolarization. Indeed, substance P release from perivascular nerve fibers was demonstrated in vitro by high potassium or capsaicin by calcium-dependent mechanisms (Moskowitz et al., 1983). (The identification of specific receptors on these axons is one important and relevant area for future study.) In vivo evidence for release may be inferred from studies demonstrating that depolarization of dural afferents causes neurogenic plasma extravasation in the dura mater (Markowitz et al., 1988), and that sensory fibers reduce the extent of norepinephrine-induced vasoconstriction and enhance plasma extravasation associated with severe hypertension and breakdown of the blood brain barrier (Moskowitz et al., 1988).

The increases in immunoreactive substance P and CGRP which reportedly occur within draining veins during unilateral trigeminal stimulation in cat and man provide evidence of transmitter release from peripheral afferents (Edvinsson et al., 1987). The contribution of perivascular afferents to this increase remains to be determined.

Neurogenic inflammation

It has been postulated that the trigeminovascular system is part of an elaborate defensive network protecting the brain both from the entry of noxious substances in the circulation and from such substances within brain (Moskowitz, 1984; Moskowitz et al., 1979). As described above, nerve fibers are situated at the interface between the circulation and the brain and surround cerebral blood vessels in close proximity to all three vessel layers. In this location, trigeminal fibers can sample continuously the microenvironment of the blood vessel wall. Like some primary sensory neurons in other organs, trigeminal nerves are critical initiators and promotors of tissue inflammation (Couture and Cuello, 1984; Jancso et al., 1967). Neural activation releases vasoactive neurotransmitters from their afferent processes, which, in turn, provoke inflammatory changes in peripheral target tissues (in this instance the cephalic blood vessel). The mechanism is similar to that described as part of the axon reflex or axon response, and presumably localizes, dilutes and clears offending toxins or foreign substances before they extend beyond their focus of origin or portal of entry.

Neurogenic inflammation accompanies antidromic electrical stimulation of sensory fibers or follows mechanical or chemical (capsaicin) stimulation of these same fibers (Couture and Cuello, 1984). Dilation and plasma leakage occur almost exclusively in those tissues possessing tachykinin-containing perivascular fibers and can be attenuated by tachykinin receptor blockers or drugs which inhibit neuropeptide release (Lembeck et al., 1982; Lembeck and Donnerer, 1985; Lundberg et al., 1983).

Utilizing ^{125}I-serum albumin as a tracer for plasma protein, extravasation was detected in the dura mater and conjunctiva, but not temporalis muscle or brain following capsaicin administration or unilateral electrical trigeminal stimulation (Markowitz et al., 1988). Plasma extravasation was C-fiber-dependent, since leakage did not develop in adult animals in which C-fibers were destroyed as neonates by capsaicin treatment. Substance P and neurokinin A but not CGRP also caused plasma extravasation in normal adult animals and animals lacking C-fibers.

The importance of neurogenic inflammation to migraine headaches remains to be determined (Hardebo, 1984), but its possible significance may be inferred from one previous report suggesting that 'sterile inflammation' develops in vessel walls during migraine headaches (Ostfeld et al., 1955), and recent data showing that ergot alkaloids useful for treating headaches block neurogenic plasma extravasation in the dura mater (Saito et al. 1987c). What initiates this response remains to be determined, but, based on the schema in Fig. 1, the appropriate stimulus may develop in or around the pial or dural circulations.

Ergot alkaloids

Ergot extracts from the fungus *Claviceps purpurea* have been prescribed for migraine headaches for more than 100 years, although these compounds were not widely used until after ergotamine tartrate had been chemically purified in 1926. Ergotamine tartrate and dihydroergotamine are the two ergot preparations most useful for treating the acute headache. Methysergide, a third ergot derivative, is effective only for prophylaxis when administered chronically. Ergot alkaloids are related chemically to LSD, lysergic acid diethylamide, and contain an indole ring structure and a peptide moiety. All three drugs act as both serotonin agonists and antagonists and effect all three putative serotonin receptor sites ($5HT_{1,2,3}$) (Richardson and Engel, 1986). Actions at adrenergic and histaminergic receptors have also been demonstrated (Berde and Schild, 1978).

When administered in clinically relevant doses, both dihydroergotamine and ergotamine tartrate blocked the development of neurogenic plasma extravasation (NPE) within the dura mater (Saito et al., 1987c). Blockade of plasma extravasation was achieved in the model following either capsaicin injection or unilateral trigeminal electrical stimulation. Blockade was not achieved by single injections of methysergide, however, but was achieved by chronic daily treatment. The ergot action could not be accounted for by vasoconstriction alone, since NPE was not blocked by angiotensin or phenylephrine, and the ergots did not block the plasma extravasation induced by administering sensory neuropeptides. Taken together, these findings are most compatible with the notion that ergots block neurogenic inflammation within intracranial vascular tissues by a C-fiber-dependent mechanism. Whether this action relates to the possible existence of presynaptic serotonin receptors on primary afferent fibers remains to be determined.

Electrophysiology

Two recent reports have helped to clarify the relationship between trigeminovascular neurons and pain mechanisms from dural blood vessels (Strassman et al., 1986; Davis and Dostrovsky, 1986). In these studies, extracellular responses were recorded from medullary trigeminal neurons predominantly within the nucleus caudalis following stimulation of cephalic blood vessels electrically or chemically (bradykinin, potassium) (Strassman et al., 1987) or mechanically (intravascular balloon dilation). Following dural shock, responses were most often elicited when the stimulus closely approximated dural blood vessels – an observation similar to headache pain in humans accompanying dural stimulation. The latency of the response was approximately 11 ms, suggesting transmission along either A-delta or C fibers. The majority of responding units were also activated by nociceptive stimulation in the cutaneous trigeminal distribution, particularly in the ipsilateral periorbital area, and were either wide-dynamic-range or nociceptive-specific in type. Responding cells were most commonly identified in laminae 1, 2 and 5 (Davis and Dostrovsky, 1986b). Visceral and somatic convergence on trigeminal nucleus caudalis neurons may provide a physiological substrate for the cutaneous referral of dural sensation.

Cutaneous nociceptive responses of trigeminal or spinal neurons can be inhibited by periaqueductal grey (PAG) stimulation and produce analgesia in a number of behavioral tests for pain. Visceral responses under PAG control are, at least in part, mediated through activation of raphe magnus neurons. The response of trigeminal cells to dural shock can be suppressed by PAG stimulation, thereby suggesting at least one mechanism by which trigeminal inputs are potentially modulated by activity within the central nervous system.

Integrating clinical and basic aspects

It seems intuitive that despite lack of exacting information regarding headache pathogenesis, headache pain must ultimately activate the trigeminovascular system. Accordingly, the perivascular primary sensory neuron may be viewed as a final common pathway subject to activation or modulation by local factors within the vessel lumen and vessel wall. At least theoretically, such a neuron may become modulated or even activated at various points along its length, from the axon terminals and axons in the blood vessel wall, to its central terminations within brain stem. Tables I and II outline a theoretical scheme for classifying triggers/modulators of vascular headaches based both on these assumptions and on recognized triggering agents. The list

TABLE I

The blood vessel wall – sensory nerve interaction

1. Biochemical modulation:	hormones
	mast cell constituents
	alcohol and drugs
	platelet contents
	food
2. Mechanical modulation:	stretch
3. Ionic modulation:	spreading depression
4. Neural modulation	opiate-containing fibers
	sympathetic
	parasympathetic

is not meant to be complete and the existence of more than a single action for each triggering agent need not be ruled out.

As noted in Table I, certain biochemical, mechanical, ionic and neural influences may raise or lower sensory fiber threshold at the blood vessel wall. Most of those listed are without direct experimental evidence at the present time. However, some modify sensory transmission in other paradigms. For example, injections of estrogen will enhance the size of the cutaneous receptive field of individual trigeminal fibers by direct effects on sensory nerve endings in the skin (Bereither et al., 1980). As another example, serotonin (platelet source?) can sensitize and potentiate the nociceptive effects of bradykinin. Severe mechanical stretch can activate the trigeminovascular system and cause pain, as demonstrated electrophysiologically and inferred from studies based on the vasomotor behavior of blood vessels following denervation (McCulloch et al., 1986; Moskowitz et al., 1988). If spreading depression is the neurophysiological event which underlies the migraine aura, then sensory fibers might depolarize passively as the result of marked changes which develop in the level of extracellular potassium, or at the end of the vasoconstriction phase which follows the spreading wave of depolarization. Adrenergic, cholinergic and peptidergic perivascular fibers may provide an additional modulating influence worthy of note. The ability of sympathetic nervous system to modulate pain is well known (Devor and Janig, 1981). That some perivascular fibers also contain a neuropeptide dynorphin (Moskowitz et al., 1987b) which modulates neurogenic inflammation and alters pain transmission may be relevant to pain mechanisms in blood vessels.

Table II lists some theoretical mechanisms which may modify trigeminovascular activity within the central nervous system. Stimulation of the periaqueductal grey has already been discussed. It seems intuitive that (a) the ability of light to provoke an attack of migraine, (b) the ability of sleep to trigger cluster headache and to relieve migraine headaches, and (c) the ability of stress to provoke headaches may relate, in part, to central modulation.

Conclusion

The better to understand and treat painful conditions, one needs to identify the cause, discover the source, and develop knowledge about aspects of peripheral and central pain transmission – and headaches are no exception. Some pathophysiological mechanisms have been proposed based on emerging principles of sensory neurobiology. The nature of vascular headaches will one day be understood when information obtained at the bedside and clinical laboratories fully integrates with emerging knowledge about pain from visceral organs.

Acknowledgements

We wish to especially acknowledge the important contributions of Dr. Raymond Maciewicz and Andrew Strassman of the Pain Physiology Laboratory at the Massachusetts General Hospital for helpful discussions. Some of the studies described in this chapter were supported by grants NS 10828 from the National Institutes of Neurological and Communicative Disorders and Stroke.

TABLE II
Central modulation of trigeminovascular transmission

1. Periaqueductal grey modulation	
2. Special senses:	light, sound
3. Altered physiological states:	sleep, stress
4. Spreading depression?	

References

Andres, K.H., von During, M., Muszynski, K. and Schmidt, R.F. (1987) Nerve fibers and their terminals of the dura mater encephali of the rat. Anat. Embryol., 175: 289–301.

Arbab, M.A.R., Wiklund, L. and Svendgaard, N.Aa. (1986) Origin and distribution of cerebral vascular innervation from superior cervical, trigeminal and spinal ganglia investigated with retrograde and anterograde WGA-HRP tracing in the rat. Neuroscience, 19: 695–708.

Berde, B. and Schild, H.O. (1978) Ergot alkaloids and related compounds, Springer-Verlag, New York.

Bereiter, D.A., Stanford, L.R. and Barker, D.J. (1980) Hormone-induced enlargement of receptive fields in trigeminal mechanoreceptive neurons. II. Possible mechanisms. Brain Res., 184: 411–423.

Blau, J.N. (1977) Migraine: a vasomotor instability of the meningeal circulation. Lancet ii: 1136–1139.

Borges, L.F. and Moskowitz, M.A. (1983) Do intracranial and extracranial trigeminal afferents represent divergent axon collaterals? Neurosci. Lett., 35: 265–270.

Couture, R. and Cuello, A.C. (1984) Studies on the trigeminal antidromic vasodilation and plasma extravasation in the rat. J. Physiol., 346: 273–285.

Davis, K.D, and Dostrovsky, J.O. (1986a) Activation of trigeminal brain-stem nociceptive neurons by dural artery stimulation. Pain, 25: 395–401.

Davis, K.D. and Dostrovsky, J.O. (1986b) Electrophysiological evidence for convergence of sagittal sinus, dural artery and cutaneous sensory information onto trigeminal brainstem neurons in the cat. Abstr. Soc. Neurosci., 230.

Devor, M. and Janig, W. (1981) Activation of myelinated afferents ending in a neuroma by stimulation of the sympathetic supply in the rat. Neurosci. Lett., 24: 43–47.

Edvinsson, L. and Uddman, R. (1982) Immunohistochemical localization and dilatory effect of substance P on human cerebral vessels. Brain Res., 232: 466–471.

Edvinsson, L., McCulloch, J. and Uddman, R. (1981) Substance P: immunohistochemical localization and effect upon cat pial arteries in vitro and in situ. J. Physiol., 318: 251–258.

Edvinsson, L., Ekman, R. and Goadsby, P.J. (1987) Release of vasoactive peptides from the trigeminovascular system of man and cat. Cephalalgia 7 (Suppl. 6): 10–12.

Graham, J.R. and Wolff, H.G. (1938) The circulation of the brain and spinal cord. Proc. A. Res. Nerv. Ment. Dis., 18: 638.

Hardebo, J.E. (1984) The involvement of trigeminal substance P neurons in cluster headache. A hypothesis. Headache, 24: 294–304.

Heyck, H. (1956) Neue Beitrage zur Klinik und Pathogenese der Migrane, Georg Thieme Verlag, Stuttgart.

Jancso, N., Jancso-Gabor, A. and Szolcsanyi, J. (1967) Direct evidence for neurogenic inflammation and its prevention by denervation and pretreatment with capsaicin. Br. J. Pharmac. Chemother., 31: 138–151.

Keller, J.T., Beduk, A. and Saunders, M.C. (1985) Origin of fibers innervating the basilar artery of the cat. Neurosci. Lett., 58: 263–268.

Lauritzen, M., Olsen, T.S., Lassen, N.A. and Paulson, O.B. (1983) Changes in regional cerebral blood flow during the course of classic migraine attacks. Ann. Neurol., 13: 633–641.

Lembeck, F., Donnerer, J. and Bartho, L. (1982) Inhibition of neurogenic vasodilation and plasma extravasation by substance P antagonists, somatostatin and [D-met^2,-pro^5]enkephalinamide. Eur. J. Pharmac., 85: 171–176.

Lembeck, F. and Donnerer, J. (1985) Opioid control of the function of primary afferent substance P fibers. Eur. J. Pharmac., 114: 241–246.

Liu-Chen, L.Y., Mayberg, M.R. and Moskowitz, M.A. (1983) Immunohistochemical evidence for a substance P-containing trigeminovascular pathway to pial arteries in cats. Brain Res., 268: 162–166.

Liu-Chen, L.Y., Gillespie, S.A., Norregaard, T.V. and Moskowitz, M.A. (1984) Co-localization of retrogradely transported wheat germ agglutinin and the putative neruotransmitter substance P within trigeminal ganglion cells projecting to cat middle cerebral artery. J. Comp. Neurol., 225: 187–192.

Liu-Chen, L.Y. Liszczak, T.M., King, J.C. and Moskowitz, M.A. (1986a) Immunoelectron microscopic study of substance P-containing fibers in feline cerebral arteries. Brain Res., 369: 12–20.

Liu-Chen, L.Y., Norregaard, T.V. and Moskowitz, M.A. (1986b) Some cholecystokinin-8 immunoreactive fibers in large pial arteries originate from trigeminal ganglion. Brain Res., 359: 166–176.

Lundberg, J.M., Brodin, E., Hua, X. and Saria, A. (1983) Vascular permeability changes and smooth muscle contraction in relation to capsaicin-sensitive substance P afferents in the guinea-pig. Acta Physiol. Scand., 120: 217–227.

Markowitz, S., Saito, K. and Moskowitz, M.A. (1988) Neurogenically mediated leakage of plasma protein occurs from blood vessels in dura mater but not brain. J. Neurosci., 7: 4129–4136.

Matsuyama, T., et al. (1984) Dual innervation of substance P-containing neuron system in the wall of the cerebral arteries. Brain Res., 322: 144–147.

Matsuyama, T., et al. (1985) Fine structure of peptidergic and catecholaminergic nerve fibers in the anterior cerebral artery and their interrelationship: an immunoelectron microscopic study. J. Comp. Neurol., 235: 268–276.

Mayberg, M.R., Langer, R.S., Zervas, N.T. and Moskowitz, M.A. (1981) Perivascular meningeal projections from cat trigeminal ganglia: possible pathway for vascular headaches in man. Science, 213: 228–230.

Mayberg, M.R., Zervas, N.T. and Moskowitz, M.A. (1984) Trigeminal projections to supratentorial pial and dural blood vessels in cats demonstrated by horseradish peroxidase histochemistry. J. Comp. Neurol. 223: 46–56.

McCulloch, J., Uddman, R., Kingman, T. and Edvinsson, L.

(1986) Calcitonin gene-related peptide: Functional role in cerebrovascular regulation. Proc. Natl. Acad. Sci. USA, 83: 5731–5735.

McMahon, M., Norregaard, T.V., Beyerl B.D., Borges, L.F. and Moskowitz, M.A. (1985) Trigeminal afferents to cerebral arteries and forehead are not divergent axon collaterals in cat. Neurosci. Lett., 60: 63–68.

Moskowitz, M.A. (1984) The neurobiology of vascular head pain. Ann. Neurol., 16: 157–168.

Moskowitz, M.A., Reinhard, J.F., Romero, J., et al. (1979) Neurotransmitters and the fifth cranial nerve: is there a relation to the headache phase of migraine. Lancet ii: 883–884.

Moskowitz, M.A., Brody, M. and Liu-Chen, L.Y. (1983) In vitro release of immunoreactive substance P from putative afferent nerve endings in bovine pia arachnoid. Neuroscience, 9: 809–814.

Moskowitz, M.A., Kuo, C., Leeman, S.E., Jessen, M.E. and Derian, C.K. (1987a) Desensitization to substance P-induced vasodilation in vitro is not shared by endogenous tachykinin neurokinin A.J. Neurosci., 7: 2344–2351.

Moskowitz, M.A., Saito, K., Brezina, L., and Dickson, J. (1987b) Nerve fibers surrounding intracranial and extracranial vessels from human and other species contain dynorphin-like immunoreactivity. Neuroscience, 23: 731–737.

Moskowitz, M.A., Wei, E.P., Saito, K. and Kontos, H.A. (1988) Pial arteriolar responses to hypertension or norepinephrine are modified by trigeminalectomy. Am. J. Physiol.

Norregaard, T.V. and Moskowitz, M.A. (1985) Substance P and the sensory innervation of intracranial and extracranial feline cephalic arteries. Brain, 108: 517–533.

O'Connor, T.P. and van der Kooy, D. (1986) Pattern of intracranial and extracranial projections of trigeminal ganglion cells. J. Neurosci., 6: 2200–2207.

Ostfeld, A.M., Reis, D.J., Goodell, H. and Wolff, H.G. (1955) Headache and hydration. Arch. Int. Med., 96: 142–152.

Penfield, W. (1935) A contribution to the mechanism of intracranial pain. Res. Nerv. Ment. Dis., 15: 399–436.

Penfield, W. and McNaughton, F. (1940) Dural headache and innervation of the dura mater. Arch. Neurol. Psychiatry, 44: 43–75.

Ray, B.S. and Wolff, H.G. (1940) Experimental studies on headache. Arch. Surg., 41: 813–856.

Richardson, B.P. and Engel, G. (1986) The pharmacology and function of 5-HT$_3$ receptors. Trends NeuroSci., 9: 424–428.

Saito, K., Greenberg, S. and Moskowitz, M.A. (1987a) Trigeminal origin of beta-preprotachykinin products in feline pial blood vessels. Neurosci. Lett., 76: 69–73.

Saito, K., Liu-Chen, L.Y. and Moskowitz M.A. (1987b) Substance P-like immunoreactivity in rat forebrain leptomeninges and cerebral vessels originates from the trigeminal but not sympathetic ganglia. Brain Res., 403: 66–71.

Saito, K., Markowitz, S. and Moskowitz, M.A. (1987c) Ergot alkaloids block neurogenic plasma extravasation in the dura mater: proposed mechanism in the treatment of vascular headaches. Abstr. Soc. Neurosci., 1669.

Saria, A., Lundberg, J.M., Skofitsch, G. and Lembeck, F. (1983) Vascular protein leakage in various tissues induced by substance P, capsaicin, bradykinin, serotonin, histamine and by antigen challenge. Naunyn-Schmiedeberg's Arch Pharmacol., 324: 212–218.

Strassman, A., Mason, P., Moskowitz, M.A. and Maciewicz, R. (1986) Response of brainstem trigeminal neurons to electrical stimulation of the dura. Brain Res., 379: 242–250.

Strassman, A., Pile-Spellman, J., Oot, R., Mason, P., Moskowitz, M. and Maciewicz, R. (1987) Responses of trigeminal nucleus caudalis neurons to mechanical and chemical stimulation of cranial blood vessels. Abstr. Soc. Neurosci., 116.

Wolff, H.G. (1948) Headache and other Head Pains, Oxford University Press, New York.

Yamamoto, K., et al. (1983) Overall distribution of substance P-containing nerves in the wall of the cerebral arteries of the guinea pig and its origins. J. Comp. Neurol., 215: 421–426.

R. Dubner, G.F. Gebhart & M.R. Bond (Eds.)
Proceedings of the Vth World Congress on Pain
© 1988 Elsevier Science Publishers BV (Biomedical Division)

CHAPTER 21

Myofascial pain syndromes of head, neck and low back

David G. Simons

Department of Physical Medicine and Rehabilitation, University of California Irvine Medical Center, Orange, CA 92668,
USA

Introduction

This communication concerns the millions of chronic pain patients throughout the world for whom no organic diagnosis can be found to account for their pain. We must either find new diseases or learn to recognize overlooked diagnoses if we are to understand and resolve their symptoms (Institute of Medicine, 1987). This paper considers overlooked diagnoses. It first examines how the patient with common myofascial trigger points (TrPs) of the head, neck and low back presents to the clinician, and then how the clinician can recognize the condition. Next it distinguishes myofascial TrPs from two closely related conditions, fibromyalgia and articular dysfunction. Finally, it notes the current surge of related research activity that helps to identify pathophysiological processes which could account for the clinical picture.

We all owe Janet Travell, M.D., a profound debt of gratitude for her life-time dedication to understanding myofascial TrPs. In 1952, she first reported many important patterns of pain referred from TrPs in muscles throughout the body (Travell and Rinzler, 1952). Her earlier study on shoulder pain in 1942 shows her longstanding interest in this field (Travell et al., 1942). Now, she has identified for us many perpetuating factors. These factors convert an acute myofascial pain syndrome (MPS) to a chronic pain syndrome. With few exceptions, both the TrPs and the factors which perpetuate them are correctable (Travell and Simons, 1983).

Myofascial TrPs are a remarkably common source of musculoskeletal pain (Simons, 1988a). Only recently has their importance begun to be widely recognized by the medical profession (Fields, 1987; Institute of Medicine, 1987). Myofascial TrPs were found to be the primary cause of pain in 85% of 283 consecutive admissions to a comprehensive pain center program (Fishbain et al., 1986). In a dental clinic for patients with chronic head and neck pain, over half of the patients (164 of 296) were found to have a primary diagnosis of MPS (Fricton et al., 1985b). In a general practice of internal medicine, 10% of all 148 English-speaking volunteer patients and 33% of the 46 patients who presented with a pain complaint had myofascial TrPs that were primarily responsible for their pain, which was usually of recent origin. In the 13 patients who received initial specific myofascial therapy, the mean visual analogue scale ratings of pain decreased from 52.7 to 21.1 (Skootsky 1986). Acute myofascial pain syndromes (MPSs) are extremely common and respond well to appropriate therapy.

Correspondence: David G. Simons, M.D., 324 12th Street, Huntington Beach, CA 92648, U.S.A.

Common myofascial trigger point syndromes

A critical step in diagnosing an acute single-muscle MPS due to TrPs is usually recognition of the referred pain pattern specific for that muscle. Presented here are examples of some common myofascial syndromes of the head, neck and low back.

Head muscles

In the head, the muscles of mastication frequently produce referred pain. Generally, local twitch responses are easily felt while injecting TrPs in the masticatory muscles but are less easily seen when examining these muscles.

Myofascial TrPs in the *masseter* muscle commonly refer pain to the side of the face and teeth, as in Fig. 1F. If unidentified, this source of tooth pain can be responsible for the extraction of innocent teeth. Another masseter pattern refers pain deep in the ear and can be frustratingly enigmatic to otolaryngologists who are unaware of this source of pain. Taut bands are readily palpated in this muscle.

The *temporalis* TrPs also commonly refer pain, thermal and mechanical hypersensitivity to normal teeth of the upper jaw and may cause unilateral temporal headache (Fig. 1A). Taut bands running in the direction of the temporalis muscle fibers are palpable at the TrPs if the muscle is placed on moderate stretch with the jaws propped open.

The referred pain from TrPs in the *lateral pterygoid* muscle (Fig. 1C) sometimes misdirects attention to the temporomandibular joint. However, the joint may also develop dysfunction because TrPs (upper arrow in Fig. 1C) are shortening fibers in the upper division of this muscle. This shortening can displace the articular disk forward. Only tenderness, and not local twitch responses or taut bands, is palpable in this deeply placed muscle.

Trigger points in the *medial pterygoid* muscle refer pain deep in the throat (Fig. 1E). Pain from this or any masticatory muscle is usually aggravated by chewing and sometimes by talking. Taut bands are palpable when the medial pterygoid is examined intraorally through the pharyngeal wall.

Local twitch responses are difficult to detect in this deep muscle.

Neck muscles

Four neck muscles characteristically refer pain upward to the head: the upper trapezius, sternocleidomastoid, splenii and suboccipital muscles. The TrPs in these muscles were the most common cause of the pain in a group of patients with chronic headache (Graff-Radford et al., 1987) and were responsible for post-partum headache following spinal analgesia (Hubbell et al. 1985). Other neck muscles refer pain downward to the neck or beyond.

The *upper trapezius* is one of the muscles most commonly afflicted with myofascial TrPs. These TrPs refer pain upward over the back of the neck ipsilaterally, and the pain often includes the temporal area and sometimes the angle of the jaw; see left-hand drawing in Fig. 1D. Taut bands are readily palpated in this muscle by grasping its anterior border between the thumb and fingers and rolling the muscle between the digits. A vigorous local twitch response of this muscle produces a movement of the head.

Pain referred from the *sternal division* of the *sternocleidomastoid* muscle (left side of Fig. 1B) surrounds the eye, may focus on the vertex and the occiput, and occasionally produces a soreness in the throat while swallowing; pain may also be referred downward to the sternum. Myofascial TrPs in this muscle sometimes disturb autonomic functions, causing uncontrollable lacrimation, coryza and/or scleral injection ipsilaterally (Travell and Simons, 1983).

Trigger points in the *clavicular division* of the *sternocleidomastoid* (right side of Fig. 1B) are one of the most common sources of musculoskeletal headache, often misdiagnosed as 'muscle tension' headache. These clavicular division TrPs can also refer pain deep in the ear and to the mastoid area behind the ear. Their referred autonomic component causes postural dizziness without deafness (Weeks and Travell, 1955; Travell and Simons, 1983). Taut bands are clearly distinguished in most of the affected sternocleidomastoid muscles, where

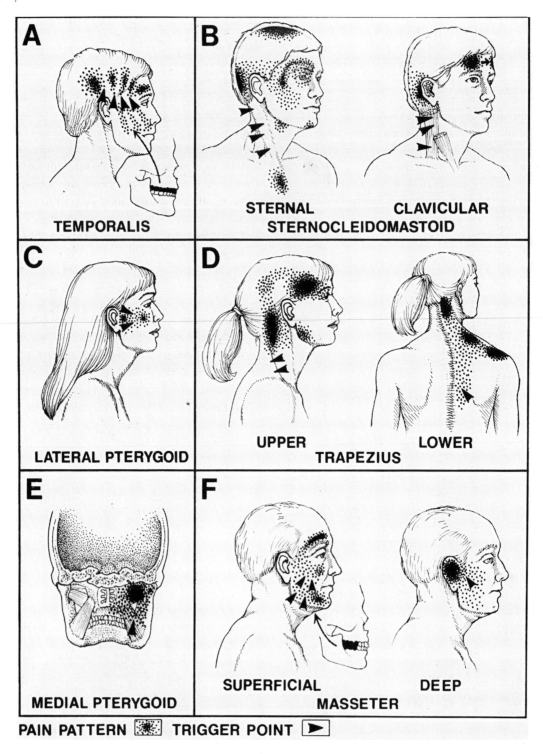

Fig. 1. Referred pain patterns (solid black and black stippling) from myofascial trigger points (arrow heads) in selected muscles of the head and neck. Reproduced, with permission, from Simons and Travell (1984).

they are accesible to palpation directly through the mobile skin of the neck. Local twitch responses of this muscle often produce a movement of the head.

Trigger points in any one of the three *scalene* muscles can refer pain distally (Fig. 2) and are a frequent cause of upper back pain along the vertebral border of the scapula. These TrPs also can refer pain down the arm to the radial side of the hand and over the front of the chest. The anterior and middle scalene muscles often entrap the lower trunk of the brachial plexus, producing neuropraxic numbness and dysesthesia in an ulnar nerve distribution (Travell and Simons, 1983). Taut bands are palpated subcutaneously against the transverse processes of the lower cervical vertebrae. Local twitch responses are rarely perceived in this group of muscles.

The *levator scapulae* is a common source of pain in the angle of the neck extending to the posterior shoulder region (Fig. 3) and it responds well to stretch and spray. When this muscle is injected for TrPs, the upper TrP is often overlooked. The upper TrP must be injected with care, directing the needle above and across but not toward the chest wall, to avoid a pneumothorax.

Back muscles

Low back pain of myofascial TrP origin is likely to arise from the quadratus lumborum, thoracolumbar paraspinal or gluteal muscles. It may also come from TrPs in the iliopsoas, rectus abdominis or intra-pelvic muscles (Simons and Travell, 1983; Travell and Simons, 1983).

The *quadratus lumborum* TrPs are among the most common sources of enigmatic low back pain, which has a variety of causes (Spangfort, 1987). The pain from these TrPs is referred unilaterally to the sacroiliac joint and various regions of the buttock and hip anteriorly and laterally, as in Fig. 4. However, these quadratus muscles are commonly involved bilaterally as antagonists, producing pain across the low back. One must carefully distinguish

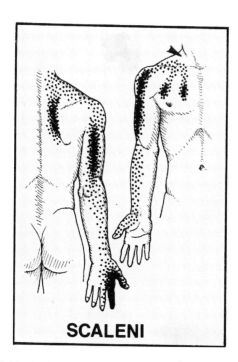

Fig. 2. Myofascial pain patterns (solid black and black stippling) referred from trigger points (arrow head) in the anterior, middle or posterior scalene muscles. Reproduced, with permission, from Simons and Travell (1984).

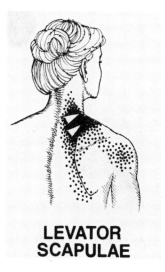

Fig. 3. Myofascial pain pattern (solid black and black stippling) referred from trigger points (arrow heads) in the levator scapulae muscle. Reproduced, with permission, from Simons and Travell (1984).

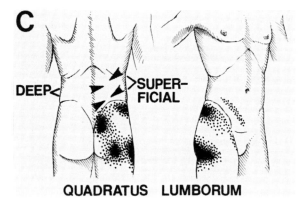

Fig. 4. Myofascial pain patterns (solid black and black stippling) referred from trigger points (arrow heads) in the deep and superficial quadratus lumborum muscle. Reproduced, with permission, from Simons and Travell (1984).

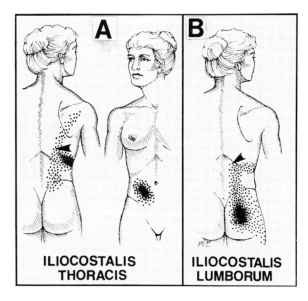

Fig. 5. Myofascial pain patterns (solid black and black stippling) referred from trigger points (arrow heads) in the iliocostalis thoracis and iliocostalis lumborum muscles. Reproduced, with permission, from Simons and Travell (1984).

between the pain referred from muscles and the pain of sacroiliac joint dysfunction which requires mobilization therapy. Both of these causes of low back pain can be relieved when diagnosed and appropriate therapy is applied. Rarely, taut bands are palpable in the lateral border of this muscle. It is usually too deep to exhibit local twitch responses.

The superficial and long-fibered paraspinal muscles, the *iliocostalis* and *longissimus*, project pain primarily downward; in the thoracolumbar region, their TrPs refer to the buttock area (Figs. 5B and 6A). Myofascial TrPs more cephalad in the iliocostalis muscles (Fig. 5A) may refer pain anteriorly as well as distally. The taut bands due to TrPs in these superficial paraspinal muscles are readily palpated and their referred pain patterns and local twitch responses are easily elicited; this is not the case in the deep paraspinal muscles. The deep short paraspinal muscles, the *multifidi* and *rotatores*, refer pain locally (Fig. 6B) often to the same segmental level; these deep paraspinal muscles refer pain to the midline, including the spinous process of the adjacent vertebra.

Trigger points in both the *gluteus maximus* (Fig. 7A) and the *gluteus medius* muscles (Fig. 7B) refer pain locally and the gluteus medius also refers to the sacrum. The gluteus maximus exhibits eloquent taut bands and local twitch responses. The *gluteus*

minimus (Fig. 7C) projects pain downward over either the posterior or the lateral thigh and may include parts of the leg. The pain referred posteriorly by TrPs in the posterior section of the gluteus minimus is frequently misdiagnosed as sciatica (Simons and Travell, 1983).

Treatment

For all of these myofascial syndromes due to TrPs, stretch and spray (Travell and Simons, 1983) and postisometric relaxation (Lewit, 1986a) provide effective treatment. Mense (1987) recently reported suppression of spinothalamic cell response to muscle nociceptors as the result of skin stimulation of convergent neurons. This is compatible with the hypothesized mechanism of the vapocoolant in the stretch-and-spray procedure (Travell and Simons, 1983). Another commonly used treatment is injection of the TrPs. Jaeger and Skootsky (1987) report that needle penetration of the TrP is the critical therapeutic requirement. The injection of fluid may also be important for washing out local sensitizing agents.

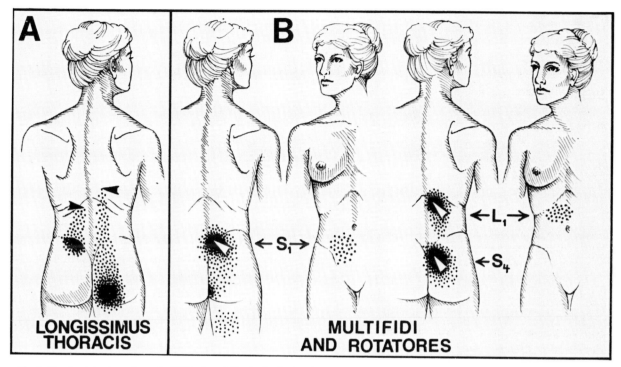

Fig. 6. Myofascial pain patterns (solid black and black stippling) referred from trigger points (arrow heads) in the superficial paraspinal muscle, the longissimus thoracis, and in the deep paraspinal muscles, the multifidi and rotatores. Reproduced, with permission, from Simons and Travell (1984).

Recognition of myofascial pain syndrome

Eight characteristics are useful for identifying MPSs due to TrPs. These eight clinical features emphasize the fact that this is primarily an affliction of muscle: (1) history of onset and cause; (2) distribution of pain; (3) restricted motion; (4) mild, muscle-specific weakness; (5) focal tenderness of a TrP which is (6) located in a palpable taut band of muscle fibers; (7) a local twitch response; and (8) reproduction of the pain pattern on mechanical stimulation of the TrP.

1. By history, the onset of pain is often sudden and associated with a clearly remembered muscular strain, but it may be gradual in onset associated with repetitive overload. A newly activated TrP may spontaneously revert to a latent TrP. However, in the presence of serious perpetuating factors newly activated TrPs persist as chronically active, or intermittently active, pain-producing TrPs. Characteristically, pain is closely related to changes in daily activity and the demands on the muscle involved.

2. Referred pain patterns are the key to identifying which muscle, or muscles, is probably causing the myofascial pain. As described above, each muscle has its own characteristic pain pattern. By having the patient point with one finger to the precise location of the pain and by the clinician's drawing of the location accurately on a body form, one identifies which muscles are the likely myofascial sources of the pain. For instance, a bilateral frontal headache pattern implicates the clavicular division of a sternocleidomastoid muscle, but the side from which it arises must be determined by physical examination (Travell and Simons, 1983). Muscle by muscle, one can piece together the puzzle of the total myofascial pain picture of a patient with TrPs in many muscles.

A TrP often refers tenderness to the zone of referred pain, which further confuses both the unwary examiner and the patient. The TrP may also refer autonomic changes which modify skin perfusion in the referred pain zone. This autonomic effect may produce thermograph changes which substantiate the history and physical findings. To date, thermographic findings have been too variable and ambiguous to make the primary diagnosis of myofascial TrPs (Simons, 1988a).

3. On examination, patients have some painful restriction of the stretch range of motion. Passive lengthening of a muscle harboring TrPs causes pain when the muscle is stretched beyond its restricted range of motion. Also, strong voluntary contraction of an involved muscle, especially in the shortened position, is usually painful.

4. The involved muscle shows some degree of weakness without atrophy. When carefully examined, it is found to inhibit maximal contraction.

5. Exquisite focal tenderness of the TrP is identified by the jump sign – vocalization and withdrawal of the patient. This spot tenderness is an essential feature of both a TrP and a tender point (TeP) (Simons, 1986; Smythe, 1986).

Algometers are becoming widely accepted as necessary to quantify TrP and TeP sensitivity in clinical studies (Jaeger and Reeves, 1986; Crook et al., 1987; Scudds et al., 1987; Tunks et al., 1987). Fischer (1986a,b; 1987a,b) designed a family of convenient spring-type pressure algometers which are commercially available. Reeves et al. (1986) established the reliability of Fischer's pressure threshold meter. Jensen et al. (1986) developed and validated an electronic strain-gauge unit which is also being produced commercially. Schiffman et al. (1987) have developed and tested the validity and reliability of an electronic strain-gauge unit with a blunt probe. When the probe is pressed across the TrP in a taut band, this unit simulates snapping palpation and returns considerable tactile feedback to the examiner. It is especially well suited to the study of local twitch responses and is expected soon to be commercially available.

6. The palpable taut band associated with a TrP is a critically important, objective finding. The TrP is the point of maximum tenderness along the course of a taut band in an involved muscle. The rope-like taut band can be palpated whenever the muscle is sufficiently close to the skin. The tension of the band's fibers is distinguished from the normally lax fibers surrounding it by stretching the muscle gently to, but not beyond, the onset of resistance. This degree of stretch maximizes the palpable differences in tension among fibers.

7. Snapping palpation across the TrP elicits a local twitch response. This response is an objective physical sign and has been observed only in response to mechanical stimulation of TrPs. It was recently studied electromyographically by Fricton et

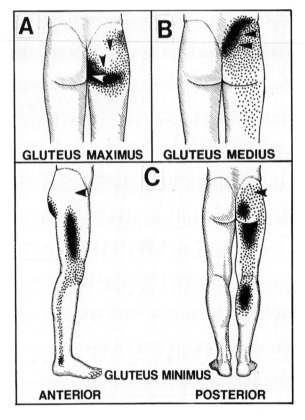

Fig. 7. Myofascial pain patterns (solid black and black stippling) referred from trigger points (arrow heads) in the three gluteal muscles. Note the difference in the distribution of the pain referred from the anterior and posterior portions of the gluteus minimus muscle. Reproduced, with permission, from Simons and Travell (1984).

al. (1985a). The totally objective local twitch response is seen as a transient dimpling of the skin near the tendinous attachment of the muscle or felt as a transient contraction of only the fibers in the taut band.

8. Mildly painful, sustained pressure on an active TrP usually reproduces or increases the referred pain caused by that TrP, if the pain is not already at maximum intensity. This confirms to both the patient and the examiner that this TrP is responsible for at least part of the patient's pain. In this way one can piece together the total pain distribution in patients with multiple TrPs and multiple referred pain patterns, each of which produces its own portion of the pain. It is noteworthy that sometimes a TrP may refer loss of sensation instead of pain (Langs, 1987).

In summary, the first four of these features are helpful in making a clinical diagnosis: the dependence of symptoms on muscular strain and activity; the recognition of referred pain patterns characteristic of specific muscles; the painful restriction of stretch range of motion; and some weakness of the involved muscles.

The last four features are essential to the identification of myofascial TrPs for research purposes. Clinically, focal exquisite TrP tenderness is always present and a taut band is palpable whenever the muscle is accessible and placed on moderate stretch. The last two features, the local twitch response and the referred pain response, are considered pathognomic of TrPs; possibly, referred pain from the TePs of fibromyalgia may prove to be an exception. The last two responses are more vigorous for more active TrPs, but may also be seen from latent TrPs.

Active TrPs are responsible for clinical pain complaints; latent TrPs do not cause a clinical complaint of pain. Although less irritable, a latent TrP may have any or all of the other characteristics of an active TrP, including local twitch responses and the reproduction of its referred pain pattern when the TrP is compressed.

Chronic myofascial pain syndromes

Thus far, presentation of common, acute single-muscle syndromes due to TrPs has been clear-cut and unambiguous. When we now consider patients with chronic musculoskeletal pain and explore underlying mechanisms, complications arise. Clinical practice and research studies become intertwined with two additional conditions, fibromyalgia and joint dysfunction. Nearly all research on muscle pain syndromes has been done on patients with chronic pain. Rarely has a study been conducted that methodically excluded the other two diagnoses from the patient population.

Acute MPSs due to TrPs usually become chronic syndromes because of preexisting perpetuating factors (Travell and Simons, 1983). Graff-Radford et al. (1987) have clearly demonstrated the importance of factors which perpetuate myofascial TrPs in the clinical management of patients with headache. Confusion arises between fibromyalgia and MPSs when, in time, perpetuating factors multiply the number of myofascial TrPs so that the pain becomes chronic and widespread.

Nearly all categories of perpetuating factors tend to increase the metabolic distress or compromise the contractile function of skeletal muscle. Mechanical stresses increase the metabolic demand. Nutritional inadequacies compromise biochemical metabolic pathways. Metabolic disturbances, such as inadequate thyroid function, directly compromise metabolism. Electrolyte disturbances such as low ionized potassium compromise muscle fiber excitability, and low ionized calcium compromises muscle fiber contractility. The importance of chronic infections and active allergies suggests that the immune system may also be involved. Anemia causes hypoxia which compromises muscle metabolism. Psychological stress is frequently expressed as increased muscle tension which mechanically overloads the muscles.

Since myofascial TrPs are often overlooked or misdiagnosed, and since fibromyalgia or fibrositis is sometimes considered largely psychogenic (Egle et al., 1987; Landrø and Winnem, 1987; Bohr, 1987), the patient wanders from health care provider to health care provider finding no one who can identify a cause of the pain or who can relieve it. Patients who suffer for months and years from undiagnosed chronic musculoskeletal pain for which no one has found a cause or effective treatment experience severe psychological trauma that is bound to produce measurable psychological and behavioral changes. Such severe unexplained suffering which is unresponsive to all treatment efforts and has an unknown prognosis is enough to cause severe psychological changes in many people. When recognized, both the perpetuating factors and MPSs are gratifyingly responsive to therapy. Most important to patients is a convincing explanation of the cause of their pain, a demonstrated response to treatment and a home exercise program that gives them control of pain relief without drugs.

Recent progress

In the last few years there has been a surge of clinical research focused on musculoskeletal pain. Four groups are contributing a remarkable fund of new knowledge. One group was sparked by Ann Bengtsson under the direction of Karl Henriksson in Linköping, Sweden; one was sparked by Bente Danneskiold-Samsøe, inspired by Rasmus Bach Anderson in Copenhagen, Denmark; another has been led by Bernadette Jaeger at the University of California, Los Angeles; and one group is headed by James Fricton at the University of Minnesota.

Closely related conditions
The pathophysiology of none of three common sources of musculoskeletal pain has yet been resolved. The three appear to be closely intertwined. To fully understand any of these, at this time, one must be aware of all three. The three are *myofascial TrPs* (Travell and Simons, 1983), *fibromyalgia* (Yunus et al., 1982; Bennett, 1987; Goldenberg, 1987) – first called fibrositis (Smythe and Moldofsky, 1977; Campbell and Bennett, 1986; Wolfe, 1986) – and *articular dysfunction* (Fisk, 1987; Lewit, 1985; Mennell, 1964). To date none of the three

conditions has an acceptable diagnostic laboratory or imaging test. Each diagnosis must be made by history and physical examination. The critical findings in each would be missed on a routine physical examination. The examiner must know what findings to look for, how to look for them and must take the time to examine the patient for them. Therefore the symptoms and findings used to distinguish one diagnosis from the other are based only on clinical experience.

In research studies, investigators may be including patients who are suffering from conditions other than the one that they wish to study. In this event, their conclusions may be more confusing than helpful. It now looks as if these conditions have different causes which can produce confusingly similar clinical pictures, but often require significantly different therapeutic approaches. Included in this circle of confusion are many conditions that may include, or be misdiagnosed as, myofascial TrPs. These terms include fibrositis (Smythe and Moldofsky, 1977; Wolfe, 1986), fibromyalgia, (Yunus et al., 1982; Goldenberg, 1987), osteochondrosis (Popelianskii et al., 1976, 1984), nonarticular rheumatism (Fassbender, 1975), muscular rheumatism (Miehlke et al., 1960) and many others (see Simons, 1975, 1976, and Reynolds, 1983).

A single-muscle *myofascial pain syndrome* due to TrPs originates as a focal disorder in muscle due to acute or repeated overload stress. It is myogenic, not psychogenic. Myofascial TrPs are distinguished clinically by referred pain and tenderness, palpable taut bands and local twitch responses. When recognized as an acute syndrome and in the absence of perpetuating factors, the pain is quickly and easily relieved. A chronic MPS which is aggravated and multiplied by perpetuating factors is another story and can look confusingly like fibromyalgia (Simons, 1986).

The second condition, *primary fibromyalgia*, is apparently a systemic disease of unknown origin that is strongly associated with a non-restorative sleep disorder (Yunus et al., 1982). It is now diagnosed chiefly by finding multiple tender points (TePs) (Goldenberg, 1987). At one time, before 'fibrositis' was redefined by Smythe and Moldofsky (1977), it was described in terms of psychogenic rheumatism (Smythe, 1972). Some authors still consider 'fibrositis' or fibromyalgia as partly, if not largely, psychogenic (Egle et al., 1987; Henriksson et al., 1987; Landrø and Winnem, 1987). Others find no psychological difference compared with other chronic painful conditions (Clark et al., 1985). Smythe and Moldofsky (1977) identified 'fibrositis' as a non-restorative sleep syndrome characterized by multiple diffuse TePs at prescribed locations. Smythe (1981) updated this definition of 'fibrositis' which has been widely adopted by rheumatologists. Yunus et al. (1982) renamed Smythe's redefinition of 'fibrositis' as primary fibromyalgia and increased the number of patients included by reducing the number of TePs required to make the diagnosis. The new term, primary fibromyalgia, is gaining wide recognition (Lund et al., 1986; Bennett, 1987; Crook et al., 1987; Goldenberg, 1987; Henrikkson et al., 1987).

Myofascial TrPs appear early in life (Bates and Grunwaldt, 1958) and occur equally in men and women (Sola et al., 1955). 'Fibrositis' is characteristically a disease of women between 40 and 60 years of age. Less than 15% of fibrositis patients are men (Wolfe, 1986).

Smythe (1986) agrees that there are essentially two different conditions characterized by tender spots in muscles: 'fibrositis', which he characterized as essentially a non-restorative sleep syndrome, and TrPs, which produced referred pain.

Trigger points have been identified as tender spots that cause referred pain when compressed (Bengtsson, 1986). Others do not mention how they distinguish TrPs (Crook et al., 1987; Tunks et al., 1987). Trigger points and TePs are always tender, but TePs do not always (if ever) refer pain. Using only the referred pain criterion for TrPs, Bengtsson et al. (1986a) found that 64% of 55 primary fibromyalgia patients had both TePs and TrPs. Eleven of the patients (20%) had at least six TrPs and no TePs. If only myofascial TrPs cause referred pain and fibromyalgic TePs do not, then this and possibly all fibromyalgia studies have included a mixed

population of patients with fibromyalgia and patients with MPSs due to TrPs. On the other hand, if fibromyalgic TePs do refer pain, then it is essential, if we are to understand these two conditions, that TrPs be unambiguously identified for experimental purposes. Trigger points should be identified not only by spot tenderness and by the capacity to refer pain, but also by their location in a palpable taut band and by their responding to snapping palpation with a local twitch response.

Indications that fibromyalgia is a systemic disease involving skin and muscle come from many sources. Both Caro (1984) and Bengtsson et al. (1986) have reported collagen changes at the dermal-epidermal junction marked by abnormal deposition of immunoglobulin G (IgG). Bartels and Danneskiold-Samsøe (1986) reported abnormal collagenous rubber-band-like constrictions of muscle fibers in non-tender muscles of fibrositis patients. Crook et al. (1987) concluded that the abnormal muscle tenderness of fibromyalgia patients is much more widespread than only the prescribed spots of muscular tenderness. They confusingly called these tender spots TrPs (Crook et al., 1987). Others have reported clear indications of an energy crisis in non-tender muscles of fibromyalgia patients (Bengtsson, 1986). Evidence includes intramuscular changes in the energy-supplying phosphates (Bengtsson et al., 1986c), reduced oxygen tension (Lund et al., 1986) and biopsy changes (Bengtsson et al., 1986b).

The third condition, *articular dysfunction*, is marked by a loss of normal joint 'play' or mobility (Mennell, 1964). Karel Lewit (1985, 1986b) emphasizes that certain articular dysfunctions are characteristically associated with tenderness and increased tension of specific related muscles. These muscular symptoms are relieved by mobilization of the restricted joint and by restoration of the normal muscle range of motion. James Fisk (1987) also emphasizes the importance of the confusingly strong interaction between joint dysfunction and muscles. Clearly, joint dysfunction can be a potent perpetuator of myofascial TrPs, if not the origin of an MPS.

A commonly overlooked painful articular dysfunction is the recently reported instability of spondylolisthetic or retro-olisthetic lumbar vertebrae. Pain is relieved by strengthening the deep spinal rotator muscles (Friberg, 1987).

Radiculopathy is often associated with myofascial TrPs (Fischer, 1986b; Rubin, 1981) and osteochondrosis (Popelianskii et al., 1984), but the myofascial component may not clear after resolution of the neuropathy unless additional specific myofascial therapy is applied to inactivate persistent TrPs. Peripheral nerve compression by tense muscles can cause symptomatic neuropraxia of muscular origin.

Nature of trigger points

Three clinical characteristics of myofascial TrPs require explanation: the local tenderness of the TrP itself, the pathways of referred pain and tenderness arising from the TrP, and the palpable hardness of the taut band. Pathophysiological mechanisms are known that can account for the clinical characteristics of myofascial TrPs. Whether they are the ones responsible remains to be firmly established.

Local tenderness and referred pain

The local tenderness of the TrP is likely due to sensitization of afferent nerve endings in the muscle (Simons, 1988a,b), as demonstrated by Mense (1977). Some likely sensitizing agents are prostaglandins, bradykinin, histamine, potassium and possibly leukotrienes. The metabolic distress to be discussed below could be the stimulus for the production of sensitizing agents. Frost (1986) reported improved relief of symptoms due to myofascial TrPs by injecting a prostaglandin inhibitor as compared with a local anesthetic. Other sensitizing agents may also be involved because non-steroidal anti-inflammatory drugs are generally ineffective in relieving the pain referred from TrPs (Travell and Simons, 1983), as recently demonstrated experimentally (Singer et al., 1987).

These same, or other, sensitized sensory nerve endings in muscle could similarly induce the modulation of referred sensation, the modulation of motor neuron excitability, and the modulation of the referred autonomic nervous system phenomena

that are so characteristic of myofascial TrPs.

There are several well-recognized mechanisms by which the nervous system can mediate referred pain (Institute of Medicine, 1987; Simons, 1988b). Four of them are: (1) convergence-projection, where an ascending nerve cell in the spinal cord receives simultaneous input from separate peripheral nociceptive cells which, in this case, would supply both the pain reference zone and the TrP; (2) convergence-facilitation, where the spinal cord receives input from one somatic region (reference zone) which is amplified (facilitated) in the spinal cord by activity originating in nociceptors (at a TrP) in another region of the body; (3) peripheral branching of axons to separate parts of the body, where the brain misinterprets the source of the sensory stimulation (Bahr et al., 1981); (4) sympathetic modulation of peripheral nociceptors, where increased sympathetic activity causes pain by releasing substances which sensitize primarily afferent nerve endings in the region of referred pain (Procacci et al., 1975).

Which of these mechanisms are responsible for phenomena that are referred from TrPs is not yet clear. The early study by Foreman et al. (1977) demonstrated convergence-projection to spinothalamic cells from visceral afferents, on one hand, and from skin and muscle afferents on the other. This observation was strongly substantiated as the rule rather than the exception in mammals by additional studies (Ammons et al., 1984; Foreman et al., 1984) and in a subsequent review (Foreman, 1986). Recent studies show that spinothalamic cells respond more vigorously to pinch of muscle afferents than to pinch of skin receptors (Foreman, personal communication, 1987). Involvement of the autonomic nervous system in the pain of patients with fibromyalgia was recently substantiated by Bengtsson and Bengtsson (1987).

Taut band

The taut band is a critically distinctive feature of a TrP and is difficult to explain. The muscle fibers of the taut band exhibit no more motor unit activity at rest than does the surrounding normal muscle, usually none. Clinically, the band feels as if the fibers passing through the TrP are shortened in the region of the TrP, but not at the far ends of the muscle.

The sarcomere, from Z band to Z band, is the contractile unit of a muscle fiber. The contractile activity of the actin and myosin filaments in the sarcomere is induced by the release of ionized calcium from the sarcoplasmic reticulum in the presence of an adequate adenosine triphosphate (ATP) energy source. Failure of return of the calcium to traumatically ruptured sarcoplasmic reticulum would sustain the contractile activity, which consumes energy. This sustained maximal contraction at the fiber level could cut off local capillary circulation, causing local ischemic hypoxia. Without an adequate ATP energy source, free calcium remains because the calcium pump fails despite repair of the sarcoplasmic reticulum. This failure sustains the continuing combination of an increased metabolic demand and ischemic hypoxia, which produces a self-sustaining energy crisis. It is noteworthy that whenever the sarcomere is lengthened sufficiently the myosin heads can no longer reach active sites on the actin. Then, contractile activity and energy consumption must stop, regardless of calcium (Simons, 1988b).

This result of elongating the sarcomere helps to explain why stretching the muscle is a universal and effective treatment for myofascial TrPs, but is not so helpful for TePs of fibromyalgia. That the contractile elements in the sarcomeres are involved in 'fibrositic nodules' (taut bands of TrPs?) is substantiated by the findings of Danneskiold-Samsøe et al. (1986). Massage of these nodules (but not of normal muscle) initially caused transient myoglobinemia which disappeared as the nodules and tenderness resolved with repeated massage treatments.

Henriksson et al. (1987) summarized a series of studies showing that an energy crisis is present in the region of TrPs and TePs in muscle biopsies of patients with fibromyalgia. Unmet metabolic demand was indicated by a decrease in high-energy phosphates and an increase in low-energy phosphates (Bengtsson et al., 1986c). Direct evidence of local vascular disturbance with hypoxia was found by subcutaneous oxymetry of the muscles (Lund et al., 1986).

Histological evidence of serious disturbance in the energy metabolism was demonstrated (Bengtsson et al., 1986b) by the presence of scattered ragged red fibers and 'moth-eaten' fibers under light microscopy in the upper trapezius muscles in 15 of 41 biopsies of patients with fibromyalgia. Thirty-one of these 41 biopsies from the upper trapezius were taken from a TeP or a TrP. A TrP was identified as a tender spot that caused referred pain when compressed. Palpable findings were not a criterion. No ragged red fibers were found in 10 control biopsies of this same muscle. The red periphery of the muscle fiber represents sick mitochondria which are essential for oxidative metabolism and are required for normal energy metabolism of the muscle.

Henriksson (personal communication, 1987) also substantiated the report of fat dusting by Miehlke et al. (1960). A longitudinal section from the same muscle as the ragged red fibers noted above, but stained with an oil red O fat stain, showed deposits of red microscopic fat droplets (fat dusting) within the muscle fibers, chiefly beneath the sarcolemma where the sick mitochondria were seen.

Substantiating this shortened-sarcomere explanation for the taut band, Kalyan-Raman et al. (1984) found occasional biopsy evidence of sarcomere shortening in the region of TePs in upper trapezius muscles in 2 of 12 patients with fibromyalgia. One would expect inconsistencies if fibromyalgia studies combined patient populations, some with myofascial TrPs and some with fibromyalgic TePs.

The applicability of the above 'fibromyalgia' findings specifically to myofascial TrPs as compared with the TePs of fibromyalgia is not clear. The possibility that some TePs as well as myofascial TrPs may refer pain has not been eliminated. No data are known that resolve this issue. As the clinical distinctions between these conditions become more widely recognized, studies based on more clearly defined patient populations will help greatly to clarify key differences in pathophysiology.

Table I summarizes diagnostic distinctions among the three closely related conditions that are commonly overlooked and which cause musculoskeletal pain. Fibrositis is characteristically a dis-

TABLE I

Diagnostic distinctions among three closely related musculoskeletal sources of pain

	Onset of symptoms	Examination of muscles
Fibrositis or fibromyalgia	Insidious; mostly women over 40	Widespread muscle tenderness – prescribed *tender* points
Myofascial trigger points	Sudden – related to movement or muscle strain; males = females	Regional myofascial *trigger* points[a]
Articular dysfunction	Sudden – related to movement	Tenderness of related muscle bellies and attachments

[a]Unambiguous identification of a trigger point requires three findings: production of referred sensory changes, an associated palpable taut band, and a local twitch response.

ease of women between 40 and 60 years of age, whereas myofascial TrPs appear equally in men and women. The history of strain of a specific muscle or muscle group helps to distinguish the pain of myofascial TrPs from the insidious onset of the diffuse widespread pain of fibromyalgia. Myofascial pain is usually asymmetrical and muscle-specific; patients with fibromyalgia are much more likely to complain of bilaterally symmetrical pain. On physical examination, three characteristics of myofascial TrPs should be considered: referral of pain, a palpable taut band, and the local twitch response.

In myofascial pain, joint mobility is restricted in the direction of elongation of the affected muscle. In articular dysfunction, the joint is likely to exhibit restricted mobility (loss of joint play) in directions other than the voluntary movement produced by

muscle contraction (Mennell, 1964). To more effectively manage the pain of the many patients with musculoskeletal problems, one must consider MPSs, fibrositis/fibromyalgia and articular dysfunctions.

Summary

Myofascial trigger points are a commonly present, but not-so-commonly recognized, source of musculoskeletal pain. They must be distinguished from the tender points of fibromyalgia and from the muscular effects of articular dysfunction. Trigger points refer pain and tenderness, are associated with taut bands that shorten the muscle, and exhibit local twitch responses. It is not known whether the tender points of fibromyalgia can also cause referred pain. Muscle biopsies and pathophysiology studies to date represent an unknown mixture of patients with fibromyalgia and myofascial trigger points. Apparently, the pain of both fibromyalgia and myofascial trigger points is associated with an intramuscular energy crisis. This crisis may be initiated by different mechanisms and is probably distributed differently throughout the muscles. Only more discriminating research will clarify these issues. With the current research studies, we are off to a most encouraging start.

Acknowledgement

The author expresses deep indebtedness to Janet G. Travell, M.D., for her great reservoir of wisdom that she has so generously contributed to this paper, and to Lois Statham Simons, R.P.T. and Bernadette Jaeger, D.D.S., for thoughtful and meticulous review of the manuscript.

References

Ammons, W.S., Blair, R.W. and Foreman, R.D. (1984) Greater splanchnic excitation of primate T_1-T_2 spinothalamic neurons. J. Neurophysiol., 51: 592–603.

Bahr, R., Blumberg, H. and Janig, W. (1981) Do dichotomizing afferent fibres exist which supply visceral organs as well as somatic structures? A contribution to the problem of referred pain. Neurosci. Lett., 24: 25–28.

Bartels, E.M. and Danneskiold-Samsøe, B. (1986) Histological abnormalities in muscle from patients with certain types of fibrositis. Lancet, i: 755–757.

Bates, T. and Grunwaldt, E. (1958) Myofascial pain in childhood. J. Pediatr., 53: 198–209.

Bengtsson, A. (1986) Primary fibromyalgia: a clinical and laboratory study. Linköping University Dissertations, No. 224, Linköping.

Bengtsson, A. and Bengtsson, M. (1987) Regional sympathetic blockage in primary fibromyalgia (PF). Pain., Suppl. 4, S295 (Abstr. No. 566).

Bengtsson, A., Henriksson, K.-G., Jorfeldt, L., Kågedal, B., Lennmarken, C. and Lindström, F. (1986a) Primary fibromyalgia – a clinical and laboratory study of 55 patients. Scand. J. Rheum., 15: 340–347.

Bengtsson, A., Henriksson, K.-G. and Larsson, J. (1986b) Muscle biopsy in primary fibromyalgia. Scand. J. Rheumatol., 15: 1–6.

Bengtsson, A., Henriksson, K.-G. and Larsson, J. (1986c) Reduced high-energy phosphate levels in painful muscle in patients with primary fibromyalgia. Arthritis Rheum., 29: 817–821.

Bennett, R. (1987) Editorial on Fibromyalgia Syndrome. J. Am. Med. Assoc., 257: 2802–2803.

Bohr, T. (1987) Painful questions about fibromyalgia. J. Am. Med. Assoc., 258: 1476.

Campbell, S.M. and Bennett, R.M. (1986) Fibrositis. Disease-a-Month, 32 (11): 653–722.

Caro, X.J. (1984) Immunofluorescent detection of IgG at the dermal-epidermal junction in patients with apparent primary fibrositis syndrome. Arthritis Rheum., 27: 1174–1179.

Clark, S., Campbell, S.M., Forehand, M.E., Tindall, E.A. and Bennett, R.M. (1985) Clinical characteristics of fibrositis: II. A 'blinded,' controlled study using standard psychological tests. Arthritis Rheum., 28: 132–137.

Crook, J., Tunks, E., Norman, G. and Kalaher, S. (1987) A comparative study of tenderness thresholds in trigger points and non-trigger points in normal and fibromyalgia patients. Pain, Suppl. 4: S307 (Abstr. No. 509).

Danneskiold-Samsøe, B., Christiansen, E. and Anderson, R.B. (1986) Myofascial pain and the role of myoglobin. Scand. J. Rheum., 15: 154–178.

Egle, U.T., Schwab, R., Rudolf, M.L., Schöfer, M., Bassler, M. and Hoffman S.O. (1987) Illness behaviour and defense mechanisms of patients with psychogenic pain: rheumatoid arthritis and fibrositis syndrome. Pain, Suppl. 4: S324 (Abstr. No. 624).

Fassbender, H.G. (1975) Non-articular rheumatism (Ch. 13). In Pathology of Rheumatic Diseases, Springer-Verlag, New York.

Fields, H.L. (1987) Pain, McGraw-Hill Book Co., New York, pp. 209–214.

Fischer, A.A. (1986a) Pressure threshold meter: its use for quantification of tender spots. Arch. Phys. Med. Rehabil., 67: 836–838.

Fischer, A.A. (1986b) Pressure tolerance over muscles and bones in normal subjects. Arch. Phys. Med. Rehabil., 67: 406–409.

Fischer, A.A. (1987a) Tissue compliance meter for objective, quantitative documentation of soft tissue consistency and pathology. Arch. Phys. Med. Rehabil., 68: 122–125.

Fischer, A.A. (1987b) Instruments for pain diagnosis in clinical practice: pressure algometers for measurement of pain sensitivity and documentation for tender points; tissue compliance meter for objective quantitative recording of muscle spasm. Pain, Suppl. 4: S292 (Abstr. No. 559).

Fishbain, D.A., Goldberg, M., Meagher, B.R., Steele, R. and Rosomoff, H. (1986) Male and female chronic pain patients categorized by DSM-III psychiatric diagnostic criteria. Pain, 26: 181–197.

Fisk, J.W. (1987) Medical Treatment of Neck and Back Pain, Charles C. Thomas, Springfield.

Foreman, R.D. (1986) Spinal substrates of visceral pain. In T.L. Yaksh (Ed.), Spinal Afferent Processing, Plenum Publishing Corp., New York, pp. 217–242.

Foreman, R.D., Blair, R.W. and Weber, R.N. (1984) Viscerosomatic convergence onto T2-T4 spinoreticular, spinoreticular-spinothalamic, and spinothalamic tract neurons in the cat. Exp. Neurol., 85: 597–619.

Foreman, R.D., Schmidt, R.F. and Willis, W.D. (1977) Convergence of muscle and cutaneous input onto primate spinothalamic tract neurons. Brain Res., 124: 555–560.

Friberg, O. (1987) Lumbar instability: a dynamic approach by traction-compression radiography. Spine, 12: 119–129.

Fricton, J.R., Auvinen, M.D., Dykstra, D. and Schiffman, E. (1985a) Myofascial pain syndrome: electromyographic changes associated with local twitch response. Arch. Phys. Med. Rehabil, 66: 314–317.

Fricton, J.R., Kroening, R., Haley, D. and Siegart, R. (1985b) Myofascial pain syndrome of the head and neck: a review of clinical characteristics of 164 patients. Oral Surg., 60: 615–623.

Frost, A. (1986) Diclofenac versus lidocaine as injection therapy in myofascial pain. Scand. J. Rheumatol., 15: 153–156.

Goldenberg, D.L. (1987) Fibromyalgia syndrome. J. Am. Med. Assoc., 257: 2782–2803.

Graff-Radford, S.B., Reeves, J.L. and Jaeger, B. (1987) Management of chronic head and neck pain: the effectiveness of altering factors perpetuating myofascial pain. Headache, 27: 186–190.

Henriksson, K.G., Bengtsson, A., Larsson, J., Lund, N. and Eneström, S. (1987) Muscle pain with special reference to primary fibromyalgia (PF). Pain, Suppl. 4: S294 (Abstr. No. 564).

Hubbell, S.L. and Thomas, M. (1985) Postpartum cervical myofascial pain syndrome: review of four patients. Obstet. Gynecol., 65: No. 3 (Suppl.) 56S–57S.

Institute of Medicine (May 1987) Pain and Disability: Clinical Behavioral and Public Policy Perspectives, National Academy Press, Washington, DC.

Jaeger, B. and Reeves, J.L. (1986) Quantification of changes in myofascial trigger point sensitivity with the pressure algometer following passive stretch. Pain, 27: 203–210.

Jaeger, B. and Skootsky, S.A. (1987) Double blind, controlled study of different myofascial trigger point injection techniques. Pain, Suppl. 4: S292 (Abstr. No. 560).

Jensen, K., Andersen, H.O., Olesen, J. and Lindblom, U. (1986) Pressure-pain threshold in human temporal region. Evaluation of a new pressure algometer. Pain, 25: 313–323.

Kalyan-Raman, U.P., Kalyan-Raman, K., Yunus, M.B. and Masi, A.T. (1984) Muscle pathology in primary fibromyalgia syndrome: a light microscopic, histochemical and ultrastructural study. J. Rheumatol., 11: 808–813.

Landrø, N.I. and Winnem, M. (1987) Psychodiagnostic evaluation of patients with myofascial pain syndrome (fibrositis). Pain, Suppl. 4: S419 (Abstr. No. 808).

Langs, H.M. (1987) Myofascial pain and analgesia. Pain, Suppl. 4: S297 (Abstr. No. 570).

Lewit, K. (1985) Manipulative Therapy in Rehabilitation of the Motor System, Butterworths, London.

Lewit, K. (1986a) Postisometric relaxation in combination with other methods of muscular facilitation and inhibition. Manual Med., 2: 101–104.

Lewit, K. (1986b) Muscular pattern in thoraco-lumbar lesions. Manual Med., 2: 105–107.

Lund, N., Bengtsson, A. and Thorborg, P. (1986) Muscle tissue oxygen pressure in primary fibromyalgia. Scand. J. Rheumatol. 15: 165–173.

Mennell, J.M. (1964) Joint Pain, Little, Brown and Company, Boston.

Mense, S. (1977) Nervous outflow from skeletal muscle following chemical noxious stimulation. J. Physiol., 267: 75–88.

Mense, S. (1987) Anatomical and neurophysiological basis of muscle pain. Pain, Suppl. 4: S209 (Abstr. No. 406).

Miehlke, K., Schulze, G. and Eger, W. (1960) Klinische und experimentelle Untersuchungen zum Fibrositissyndrom. Z. Rheumaforsch., 19: 310–330.

Popelianskii, Ia. Iu., Bogdanov, E.I. and Khabirov, F.A. (1984) [Algesic trigger zones of the gastrocnemius muscle in lumbar osteochondrosis (clinicopathomorphological and electromyographic analysis)] (Russian). ZH Nevropatol. Psikhiatr., 84: 1055–1061.

Popelianskii, Ia. Iu., Zaslavskii, E.S. and Veselovskii, V.P. (1976) [Medicosocial significance, etiology, pathogenesis and diagnosis of nonarticular disease of soft tissues of the limbs and back.] (Russian) Vopr. Revm., 3: 38–43.

Procacci, P., Francini, F., Maresca, M. and Zoppi, M. (1975) Cutaneous pain threshold changes after sympathetic block in reflex dystrophies. Pain, 1: 167–175.

Reeves, J.L., Jaeger, B. and Graff-Radford, S.B. (1986) Reliability of the pressure algometer as a measure of myofascial trigger point sensitivity. Pain, 24: 313–321.

Reynolds, M.D. (1983) The development of the concept of fibrositis. J. Hist. Med. Allied Sci., 38: 5–35.

Rubin, D. (1981) An approach to the management of myofascial trigger point syndromes. Arch. Phys. Med. Rehabil., 62: 107–110.

Schiffman, E., Fricton, J., Haley, D. and Tylka, D. (1987) A pressure algometer for myofascial pain syndrome: reliability and validity. Pain, Suppl. 4: S291 (Abstr. No. 558).

Scudds, R.A., McCain, G.A., Rollman, G.B. and Harth, M. (1987) Changes in pain responsiveness in fibrositis patients after successful treatment. Pain, Suppl. 4: S353 (Abstr. No. 677).

Simons, D.G. (1975, 1976) Muscle pain syndromes–Parts I and

II. Am. J. Phys. Med., 54: 289–311 and 55: 15–42.

Simons, D.G. (1986) Fibrositis/fibromyalgia: a form of myofascial trigger points? Am. J. Med., 81 (Suppl. 3A): 93–98.

Simons, D.G. (1988a) Myofascial pain syndromes: Where are we? Where are we going? Arch. Phys. Med. Rehabil., 69: 207–212.

Simons, D.G. (1988b) Myofascial pain syndrome due to trigger points. Chapter In J. Goodgold (Ed.), Rehabilitation Medicine, C.V. Mosby Co., St. Louis, in press.

Simons, D.G. and Travell, J.G. (1983) Myofascial origins of low back pain. Parts 1,2,3. Postgrad. Med., 73: 66–108.

Simons, D.G. and Travell, J.G. (1984) Myofascial pain syndromes, Ch. 2.A.7. In P.D. Wall and R. Melzack (Eds.), Textbook of Pain, Churchill Livingstone, London, pp. 263–276.

Singer, E.J., Sharav, Y., Dubner, R. and Dionne, R.A. (1987) The efficacy of Diazepam and Ibuprofen in the treatment of chronic myofascial orofacial pain. Pain, Suppl. 4: S83 (Abstr. No. 161).

Skootsky, S. (1986) Incidence of myofascial pain in an internal medical group practice. Presented to the American Pain Society, Washington, DC, November 6–9.

Smythe, H.A. (1972) Non-articular rheumatism and the fibrositis syndrome. In J.L. Hollander and D.J. McCarty, (Eds.), Arthritis and Allied Conditions, 8th Edn., Lea & Febiger, Philadelphia.

Smythe, H. (1986) Tender points: evolution of concepts of the fibrositis/fibromyalgia syndrome. Am. J. Med., (Suppl. 3A) 81: 2–6.

Smythe, H.A. and Moldofsky, H. (1977) Two contributions to understanding of the 'fibrositis' syndrome. Bull. Rheum. Dis., 28: 928–931.

Sola, A.E., Rodenberger, M.L. and Gettys, B.B. (1955) Incidence of hypersensitive areas in posterior shoulder muscles. Am. J. Phys. Med., 34: 585–590.

Spangfort, E. (1987) The low back pain problem. Pain, Suppl. 4: S111 (Abstr. No. 210).

Travell, J. and Rinzler, S.H. (1952) The myofascial genesis of pain. Postgrad. Med., 11: 425–434.

Travell, J.G., Rinzler, S.H. and Herman, M. (1942) Pain and disability of the shoulder and arm. Treatment by intramuscular infiltration with procaine hydrochloride. J. Am. Med. Assoc., 120: 417–422.

Travell, J.G. and Simons, D.G. (1983) Myofascial Pain and Dysfunction: The Trigger Point Manual, Williams & Wilkins, Baltimore, MD.

Tunks, E., Norman, G., Kalaher, S. and Crook, J. (1987) Validity and reliability of the clinical use of a pressure algometer in the study of trigger points. Pain, Suppl. 4: S307 (Abstr. No. 590).

Weeks, V.D. and Travell, J. (1955) Postural vertigo due to trigger areas in the sternocleidomastoid muscle. J. Pediatr., 47: 315–327.

Wolfe, F. (1986) The clinical syndrome of fibrositis. Am. J. Med., 81 (Suppl. 3A): 7–14.

Yunus, M., Masi, A.T., Calabro, J.J. and Shah, I.K. (1982) Primary fibromyalgia. Am. Fam. Physician, 25: 115–121.

R. Dubner, G.F. Gebhart & M.R. Bond (Eds.)
Proceedings of the Vth World Congress on Pain
© 1988 Elsevier Science Publishers BV (Biomedical Division)

CHAPTER 22

Peripheral and central electrophysiological mechanisms of joint and muscle pain

Gisèle Guilbaud

I.N.S.E.R.M. Unité 161, 2 Rue d'Alesia, 75014 Paris, France

Introduction

Although most studies dealing with pain mechanisms have concentrated on the processing of noxious stimuli applied to the skin, pain from joints and skeletal muscles is more commonly encountered in clinical situations than is cutaneous pain. Comparable mechanisms could underly the various somatic pains, but deep pain might present some unique characteristics. Pain from deep tissues is often reported to have a dull, aching quality, to be poorly localized, diffuse, with simultaneous projected and referred pain. However it can also be sharp, lancinating and well localized. This might relate to anatomical considerations: if the pain originated in joints and in muscular fascia directly underneath the skin, it could be more precisely localized by contrast to the more diffuse pain from deeper tissues (Lewis, 1942, and ref. in Mense, 1986). Differences in innervation density might also be of importance (Feindel et al., 1948). Although less extensive than studies on cutaneous pain, relatively recent electrophysiological investigations are now providing some clues for a better knowledge of the physiological processing of joint and muscle pain.

There is now evidence that some thin peripheral fibres can convey noxious inputs originating in muscles and joints, and that these messages can reach upper levels of the central nervous system, such as the thalamus and the somatosensory cortex, after a relay in the dorsal horn of the spinal cord. Interestingly these data have been obtained not only with normal animals, but also, if not mainly, in experimental models of muscular and arthritic pain. In addition, the use of one of these models, polyarthritic rats, even if it does not provide conclusive arguments, relates to the question of a putative selective system partly devoted to deep pain. Indeed, with this model it was revealed that in these pathological conditions, neuronal populations and ascending pathways involved in the transmission of messages elicited from the inflamed joints (giving rise to the nociceptive manifestations seen in the freely moving animal) seem to be to some extent different from those involved in the transmission of noxious cutaneous inputs in normal animals. The involvement of the peripheral nerve fiber in these changes is clearly demonstrated. However, it is also possible that the dramatic changes in the neuronal responsiveness of several CNS areas seen in the chronic animals might be relevant to central modulation exerted on the somatic inputs at various levels of the CNS. Indeed, there is also evidence that the reactivity of endogenous opioid systems is greatly changed in animals with persistent pain. These various aspects will be successively considered in this review.

Activation of thin afferent fibres by noxious stimulation of deep tissues

Muscle receptors

In a muscle nerve, there is a large proportion of fine afferent fibres, either myelinated (group III) or un-myelinated (group IV) (ref. in Mense, 1986), and it has been clearly demonstrated that these fibres can innervate both the belly and tendons of a muscle (Anders et al., 1985). By analogy with cutaneous nerve fibres involved in the transmission of noxious messages originating in the skin, it was logically suggested that these fine afferent fibres could con-tribute to muscular pain, especially to intermittent claudication, which attracted much interest (see ref. in Mense, 1986). Before the development of the sin-gle-unit recording technique, Bessou and Laporte (1958), using the method of antidromic collision,

concluded that non-myelinated afferent fibers of a muscle nerve might be involved in the production of an ischemic muscular pain. Paintal (1960) was the first to record, in single muscular group III fi-bres, activity induced by noxious stimulation, such as a strong local pressure or an injection of hyper-tonic saline. There were subsequently several stud-ies by other pioneers of single-unit recordings (Bes-sou and Laporte, 1961; Iggo, 1961) showing that group III and IV afferents could be activated by a variety of mechanical, thermal and chemical stimuli when their intensity reached the noxious range. The next wave of systematic and extensive studies was in the 1970s. Recordings from a great number of muscular fibres demonstrated that several algogenic substances injected into the muscle artery, usually released in the inflammatory exudate (histamine, bradykinin, serotonin, potassium), greatly activat-

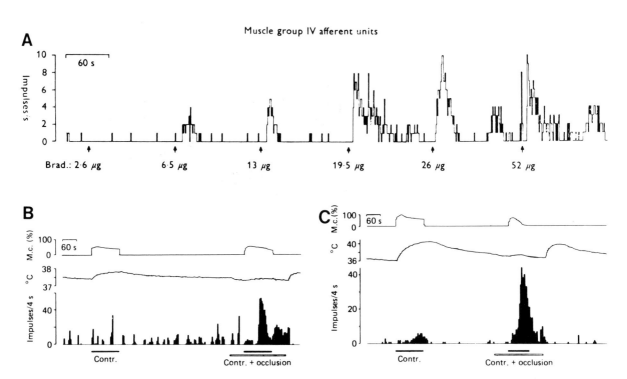

Fig. 1. Responses of a single group IV muscle afferents in A, to increasing doses of bradykinin, indicated by the arrows, with the appearance of after-discharges at the highest doses. The ordinate shows the number of impulses per second, the abscissa the dose of bradykinin injected into the muscle artery; in B and C, to a normal and to an ischemic contraction. Ordinate, from the bottom to top: number of impulses per 4 s, temperature of the muscle, intensity of the muscle contraction expressed as percentage of the maxi-mal contraction. (Adapted from Mense, 1986; and Mense and Stahnke, 1983).

ed the thin afferents, whereas large fibres (corresponding to muscle spindles and tendon organs) did not exhibit such marked activation (Mense and Schmidt, 1974; and ref. in Mense, 1986). In several studies, group III and IV endings were subjected to graded stimuli. As shown in Fig. 1, where increasing doses of bradykinin were successively intra-arterially injected close to the receptive field, a relationship between the response and the stimulus intensity could be observed. Two other interesting features observed for many of these receptors were their ability to be sensitized, and the ability of peripheral analgesics to depress their responses. The thresholds to mechanical stimulation of receptors requiring intense and noxious pressure for activation are greatly lowered after infiltration of their receptive field with bradykinin, so that they can be driven by light touch and gentle pressure (Mense, 1986). Responses of these receptors to bradykinin can be significantly reduced by aspirin (Mense, 1982). Finally, another unambiguous demonstration of the role of the thin muscular afferent fibres in muscular pain came from a study by Mense and Stahnke (1983), analysing their responses during muscular contraction with intact blood supply or after occlusion of the muscle artery. During ischemic contractions some receptors (all belonging to group IV) which did not respond to a normal contraction exhibited vigorous activation during ischemic work (Fig. 1). A more recent study also emphasized changes in the activities of the thin afferent fibres of a muscle, during the inflammatory process produced by the injection of carrageenan (Berberich et al., 1986). There are thus, in the periphery, several neurophysiological correlates for several types of muscular pain, such as hyperalgesia and allodynia of an inflamed muscle, or ischemic pain during arterial occlusion. Finally, evidence of involvement of the muscular thin afferent fibres in muscular pain was provided by Torebjörk et al. (1984), where painful sensation could be correlated with the characteristics of the electrical intraneural stimulation of muscle fascicles in the median nerve of healthy subjects.

Joint receptors

In the nomenclature of Freeman and Wyke (1967) for the different joint receptors, it appears that group III fibres give rise to the unmyelinated plexuses in the inner zone of the fibrous capsule, and group IV fibres to free nerve endings which are numerous in the joint capsule. In a more recent systematic investigation of the cat's knee joint via the medial and the posterior articular nerves, it appeared that fine myelinated and unmyelinated fibres are at least six times as frequent as thick myelinated ones (Langford et al., 1984). In the first single-fibre investigations on joint knee receptors in cat (Burgess and Clark, 1969; Clark, 1975; Grigg, 1975), very few were described as having a very high threshold to mechanical stimuli, and even in these cases they were 'weakly activated'. In a recent study, also on the cat knee joint, Schaible and Schmidt (1983) distinguished several categories of receptors of group III and IV. Amongst them were fibres weakly activated by non-noxious movements, but responding strongly to noxious movements, and units responding only to noxious ones. A great proportion of the thin afferent fibres could not be activated by any kind of mechanical stimulation. In sharp contrast, after a close injection of bradykinin (Kanaka et al., 1985) or during inflammation of the knee joint by injection of carrageenan conjugated with kaolin, this proportion of inactive units dramatically fell (Coggeshall et al., 1983). In the case of an inflamed joint, the proportion of thin fibres which could be driven by innocuous movements was increased (from 31 to 90% in group III, and from 13 to 73% in group IV) (Coggeshall et al., 1983; Grigg et al., 1986). This indicates that units are likely to have been sensitized by the inflammatory process. In addition, it was shown that prostaglandins, well known to be released in the inflammatory exudate, could induce a sensitizing action on articular group III units, with both a lowering of threshold and a more forceful response to movement, with this effect being depressed by indomethacin (Heppelmann et al., 1985).

Comparable data have been obtained in the rat, in a situation of chronic articular inflammation

(Guilbaud et al., 1985a). In this case, the rats were rendered polyarthritic by Freund's adjuvant injected at the base of the tail (Pearson and Wood, 1959), 3–4 weeks before the investigation. In these rats, the ankles are especially inflamed, and behavioural studies have shown that they can be an effective source of noxious input in conscious rats (Pircio et al., 1975; De Castro Costa et al., 1981; Kayser and Guilbaud, 1983; Calvino et al., 1987b). In particular the animals exhibit a clear decrease in the vocalization threshold to paw pressure. In these

conditions the characteristics of the receptors in the ankle joint capsule differ greatly from those observed for the capsule receptors recorded in normal ankles (Guilbaud et al., 1985). A resting discharge, absent in normal rats, was frequent in arthritics; there was a profound decrease of the mechanical threshold of the unit responses in arthritic in comparison with normal animals (Fig. 2); pressure on the ankle or small degrees of flexion or extension produced a high rate of discharge in receptors of arthritic rats, while similar stimuli were ineffective in

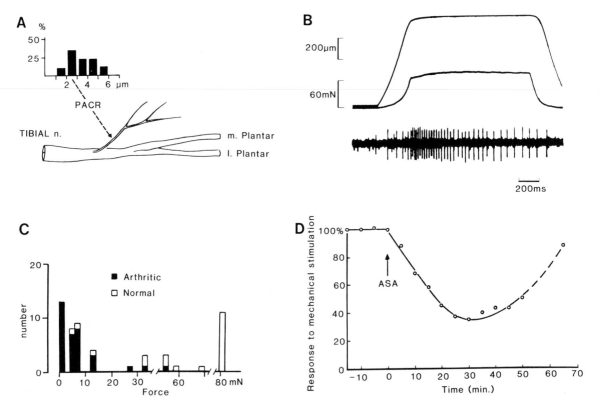

Fig. 2. A. Schematic diagram of the tibial nerve, showing the primary articulo-cutaneous ramus (PACR) arising from the medial plantar division of the tibial nerve and giving rise to three branches. The histogram illustrates the percentage of the PACR nerve fibers according to their diameter. B. Response of a joint capsule receptor to a controlled indentation in an arthritic rat. In each descending record are displayed the indentation applied to the capsule (expressed in μm), the force developed (in mN) and the afferent discharge in the PACR. C. Number of joint capsule receptors according to their activation threshold values, measured with Von Frey hairs, for mechanical stimulation, in normal (open bars) and arthritic (filled bars) rats. D. The effect of topical application to the exposed joint capsule of an arthritic rat of a solution containing 100 μg lysine acetylsalicylate on the responses of a single joint capsule receptor to a controlled mechanical stimulation. A decline in sensitivity is apparent within 5 min, and continues for the next 30 min, to reach a minimum of 35% of control values. Recovery then began and was almost complete at 65 min. (Adapted from Guilbaud et al., 1985 and Guilbaud and Iggo, 1985.)

normals. These electrophysiological features correlate well with the clinical observations performed in
these rats and in patients with arthritis. In addition,
the responses of the capsule afferents recorded in
arthritic rats are strongly depressed by aspirin
(Guilbaud and Iggo, 1985) (Fig. 2).

Activation of central neurones by noxious stimulation of deep tissues

There are several controversies concerning the spinal termination of muscular nerves, particularly
with regard to the thin afferent fibres (see ref. in
Mense, 1986). However, from data using restricted
application of horseradish peroxidase to a feline
muscle nerve, its central terminations were found in
lamina I and V of the dorsal horn, but not in lamina
II, III or IV. This was confirmed by a study which
combined neurophysiological and histochemical
methods, to visualize functionally identified fibres.
Again it was found that the axons from the deep
nociceptors (only group III were studied) terminate
either in lamina I and/or in lamina IV/V (Mense,
1986). Thus, it appears that there is an anatomical
substrate for a direct nociceptive input from the
deep tissues to some dorsal horn neurones.

Spinal level and supraspinal level in normal animals
Contrasting with the numerous studies dealing with
the activation of dorsal horn neurones by noxious
stimulation of the skin, those concerned with the
noxious stimulation of the deep tissues appear scarce. In fact it has been shown by various groups that
neurones found in or near lamina V, and also in lamina I, could either receive input from muscular or
articular group III fibres, or be activated by various
chemical and mechanical algesic stimulations of a
muscle (Pomeranz et al., 1968; Cervero et al., 1976;
Foreman et al., 1977, 1979; Hong et al., 1979; Craig
and Kniffki, 1982; Schaible et al., 1987a) (Fig. 3).

In several of these studies it was simultaneously
observed that many of the dorsal horn neurones so
activated in fact receive both cutaneous, articular
and muscular, and even visceral inputs (Pomeranz

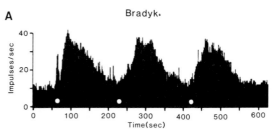

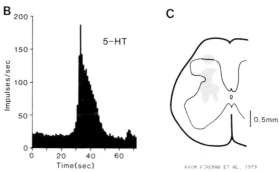

Fig. 3. Excitatory action in A and B of algesic chemicals injected
into the arterial circulation of the triceps surae muscles in anesthetized monkey (successive injections of bradykinin or of 5-
hydroxytryptamine (5-HT), on spinothalamic tract neurones at
locations shown in C. (Adapted from Foreman et al., 1979.)

et al., 1968; Willis et al., 1974; ref. in Foreman et
al., 1979, ref. in Menetrey et al., 1980; Schaible et
al., 1987a). The proportion of such neurones has
not been clearly established so far, but it appears
that it is relatively high, so only a few neurones are
exclusively activated by noxious deep input (Craig
and Kniffki, 1982). Nevertheless, the existence of
the convergence between cutaneous and deep messages on the same neurone has been considered as
an explanation of the projected cutaneous pain and
hyperalgesia which often accompany muscular
pain. In fact, such convergence has been reproduced in investigations in humans, using either saline injection into an interspinus ligament, or micro-
electrical stimulation of a nerve muscular fascicule
(Hockaday and Whitty, 1967; Torebjörk et al.,
1984). Moreover, it was clearly demonstrated in
cat, rat and monkey that some of the dorsal horn
neurones receiving deep noxious inputs could project, directly or otherwise, to the thalamus either via
the spinocervico- or the spinothalamic tract (Fore-

man et al., 1979; Craig and Kniffki, 1982; Menetrey et al., 1977; Schaible et al., 1987a,b). In addition, in the rat, there is evidence that inputs due to strong pressure on deep tissues or to joint movement could be conveyed through the spinoreticular tract (Menetrey et al., 1980).

Thus, there is no doubt that responses elicited from deep tissues, and perceived as nociceptive, are conveyed to supraspinal structures. However, little is known about the next step in their integration. In appeared from a study using gross potentials evoked in the ventrobasal complex of the cat, by electrical stimulation of muscular nerves, that high-threshold input driven by group III fibres could reach the thalamus (Mallart, 1968). The same difficulties arose with regard to the more general problem of pain processing at the thalamic level (see ref. in Guilbaud et al., 1985b). Recently, two groups simultaneously described cat nociceptive neurones driven by slowly conducting cutaneous and muscular afferent fibres and located in the ventral and dorsolateral periphery of the ventroposterolateral nucleus, and in the transitional zone between this nucleus and the ventrolateral nucleus (Honda et al., 1983; Kniffki and Mizumura, 1983). This region is, in cat, one of the areas which seem to receive axon terminals of spinothalamic cells (see ref. in Kniffki, 1987). In cat, a small fraction of the units in somatosensory cortex area 3a were found to be activated by stimulation of group III and IV fibres, strong pressure of a muscle, or injection of algogenic agents (Iwamura et al., 1981). In rats there are only a few neurones in the somatosensory cortex which are specifically activated by noxious deep stimuli (Lamour et al., 1983a).

In fact, in normal animals, data are very scarce on the processing of deep pain input at the supraspinal level. Recently, studies using arthritic rats have shed light on this question.

Spinal and supraspinal neurones implicated in the transmission of joint inputs in models of experimental articular pain

The various systematic electrophysiological investigations performed in polyarthritic rats, at various levels of the central nervous system, have demonstrated that inputs elicited from the inflamed joints reach these various CNS sites. In addition they have emphasized profound changes in the responsiveness of the somatosensory neurones. A great majority of them (the exact proportion depends on the area considered) could be maximally activated when apparently gentle stimuli were applied to the joints or surrounding cutaneous areas.

Spinal level In the first study (Menetrey and Besson, 1982) considering responses of dorsal horn neurones in unanesthetized arthritic rats, the rats were decerebrated and spinalized at C2. This particular study was mainly devoted to the modifications of neuronal responses due to cutaneous inputs. For the superficial dorsal horn cells (in lamina I and II), there were neurones driven from the non-edematous skin of the paw, with properties similar to those observed in healthy animals, and other neurones driven from inflamed skin, characterized by novel electrophysiological properties. A first striking observation was the relatively high level of background activity with a frequent bursting pattern (Fig. 4A), which sharply contrasted with the almost total absence of background activity for neurones located in the superficial laminae in normal animals. Also striking was the high degree of responsiveness of these superficial neurones to light mechanical stimuli. None of them was exclusively driven by intense stimuli such as pinch. Modifications of responsiveness were also observed for some neurones located in deeper laminae of the dorsal horn. Beside neurones with apparent 'normal' characteristics, a large proportion exhibited curious properties. Neurones receiving both $A\alpha\beta$ and $A\delta$ or C inputs (thus akin to the classical wide-dynamic-range cells) were maximally activated by moderate mechanical stimulation, without subsequent increase in discharge in response to intense pinch (Fig. 4B). Their background discharge was also high, and frequently included bursting patterns.

In the second investigation on responsiveness of dorsal horn units (Calvino et al., 1987a), rats were not spinalized, but were under a moderate and stab-

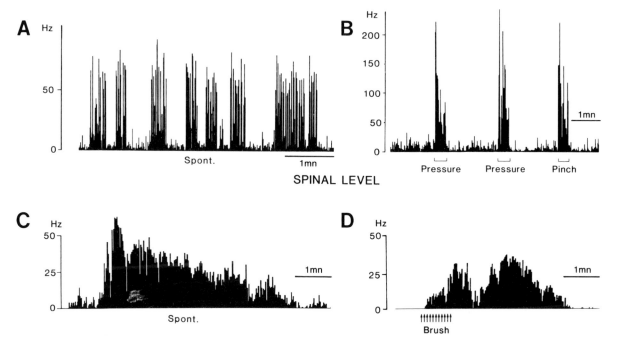

Fig. 4. Activity of spinal dorsal horn neurones recorded in arthritic rats spinalized (in A and B), or anesthetized (in C and D). Responses elicited by moderate stimulation of the receptive field, (joint or surrounding skin in B and D), without further increases in discharge when a pinch was applied (B). Activity occurring wihout intentional stimulation in A and C. (A and B are adapted from Menetrey and Besson, 1982; C and D from Calvino et al., 1987.)

le gaseous anesthesia. Again, atypical responses were observed. In addition, it was clearly observed that half of the neurones excited by somatic stimuli responded to moderate pressure or movement of the inflamed ipsilateral ankle, and that the responses so elicited often exhibited after-discharges of variable but long duration (Fig. 4D). Numerous paroxysmal discharges occurred without intentional stimulation (Fig. 4C).

Interestingly, a comparable 'sensitization' of dorsal horn responses was also observed during acute inflammation, induced by injection of kaolin together with carrageenan, in the cat knee joint (Schaible et al., 1987b). It was shown that spinal dorsal horn neurones, which initially showed little or no response to the knee flexion, developed large responses within 2–3 h after inflammation of the joint.

Supraspinal level The first systematic electrophysiological investigation performed at this level in ar-

thritic rats concerned the ventrobasal complex of the thalamus (VB) (Gautron and Guilbaud, 1982). This structure, in the rat, was known to receive, in addition to the lemniscal ascending pathway specific for touch, direct projections from dorsal horn neurones activated by noxious stimulation (ref. in Guilbaud et al., 1985b). In a previous extensive investigation of the VB complex of normal rat, it was shown that numerous neurones exclusively activated by noxious stimuli were intermingled with the classical neurones involved in the transmission of light touch information (Guilbaud et al., 1980).

Among the population of 168 somatosensory VB neurones which have been analysed in arthritic rats, we first observed that few of them (only 25%) responded with electrophysiological characteristics reminiscent of those described for VB neurones in normal rats. Moreover, their separation into various functional groups was different. For instance, the proportion of neurones exclusively driven by pinch was especially small (only 12%), and the responses of these neurones to intense stimuli habituated when the stimulus was repeated.

Secondly, for the other somatosensory neurones (65% of the whole population), unusual properties were noted. A large proportion of these neurones were driven by gentle movement and/or mild lateral pressure of an inflamed joint, a stimulus which is usually inefficient, or only induces a phasic response of short duration for the VB neurones in normal animals. In sharp contrast, in arthritic rats, the effective movement, either an extension, a flexion, or both, induced an immediate and sustained increase in the neuronal discharge, which outlasted by several-fold (2 to 12 times) that of the stimulation. The mean duration of the after-discharge calculated for responses of 44 neurones, elicited by a joint movement maintained for 15 s, was 49.5 ± 4.6 s. Very light tactile stimulation such as brushing or light repetitive touch, applied to the cutaneous areas surrounding the inflamed joints, could be sufficient to elicit responses of such long duration, as shown in Fig. 5. This response pattern is very unusual. The

VB neurones recorded in the normal animal, specific to light touch, exhibit a response which is rapidly adapting, without any after-discharge at all (Fig. 5). Another striking feature was the large proportion of neurones which displayed paroxysmal discharges lasting several seconds or minutes, occurring without intentional stimulation.

The pattern and circumstances of the neuronal responses recorded in the VB of arthritic rats are strongly reminiscent of the characteristics of behavior exhibited by the arthritic animal when it is freely moving, and of the painful sensations presented by patients with arthritis. In addition, the functional implication of such neuronal activity was confirmed by another study, which clearly showed that VB neuronal responses induced by stimulation of inflamed joints were strongly depressed by aspirin (Guilbaud et al., 1982). This depressive action likely reflects the peripheral effect of aspirin, as described above (Guilbaud and Iggo, 1985).

Subsequent investigations performed in other thalamic nuclei known to be involved in the trans-

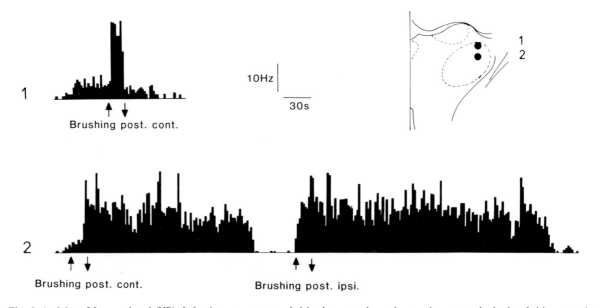

Fig. 5. Activity of 2 ventrobasal (VB) thalamic neurones recorded in the same electrode tract in an anesthetized arthritic rat, as in C and D of Fig. 4. Response of neurone 1 is comparable to responses recorded in the VB of normal rat; responses of neurone 2 elicited by application of light brushing to both inflamed wrists, exhibiting unusual patterns with long after-discharges. Inset shows location of neurone 1 and 2 in VB.

ARTHRITIC

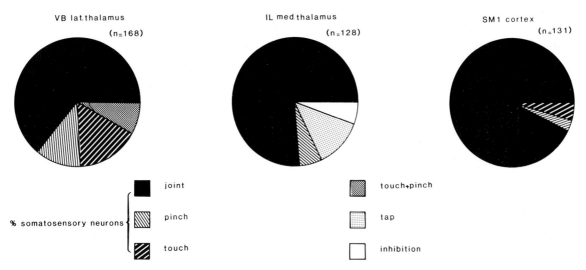

VB lat.thalamus
(n=168)

IL med.thalamus
(n=128)

SM1 cortex
(n=131)

% somatosensory neurons

- joint
- pinch
- touch
- touch+pinch
- tap
- inhibition

Fig. 6. Schematic representation of the proportion of neurones activated by various somatic stimuli in the structures which have been systematically explored. Notice the great proportion of neurones which are activated by moderate stimulation of the inflamed joints. VB = ventrobasal, IL = intralaminar, SM1 cortex = somatosensory cortex.

mission of noxious messages confirmed that the joint input was predominant in these arthritic rats. Indeed the proportion of somatosensory neurones responding to lateral pressure or movement of one or several inflamed joints was a common feature of all the studies performed in these rats (Fig. 6); either in the somatosensory cortex (Lamour et al., 1983), or in the intralaminar and medial thalamic nuclei (Kayser and Guilbaud, 1984; Dostrovsky et al., 1987). An effect of aspirin on responses in some of these structures was present (Fig. 7), with a time course comparable to its effects at the peripheral level.

Thus, it is likely that the increased responsiveness of CNS neurones to moderate stimulations of the inflamed joints is partly due to the changes in the responsiveness of articular receptors reported in the previous section. However, additional observations suggest a more complex interaction between peripheral and central processes, which could be responsible for the modifications noted in these arthritic rats. In addition these central phenomena could more or less account for several characteristics of clinical deep pain.

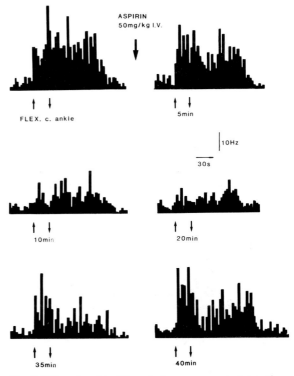

ASPIRIN
50mg/kg I.V.

FLEX. c. ankle

5min

10Hz

30s

10min

20min

35min

40min

Fig. 7. Effect of aspirin (50 mg/i.v.) on responses to joint stimulation recorded in the sub-medius nucleus of an arthritic rat. Flex. C. ankle = flexion of the contralateral ankle.

Central phenomena which might contribute to the change in the responsiveness of the somatosensory neurones seen in arthritic rats: their relationship to clinical observations on deep pain

Referred pain – segmental, heterosegmental and/or supraspinal 'spread of excitation'

Previous observations on the distribution of referred pain, especially frequent in the pathology of deep tissues, pointed out that some were experienced within an area belonging partly to one segment (ref. in Hardy et al., 1967; Simons and Travell, 1985; Chapter 28 of this volume). However, some pains do not follow a simple 'segmental' pattern. This was reported in numerous clinical observations (ref. in Hardy et al., 1967) and shown in several experimental human investigations, using either an injection of hypertonic saline in an interspinal ligament (see ref. in Hockaedey and Whitty, 1967), or electrical stimulation of a muscle nerve fascicle (Torebjörk et al., 1984). In addition to the local pain elicited by the initial stimulus, several types of referred pain extending sometimes to muscular areas with a different segmental innervation could occur. For instance, it is possible for pain to be experienced on the side opposite to the site of the noxious stimulation. In these circumstances, spread of the effects of noxious stimulation associated with deep pain, based solely on anatomical arrangements within the spinal cord or brain stem, or even supraspinal areas, has also been suggested (Hardy et al., 1967; Simons and Travell, 1985; ref. in Torebjörk et al., 1984).

Data reported from several animal experiments using models of localized articular and cutaneous inflammatory pain might be related to these clinical observations. After the initiation of hyperalgesic inflammation, it is indeed possible to observe changes in withdrawal threshold, by stimulating areas remote from the initial injury (see ref. in Kayser and Guilbaud, 1986). Neurophysiological correlates have been described recently in such models. After the induction of a localized inflammation, changes in the neuronal responses, either at the spinal (Schaible et al., 1987b) or thalamic level (Guilbaud et al., 1986a), have been observed by stimulating the injury site, and also part(s) of the body, distant from the initial receptive field (namely the opposite posterior and even the anterior paws, where the lesion was on one posterior paw). In these cases, the

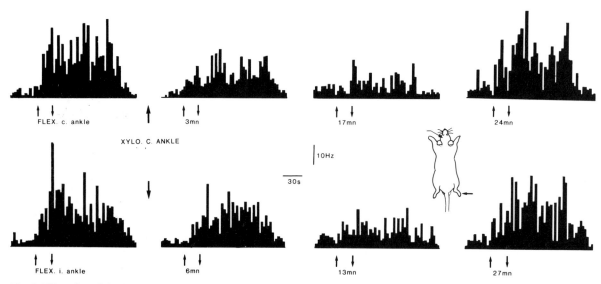

Fig. 8. Effect of one injection (indicated by the two thick arrows) of 0.05 ml lidocaine/epinephrine hydrochloride solution (respectively, 1 and 0.0025% in saline), in the contralateral (the right) inflamed ankle (Xylo. C. Ankle) on the responses elicited from the two ankles, and recorded in the left VB. Flex. c. ankle, Flex. i. ankle = flexion of the contra- and ipsilateral ankle.

injection of a local anesthetic at the site of injury altered the responses in the lesioned and non-lesioned distant areas (Guilbaud et al., 1986a). These phenomena suggest that central processes have been triggered by the local inflammation, and, whatever their origin in the CNS, could be responsible for the 'remote' modifications that we roughly equate to distant 'referred pain'. This type of observation was also recently made in polyarthritic rats. In this experimental situation responses of a VB neurone with a bilateral receptive field were studied. The injection of a local anesthetic in one ankle depressed the responses elicited from both inflamed ankles (Fig. 8). Thus, in arthritic rats, not only is the responsiveness of the receptors changed, but also, indirectly, there is an alteration in the responsiveness of several pools of central neurones remote from the stimulation site. Thus, several phenomena, segmental, heterosegmental and/or supraspinal, could contribute to the predominance of joint input in the central nervous structures of arthritic rats.

Projected hyperalgesia and tenderness – convergence of several somatic inputs on the same neurone – does a selective system exist for nociceptive joint inputs?
As mentioned previously, the existence of convergence of noxious inputs from various origins (cutaneous, muscular, articular, visceral), on the same neurone, has been seen at spinal and supraspinal

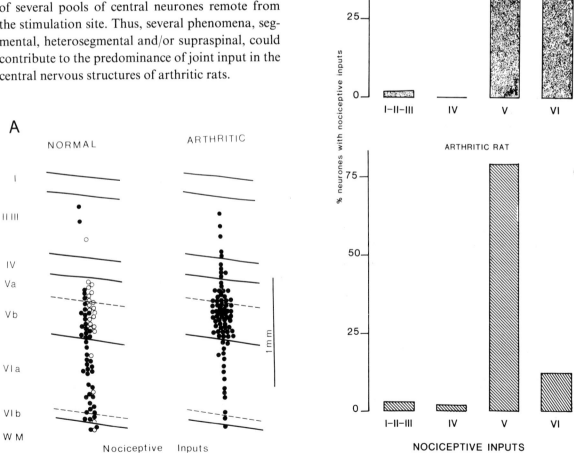

Fig. 9. A shows the localization in the different cortical laminae of the somatosensory cortical neurones receiving nociceptive inputs, in normal and arthritic rats. In B, the classification is expressed as a percentage of the number of neurones receiving nociceptive inputs.

levels of the CNS (ref. in Foreman et al., 1979; Guilbaud et al., 1980; Schaible et al., 1987a; Kniffki and Mizumura, 1983). This has provided an interesting neurophysiological basis for explaining the projected tenderness and hyperalgesia which are frequently associated with articular and muscular pain, and which fits well with the well-known proposition of Ruch (1946) in the case of visceral pain. We initially suggested that VB neurones activated by joint stimuli in arthritic rats belong to the same neuronal population as those which were driven by intense cutaneous pinch in normal animals (Gautron and Guilbaud, 1982; Guilbaud et al., 1983). However, several observations in recent electrophysiological investigations in arthritic rats have cast doubt on this initial suggestion. In normal rats, somatosensory cortical neurones activated by noxious stimuli, and receiving input from the VB, were not found in lamina IV, but located in the deeper laminae, including VIa and VIb (Lamour et al., 1983b). In contrast, in arthritic rats, neurones driven from the inflamed joints had the tendency to be more superficial (mainly in the lamina Va, and even in lamina IV) (Fig. 9). This suggestion that neuronal populations involved in both situations could partly differ was confirmed in the study of intralaminar thalamic nuclei. In normal rats, few somatosensory neurones, mainly the nociceptive neurones, can be recorded in the ascending branch of the nucleus centralis lateralis, a part of the thalamic intralaminar nuclei (Peschanski et al., 1981). In sharp contrast, it appears that in arthritic rats numerous neurones located in this zone could be strongly activated from the inflamed joints (Fig. 10). Also, in these pathological conditions, the ascending pathways conveying nociceptive messages from the inflamed joints to the VB complex of the thalamus seem to differ in comparison with those involved in normal rats. In healthy animals, the lateral spinothalamic tract seems to have the major role in conveying noxious messages from that half of the body relaying input to the contralateral VB complex, while additional pathways (such as the ipsilateral component of the spinoreticular) appear likely to be involved in noxious joint inputs in ar-

thritic animals (Peschanski et al., 1985; Guilbaud et al., 1986b). Thus, these different observations tend to indicate that the central neurones exclusively driven by intense stimulation in the normal animal, and those excited by inflamed joints, belong, at least in part, to different neuronal populations, and that the nociceptive inputs may be partly conveyed by distinct ascending pathways.

Support for this hypothesis comes from data from normal cat, where some neurones of several CNS structures have been reported to be specifi-

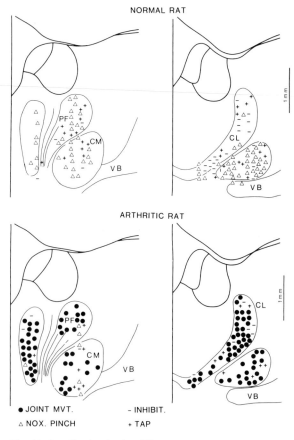

Fig. 10. Localization in the different intralaminar thalamic nuclei of the somatosensory neurones receiving nociceptive inputs in normal and arthritic rats. PF = parafascicularis, CM = centre median, CL = centralis lateralis, VB = ventrobasal. These neurones were activated by a movement of a joint (Joint Mvt.), a nociceptive pinch (Nox. Pinch), a brisk tap (Tap), or were inhibited (Inhibit.).

cally driven by deep stimulation (Craig and Kniffki, 1985). An ascending tract with an exclusive input from joint may exist through the CNS, but it appears that the information is from large afferent fibres, likely to be non-nociceptive (Gardner et al., 1949; Burgess and Clark, 1969; Kuno et al., 1973; ref. in Schaible et al., 1987a). If a more or less selective pathway exists for noxious joint inputs, it appears from the data reported here that it is relatively 'silent' in normal conditions, and is sensitized by the inflammatory process. The 'sensitization' observed at the central level not only reflects that described at the periphery but includes an additional change in CNS activity.

The possible implication of different neurones and pathways in conveying noxious articular messages does not explain another striking observation seen with experiments on arthritic rats. Either at the spinal level, or in various supraspinal CNS structures of arthritic rats, there are few neurones exclusively driven by intense cutaneous stimuli, when compared to the proportion found in normal animals (Menetrey and Besson, 1982; Gautron and Guilbaud, 1982; Lamour et al., 1983; Kayser and Guilbaud, 1984; Dostrovsky et al., 1987). We first thought that this was due to convergence, and that in fact the same population of neurones was involved in both situations. It turns out that this is not entirely the case. Even if a putative selective system really exists for the nociceptive joint inputs, it

cannot explain why neurones exclusively driven by intense cutaneous stimuli are so rare or exhibit habituation as described at several levels of the CNS (Menetrey and Besson, 1982; Gautron and Guilbaud, 1982). Nor can it explain why neurones responding specifically to light touch inputs are so scarce at the cortical level (Fig. 6) in arthritic rats. Since these observations do to seem directly due to alteration of the peripheral input (Guilbaud et al., 1985a), we suggest that some spinal and/or supraspinal controls might differentially modulate the various peripheral somatic inputs, leading to the great predominance of noxious joint messages, which seem to activate the whole brain. For instance, it can be speculated that control(s), excited by endogenous opioid systems could be different in these rats as compared to normals, consistent with the modification of this system in conditions of persistent pain (see Chapter 8 of this volume). Thus, it is still unknown to what extent central phenomena triggered by peripheral sensitization participate in the changes in neuronal responsiveness seen in various areas of the CNS.

Acknowledgements

The author wishes to thank Dr. A.H. Dickenson for English revision, and Mme. M. Gautron and Mr. E. Dehausse for the illustrations.

References

Andres, K.H., Düring, M. von and Schmidt, R.F. (1985) Anat. Embryol., 172: 145–156.

Berberich, P., Hoheisel, U. and Mense, S. (1986) Discharges properties of group II and IV receptors in an inflamed muscle. Proc. German Physiol. Soc., April 1986.

Bessou, P. and Laporte, Y. (1958) C.R. Soc. Biol. Paris, 152: 1587–1590.

Bessou, P., Laporte, Y. (1961) Étude des rècepteurs musculaires innervés par les fibres afférentes du groupe III (fibres myelinisées fines) chez le chat. Arch. Ital. Biol., 99: 293–321.

Burgess, P.R. and Clark, F.J. (1969) Characteristics of knee joint receptors in the cat. J. Physiol. (Lond.), 203: 317–335.

Calvino, B., Villanueva, L. and Lebars, D. (1987) Dorsal horn (convergent) neurones in the intact anesthetized arthritic rat: I: Segmental excitatory influences. Pain, 28: 81–98.

Calvino, B., Crepon-Bernard, M.O. and Lebars, D. (1987) Parallel clinical and behavioural studies of adjuvant-induced arthritis in the rat: possible relationship with 'chronic pain'. Behav. Brain Res., 24: 11–29.

Cervero, F., Iggo, A. and Molony, V. (1976) Nociceptor-driven dorsal horn neurones in the lumbar spinal cord of the cat. Pain, 2: 5–24.

Clark, F.J. (1975) Information signaled by sensory fibers in medial articular nerve. J. Neurophysiol., 38: 1464–1472.

Clark, F.J., Landgren, S. and Silfvenius, H. (1973) Projections to the cat's cerebral cortex from low threshold joint afferents. Acta Physiol. Scand., 89: 504–521.

Coggeshall, R.E., Hong, K.A.P., Langford, L.A., Schaible, H.G. and Schmidt, R.F. (1983) Discharge characteristics of fine medial articular afferents at rest and during passive movements of inflamed knee joints. Brain Res., 272: 185–188.

Craig, A.D. and Kniffki, K.D. (1985) Spinothalamic lumbosacral lamina I cells responsive to skin and muscle stimulation in the cat. J. Physiol. (Lond.), 365: 197–221.

De Castro-Costa, M., De Sutter, P., Gybels, J. and Van Hees, J. (1981) Adjuvant-induced arthritis in rats as a possible model of chronic pain. Pain, 10: 173–186.

Dostrovsky, J.O., Guilbaud, G. and Gautron, M. (1987) Nociceptive neurons in nucleus submedius of the arthritic rat. Vth World Congress on Pain of the IASP.

Feindel, W.H., Weddel, G. and Sinclair, D.C. (1948) Pain sensibility in deep somatic structures. J. Neurol. Neurosurg. Psychiatry, 11: 113–117.

Foreman, R.D., Schmidt, R.F. and Willis, W.D. (1977) Convergence of muscle and cutaneous input onto primate spinothalamic tract neurons. Brain Res., 124: 550–560.

Foreman, R.D., Schmidt, R.F. and Willis, W.D. (1979) Effects of mechanical and chemical stimulation of fine muscle afferents upon primate spinothalamic tract cells. J. Physiol. (Lond.), 286: 215–231.

Freeman, M.A.R. and Wyke, B. (1967) The innervation of the knee joint. An anatomical and histological study in the cat. J. Anat. (Lond.) 101: 505–532.

Gardner, E., Latimer, F. and Stilwell, D. (1949) Central connections for afferent fibers from the knee joint of the cat. Am. J. Physiol., 159: 195–198.

Gautron, M. and Guilbaud, G. (1982) Somatic responses of ventrobasal thalamic neurones in polyarthritic rats. Brain Res., 237: 459–471.

Grigg, P. (1976) Response of joint afferent neurons in cat medial articular nerve to active and passive movements of the knee. Brain Res., 118: 482–485.

Grigg, P., Schaible, H.G. and Schmidt, R.F. (1986) Mechanical sensitivity of group III and IV afferents from posterior articular nerve in normal and inflamed cat knee. J. Neurophysiol., 55: 635–643.

Guilbaud, G., Peschanski, M., Gautron, M. and Binder, D. (1980) Neurones responding to noxious stimulation in VB complex and caudal adjacent regions in the thalamus of the rat. Pain, 8: 303–318.

Guilbaud, G., Benoist, J.M., Gautron, M. and Kayser, V. (1982) Aspirin clearly depresses responses of ventrobasal thalamus neurones to joint stimuli in arthritic rats. Pain, 13: 153–163.

Guilbaud, G., Gautron, M., Benoist, J.M. and Kayser, V. (1983) Characteristics of some ventrobasal thalamic neurons in polyarthritic rats. Effects of acute injection of Aspirin on neuronal responses to joint stimulation. In J.J. Bonica et al. (Eds.), Advances in Pain Research and Therapy, Raven Press, New York, pp. 393–400.

Guilbaud, G. and Iggo, A. (1985) The effect of lysine acetylsalicylate on joint capsule mechanoreceptors in rats with polyarthritis. Exp. Brain Res., 61: 164–168.

Guilbaud, G., Iggo, A. and Tegner, R. (1985) Sensory receptors in ankle joint capsules of normal and arthritic rats. Exp. Brain, Res., 58: 29–40.

Guilbaud, G., Peschanski, M. and Besson, J.M. (1985) Experimental data related to nociception and pain at the supra spinal level. In P.D. Wall and R. Melzack (Eds.), Textbook of pain, Churchill Livingston, Edinburgh, pp. 110–118.

Guilbaud, G., Kayser, V., Benoist, J.M. and Gautron, M. (1986) Modifications of the responsiveness of rat ventrobasal thalamic neurons at different stages of carragenin-inflammation. Brain Res., 385: 86–98.

Guilbaud, G., Peschanski, M., Briand, A. and Gautron, M. (1986) The organization of spinal pathways to ventrobasal thalamus in an experimental model of pain (the arthritic rat). An electrophysiological study. Pain, 26: 301–312.

Hardy, J.D., Wolff, H.G., Goodell, B.S. and Boring, E.G. (1967) Pain Sensations and Reactions, 2nd edn., The Williams & Wilkins Company, New York, pp. 435.

Heppelmann, B., Schaible, H.G. and Schmidt, R.F. (1985) Effects of prostaglandins E1 and E2 on the mechanosensitivity of group III afferents from normal and inflamed cat knee joints. In H.L. Fields et al. (Eds.), Advances in Pain Research and Therapy, Raven Press, New York, pp. 91–101.

Hockaday, J.M. and Whitty, C.W.M. (1967) Patterns of referred pain in the normal subject. Brain, 90: 481–496.

Hong, S.K., Kniffki, K.D., Mense, S., Schmidt, R.F. and Wendisch, M. (1979) Descending influences on the responses of spinocervical tract neurones to chemical stimulation of fine muscle afferents. J. Physiol. (Lond.), 290: 129–140.

Honda, C.N., Mense, S. and Perl, E.R. (1983) Neurons in ventrobasal region of cat thalamus selectively responsive to noxious mechanical stimulation. J. Neurophysiol., 49: 662–673.

Iggo, A. (1961) Non-myelinated fibres from mammalian skeletal muscle. J. Physiol. (Lond.), 155: 52–53P.

Iwamura, Y., Kniffki, K.D., Mizumura, K. and Wilberg, K. (1981) Responses of feline S1 neurones to noxious stimulation of muscle and tendon. Pain, Suppl. 1: S213.

Kanaka, R., Schaible, H.G. and Schmidt, R.F. (1985) Activation of fine articular afferent units by bradykinin. Brain Res., 327: 81–90.

Kayser, V. and Guilbaud, G. (1983) Effects of morphine, but not those of the enkephalinase inhibitor, Thiorphan, are enhanced in arthritic rats. Brain Res., 267: 131–138.

Kayser, V. and Guilbaud, G. (1984) Further evidence for changes in the responsiveness of somatosensory neurons in arthritic rats: a study in the posterior intralaminar region of the thalamus. Brain Res., 323: 144–147.

Kayser, V. and Guilbaud, G. (1987) Local and remote modifications of nociceptive sensitivity during carrageenan-induced inflammation in the rat. Pain, 28: 99–108.

Kniffki, K.D. and Mizumura, K. (1983) Responses of neurons in VPL and VPL-VL region of the cat to algesic stimulation of muscle and tendon. J. Neurophysiol. 49: 649-661.

Kniffki, K.D. and Vahle-Hinz, C. (1987) The periphery of the cat's ventroposteromedial nucleus (VPMp) nociceptive neurones. In J.M. Besson, G. Guilbaud, M. Peschanski, (Eds.), Thalamus and Pain, Elsevier, Amsterdam, pp. 245–257.

Kuno, M., Munoz-Martinez, E.J. and Randic, M. (1973) Sensory inputs to neurones in Clarke's column from muscle, cutaneous and joint receptors. J. Physiol., 228: 327–342.

Lamour, Y., Willer, J.C. and Guilbaud, G. (1983) Rat somatosensory (Sm1) cortex: I. Characteristics of neuronal responses to noxious stimulation and comparison with responses to non-noxious stimulation. Exp. Brain Res., 49: 35–45.

Lamour, Y., Guilbaud, G. and Willer, J.C. (1983) Altered properties and laminar distribution of neuronal responses to peripheral stimulation in the SmI cortex of the arthritic rat. Brain Res., 273: 183–187.

Langford, L.A., Schaible, H.G. and Schmidt, R.F. (1983) Structure and function of fine joint afferents: observations and speculations. In W. Hamman and A. Iggo (Eds.), Sensory Receptor Mechanisms, World Scientific Publ. Co., Singapore, pp. 241–252.

Lewis, T. (1942) Pain, Macmillan, London, (Facsimile edition 1981).

Mallart, A. (1968) Thalamic projection of muscle nerve afferents in the cat. J. Physiol. (Lond.), 194: 337–353.

Menétrey, D. and Besson, J.M. (1982) Electrophysiological characteristics of dorsal horn cells in rats with cutaneous inflammation resulting from chronic arthritis. Pain, 13: 343–364.

Menétrey, D., Giesler, G.J. and Besson, J.M. (1977) An analysis of response properties of spinal cord dorsal horn neurones to nonnoxious and noxious stimuli in the spinal rat. Exp. Brain. Res., 27: 15–33.

Menétrey, D., Chaouch, A. and Besson, J.M. (1980) Location and properties of dorsal horn neurons at origin of spinoreticular tract in lumbar enlargement of the rat. J. Neurophysiol., 44: 862–877.

Mense, S. (1982) Reduction of the bradykinin-induced activation of feline group III and IV muscle receptors by acetylsalicylic acid. J. Physiol. (Lond.), 326: 269–283.

Mense, S. (1986) Slowly conducting afferent fibers from deep tissues: Neurobiological properties and central nervous actions. Prog. Sens. Physiol., 6: 139–219.

Mense, S. and Schmidt, R.F. (1974) Activation of group IV afferent units from muscle by algesic agents. Brain Res., 72: 305–310.

Mense, S. and Stahnke, M. (1983) Responses in muscle afferent fibers of slow conduction velocity to contractions and ischemia in the cat. J. Physiol. (Lond.), 342: 383–397.

Paintal, A.S. (1960) Functional analysis of group III afferent fibers of mammalian muscles. J. Physiol. (Lond.), 152: 250–270.

Pearson, C.M. and Wood, F.D. (1959) Studies of polyarthritis and other lesions induced in rats by injection of mycobacterial adjuvant. I. General clinical and pathological characteristics and some modifying factors. Arthritis Rheum., 2: 440–459.

Peschanski, M., Guilbaud, G. and Gautron, M. (1981) Posterior intralaminar region in rat: neuronal responses to noxious and non-noxious cutaneous stimuli. Exp. Neurol., 72: 226–238.

Pircio, A.W., Fedele, C.T. and Bierwagen, M.E. (1975) A new method for the evaluation of analgesic activity using adjuvant-induced arthritis in the rat. Eur. J. Pharmacol., 31: 207–215.

Pomeranz, B., Wall, P.D. and Weber, W.V. (1968) Cord cells responding to fine myelinated afferents from viscera, muscle and skin. J. Physiol. (Lond.), 199: 511–532.

Ruch, T.C. (1946) Visceral sensation and referred pain, Howell's Textbook of Physiology, Saunders, London.

Schaible, H.G. and Schmidt, R.F. (1983) Activation of groups III and IV sensory units in medial articular nerve by local mechanical stimulation of knee joint. J. Neurophysiol., 49: 35–44.

Schaible, H.G. and Schmidt, R.F. (1983) Responses of fine medial articular nerve afferents to passive movements of knee joint. J. Neurophysiol., 49: 1118–1126.

Schaible, H.G., Schmidt, R.F. and Willis, W.D. (1987) Convergent inputs from articular, cutaneous and muscle receptors onto ascending tract cells in the cat spinal cord. Exp. Brain Res., 66: 479–488.

Schaible, H.G., Schmidt, R.F. and Willis, W.D. (1987) Enhancement of the responses of ascending tract cells in the cat spinal cord by acute inflammation of the knee joint. Exp. Brain. Res., 66: 489–499.

Simons, D.G. and Travell, G. (1985) Myofascial pain syndromes. In Textbook of Pain, Churchill Livingstone, Edinburgh, pp. 263–276.

Torebjörk, H.E., Ochoa, J.L. and Schady, W. (1984) Referred pain from intraneural stimulation of muscles fascicles in the median nerve. Pain, 18: 145–156.

R. Dubner, G.F. Gebhart & M.R. Bond (Eds.)
Proceedings of the Vth World Congress on Pain
© 1988 Elsevier Science Publishers BV (Biomedical Division)

CHAPTER 23

Visceral pain

Fernando Cervero

Department of Physiology, Medical School, University of Bristol, University Walk, Bristol, BS8 1TD, U.K.

There is currently a renewed interest among basic scientists and clinicians in the mechanisms of deep and visceral pain (Cervero and Morrison, 1986). Scientists involved in pain research have realized that the neural organization of sensory systems cannot be fully understood without giving due consideration to the so far neglected inputs from deep somatic and visceral organs. Moreover, visceral pain is the most common form of pain produced by disease and clinicians know only too well that neurological models based entirely on the organization of acute cutaneous pain can offer little help in the understanding and treatment of pain of visceral origin. It is therefore encouraging to see a new surge of experimental and clinical work specifically aimed at improved our knowledge of the basic mechanisms of visceral pain.

The aims of this review are to highlight those aspects of visceral pain research that are the targets of current investigation and to discuss the clinical relevance of the new findings. This will not cover all possible angles of the problem but may help to point out the areas in need of further work. As it is a new and developing field, there are still many unresolved questions and some that are the subject of disputed interpretations. Whenever appropriate, these will be presented and discussed within the context of the available experimental evidence.

Clinical features of visceral pain

Neurophysiological thinking about pain in general has been dominated by Sherrington's approach to pain as the 'psychical adjunct of a protective reflex' (Sherrington, 1906). This concept has given credibility to experimental pain models based on anaesthetized or decerebrated animal preparations in which the 'pain' variable was measured by reference to the physical parameters of the protective reflex (i.e. tail flicks, motoneuronal activity, EMG). This approach is extremely useful when dealing with acute cutaneous pain, as it reflects the survival value of skin pain and the close relationship between this form of pain and the withdrawal reflex. However, pain of visceral origin shows a number of clinical features that make it quite different from acute cutaneous pain and do not validate Sherrington's definition based on a utilitarian approach to pain.

Visceral pain cannot be evoked from all viscera

The fact that pain cannot be triggered by stimulation of all internal organs is the strongest argument against a survival role for visceral pain. Moreover, it is not immediately clear why pain should be evoked by certain internal stimuli, such as renal or biliary calculi, in situations that cannot be improved by any form of natural therapy.

Visceral pain is usually evoked by stimuli that cause strong contractions of smooth muscle and/or ischaemia of the viscus. Nevertheless, extensive destruction by injury or malignant growth of organs such as the liver, the kidneys or the lungs does not evoke any sensory feed-back to the individual unless adjacent structures are also affected (MacKenzie, 1909; Morley, 1931). It is difficult to find a rational justification for the fact that no sensations can be evoked from some very important internal organs. The lack of a protective, and hence useful, role for visceral pain has puzzled mankind for centuries and it is probably the reason why visceral pain has been regarded in the western world as a curse of supernatural origin: 'in sorrow thou shalt bring forth children' (Genesis 3, 16).

Visceral pain is not linked to internal injury

As pointed out in the previous paragraphs, extensive injury of some internal organs can be painless whereas smooth muscle spasms not involving tissue damage are extremely painful. As far as visceral pain is concerned there is not a clear cut relationship between internal injury and pain. Some forms of injury, such as persistent ischaemia, or some of the consequences of injury, such as inflammation, can indeed evoke visceral pain. However, even these stimuli will not always trigger pain sensations when applied to certain viscera.

The traditional view is that visceral pain can be evoked by the following stimuli: (i) spasm of the smooth muscle in hollow viscera, (ii) distension of hollow viscera, (iii) ischaemia, (iv) inflammatory states, (v) chemical stimuli, and (vi) traction, compression and twisting of the mesenteries (Ayala, 1937). Notoriously absent from this list are forms of injury such as cutting, crushing or burning, which are capable of producing extensive internal damage and are also very general stimuli for cutaneous pain.

The most immediate consequence of this lack of correlation between injury and visceral pain is that the concept of 'noxious' stimulus needs to be redefined in so far as visceral pain is concerned. When studying the neurophysiological mechanisms of visceral pain, a noxious visceral stimulus is not the stimulus that produces (or can produce) injury but the stimulus that evokes (or can evoke) pain. Not all visceral stimuli that produce injury are necessarily noxious, since not all visceral injury is painful. It is therefore proposed that the association between noxious stimulus and injury is not intrinsic to the biological meaning of noxious stimulus but applies only to cutaneous stimulation.

Visceral pain can be referred to other locations

Many forms of visceral pain are felt in regions of the body other than the organ whose stimulation caused the pain (Head, 1893). The pain of angina is a characteristic example of a pain produced by cardiac ischaemia and felt as a crushing sensation extending from the thorax into the left shoulder and arm. This referral is one of the most representative features of deep and visceral pain and provides a valuable diagnostic tool to trace the source of the originating pain.

Visceral pain is diffuse and poorly localized

All forms of visceral pain are poorly localized and most are felt in areas considerably larger than the size of the originating viscus. It is also a common experience that as the pain becomes more intense, so the somatic area in which the pain is felt becomes larger (MacKenzie, 1909). These properties of visceral pain show that its localization is very poor and that the representation of internal organs within the central nervous system is very imprecise. If we consider the small intestine alone, the total surface area of this organ is more than an order of magnitude greater than the area of skin that covers the abdomen; yet, while cutaneous abdominal pain can be localized accurately within a few centimetres, intestinal pain is felt vaguely over the entire abdomen.

A classical exception to the poor localization of visceral pain is the pain of gastro-duodenal peptic ulcer, which some patients are able to pinpoint to the epigastrium with a fingertip. This form of pain, although very restricted, is nevertheless not localized to the stomach or duodenum, as can be easily demonstrated by the fact that displacing the contents of the abdomen by means of deep respiratory movements does not alter the locus of the pain (MacKenzie, 1909).

Some forms of visceral pain are known as 'true' visceral pains, implying a precise localization of the sensation to the diseased viscus (Procacci et al., 1986). The better-localized forms of 'true' visceral pain are usually due to the spread of the visceral lesion and the activation of somatic nerves close to the injured or diseased organ (i.e. those innervating peritoneum, muscles or ligaments). In other cases, the feeling of abdominal pain as a sensation originating from inside the body rather than from its surface is probably the consequence of the spatio-temporal pattern of activation of somatosensory pathways by visceral afferent fibres.

The lack of evidence for a sensory channel specifically concerned with the transmission of visceral sensory impulses and the considerable amount of experimental data on viscero-somatic convergence in the central nervous system are powerful arguments against the existence of a specific visceral mechanism for the so-called 'true' visceral pain (Cervero and Tattersall, 1986).

Visceral pain is accompanied by intense motor and autonomic reflexes

All forms of pain, cutaneous and visceral, are part of a general neurophysiological response which also includes motor and autonomic reflexes. These reflex responses are the 'pseudaffective' reactions (Sherrington, 1906), whose presence is often used experimentally to assess the noxious nature of the triggering stimulus. What is peculiar to pain of internal origin is the disproportion between the nature of the visceral stimulus and the intensity and duration of the pseudaffective reflexes.

Visceral pain is frequently accompanied by skeletal muscle contractures and spasms which last for a considerable amount of time and which contribute greatly to the patient's discomfort. The contracture of the abdominal wall during acute abdomen episodes is a characteristic example of such reactions. Equally, many forms of visceral pain are accompanied by intense autonomic reflexes such as persistent increases in heart rate and blood pressure, sweating and changes in the pattern of motility and secretion of other viscera, all of which can result in profound local and systemic alterations of normal autonomic tone. All these reactions are clear indications of a substantial increase in the excitability of the central nervous system following the arrival of a visceral nociceptive message. The central actions generated by visceral nociceptive impulses are thus of a more general and diffuse nature than those evoked by a restricted cutaneous stimulus.

Very few of these pseudaffective reactions can help the general state of the individual or can deal effectively with the originating cause of the pain. Therefore, their presence makes the patients more ill than they would be without them. The fact that some of these reflexes can be of considerable diagnostic value should not prevent the physician from making a quick intervention to relieve the pain and reduce the motor and autonomic responses.

Visceral nociceptors

One of the most fundamental questions of sensory physiology relates to the mode of encoding of peripheral stimuli by sensory receptors. The two main theories of pain mechanisms that have dominated scientific thinking this century – the specificity theory and the pattern theory – were radically different in their proposed encoding principles for peripheral receptors. The specificity interpretation is based on the existence of a specific category of 'pain receptor' or nociceptor, whereas the pattern approach proposes that pain is signalled by the temporal and spatial components of the response patterns of non-specific receptors (see Willis (1985) for a detailed review).

The existence of specific nociceptors in the skin, muscles, joints and other somatic structures is now beyond question (Torebjörk, 1985). The functional properties of cutaneous nociceptors have been studied in many animal species, including man. Micro-neurographic examination of afferent fibres in human nerves has provided definitive evidence showing a distinct correlation between electrical activity in afferent fibres connected to nociceptors and the perception of elementary sensations of pain (Torebjörk and Ochoa, 1983). While the pattern of the afferent discharge may encode the intensity of a sensory experience, the signalling of normal skin pain to the nervous system is mediated by activity in specific nociceptive afferent fibres.

In so far as visceral pain is concerned, the problem of sensory encoding by visceral afferent fibres has not yet been resolved. Several different opinions coexist in the current literature and the experimental evidence behind these notions is neither uniform nor conclusive.

An added level of complexity in this argument originates from the fact that the activation of many visceral afferent fibres does not result in the conscious perception of a specific sensation. Many of these visceral fibres (such as those connected to arterial baroreceptors and chemoreceptors, lung stretch receptors or intestinal chemoreceptors) are not 'sensory' fibres, since their activation does not evoke a sensory response, but only 'afferent' fibres concerned with the homeostatic regulation of the internal environment (Cervero, 1983, 1985). This distinction between 'afferent' and 'sensory' innervation does not apply to skin fibres, since all cutaneous afferents have the potential to evoke sensations. In contrast, some of the messages carried by visceral afferent fibres will never reach the level of a conscious sensory perception, whereas others will become sensory signals. Since discomfort and pain are the most common (and often the only) sensations evoked from viscera, the process of discrimination between sensory and non-sensory signals will have to differentiate visceral stimuli that evoke no sensation from those that evoke pain.

There are essentially three possible ways for visceral sensory receptors to encode nociceptive events (Fig. 1):

(i) By specific visceral nociceptors. This is an extension to the visceral domain of the concept of cuta-

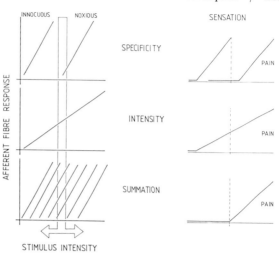

Fig. 1. Diagrammatic representation of three possible encoding mechanisms of noxious events (specificity, intensity and summation) by visceral sensory receptors. The relationship between stimulus intensity and afferent fibre response is represented for each of the three hypotheses and is correlated with the perception of pain sensations.

neous nociceptor. It requires the existence within those viscera from which pain can be evoked of two separate populations of sensory receptors, one responding to innocuous stimuli and the other to noxious stimuli. There is some experimental evidence for the existence of a separate category of visceral nociceptor in organs such as the heart, the lungs, the gall bladder and biliary ducts, the testes and perhaps the uterus (Baker et al., 1980; Cervero, 1982; Widdicombe, 1974; Kumazawa, 1986; Robbins et al., 1987).

(ii) By non-specific 'intensity'-encoding receptors. This is a straightforward extension of the 'pattern' theory (Sinclair, 1967), which postulates the existence of a single and homogeneous population of sensory receptors. These receptors could encode the nature of the stimulus in the 'intensity' of their responses, so that low intensities of stimulation would evoke low firing rates (and no sensation) and noxious intensities of stimulation would evoke high firing rates (and pain). This interpretation has been defended recently by Jänig and Morrison (1986). However, the experimental data on which they base their arguments (largely from studies on the affe-

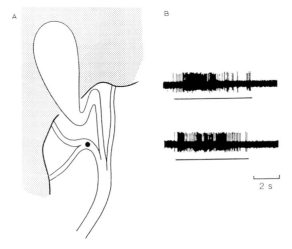

Fig. 2. Receptive field (spot) of a visceral nociceptor located on one of the hepatic ducts of a ferret. The responses of the afferent fibre to probing are shown in B. (From Cervero, 1982.)

rent innervation of the bladder and colon) seem to fit better with the third option described below.

(iii) By peripheral recruitment of receptors showing a wide range of thresholds (summation). This interpretation denies the existence of two distinct and separate populations of sensory receptor (nociceptors and non-nociceptors) but does not support the notion of a single population of afferent fibres with a narrow range of excitability thresholds. Instead, it is based on the existence of different kinds of afferent fibres whose thresholds form a continuum ranging from innocuous to noxious levels. Thus, as the stimulus intensity increases, more and more of these receptors will be activated and pain will be felt by a process of central summation. The data from Jänig and Morrison's studies (1986) fit better with the idea of a continuum of thresholds rather than with the notion of a homogeneous population of afferent fibres which can be activated within a narrow range of stimulus intensities.

It is important to point out that the sensory innervation of viscera has so far been studied in very few organs and that there are still many viscera for which we have few or no data regarding the functional properties of their afferent fibres. Under these circumstances it seems rather premature to make generalizations as to whether visceral pain is

mediated by a unique class of visceral receptor. In addition, visceral pain is often the consequence of irritation and inflammation of the mucosa of internal organs, and recent studies using these models are beginning to show that the properties of visceral afferents from inflamed tissue are different from those of normal tissue (Bahns et al., 1987). It is possible that both specific and non-specific visceral nociceptors act in parallel, conveying information to the central nervous system about noxious visceral events. Also, it could be that the activation of specific visceral nociceptors results in more restricted and clear-cut forms of visceral pain, whereas the vague and dull forms of abdominal discomfort are due to general stimulation of non-specific gut receptors.

Some gastrointestinal sensations, such as those evoked by colorectal distension, begin as non-painful feelings of distension and evolve towards an uncomfortable and painful sensation as the distension progresses. These properties can be paralleled by the electrophysiological properties of some colonic receptors (Haupt et al., 1983) which respond with greater impulse frequencies to colonic distensions of increasing magnitude. On the other hand, viscera such as the gall bladder and the biliary ducts from which pain is the only sensation that can be evoked appear to be innervated by specific visceral nociceptors (Cervero, 1982, 1985) (Fig. 2). In any case, it is a dangerous oversimplification to relate the final perception of a visceral sensation to the properties of the peripheral sense organ at the origin of the sensory pathway. The final conscious perception of pain depends on the way in which the central nervous system integrates the afferent visceral inflow, regardless of the peripheral encoding mechanism.

Neurophysiological mechanisms of visceral pain

Most internal organs have a dual afferent innervation. Some afferent fibres join sympathetic nerves (such as the splanchnic and hypogastric nerves), whereas other afferent fibres from the same viscera course in parasympathetic nerves (such as the vagus and pelvic nerves). It has been standard opinion in textbooks and reference monographs that visceral pain is mediated by afferent fibres in sympathetic nerves and that the activation of afferent fibres running in parasympathetic nerves does not evoke visceral sensations and is concerned only with the reflex regulation of visceral function (Ruch, 1946).

This notion is well supported by clinical evidence. It has been known for some time that stimulation of the splanchnic nerves in conscious humans under local anaesthesia elicits severe pain (Leriche, 1939). Also, clinical studies using a combination of stimulation and blocking techniques have repeatedly shown that abdominal pain is evoked by stimulation of sympathetic but not of parasympathetic nerves, and is relieved by section or blockade of sympathetic but not of parasympathetic nerve trunks (White, 1943). Recently, further clinical evidence has been obtained showing that splanchnic nerve blockade during major abdominal surgery under general anaesthesia prevents endocrine-metabolic responses to the visceral surgical procedure and helps post-operative recovery (Shirasaka et al., 1986). This shows that the pseudaffective components of the visceral nociceptive response are also mediated by afferent impulses in sympathetic nerves. Therefore, it can be concluded that many forms of visceral pain are signalled by sympathetic nerves (splanchnic and hypogastric nerves) and that the afferent innervation of some internal organs mediated by parasympathetic nerves is not concerned with the signalling and transmission of visceral pain.

Visceral afferent fibres running in sympathetic nerve have their cell bodies in thoraco-lumbar spinal ganglia and their central projections enter the spinal cord at levels between T2-3 and L2-3. It has been known for some time that the total number of primary afferent fibres involved in the transmission of visceral nociceptive information is quite small (Procacci, 1969). This low density of innervation is very striking when one takes into account the large surface area of some internal organs, particularly those of the gastro-intestinal tract, and is probably the reason for the diffuse nature of gastro-intestinal

pain. Recent studies, using neuronal tracing and labelling methods, have established that visceral afferent fibres constitute less than 10% of the total afferent inflow to the thoraco-lumbar spinal cord (Cervero et al., 1984).

It must be noted that this region of the spinal cord receives its somatic input from the body areas with the poorest sensory discrimination (i.e. the back and the abdomen), whereas the visceral input to the thoraco-lumbar cord mediates pain from all upper abdominal organs, including the stomach, the duodenum, the biliary tract, the pancreas and the small intestine. Yet the somatic sensations require 90% or more of the total afferent input to the thoraco-lumbar spinal cord, whereas all visceral pain from the upper abdomen is mediated by less that 10% of all spinal afferents.

It is, then, abundantly clear that the gastrointestinal tract has an extremely low density of sensory innervation, particularly by those afferent fibres that mediate the sensations of visceral pain. This explains why large areas of the gut appear to be insensitive or require considerable stimulation before giving rise to pain. One such form of stimulation is the intense and persistent contraction of the intestinal wall that evokes colic pain. These contractions activate maximally and simultaneously the few nociceptive afferent fibres present in a given loop of intestine, and in this way evoke painful sensations in synchrony with the motor events. Smaller, irregular or less persistent contractions are probably insufficient to excite enough afferents with the intensity or synchrony necessary to activate nociceptive pathways in the central nervous system.

Visceral afferent fibres reach the dorsal horn of the spinal cord via Lissauer's tract and join medial and lateral bundles of fine fibres that run along the edges of the dorsal horn. Fibres from these bundles penetrate the grey matter and terminate within laminae I and V of the dorsal horn (De Groat, 1986). Many of the fine afferents which terminate in the deep dorsal horn (lamina V) contain substance P and have been shown to be largely of visceral afferent origin (Sharkey et al., 1987). The substantia gelatinosa (lamina II) does not receive a direct visceral projection. Since the majority of visceral afferent fibres are unmyelinated, this observation calls into question the generally accepted belief that most unmyelinated afferent fibres terminate in the substantia gelatinosa of the dorsal horn. It would appear that neurones within this superficial region are only responsible for the integration of cutaneous sensory signals and not for the relay and processing of all sensory messages carried by unmyelinated afferent fibres.

The fact that visceral pain is diffuse, ill-localized and sometimes referred to somatic structures has always been taken into account when proposing neurological mechanisms of visceral pain. Central to all the proposals is the clinical observation that the referral of visceral pain usually takes place to a somatic area innervated by the same spinal cord segments receiving the input from the originating viscus. Therefore, all neurophysiological interpretations of visceral pain are based on viscero-somatic integration, that is, the convergence of inputs from viscera and from somatic structures onto sensory neurones whose activation leads to the experience of somatic pain.

The simplest form of viscero-somatic convergence would be primary afferent fibres with multiple endings in skin, muscle and viscera (Pierau et al., 1984). Such primary afferents have been described in several animal species but their numbers are so low that it is hard to believe that all manifestations of referred visceral pain are due to such prespinal convergence.

It is therefore more likely that the referred and diffuse properties of visceral pain are due to viscero-somatic convergence on central nervous system neurones and by extensive integration of somatic and visceral sensory signals. MacKenzie (1909) provided a comprehensive model of viscero-somatic convergence by suggesting that visceral impulses arriving at the spinal cord could produce an 'irritable focus' within the grey matter. Such an area of irritation would be responsible for the activation of somatic sensory neurones (and hence the referred sensation) and for the triggering of somatic and visceral reflexes. This proposal was elaborated further in Ruch's (1946) 'convergence-projection' theory of referred pain in which he suggested that the referral of the sensation was due to viscerosomatic convergence onto neurones of the spinothalamic tract and subsequent 'faulty' localization because of previously learned experiences. This hypothesis has received considerable experimental support in recent years, particularly those aspects of the theory that predicted the existence of viscerosomatic convergence in the spinal cord (see Cervero and Tattersall (1986) for a recent review).

Viscero-somatic convergence in the spinal cord

More than 75% of all neurones in the thoracic spinal cord are viscero-somatic, that is, receive convergent inputs from viscera and from the skin. Since the actual number of visceral afferent fibres entering the spinal cord is very small, this figure is an expression of the considerable amount of central divergence of the visceral sensory input to the cord. Many of these viscero-somatic neurones are probably not concerned with the sensory components of visceral nociception but with the handling of the general increase in excitability produced by the arrival in the nervous system of a visceral nociceptive volley which results in motor and autonomic activity.

Examination of the input properties of viscerosomatic neurones, their ascending projections and the nature and strength of their supraspinal control has revealed several categories of viscero-somatic neurones, which can be reduced to two very broad groups:
(i) Viscero-somatic neurones with a restricted visceral input and subject to descending inhibitory control. These neurones are a minority among viscero-somatic neurones and are located mainly in the superficial dorsal horn. They are activated by ipsilateral visceral afferent fibres and have restricted somatic receptive fields from which they can only be driven by noxious stimulation of the skin (Fig. 3). Neurones in this region of the dorsal horn are known to project to the brain via spino-thalamic

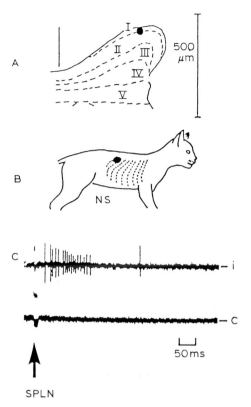

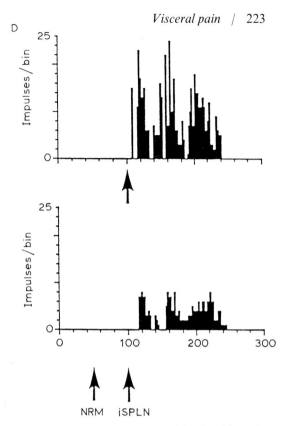

Fig. 3. A viscero-somatic neurone of the thoracic spinal cord of the cat. A: location of the cell in lamina I of the dorsal horn. B: restricted cutaneous receptive field from which the cell could only be activated by noxious stimuli (nociceptor-specific). C: this cell responded to electrical stimulation of the ipsilateral (i) splanchnic nerve (SPLN) but not of the contralateral (c) splanchnic nerve. D: inhibition of the visceral response by electrical stimulation in the nucleus raphe magnus (NRM).

pathways and seem to be part of the nociceptive-specific system of the superficial dorsal horn (Cervero and Tattersall, 1987).

These cells are subject to segmental inhibitory controls and to descending inhibition of supraspinal origin (Tattersall et al., 1986a,b). They can be inhibited by electrical stimulation in the nucleus raphe magnus (NRM) (Fig. 3) and it is likely that this inhibition originates from NRM cell bodies. These cells are good candidates for a transmission system that could mediate the more immediate sensory effects resulting from visceral noxious stimulation.

(ii) Viscero-somatic neurones with a diffuse visceral input and subject to descending excitatory and inhibitory control. These are neurones located in the deep dorsal horn and in the ventral horn and driven by bilateral visceral inputs. They are the most nu-

merous group of viscero-somatic neurones, have large and multireceptive somatic receptive fields often involving inputs of deep somatic origin and their visceral inputs are mediated or reinforced by supraspinal loops (Tattersall et al., 1986a,b). A proportion of them project to the reticular formation of the brain stem and it seems that their descending excitation originates from rostral medullary centres.

These cells will have their excitability increased by visceral nociceptive stimulation and will remain in a highly excitable state as a consequence of their spinal-bulbo-spinal positive-feedback loops. It is therefore conceivable that they are concerned with the integration of the non-sensory components of visceral pain, i.e. the persistent increases in motor and autonomic reflex activity which are so characteristic of visceral nociception.

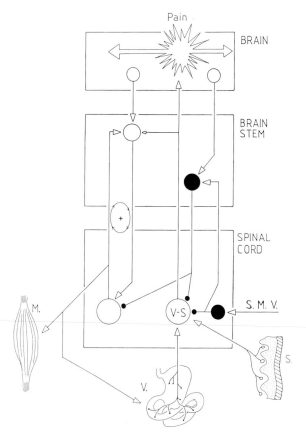

Fig. 4. Neuronal model of the way in which visceral nociceptive signals are processed by the central nervous system. The perception of visceral pain depends on the activation of viscerosomatic (VS) convergent pathways whose activity can be modulated by segmental interactions with inputs from the skin (S), muscle (M) or other viscera (V) or by suprasegmental inhibitory systems. These inhibitory pathways are shown by the black neurones. In addition, excitatory loops between the spinal cord and the brain stem help to maintain activity within the system, resulting in enhanced motor and autonomic reflexes and persistent pain.

A neurophysiological model of visceral pain

The neurophysiological model illustrated in Fig. 4 represents an attempt to depict the spinal and supraspinal integration of visceral pain in a simple and diagrammatic form. This model is based on the postulates of the 'convergence-projection' theory of visceral pain and relies on experimental evidence obtained from animal studies over the last decade.

The central element of the model is a viscerosomatic convergent pathway with rostral projections which eventually reach brain areas concerned with the perception of a pain experience. The somatic input to this pathway is restricted to the corresponding dermatome but the visceral input arises from a large surface area which takes into account the scarce innervation of internal organs. This sensory pathway is subject to inhibitory influences of segmental and suprasegmental origin, the latter originating from the NRM. These inhibitory influences are responsible for the sensory modulation of the convergent pathway.

The other element of the model is the spinal-bulbo-spinal positive-feedback loop, which maintains excitability within the sensory channel and is probably related to motor and autonomic outflow. The balance between this excitatory system and the inhibitory modulation of the sensory pathway could therefore determine the intensity of the final perception of pain and the persistence and magnitude of the accompanying non-sensory reactions.

Clinical procedures targeted on breaking the positive-feedback loop between the spinal cord and the brain stem or on enhancing the endogenous inhibitory system would therefore result not only in the relief of pain but also in the prevention of the longer-lasting motor and autonomic reactions. There is already clinical evidence showing the beneficial effects of splanchnic nerve blockade during major abdominal surgery under general anaesthesia (Shirasaka et al., 1986). Such procedures prevent the metabolic responses due to the surgical stress and help post-operative recovery. The rationale behind this clinical approach is based on the neurophysiological mechanisms presented, in a simple form, in the proposed model (Fig. 4).

Summary and conclusions

Pain of visceral origin is the most common form of pain produced by disease and is often the critical symptom that brings patients to seek medical attention. In spite of the immediate medical relevance of visceral pain and of the fact that it accounts for a substantial proportion of recurrent and persistent pain syndromes, little is known about the basic neurophysiological mechanisms responsible for the generation and perception of visceral pain. Such knowledge would greatly help the development of new therapies for the relief of pain of internal origin.

Pain mechanisms have traditionally been studied by examining the immediate reactions of the central nervous system to an acute skin injury. This experimental approach has produced a considerable amount of information on the signalling and transmission of acute cutaneous pain but has provided little help for the understanding of pain of internal origin. This latter form of pain shows clinical characteristics which are markedly different from those of superficial acute pain. Visceral pain is dull, aching, badly localized and often referred to a part of the body away from the diseased organ. Visceral pain can vary in intensity with time but seldom disappears completely within a short period of time. In most cases, visceral pain is accompanied by a general increase in the excitability of the central nervous system, as shown by tenderness of the skin, general discomfort, muscle spasms and increased autonomic reflexes (e.g. sweating, cardiovascular changes, altered gastro-intestinal motility). These characteristics of visceral pain show that the central nervous system reacts to internal injury in a different way than to external injury, the latter usually resulting in a bright, well-localized and acute pain rarely accompanied by persistent general reactions.

Visceral pain is normally mediated by the activation of visceral afferent fibres running in sympathetic nerves. It is now known that these fibres consti-

tute a very small proportion (10% or less) of the total afferent input to the spinal cord. Such a low density of sensory innervation is probably one of the main reasons for the diffuse nature of visceral pain. The receptor endings of these fibres respond to mechanical and chemical stimulation of viscera but there is still some controversy as to whether there is a category of visceral receptor akin to the cutaneous nociceptor (i.e. responding solely to noxious intensities of stimulation).

Within the spinal cord visceral afferent fibres converge onto neurones driven by somatic nociceptive inputs, including those cells whose axons project through nociceptive pathways such as the spinothalamic tract. Convergence of visceral and somatic afferent fibres onto nociceptive pathways has been interpreted as the neurophysiological basis of referred visceral pain. Many neurones in the spinal cord respond to stimulation of visceral afferent fibres via long excitatory loops that involve a supraspinal relay. This positive feedback between brain stem and spinal cord areas involved in somatic and autonomic reactions to injury could provide a mechanism for the long-lasting increases in central excitability that follow noxious visceral stimulation. In addition, a descending inhibitory system from the brain stem to the spinal cord can modulate the transmission of nociceptive signals through the cord and so alter the final perception of the sensory signal.

The organization of visceral nociceptive systems is similar to that of a general alarm mechanism triggered by a few peripheral sensors but capable of extensive central reactions. This type of organization is, however, unsuitable for providing well-localized and finely discriminated sensory information.

References

Ayala, M. (1937) Douleur sympathique et douleur viscerale. Rev. Neurol., 68: 222–242.

Bahns, E., Habler, H.J., Jänig, W. and Koltzenburg, M. (1987) Properties of mechano- and chemosensitive primary afferents from urinary bladder. Pain, Suppl. 4: S20.

Baker, D.G., Coleridge, H.M., Coleridge, J.C.G. and Nerdrum, T. (1980) Search for a cardiac nociceptor: stimulation by bradykinin of sympathetic afferent nerve endings in the heart of

the cat. J. Physiol., 306: 519–536.

Cervero, F. (1982) Afferent activity evoked by natural stimulation of the biliary system in the ferret. Pain, 13: 137–151.

Cervero, F. (1983) Mechanisms of visceral pain. In S. Lipton and J. Miles (Eds.), Persistent Pain, Grune and Stratton, London, Vol. IV, pp. 1–19.

Cervero, F. (1985) Visceral nociception: peripheral and central aspects of visceral nociceptive systems. Phil. Trans. R. Soc. Series B, 308: 325–337.

Cervero, F., Connell, L.A. and Lawson, S.N. (1984) Somatic

and visceral primary afferents in the lower thoracic dorsal root ganglia of the cat. J. Comp. Neurol., 228: 422–431.

Cervero, F. and Morrison, J.F.B. (Eds.) (1986) Visceral Sensation, Progr. Brain. Res., Vol. 67, Elsevier, Amsterdam, pp. 324.

Cervero, F. and Tattersall, J.E.H. (1986) Somatic and visceral sensory integration in the thoracic spinal cord. In F. Cervero and J.F.B. Morrison (Eds.), Visceral Sensation, Progr. Brain Res. Vol. 67, Elsevier, Amsterdam, pp. 189–205.

Cervero, F. and Tattersall, J.E.H. (1987) Somatic and visceral inputs to the thoracic spinal cord of the cat: marginal zone (lamina I) of the dorsal horn. J. Physiol., 388: 383–395.

De Groat, W.C. (1986) Spinal cord projections and neuropeptides in visceral afferent neurones. In F. Cervero and J.F.B. Morrison (Eds.), Visceral Sensation, Progr. Brain Res. Vol. 67, Elsevier, Amsterdam, pp. 165–187.

Haupt, P., Jänig, W. and Kohler, W. (1983) Response pattern of visceral afferent fibres, supplying the colon, upon chemical and mechanical stimuli. Pflugers. Arch., 398: 41–47.

Head, H. (1893) On disturbances of sensation with special reference to the pain of visceral disease. Brain, 16: 1–133.

Jänig, W. and Morrison, J.F.B. (1986) Functional properties of spinal visceral afferents supplying abdominal and pelvic organs with special emphasis on visceral nociception. In F. Cervero and J.F.B. Morrison (Eds.), Visceral Sensation, Progr. Brain Res. Vol. 67, Elsevier, Amsterdam, pp. 87–114.

Kumazawa, T. (1986) Sensory innervation of reproductive organs. In F. Cervero and J.F.B. Morrison (Eds.), Visceral Sensation, Progr. Brain Res. Vol. 67, Elsevier, Amsterdam, pp., 115–131.

Leriche, R. (1939) The Surgery of Pain, Bailliere, Tindall and Cox, London.

MacKenzie, J. (1909) Symptoms and Their Interpretation, Shaw and Sons, London, p. 297.

Morley, J.A. (1931) Abdominal Pain, E. and S. Livingstone, Edinburgh.

Pierau, F.K., Fellmer, G. and Taylor, D.C.M. (1984) Somatovisceral convergence in cat dorsal root ganglion neurones demonstrated by double-labelling with fluorescent tracers. Brain Res., 321: 63–70.

Procacci, P. (1969) A survey of modern concepts of pain. In P.J. Vinken and G.W. Bruyn (Eds.), Handbook of Clinical Neurology, Vol. I, Elsevier, Amsterdam, pp. 114–146.

Procacci, P., Zoppi, M. and Maresca, M. (1986) Clinical approach to visceral sensation. In F. Cervero and J.F.B. Morrison (Eds.), Visceral Sensation, Progr. Brain Res. Vol. 67, Elsevier, Amsterdam, pp. 21–28.

Robbins, A., Sato, Y., Hotta, H. and Berkley, K.J. (1987) Response of uterine afferent fibers in the rat to sodium ajamide and CO_2. Pain, Suppl. 4: S.20.

Ruch, T.C. (1946) Visceral sensation and referred pain. In J.F. Fulton (Ed.), Howell's Textbook of Physiology, 15th edn., Saunders, Philadelphia, pp. 385–401.

Sharkey, K.A., Sobrino, J.A. and Cervero, F (1987) Evidence for a visceral afferent origin of Substance P-like immunoreactivity in Lamina V of rat thoracic cord. Neuroscience (in press).

Sherrington, C.S. (1906) The Integrative Action of the Nervous System, C. Scribner and Sons, New York.

Shirasaka, C., Tsuji H., Asoh, T. and Takeuchi, Y. (1986) Role of the splanchnic nerves in endocrine and metabolic response to abdominal surgery. Br. J. Surg., 73: 142–145.

Sinclair, D. (1967) Cutaneous Sensation, Oxford University Press, London.

Tattersall, J.E.H., Cervero, F. and Lumb, B.M. (1986a) Effects of reversible spinalization on the visceral input to viscero-somatic neurones in the lower thoracic spinal cord of the cat. J. Neurophysiol., 56: 785–796.

Tattersall, J.E.H., Cervero, F. and Lumb, B.M. (1986b) Viscerosomatic neurones in the lower thoracic spinal cord of the cat: excitations and inhibitions evoked by splanchnic and somatic nerve volleys and by stimulation of brain stem nuclei. J. Neurophysiol., 56: 1411–1423.

Torebjörk, H.E. (1985) Nociceptor activation and pain. Phil. Trans. R. Soc. B., 308: 227–234.

Torebjörk, H.E. and Ochoa, J.L. (1983) Selective stimulation of sensory units in man. Adv. Pain Res. Ther., 5: 99–104.

White, J.C. (1943) Sensory innervation of the viscera: studies on visceral afferent neurones in man based on neurosurgical procedures for the relief of intractable pain. Res. Pub. Assoc. Res. Nerv. Mental Dis., 23: 373–390.

Widdicombe, J.G. (1974) Enteroceptors. In J.I. Hubbard (Ed.), The Peripheral Nervous System, Plenum Press, New York, pp. 455–485.

Willis, W.D. (1985) The Pain System, Karger, Basel.

R. Dubner, G.F. Gebhart & M.R. Bond (Eds.)
Proceedings of the Vth World Congress on Pain
© 1988 Elsevier Science Publishers BV (Biomedical Division)

CHAPTER 24

Differential modulation of thoracic and lumbar spinothalamic tract cell activity during stimulation of cardiopulmonary sympathetic afferent fibers in the primate. A new concept for visceral pain?

Robert D. Foreman, Stuart F. Hobbs, Uh-Taek Oh and Margaret J. Chandler

*University of Oklahoma, Health Sciences Center, Department of Physiology and Biophysics,
Oklahoma City, OK 73190, USA*

Summary

The major implication of this study is that there may be as yet undescribed neural mechanisms underlying the phenomenon of visceral pain. Our evidence indicates that the spinal cord can differentially control the information coming into it depending upon the segment being excited. These results raise the possibility that inhibition of some segments of the spinal cord should increase contrast between cells that are excited and those that are not excited by the noxious input. That is, the signal-to-noise ratio for cells excited by noxious input may be improved by this process. Further work is required to determine how this information can be transmitted, enhanced and controlled.

Introduction

Pain accompanying myocardial ischemia, i.e., angina pectoris, is generally sensed as arising from the chest, shoulders or arms (Harrison and Reeves, 1968; Procacci and Zoppi, 1985). Ruch (1961) proposed in the convergence-projection theory that this pain referral results from convergence of excitatory visceral and somatic inputs onto the same cell. Several studies support the theory that pain originating from visceral organs is referred to somatic structures as a result of convergence of visceral and somatic afferent fibers onto spinothalamic tract (STT) cells (Blair et al., 1981; Ammons et al., 1985a,b). Electrical stimulation of the cardiopulmonary afferent fibers (Blair et al., 1981), coronary artery occlusion (Blair et al., 1984b) and intracardiac injection of bradykinin (Blair et al., 1982, 1984a; Ammons et al., 1985b) activate $T_1–T_5$ STT neurons that also respond to somatic stimulation of the chest and forearm.

Pain resulting from urinary bladder distension is referred to the lower abdomen and groin (Smith, 1972; Applebaum et al., 1980). The location of the pain suggests that afferent fibers from the urinary bladder excite a different group of STT neurons than afferents of cardiopulmonary origin. The convergence-projection theory of Ruch (1961) also supports this referral of pain. An electrophysiological study supported this theory because STT cells in the $L_6–S_2$ segments of the spinal cord are excited by somatic afferent input from the hindlimbs and by urinary bladder distension (Milne et al., 1981). In contrast, urinary bladder distension inhibits the activity of STT cells located in the T_1–T_5 segments of the spinal cord (Hobbs et al., 1986; Oh et al., 1986). These results indicate that stimulation of visceral afferents excites cells in spinal cord segments which directly receive the projections of these afferents. However, stimulation of these afferents also has the potential for inhibiting activity of cells in distant segments which do not receive direct projections from these fibers. Since T_1–T_5 STT cells are excited by cardiopulmonary afferent input and are inhibited by urinary bladder distension, we hypothesized that stimulation of the cardiopulmonary afferents should inhibit cells of the lumbosacral segments of the spinal cord which are excited by urinary bladder distension. To test this hypothesis, we recorded spontaneous and evoked activity from STT cells in the lumbosacral region of the spinal cord and electrically stimulated the cardiopulmonary afferent fibers to determine whether these STT cells could be inhibited. Activity in these cells was evoked by urinary bladder distension and hindlimb pinch.

Methods

Experiments were performed on 11 monkeys (*Macaca fascicularis*) tranquilized with ketamine (10–20 mg/kg i.m.) and anesthetized with α-chloralose (60–80 mg/kg i.v.). α–Chloralose was infused at the rate of 3.0–6.0 mg/kg/h and pancuronium bromide was infused at the rate of 115–230 μg/kg/h to maintain the level of anesthesia and muscle paralysis, respectively. Catheters were placed in the femoral vein for fluid and drug injection and in the femoral artery for monitoring blood pressure. Artificial ventilation was used to maintain the expiratory CO_2 between 4.0 and 5.0%. Body temperature was kept at $37 \pm 1°C$ with a servo-controlled heat lamp.

A thoracotomy was made in the second or third intercostal space of the left side. A bipolar platinum electrode was placed on the caudal ansa subclavia and the sympathetic chain between the T_2 and T_3 rami communicantes to stimulate the cardiopulmonary sympathetic afferents.

A midline suprapubic incision was made to expose the urinary bladder. A small incision was made in the dome of the urinary bladder, and a balloon attached to a double-lumen plastic tube 1 cm in diameter was inserted into the bladder. The outer tubing was connected both to a water-filled reservoir which could be raised above the level of the bladder to distend it isotonically (constant pressure) and to a syringe to evoke isovolumic (constant volume) bladder distension. Urinary bladder pressure was measured with a pressure transducer connected to an inner cannula of tubing that ended in the balloon.

After animals had been placed in a stereotaxic frame, a laminectomy was performed to expose the L_6–S_2 spinal segments for recording STT cells. To excite neurons antidromically from the thalamus, a craniotomy was performed, and a concentric bipolar electrode was placed in the right ventral posterior lateral nucleus (Blair et al., 1981).

The left side of the spinal gray matter was searched with a carbon-filament glass microelectrode while the thalamus was stimulated (10 Hz, 2 mA, 100 μs duration). Standard criteria were used to demonstrate that all cells were activated antidromically (Trevino et al., 1973). After a cell had been isolated within a window discriminator and identified as an STT neuron, the somatic receptive field of each cell was determined as described previously (Blair et al., 1981; Ammons et al., 1985a). Each cell was also tested for its response to visceral input from the cardiopulmonary region by stimulating the cardiopulmonary sympathetic fibers (1–34 V, 100–500 μs, 20 Hz). Responses were studied during spontaneous activity, pinching the somatic receptive field, and urinary bladder distension.

After each cell had been studied completely, DC current (50 μA, 20 s) was passed through the electrode to mark the recording location. Thalamic sites were determined from small lesions (20 μA, 20 s) made at the completion of the experiment. Brain and spinal segments were fixed in a 10% formalin solution. The tissue was frozen and cut into 60-μm sections to determine the location of the recording and stimulation sites. All thalamic sites were in the ventral posterior lateral nucleus.

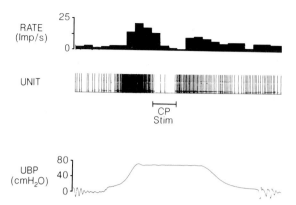

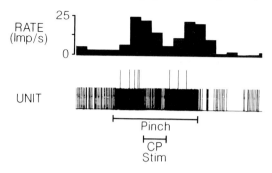

Fig. 1. Effects of distending the urinary bladder and electrically stimulating the cardiopulmonary (CP) afferent fibers on a lumbosacral (S_1) spinothalamic tract cell. The horizontal bar is the period of CP afferent stimulation. Traces from top to bottom are: rate in impulse/s; unit, where each line represents a single extracellular action potential; and UBP is urinary bladder pressure in cmH_2O.

Fig. 2. Responses of a lumbosacral (L_6) spinothalamic tract cell to electrical stimulation of the cardiopulmonary (CP) afferent fibers during a noxious pinch of the left hindlimb (LHL). The hindlimb was pinched as indicated by the long horizontal bar just below the unit tracing. The short horizontal bar indicates the period of electrical stimulation of the CP afferents (34 V, 500 μs, 20 Hz).

Results

Recordings were made from 17 L_6–S_2 STT neurons. Urinary bladder distension excited 7, inhibited 3 and did not affect 7 STT cells. All of these neurons were activated by somatic manipulation of the hindlimb or tail. Cells were classified according to the type of somatic stimuli required to activate them. Ten wide-dynamic-range cells were excited slightly during hair movement, but increased their discharge rate during a noxious pinch. One high-threshold cell was excited only during a noxious pinch, and six high-threshold inhibitory cells required a pinch to activate them, but hair movement inhibited the spontaneous activity. Cells were found primarily in laminae I, IV, V and X.

Responses of lumbosacral STT cells to cardiopulmonary stimulation
Electrical stimulation of cardiopulmonary sympathetic afferent fibers inhibited spontaneous activity of 13 (76%) lumbosacral STT cells. We wanted to determine whether, in addition to inhibiting spontaneous activity, cardiopulmonary afferent fibers could inhibit activity of lumbosacral STT cells when they were activated during urinary bladder distension. Fig. 1 shows the excitatory effect of urinary bladder distension on an S_1 STT cell. Stimulation of cardiopulmonary afferents markedly reduced the increased activity recorded during urinary bladder distension. After cessation of electrical stimulation, cell activity again increased, but not back to control levels. This post-stimulus reduction in evoked activity is explained by the fact that activity of STT neurons often adapts during maintenance of urinary bladder distension. These results demonstrate that cardiopulmonary afferent stimulation inhibits spontaneous and evoked activity of lumbosacral STT cells.

Since cardiopulmonary stimulation inhibited the responses of cells to visceral input, we wanted to determine whether this stimulus could also suppress cell activity evoked from pinching somatic receptive fields. Fig. 2 shows the excitatory response of an L_6 STT cell to noxious pinch of the left hindlimb. During the pinch, electrical stimulation of the cardiopulmonary afferents markedly suppressed cell activity. Activity returned to control levels after the cardiopulmonary afferent stimulation had ceased.

Differential inhibition
Comparison of the results described here to the responses of T_2–T_5 STT cells during urinary bladder distension and hindlimb pinch (Hobbs et al., 1986;

TABLE I

Comparison of inputs at different segments of the spinal cord

	Stimulus			
	Visceral		Somatic	
	CP aff. elec. stim.	Urinary bladder distension	LT triceps pinch	LHL pinch
T_2–T_5	+ + +	– – –	+ + +	– – –
L_6–S_2	– – –	+ + +	– – –	+ + +

The plusses ($+ + +$) indicate excitation and the minuses ($– – –$) indicate inhibition CP aff. elec. stim. – cardiopulmonary afferent electrical stimulation; LT triceps pinch – left triceps pinch; LHL pinch – left hindlimb pinch.

Oh et al., 1986) emphasizes the differential responses of STT cells to stimulation of visceral and somatic input and is illustrated schematically in Table I. Electrical stimulation of the cardiopulmonary afferent fibers excited the T_2-T_5 STT cells, but inhibited the cells in the L_6–S_2 segments. In contrast, urinary bladder distension, which excites pelvic afferent fibers, inhibited cells in the T_2–T_5 segments of the spinal cord, but primarily excited the L_6–S_2 STT neurons. A comparison of the somatic input shows that noxious pinch of the left forelimb triceps excited cells in the T_2–T_5 segments which receive direct projections from the forelimb but inhibited the STT cells of the L_6–S_2 segments. In contrast, noxious pinch applied to the left hindlimb inhibited cells distant from the lumbosacral input, i.e., the T_2-T_5 cells, but excited the L_6–S_2 neurons. This table illustrates that visceral and somatic afferent inputs generally excite cells in the segments to which these afferents project directly, but inhibit cells located in distant segments.

Discussion

This study is the first to demonstrate that cardiopulmonary sympathetic afferent input can inhibit STT cells of the L_6–S_2 segments of the spinal cord.

A reciprocal response exists when the urinary bladder is distended because it inhibits STT cells of the thoracic segments. The responses to somatic stimuli show the same characteristics. Noxious input from the thoracic receptive fields produces inhibition of the lumbosacral STT cells and noxious input from the lumbar receptive field can inhibit cells of the thoracic cord. These results led to the suggestion that noxious stimulation of a visceral organ excites STT cells in cord segments which receive direct afferent projections from the organ, but inhibits STT cells outside these segments.

Activation of cells in the segments directly receiving afferent input and inhibition outside the excitatory receptive field has been demonstrated for the somatic system. LeBars et al. (1979a,b) and Gerhart et al. (1981) have demonstrated that a noxious pinch applied to numerous sites outside a cell's excitatory field produces inhibition. Also, Dickenson et al. (1980) showed that there is differential inhibition of lumbosacral dorsal horn cells and trigeminal nucleus caudalis neurons to somatic input depending upon the segment being stimulated. We advanced this concept by showing that visceral inputs also produce differential inhibition. For example, noxious afferent input to the thoracic segments from the cardiopulmonary region or forelimb and chest inhibits activity of lumbosacral STT cells. The opposite response occurs when cell activity is recorded in the thoracic segments, and receptive fields of the hindlimb and the afferents from the urinary bladder are stimulated. These results raised the possibility that the STT cells responding to visceral and somatic inputs are inhibited differentially depending upon the location of the noxious stimulus.

The differential effects of noxious afferent input on STT cells raises the following question: what central pathways may be involved in mediating this viscerotopic, as well as somatotopic, inhibition? Previous work has suggested that noxious stimulation of skin outside of the excitatory receptive field requires supraspinal pathways to produce inhibition (LeBars et al., 1979a,b). The results of Gerhart et al. (1980) are somewhat different because in most cases transection of the cervical spinal cord reduced the effects of a noxious inhibitory stimulus. Therefore, there is a possibility that propriospinal as well as supraspinal pathways are involved in producing this kind of differential inhibition. Preliminary experiments in our laboratory showed that inhibition of lumbosacral STT cell response to stimulation of cardiopulmonary sympathetic afferent fibers and to pinch of the forelimbs remains after the C_1 cord has been transected (Oh et al., 1987). Further documentation is required to clarify these results. The exact

pathways and mechanisms for producing these complex interactions are still in question.

Acknowledgements

The authors thank Diana Holston for her expert technical assistance and Charlene Clark for typing the manuscript. This work was supported by National Institutes of Health grants HL07430 (S.F.H.), NS08150 (M.J.C.) and HL22732.

References

Ammons, W.S., Girardot, M.-N. and Foreman, R.D. (1985) T_2–T_5 spinothalamic neurons projecting to medial thalamus with viscerosomatic input. J. Neurophysiol., 54: 73–89.

Ammons, W.S., Girardot, M.-N. and Foreman, R.D. (1985b) Effects of intracardiac bradykinin on T_2–T_5 spinothalamic cells. Am. J. Physiol., 249: R147–R152.

Applebaum, A.E., Vance, W.H. and Coggeshall, R.E. (1980) The segmental localization of sensory cells that innervate the bladder. J. Comp. Neurol., 192: 203–210.

Blair, R.W., Weber, R.N. and Foreman, R.D. (1981) Characteristics of primate spinothalamic tract neurons receiving viscerosomatic convergent inputs in T_3–T_5 segments. J. Neurophysiol., 46: 797–811.

Blair, R.W., Weber, R.N. and Foreman, R.D. (1982) Responses of thoracic spinothalamic neurons to intracardiac injection of bradykinin in the monkey. Circ. Res., 51: 83–94.

Blair, R.W., Weber, R.N. and Foreman, R.D. (1984a) Responses of spinoreticular and spinothalamic cells to intracardiac bradykinin. Am. J. Physiol., 246: H500–H507.

Blair, R.W., Ammons, W.S. and Foreman, R.D. (1984b) Responses of thoracic spinothalamic and spinoreticular cells to coronary artery occlusion. J. Neurophysiol., 51: 636–648.

Dickenson, A.H., LeBars, D. and Besson, J.-M. (1980) Diffuse noxious inhibitory controls (DNIC). Effects on trigeminal nucleus caudalis neurones in the rat. Brain. Res., 200: 293–305.

Gerhart, K.D., Yezierski, R.P., Giesler, G.J. Jr. and Willis, W.D. (1981) Inhibitory receptive fields of primate spinothalamic tract cells. J. Neurophysiol., 46: 1309–1325.

Harrison, T.R. and Reeves, T.J. (1968) Patterns and causes of chest pain. In Principles and Problems of Ischemic Heart Disease, Year Book Medical Publishers, Chicago, pp. 197–204.

Hobbs, S.F., Brennan, T.J., Oh, U.T., Garrison, D. and Foreman, R.D. (1986) Urinary bladder distension inhibits somatic inputs to T_2–T_5 spinothalamic tract neurons in the primate. Neurosci. Abstr., 12:30.

LeBars, D., Dickenson, A.H. and Besson, J.-M. (1979a) Diffuse noxious inhibitory controls (DNIC). I. Effects on dorsal horn convergent neurons in the rat. Pain, 6: 283–304.

LeBars, D., Dickenson, A.H. and Besson, J.-M. (1979b) Diffuse noxious inhibitory controls (DNIC). II. Lack of effect of nonconvergent neurons, supraspinal involvement and theoretical implications. Pain, 6: 305–327.

Milne, R.J., Foreman, R.D., Giesler, G.J. and Willis, W.D. (1981) Convergence of cutaneous and pelvic visceral nociceptive inputs onto primate spinothalamic neurons. Pain, 11: 163–183.

Oh, U.T., Brennan, T.J., Hobbs, S.F. and Foreman, R.D. (1986) Effects of urinary bladder distension (UBD) on the T_2–T_5 spinothalamic tract (STT) cells of the primate. Neurosci. Abstr., 12: 375.

Oh, U.T., Hobbs, S.F., Chandler, M.J. and Foreman, R.D. (1987) Viscerosomatic inhibition of lumbosacral spinothalamic tract (STT) cells in monkeys: role of C_1–C_2 spinal cord. Neurosci. Abstr., 13.

Procacci, P. and Zoppi, M. (1985) Heart pain. In P.D. Wall and R. Melzack (Eds.), Pain, Churchill Livingstone, Edinburgh, pp. 309–318.

Ruch, T.C. (1961) Pathophysiology of pain. In T.C. Ruch, H.D. Patton, J.W. Woodbury and A.L. Towe (Eds.), Neurophysiology, Saunders, Philadelphia, pp. 350–368.

Smith, D.R. (1972) General Urology, Lange, Los Altos, pp. 30, 215.

Trevino, D.L., Coulter, J.D. and Willis, W.D. (1973) Location of cells of origin of spinothalamic tract in lumbar enlargement of the monkey. J. Neurophysiol., 36: 750–761.

R. Dubner, G.F. Gebhart & M.R. Bond (Eds.)
Proceedings of the Vth World Congress on Pain
© 1988 Elsevier Science Publishers BV (Biomedical Division)

CHAPTER 25

Muscle pain with special reference to primary fibromyalgia (PF)

K.G. Henriksson[1] and Ann Bengtsson[2]

[1]Neuromuscular Unit and [2]Division of Rheumatology, Department of Internal Medicine, University Hospital, Linköping, Sweden

Introduction

Chronic diffuse muscle pain in patients without overt neuromuscular disorder or inflammatory joint disease is a common pain problem. The chronic muscle pain syndrome has several designations, e.g. diffuse fibrositis and diffuse myofascial syndrome. Yunus et al. preferred the term fibromyalgia in a study where they also proposed diagnostic criteria; primary fibromyalgia (PF) when no other cause is found and secondary when the muscle pain is present in conjunction with diseases such as hypothyreosis or rheumatoid arthritis (Yunus et al., 1981). These criteria are similar to those presented in IASP's classification of chronic pain (Merskey, 1986). Yunus et al. regarded the absence of other diseases and the presence of normal laboratory tests as an obligatory criterion for PF. Also in the IASP's classification the absence of laboratory evidence of inflammation or muscle damage is included among the diagnostic criteria. These diagnostic criteria are challenged by the results described in this paper. The relevance of these studies to the diagnosis and etiology of fibromyalgia is also discussed. Here we deal only with the muscular symptoms and signs in the fibromyalgia syndrome, and the only laboratory studies reported are those related to muscle tissue. All patients in the different studies fulfilled the diagnostic criteria proposed by Yunus et al.

Muscle morphology

Muscle biopsies from the trapezius and brachioradial muscles where the PF patients had pain and tender or trigger points (TPs) were compared with biopsies from the same muscles in healthy volunteers (Bengtsson et al., 1986a). In the patient group, biopsies were also studied from other muscles (deltoid, anterior tibial, etc).

Method

For routine histopathology serial sections of formaldehyde-fixed tissue were used: stains; Htx-eosin, van Gieson, Ladewig stain. For histochemistry tissue frozen in liquid nitrogen was used: staining for myofibrillar ATPase (preincubation at pH 9.4 and 4.6), NADH-tetrazolium reductase, phosphorylase, acid phosphatase, glycogen (PAS) and lipids (Oil-red-O). Gomori-trichrome, Htx-eosin and van Gieson stains were also employed. Capillary density was measured in trapezius muscle (amylase-PAS method).

Type 1 fibers: weak ATPase reaction at pH 9.4.

Correspondence: K.G. Henriksson, Neuromuscular Unit, University Hospital, S-581 85 Linköping, Sweden

Type 2 fibers: strong ATPase reaction at pH 9.4. Moth-eaten (ME) fibers: multifocal loss of activity in staining for oxidative enzymes. Ragged-red (RR) fibers: subsarcolemmal zones of bright-red or reddish-blue material when staining with Gomori-trichrome and an accumulation of formazan particles in the same area when staining for NADH-tetrazolium reductase. The fibers also have a ragged appearance.

Results

Trapezius muscle: the frequency of type 1 and type 2 fibers, the mean fiber area of type 1 and type 2 fibers and capillary density did not differ between patients and controls. Fibers with 'moth-eaten' appearance were type 1 fibers. In both patients and controls ME fibers were significantly larger than other type 1 fibers. In PF patients 11.9% of type 1 fibers had a 'moth-eaten' appearance. The corresponding figure for normal controls was 9.2%. The results of the histopathological and histochemical studies are presented in Table I. Electron microscopy (10 patients) revealed abnormalities in all, namely, mitochondrial abnormalities (such as elec-

tron-dense inclusions and lack of inner membrane), Z-streaming and cytoplasmic bodies. There was an abnormal ratio of mitochondria and myofibrils.

Comments

The most commonly found changes in the most painful muscles (shoulder muscles) were disruption of the intermyofibrillar network (ME fibers) (Fig. 1) and changes related to mitochondrial damage (RR fibers) (Fig. 2). It should be noted that the 'ragged-red' changes of a fiber may be segmental. The number of RR fibers registered in a biopsy therefore depends on the number of sections analysed. The ME fibers were a consistent finding in all control muscles. In our original control material no RR fibers were found in the trapezius muscle. In a more recent study we also found RR fibers in biopsies from some persons without muscular pain. Kalyan-Raman et al. (1984) found ME fibers in 5 of 12 biopsies from the trapezius muscle taken from PF patients. They did not report RR fibers.

The trapezius muscle, which is painful and contains TPs in nearly all PF patients, is also often the site of localized chronic muscular pain caused by

TABLE I

Light microscopical and histochemical changes in 77 muscle biopsies from 57 PF patients and 17 biopsies from 9 healthy controls

	M. trapezius		M. deltoideus:	M. brachioradialis		M. tibialis anterior:	M. quadriceps:	M. vastus lat. or med.:
	Patients (*n*=41)	Controls (*n*=10)	Patients (*n*=9)	Patients (*n*=6)	Controls (*n*=7)	Patients (*n*=16)	Patients (*n*=1)	Patients (*n*=4)
Normal borderline	18	9	4	6	5	10	1	3
Occasional degeneration regeneration	9	1			1	1		1
Infiltrates	3		1			5		
'Moth-eaten' fibers	35	9	3					
Ragged-red fibers	15		2		1			

Normal/borderline: biopsies showing occasional findings of internally placed nuclei, atrophic fibers, split fibers and variations in fiber diameter. Regeneration: basophilic sarcoplasm and vesicular nuclei containing nucleoli. Inflammatory cell infiltrates: lymphocytes with perivascular localization. *n* = number of biopsies.

overload in connection with static contractions, e.g. in persons with assembly work. We have recently studied biopsies from the trapezius muscle in 10 patients with localized shoulder pain due to overload (Larsson et al., 1988). In 8 of these biopsies RR fibers were found as well as an increased frequency of type 1 fibers (slow oxidative fibers) compared with controls. In this context it is of interest to note that Mattila et al. (1986) when studying the multifidus muscle in patients with low back pain found ME fibers in 27 of 41 patients. Only in 1 of 12 control patients were ME fibers found.

The changes in the interfibrillar network and the changes of mitochondria may not be related to pain but rather to static overload with an intensity high enough to induce partial hypoxia. In an experimental study Heffner and Barron (1978) found that ME appeared before RR fibers in ischaemic rat muscle. Measurements of muscle tissue oxygen pressure (see below) support the suggestion that hypoxia is present in painful muscles of PF patients.

Muscle tissue oxygen

Ten patients and 8 healthy volunteers were studied. Oxygen tissue pressure was measured with a multipoint oxygen electrode (MDO electrode) (Lund et al., 1986). Measurements were made on the surface of resting but painful muscles; trapezius muscle, 10 patients, 8 controls; brachioradial muscle, 4 patients and 5 controls. The measurements were performed with the patient or control person sitting as relaxed as possible.

The catchment zone of the electrode is 20 μm, which is equivalent to half a muscle fiber. Results are presented as histograms. The normal histogram has a gaussian curve form. During pathological conditions histograms can be of either 'scattered' or 'slope' type. The 'slope' histogram (all values low) is found during tissue hypoxia. A scattered histogram is probably an indication of maldistribution of capillary blood flow (Lund et al., 1980).

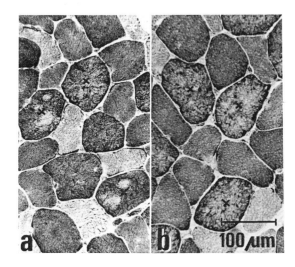

Fig. 1. (a) Moth-eaten muscle fibers (x). Patient with fibromyalgia; trapezius muscle. Stain for NADH-tetrazolium reductase. (b) Moth-eaten muscle fibers (x). Trapezius muscle, healthy control. Stain for NADH-tetrazolium reductase.

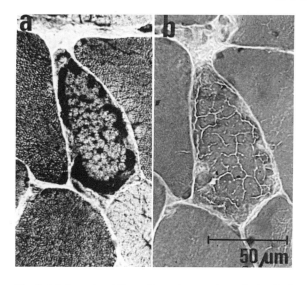

Fig. 2. (a) Ragged-red fibers. Trapezius muscle, patient with fibromyalgia. Stain for NADH-tetrazolium reductase. (b) As in (a) but Gomori-trichrome stain.

Results

The measurements on the trapezius muscle disclosed abnormal histograms in all PF patients, and were of either scattered or slope type. All controls were normal. The measurements on the brachioradial muscle of patients showed that 3 out of 4 histograms were abnormal. One histogram of the five normal controls was abnormal.

Comments

The pathological findings reported above are an indication of maldistribution of capillary blood flow. There is no difference in capillarization in painful muscle compared to controls (Bengtsson et al., 1986a) and lactate values are not increased (see below). The maldistribution of capillary blood flow may not affect the whole muscle but may be focal.

Chemical analyses of high-energy phosphates

Fifteen biopsies taken from the TP area in the trapezius muscle in PF patients were studied (Bengtsson et al., 1986b). For comparison, 6 biopsies from anterior tibial muscle in PF patients were investigated. There were no TPs in the anterior tibial muscle. Biopsies from trapezius muscle taken from 8 healthy volunteers served as controls. The method used for chemical analyses was as previously described (Harris et al., 1974).

Results

There was no difference in fiber type frequency between patients and healthy controls. The trapezius muscle of the patient group had lower mean values for adenosine triphosphate (ATP) (17% decrease, $P < 0.001$), and phosphocreatine (PC) (21% decrease, $P < 0.001$). The energy charge potential (Atkinsson and Walton, 1967) was decreased in patients ($P < 0.02$). Lactate, pyruvate and glycogen values did not differ significantly between patients and controls. In the anterior tibial muscle ATP and PC values were normal.

Comments

The most striking finding is the decreased level of ATP and PC. Similar changes in energy metabolite values have also been found in rheumatoid arthritis

(Nordemar et al., 1974). The results represent mean values of the whole biopsy and do not rule out a more pronounced decrease of energy metabolism in some fibers. The low ATP values are difficult to explain as a result of intensive muscle work or the result of ischaemia, as there is no indication of glycogen decrease or of increased inosine monophosphate or lactate values. The changes in muscle chemistry rather point to defective ATP production by oxidative phosphorylation in some fibers. This assumption would agree with the morphological finding of RR fibers. A hypothetical possibility is that long periods of partial hypoxia occur in painful muscles, and that free radicals could possibly damage the mitochondrial membranes.

Activity of muscle sympathetic nerves

Eight PF patients received a stellate ganglion blockade with bupivacaine and 14 days later an intervenous regional sympathetic blockade with guanethidine. Twenty patients served as controls. Ten received a sham (placebo) injection with physiologic saline superficial to the stellate ganglion and 10 received bupivacaine (Bengtsson et al., 1988).

Methods

The efficiency of the stellate ganglion blockade was evaluated, the pain was recorded and the number of TPs counted. Before and during the guanethidine blockade 8 PF patients were tested neurophysiologically (hand grip strength, fatiguability, relaxation rate) (Bäckman et al., 1988).

Results

During the stellate ganglion blockade there was a significant reduction in pain and number of TPs. The guanethidine blockade reduced the number of TPs but had no effect on rest pain. No significant effects were achieved in the control groups. The PF patients demonstrated a lower hand grip strength, an increased fatiguability and a slower relaxation rate than the control persons. Guanethidine blockade diminished fatiguability and enhanced the relaxation rate in the PF patients.

Comments

Can the disappearance of pain and TPs after blocking of sympathetic nerves be a placebo effect? This is unlikely, since only the sympathetic blockade gave a significant reduction in pain and TPs. A true placebo is difficult to achieve, since the effects of the sympathetic blockade are obvious to both the patient and the observer. The effect of guanethidine blockade on pain and TPs was less pronounced than the effect of stellate blockade with lidocaine. This may be explained by the fact that a guanethidine blockade is less complete than a stellate blockade and by the fact that the pain and TPs are less pronounced in the distal parts of the extremities as compared to more proximal parts. Guanethidine blockade only affects the distal parts of the arm.

Static muscle contraction of a muscle group causes activity in the sympathetic nerves of resting muscles (Mark et al., 1985). This activity continues as long as there is ischaemia in the working muscle. Pain may increase muscle tension, which in turn increases vasoconstrictor sympathetic activity. This increases or maintains the muscle hypoxia induced by the increase in muscle tension. A vicious circle leading to pain may be established.

The neurophysiological studies support the proposition that muscle fatiguability has both a central and a peripheral component. The relaxation rate is dependent on muscular temperature. The increased relaxation rate after guanethidine blockade in PF patients could be due to decreased activity in muscle sympathetic nerves and/or increased intramuscular temperature.

Other investigations

Another investigation to be mentioned is a Danish study (Bartels and Danneskiold-Samsoe, 1986) of biopsy specimens from the quadriceps muscle. The study was performed on glycerinated muscle fibers. In muscles from patients with fibromyalgia (fibrositis) rubber-like structures were found around the muscle fibers, and thin threads (elastic fibers?) were seen between the muscle fibers. The authors speculate that the elastic fibers create a pull between neighbouring muscle fibers and that this could result in pain.

General conclusions

Fibromyalgia (primary and secondary) is a chronic pain syndrome. In addition to muscular symptoms (pain, tenderness, stiffness and fatiguability) the patients have other symptoms which are less specific and similar to those seen in psychosomatic disorders and other chronic pain conditions.

Both our own studies and the other studies referred to above show that muscle metabolism, muscle physiology and muscle morphology are changed in painful muscles as compared to non-painful muscles. Additionally our results provide evidence that activity in the muscle sympathetic nerves may play a part in the etiology of the pain.

The results of our studies suggest that pain in PF could be nociceptive. This does not rule out the possibility that central mechanisms could also be of importance for the development of chronic pain in the muscles.

The diagnostic sensitivity and specificity of different laboratory methods (e.g. muscle biopsy) have not yet been established. The results suggest that the PF syndrome should be defined not solely by clinical symptoms and signs, but also by findings in laboratory investigations of painful muscles. It is time to exclude 'absence of pathological findings' as a diagnostic criterion for the fibromyalgia syndrome.

References

Atkinson, E.E. and Walton, G.M. (1967) Adenosine triphosphate conservation in metabolic regulation. J. Biol. Chem., 242: 3239–3241.

Bäckman, E., Bengtsson, A., Bengtsson, M., Lennmarken, C. and Henriksson, K.G. (1987) Skeletal muscle function in primary fibromyalgia. Effect of regional sympathetic blockade with guanethidine. Acta Scand. Neurol., Sept 3: 3227.

Bartels, E.M. and Danneskjold-Samsoe, B. (1986) Histological abnormalities in muscle from patients with certain types of fibrosis. Lancet, i: 755–757.

Bengtsson, A., Henriksson, K.G. and Larsson, J. (1986) Muscle biopsy in primary fibromyalgia. Scand. J. Rheumatol., 15: 1–6.

Bengtsson, A., Henriksson, K.G. and Larsson, J. (1986) Reduced high-energy phosphate levels in the painful muscles of patients with primary fibromyalgia. Arthritis Rheum., 24: 817–821.

Bengtsson, A. and Bengtsson, M. (1988) Regional sympathetic blockade in primary fibromyalgia (PF). Pain, in press.

Harris, R.C., Hultman, E. and Nordesjö, L.O. (1974) Glycogen, glycolytic intermediates and high-energy phosphates determined in biopsy samples of musculus quadriceps femoris of man at rest: methods and variance of values. Scand. J. Clin. Lab. Invest., 33: 109–120.

Heffner, R. and Barron, S.A. (1978) The early effects of ischemia upon skeletal muscle mitochondria. J. Neurol. Sci., 38: 295–315.

Kalyan-Raman, U.P., Kalyan-Raman, K., Yunus, M.B. and Masi, A.T. (1984) Muscle pathology in primary fibromyalgia syndrome: a light microscopic histochemical and ultrastructural study. Rheumatology, 11: 808–813.

Kessler, M. and Lübbers, D.W. (1966) Aufbau und Anwendungsmöglichkeit verschiedener pO_2-elektroden. Pflügers Arch., 291: R82.

Larsson, S-E., Bengtsson, A., Bodegård, L., Henriksson, K.G. and Larsson J. (1988) Light microscopical and biochemical muscle changes in workrelated chronic myalgia. Acta Ortopaed. Scand., in press.

Lund, N., Bengtsson, A. and Thorborg, P. (1986) Muscle tissue Oxygen pressure in primary fibromyalgia. Scand. J. Rheumatol., 15: 165–173.

Lund, N., Jorfeldt, L., Lewis, D.H. and Ödman, S. (1980) Skeletal muscle oxygen pressure fields in artificially ventilated critically ill patients. Acta Anesth. Scand., 24: 347–353.

Mark, A.L., Victor, R.G., Neshed, C. and Wallin, B.G. (1985) Microneurographic studies of the mechanisms of sympathic nerve responses to static exercise in humans. Circ. Res., 57: 461–469.

Mattila, M., Hurme, M., Alaranta, H., Paljärvi, L., Kalimo, H., Falck, B., Lehto, M., Einola, S. and Järvinen, M. (1986) The multifidus muscle in patients with lumbar disc herniation: a histochemical and morphometric analysis of intraoperative biopsies. Spine, 11: 732–738.

Merskey, H. (Ed.) (1986) Fibrositis or diffuse myofascial pain syndrome. In classification of chronic pain. Pain, Suppl. 3: 833–835.

Nordemar, R., Lövgren, O., Harris, R.C. and Hultman, E. (1974) Muscle ATP in rheumatoid arthritis: a biopsy study. Scand. J. Clin. Lab. Invest., 34: 185–191.

Yunus, M.B., Masi, A.T., Calabro, J.L., Miller, K.A. and Figenbaum, S.L. (1981) Primary fibromyalgia (fibrositis): clinical study of 50 patients with matched normal controls. Semin. Arthritis Rheum., 11: 151–171.

R. Dubner, G.F. Gebhart & M.R. Bond (Eds.)
Proceedings of the Vth World Congress on Pain
©1988 Elsevier Science Publishers BV (Biomedical Division)

CHAPTER 26

The low back pain problem

Erik Spangfort

Department of Orthopaedic Surgery, Huddinge University Hospital, S-14186 Huddinge, Sweden

The problem

Low back pain (LBP) is one of the most complex and frustrating problems we encounter in clinical practice. An elementary survey of this subject usually takes at least one week, and would require an impressive panel of qualified specialists from a wide range of different scientific fields to achieve it. This paper is limited to some plain and basic reflections from the workshop floor, from the rank and file, and primarily concerns the topic of 'non-specific' or 'idiopathic' LBP from a clinical point of view.

It is obviously a truism that LBP is a subjective symptom and not a specific patho-anatomical diagnosis. The concept of LBP as a nosological entity, or a specific disease, has been called 'the Uniformity Myth'. This myth still seems to be very much alive and to confound many discussions and studies of the LBP problem. In fact, 'LBP patients' have one feature in common — and only one: they have, they believe they have, or they claim they have a pain in the back.

There is good reason to believe that almost all patients with a low back complaint experience some degree of pain with a physical origin, but in the majority the true site and origin of the pain are never established and therefore most cases of LBP are 'non-specific' pain problems.

Fig. 1 shows the simplistic model we prefer to use when dealing with the LBP problem. In this example the pathology is a ruptured disc. Myelography/ CT shows the herniation, and clinical signs and symptoms are almost pathognomonic. The solution of the problem is just as simple. The herniation is removed by a fairly easy operation, normal anatomy is restored, the herniation disappears from the X-ray pictures, the patient becomes pain-free, and everybody is happy! This situation does occur, as shown by Mixter and Barr (1934) more than 50 years ago, but in the daily clinical setting it is really quite rare, occurring in no more than a few per cent of all patients with disabling LBP. The misuse of the diagnosis 'lumbar disc herniation' and similar terms for all kinds of segmental pain problems is one example of 'the uniformity myth', and the orthodox chiropractors' 'subluxation' is another.

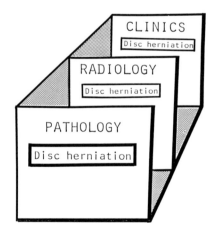

Fig. 1.

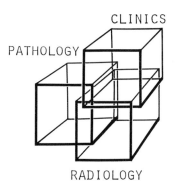

Fig. 2.

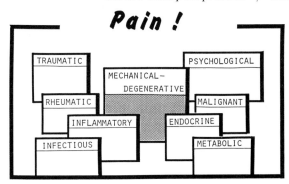

Fig. 3.

Fig. 2 is a better illustration of the LBP problem. 'Pathology', 'radiology' and 'clinics' represent three different 'information systems' that do not fit together: the LBP problem is multi-dimensional. Many pathological features have been studied and demonstrated in the lumbar spine, but in the large number of 'non-specific' LBP patients the correlation between objective pathology and clinical symptoms is weak or absent. The same is true of the 'image-system': radiology, myelography, CT and recently MRI. It may be important to exclude malignancy or fractures, but in most LBP patients the pictures add little or nothing to the clinical diagnosis. Instead, X-ray pictures may be misleading, although they often seem so convincing. It is easy to assume that an old spondylolisthesis, indisputably demonstrated by X-ray at the age of 40, is also the true source of segmental pain, even if the condition has been completely quiet since childhood and has nothing to do with the patient's pain problem.

The patient presents a different system of clinical symptoms and signs to the clinician, and to the patient the low back problem is predominantly a pain problem. In fact, functional impairment of the lumbar spine without pain is rarely perceived as disabling by the patient, who does not consider improving the mechanical function of the spine without relieving pain to be successful treatment.

When specific pathology has been ruled out, we face a musculo-skeletal pain problem without much support from pathology, radiology or laboratory techniques in diagnosis, prognosis or choice of

treatment (Fig. 3). In this common situation the objective must be to identify the main mechanism(s) behind the patient's experience of LBP and to determine the basic etiology of the complaints. This is the key to the choice of treatment. To do so, at a reasonable level of probability, is often time-consuming and may, indeed, require considerable clinical experience and a good understanding of anatomy, biomechanics, pathology, ergonomics and psychology.

I do not doubt that a substantial improvement in the evaluation, care and treatment of 'non-specific' LBP-patients is a very realistic possibility, but progress in this complex field depends on a systematic and structured approach to the problem. A meticulous recording of the medical history, a systematic and detailed analysis of the pain condition and a full physical examination are required. There is no easy short-cut to the solution of this problem, but it is quite possible to reorganize and simplify the clinical routines, which unnecessarily consume so much time and energy.

The patient

When disability is caused by a pain condition with little or no objective medical impairment, the assessment, quantification and scaling of the disability becomes a key problem in clinical work, in the court-room and in research. Definition of the terms and concepts we apply in this context – Impairment, Disability and Handicap – is crucial but controversial. In fact, no single set of definitions has universal applicability, as these concepts cannot always be defined within the same frames of reference. Nevertheless, is is necessary to agree on some fairly simple definitions, before looking at the individual LBP patient. The definitions given below are related mainly to the International Classification suggested by WHO (1980).

Impairment: any loss or abnormality in body structure or function
The term refers to deviations from generally accepted standards of biomedical status, e.g. an amputation or decreased range of motion in a joint. This is the true working field for physicians, who are traditionally trained to judge physical and mental function at the organ-system level according to accepted medical standards.

Disability: impaired performance as a human being
The term refers to the integrated activities expected from the individual as 'a whole man' without consideration of environmental variables, such as his social, geographical or cultural situation.

Handicap: the total disadvantage in the individual's particular environment and social situation
The handicap usually results from impairment or disability, but the state of being handicapped is relative to other people, the valuation is dependent on the environment and cultural norms, and even normal physiological features may constitute a handicap, e.g. skin-colour or age. A scar across a man's

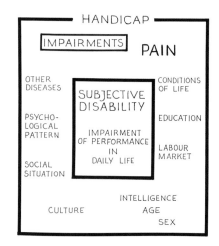

Fig. 5.

face is a handicap in some cultures, a desirable advantage in others.

Fig. 4 shows that the three concepts partially overlap. Therefore the definitions are not mutually exclusive, and this adds to the complexity of classification and assessment. Impairments do not always cause disability, and the same impairment may cause disability in one patient but not in another. On the other hand, it is difficult to imagine a disability which is not caused by impairment. However, handicap may be caused by an impairment which is not disabling, and also by normal physiological conditions.

Considering the LBP patient and applying our definitions, the outer frame of Fig. 5 represents the patient's total handicap. The central square represents the patient's own perception of disability – the 'subjective' disability, if you can accept the term.

'Subjective' disability is, of course, highly influenced by the possible occurrence of objective, physical impairments, but in 'non-specific' LBP patients physical impairments are scarce or absent. The experience of pain is the main cause of 'subjective' disability, and the patients' perception of disability is, therefore, modified by a large number of well-known variables, such as life conditions, education, the state of the labour market, age, sex, culture, social conditions, psychological pattern, etc.

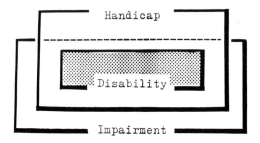

Fig. 4.

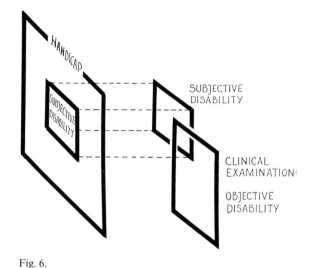

Fig. 6.

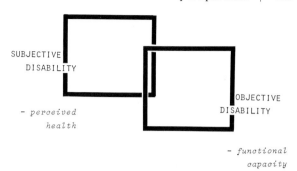

Fig. 7.

From the orthopaedic point of view most of these variables are confounding.

In Fig. 6 the patient is shown presenting his problem to the doctor as 'subjective' disability. In the conventional clinical setting, the doctor performs a clinical examination in order to identify impairments for diagnosis and assessment of the 'objective' disability. His ambition is to cover the 'subjective' square with his 'objective' square to explain the patient's perception of disability, and, hopefully, do something about it. In some situations there is perfect matching of the two squares, a complete agreement between the patient and the doctor in assessment of the disability, e.g. in a case of traumatic fracture with severe cord damage. Appropriate treatment may still be a clinical problem, but there is no conflict between different concepts of disability. In 'non-specific' LBP patients (Fig. 7) it is usually impossible to achieve a complete matching of the squares by clinical examination – in some cases the squares do not even touch each other. The resulting reactions of disappointment, frustration and anger are a threat to the patient-doctor relationship in this situation. Evidently this problem is multi-dimensional, and an improvement of the present unsatisfactory state of affairs requires a multidisciplinary approach, which is also the conclusion from many clinical studies.

As an orthopaedic clinician I must, however, stress the point that part of the discrepancy in the presentation of subjective symptoms and objective signs is often caused by deficiencies in the clinical examination. Enlarging the 'objective' square by improving the clinical examination is one way to reduce discrepancy between 'subjective' and 'objective' disability. All components of physical disease in the condition must be identified and assessed separately, as the indication for surgical intervention is a treatable physical disorder. Unusual pain behaviour should not be punished by refusal of appropriate surgery, and the desperate claim that 'something must be done' about the pain is not a proper indication for surgery.

The treatment

Conflicting claims exist for almost all types of LBP treatment, and we are constantly required to provide scientific evidence for or against different methods of treatment, both conservative and surgical. In this context the term 'scientific' usually refers to the established pharmacological model of clinical trial – the controlled, prospective, randomized, placebo, double-blind, 'wash-out and cross-over' design that apparently allows indisputable conclusions about the benefits and side-effects of the drug on trial. The conditions used for pharmacological trials apply also to LBP trials, but, unfortunately, nobody has been able to design and perform acceptable clinical trials of LBP treatment in these terms. The methodological difficulties are considerable, and I shall address only one of the key problems: the assessment of treatment outcome.

The outcome of treatment may be measured as the total change before and after a specified type of treatment (Fig. 8). However, it is well known that the rate of spontaneous recovery in LBP patients may be as high as 90% within two months, particularly if patients with a short duration of LBP are selected for study. Spontaneous recovery is not a result of treatment and sometimes it occurs in spite of the treatment. Elementary as this may seem, the inclusion of spontaneous recovery is still a common source of error in treatment claims. In theory the error is avoided by assessment of spontaneous recovery in a randomized control group without treatment. Organizing an acceptable control group in LBP trials is extremely difficult. Some intervention is unavoidable, and disruption of all treatment with the patient's consent according to randomized decision may actually cause a negative effect, a nocebo effect.

The placebo effect is a result of treatment, but only to the extent that improvement is caused by the patient's own expectation of benefit from treatment. The error caused by placebo effect is assessed by placebo treatment, but in the study of methods involving physical handling of the patient, which is the case in most types of physical therapy, no reliable placebo treatment has yet been devised, and sham-operations are not acceptable. The problem is virtually insoluble, but possibly it may be approached by psychological methods.

The real effect of treatment is the combined result of care effects and specific cure effect, and, at best, this total real effect of treatment may be assessed in a single-blind model. In the term 'care effects' are included the effects of the therapist's attitude, of listening to the patient, of a careful medical examination, intelligible information about the mechanism of pain and the prognosis, low back education, vocational and ergonomic advice, relaxation, etc. In a strictly biomedical sense these effects may be 'unspecific', as they do not result from correction of an organic disorder, but they are certainly not placebo effects. As pain, distress, anxiety, illness behavior and social dysfunction are also important variables in disability caused by non-specific LBP, the 'care effects' may, indeed, account for most of the total real treatment effects.

In some cases it is possible to demonstrate, beyond doubt, the specific cure of physical disorders causing LBP, particularly if the pathological condition can be identified by surgical exposure. In non-specific LBP patients it has not been possible to provide direct evidence of specific cure by physical therapy, which presumably occurs in some cases. This is really not surprising, as we still cannot identify and demonstrate the true physical mechanism of pain in most patients. Consequently, we may be able to assess the total real effect of treatment, that is, the combined care and cure effects, or at least the relative merits of different treatment approaches. However, we cannot provide direct evidence of possible specific effects.

This does not mean that we can afford to abstain from clinical LBP research whilst waiting for the solution of insoluble problems. It means that there is a need to develop and apply methods most suitable for the task.

There is no doubt that the clinical description of LBP can be improved and LBP syndromes can be

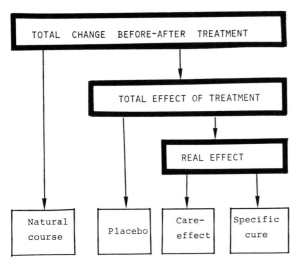

Fig. 8.

identified more satisfactorily by methods of 'pattern recognition' and multivariate analysis. However, this implies collection, handling and careful interpretation of large amounts of very 'soft' data. Therefore, clinical LBP research is difficult, time-consuming and expensive, and it requires meticulous and rigorous planning, clinical knowledge and experience, and multidisciplinary co-operation.

Modern computer techniques are powerful tools for this purpose, but it is also true in clinical LBP research that 'garbage in is garbage out'. The quality of basic medical data is inborn, and sick primary data cannot be cured by sophisticated statistical manipulations. For analysis by computers, the complex clinical information we work with must be analysed and broken down to well-defined elements. This is a difficult, and perhaps tedious, job, but it must be done to improve the quality of clinical LBP research, to facilitate multicenter studies, and allow direct comparisons across different trials.

References

Mixter, W.J. and Barr, J.S. (1934) Rupture of the intervertebral disc with involvement of the spinal canal. N. Engl. J. Med., 211: 210–215.

World Health Organization (1980) International Classification of Impairments, Disabilities and Handicaps, Geneva.

R. Dubner, G.F. Gebhart & M.R. Bond (Eds.)
Proceedings of the Vth World Congress on Pain
© 1988 Elsevier Science Publishers BV (Biomedical Division)

CHAPTER 27

Genesis of the failed back syndrome

Donlin M. Long

Department of Neurological Surgery, The Johns Hopkins Hospital, 600 N. Wolfe Street, Baltimore, MD, 21205, USA

Introduction

The most common cause of incapacitating chronic pain in the USA is the so-called 'failed back syndrome'. This inaccurate title obscures a large heterogeneous group of patients. Of 1541 patients admitted to our multidisciplinary inpatient treatment program 878 had an admitting diagnosis of failed back syndrome. The nonspecific nature of the diagnosis and the heterogeneity of the population led us to undertake a retrospective longitudinal study of the development of the syndrome and its evaluation and therapy in order to specify factors important in the genesis and maintenance of the problem.

During the period 1976 to 1982, 494 patients with chronic pain were personally managed by the author in the context of an inpatient multidisciplinary chronic pain treatment program. The program included an extensive diagnostic regimen aimed at elucidating the cause of the pain; a thorough psychosocial evaluation and a treatment program based upon detoxification, behavioral modification and pain therapy. The specific diagnostic regimen was tailored to the patient's needs. All of these patients were examined independently by a neurosurgeon and an orthopedist. Imaging and electrodiagnostic studies pertinent to the problem and sufficient to establish a diagnosis were undertaken, but were individualized. All patients were seen by a clinical psychologist, a psychiatrist and a psychiatric social worker. An extensive psychosocial history was taken encompassing all aspects of the patient's function. In addition to these clinical examinations a routine battery of psychometric studies were done, including intelligence testing, the Minnesota Multiphasic Personality Inventory, the California Personality Inventory, the Adjective CheckList, the McGill Pain Questionnaire, the Folstein Mini Mental Examination, and the Hendler Pain Questionnaire. Extensive drug histories were obtained and verified by toxicology screens. All patients were withdrawn from tranquilizing and narcotic medications and the history and testings were repeated. These data were collated at a meeting of the pain treatment team, which included the pain manager, the consulting psychiatrist, the clinical psychologist, the psychiatric social worker and the nurse therapist. The physical diagnosis or lack thereof was established at this meeting, as was the most appropriate psychiatric diagnosis.

All 494 patients were evaluated in the same way. From this group 78 patients were extracted because all previous medical records and all actual X-rays ever performed in their care could be obtained for review. This group was different from the larger group in no other way. The availability of all records and images allowed a longitudinal reconstruction of the patient's original complaint and findings and the subsequent clinical course. The history was reconstructed separately by the pain manager and a single orthopedic consultant. All of the X-rays were then reviewed independently by both individuals and the findings were recorded. These findings were applied to the historical data line and a series of decision-making points were examined. The history and physical examination at the time of the first complaint and the images at that time were reviewed and the best retrospective diagnosis was made (Mayfield, 1976). The indications for intervention approved by the American Association of Neurological Surgeons and the American Academy of Orthopedics were applied to determine the patient's suitability for first surgery. Subsequent studies were reviewed to determine surgical complications and for comparison with outcome. This process was repeated for each new medical contact and each intervention. The criteria for surgery were applied to the patient's recorded status at the time of each intervention. Finally, all of these data were collated with the extensive data of the pain treatment program to determine both the outcome of therapy and, insofar as possible, a retrospective analysis of the premorbid psychosocial status.

Results

The spinal diagnoses are given in Table I. These were made at the time of Pain Treatment Center discharge and best describe the patients' status then. Three general factors appear to be important in the maintenance of the pain complaint. These were controlled substance use, depression, and premorbid psychosocial status. 74% of the patients were using narcotics on a regular basis. 12% demonstrated intoxication or definite drug-seeking behavior. 66% utilized tranquilizing medication and 12% were considered to be intoxicated from one of these drugs. Depression was extremely common, occurring in 85% of patients. This incidence is the same as that found in all of our examinations of patients suffering from the chronic pain syndrome. The psychosocial history, psychiatric examination and psychological testing indicated the presence of overt psychiatric disease in 44 patients. In all of these patients the disease appeared to antedate the pain-producing event. Thirty-four of these patients were diagnosed as having a personality disorder and in all of these patients the history suggested that the personality disorder predated the pain ictus.

Review of the historical and physical data coupled with imaging and comparison of these data with the accepted indications for intervention was most interesting. At the time of first surgery, 55% did not meet the accepted criteria for intervention. 26% fulfilled all of the criteria. At the time of a second operative procedure, 40% fulfilled the criteria. All operations beyond the second were for some effect of a previous procedure and all such patients were considered operative candidates by virtue of imaging abnormalities.

The origins of the apparent failed back syndrome in these patients were diverse. A small number had been erroneously diagnosed. However, a major error in physical diagnosis was unusual. A larger number, 13%, had an overt psychiatric disease and there were no apparent physical findings to explain the pain complaint. Another group, 34%, all suffered from an identifiable complication of one or more previous operations. The largest group, 44%, were characterized by a premorbid personality disorder, a complaint of back pain not substantiated by physical examination or imaging studies and one or more failed operative procedures which were undertaken in the absence of the criteria for intervention accepted by national neurosurgical and orthopedic groups.

Another sizable group of patients, 35%, had no physical or imaging evidence of significant spine disease even though the complaint of incapacitating

TABLE I

Normal examinations	16
Minor spondylitic or operative changes	16
Epidural scar	11
Arachnoiditis	10
Traumatic neuritis	5
Spondylosis	4
Spinal stenosis	4
Compression fracture	1
Pseudomeningocoele	1
Foraminal stenosis	1
Herniated lumbar disc	1
Non-spinal pain	8

back pain was at least several years old. Virtually all of these patients had evidence of a personality disorder (Burton et al., 1981).

Discussion

One of the major problems in dealing with the so-called failed back syndrome is the heterogeneity of the population. Failure to recognize the multiple factors involved in the complaint of back pain at its onset and throughout subsequent therapy has two major consequences: patients may not be given appropriate psychiatric assistance and surgery may be inappropriately undertaken for the complaint of unremitting pain after a failure of appropriate conservative care.

There are several problems in generalizing the results of a study such as this. The numbers are small compared to the overall pain population. Only a larger study will answer the question of possible bias in patient selection. The extreme difficulty in getting all of the images done in such patients makes it unlikely that a larger retrospective study can be undertaken. It required seven years and 1500 patients to obtain this relatively small sample. A prospective study probably would be more effective (Spangfort, 1972).

Nevertheless, the specification of these patients suffering from chronic low back syndrome can be useful in helping the clinician to modify current concepts and practices when evaluating and treating low back pain. The majority of patients suffering from disabling low back pain were in one of two large groups. There were those with a spinal problem which had been inadequately diagnosed, inadequately treated or complicated by treatment. It is very important to recognize this group, and to diagnose and treat them appropriately. An even larger group had no significant physical abnormalities through multiple evaluations, or at least, before first intervention. These patients were uniformly characterized by psychiatric abnormalities which were readily diagnosable. The presence or absence of drug misuse and the presence of depression did

not serve to differentiate these two groups of patients.

The size of the group of patients continuing to be incapacitated by back pain in the absence of physical or imaging abnormalities who had not undergone multiple surgical procedures suggests that simply restricting surgery in these patients will not lessen the disability. However, stringent criteria for the surgical treatment of low back and leg pain present in the absence of typical signs and symptoms can reduce medical costs and reduce the change of injury from surgical complication. Another complicating feature of this whole complex problem is the fact that the criteria for intervention for lumbar disc disease are empirical, drawn from the experience of many spine surgeons. Their prognostic significance has never been validated by a study. Nevertheless, this reconstruction of care in patients suffering from failed back syndrome certainly suggests that, in a significant number, ineffective surgery was based upon inadequate criteria for intervention. Obviously this is an extremely small sample and the data cannot be extrapolated to describe surgery for lumbar disc disease in general. (White and Gordon, 1982; Weber, 1983).

The failed back syndrome is a virtually useless diagnosis which has been used to obscure a heterogeneous population. If we are to make progress in the treatment of these individuals it is mandatory that the diagnosis be individualized and accurately describe the patient. This broad non-specific diagnostic term has pejorative connotations and does a great disservice to many patients. These preliminary data indicate that a first-order division of the failed back syndrome can be made into four main categories: a small group of patients with an erroneous diagnosis; a larger group of patients with a complication of an indicated surgical procedure; a group of patients with overt psychiatric disease without significant physical abnormalities; and a group of patients more disabled than is justified by the findings who share the common characteristic of personality dysfunction. The latter two groups are further distinguished by the likelihood that they would have undergone an ineffective series of operations based upon complaints of pain, not objective physical findings. Undoubtedly there will be additional homogeneous subgroups which can be defined within these various categories. Their definition is the next step in the investigation of this, the major chronic pain problem in the USA.

References

Burton, C.V., Kirkaldy-Willis, W.H., Yong-Hing, K. and Heithoff, K.B. (1981) Causes of failure of surgery on the lumbar spine. Clin. Orthop. Rel. Res., 157: 191–199.

Mayfield, F.H. (1976) Complications of laminectomy. Clin. Neurosurg., 23: 435–439.

Spangfort, E.V. (1972) The lumbar disc herniation: A computer-aided analysis of 2504 operations. Acta Orthop. Scand., (Suppl.) 142: 1–71.

Weber, R.H. (1983) Lumbar disc herniation: A controlled prospective study with ten years of observation. Spine, 8: 131–140.

White, A. and Gordon, S. (1982) The American Academy of Orthopaedic Surgeons Symposium on Idiopathic Low Back Pain, C.V. Mosby Co., St. Louis.

Psychological Aspects of Chronic Pain

R. Dubner, G.F. Gebhart & M.R. Bond (Eds.)
Proceedings of the Vth World Congress on Pain
© 1988 Elsevier Science Publishers BV (Biomedical Division)

CHAPTER 28

Assessing the psychological profile of the chronic pain patient

Laurence A. Bradley

Bowman Gray School of Medicine, Wake Forest University, NC, USA

Introduction

Few guidelines were available when I first became interested in evaluating chronic pain patients in 1975. Sternbach (1974) had developed a typology of MMPI profiles and a list of 'pain games' associated with these patients. Fordyce and his colleagues had begun to demonstrate how operant conditioning could increase or reduce pain behavior (Fordyce et al., 1968, 1973). However, many health care professionals were still unaware of the work of these investigators.

Fortunately, hundreds of studies regarding the psychological assessment of chronic pain patients have appeared since 1975. I will summarize the progress that has been made in this area and describe the assessment procedures that should be available to all persons who study or provide health care to chronic pain patients. In addition, I will note the assessment issues toward which future research efforts should be directed.

Given the multidimensional nature of pain (IASP Subcommittee on Taxonomy, 1979), it has been suggested that psychological assessment of chronic pain patients should include the evaluation of overt motor behaviors, cognitive-verbal responses and physiological responses (Keefe, 1982). I will discuss the assessment of overt motor behaviors and cognitive-verbal responses. Von Knorring (1987) describes several physiological assessment strategies in Chapter 29.

Measurement of overt motor behaviors

Fordyce and his colleagues (Fordyce et al., 1973, 1984; Fordyce, 1976) have produced an important series of papers which have demonstrated the benefits of using overt motor behaviors as measures of pain. The primary benefit associated with the evaluation of overt motor or pain behaviors is that it provides the clinician with quantifiable data regarding the disability shown by patients in physical mobility and other activities which are directly related to functioning in vocational, social and leisure endeavors (White et al., 1985).

Direct behavioral observations
Two groups of investigators have recently developed standardized protocols for measuring behaviors such as grimacing, bracing, guarded movement and rubbing of painful body parts. Keefe and Block (1982) produced the first of these protocols, which required chronic low back pain patients to perform for video recording a 10-min standardized series of activities (i.e., walking, sitting, reclining and standing). Two trained observers independently viewed

Correspondence: Dr. Laurence A. Bradley, Section on Medical Psychology, Bowman Gray School of Medicine of Wake Forest University, Winston-Salem, NC 27103, U.S.A.

the video recordings and noted the frequencies of guarding, bracing, rubbing, grimacing and sighing behavior during 20-s observation periods.

Our research team has successfully modified the protocol for use with rheumatoid arthritis (RA) patients (McDaniel et al., 1986; Anderson et al., 1987a, 1987b). We have shown that RA patients' pain behaviors are correlated with self-reports of functional disability (McDaniel et al., 1986) as well as with subjective and objective measures of disease activity (Anderson et al., 1987a); unlike self-reports of pain intensity, however, the pain behaviors are independent of self-reports of depression (Mc Daniel et al., 1986; Anderson et al., 1987b) (see Table I).

Keefe and his colleagues recently have modified their original protocol for use with osteoarthritis patients (Keefe et al., 1987a) and patients with head and neck cancer (Keefe et al., 1985). They also have shown that direct observations of pain behavior are associated with patients' responses to the Illness Behavior Questionnaire (Keefe et al., 1986) and a Coping Strategies Questionnaire (Keefe et al., 1987b) independently of medical status variables. Additional work should be performed regarding the relationships among pain behavior and various measures of cognitive-verbal responses. Moreover, there is a need to determine whether pain behavior may be observed in a reliable manner in patients'

TABLE I

Correlations between RA patients' pain behaviors and measures of disease activity and self-reports of pain, disability and depression

Criterion measures	Total pain behavior
Total McGill Pain Questionnaire	0.45[c]
Modified Health Assessment Questionnaire (functional disability)	0.49[c]
Depression Adjective Checklist	0.11
Grip strength	−0.24[a]
Number of painful joints	0.41[c]
Rheumatoid Activity Index	0.37[b]

These data were originally reported by Anderson et al. (1987a) and McDaniel et al. (1986).
[a] $P < 0.05$, [b] $P < 0.01$, [c] $P < 0.001$.

home and work environments. Finally, it is necessary to determine whether observations of pain behaviors are sensitive to change following the administration of pharmacological or surgical treatments. In this regard, our research group is currently studying changes in pain behavior shown by RA patients after receiving either non-steroidal anti-inflammatory medication or placebo tablets.

Self-monitored observations

Another commonly used assessment method is patient self-monitoring of their behavior (White et al., 1985). It has two major advantages over the direct observation techniques described earlier. First, self-monitoring requires little additional training of health care staff members and patients. Furthermore, self-monitoring allows for the continuous recording of a wider variety of behaviors in environments other than the hospital (White et al., 1985).

The majority of the self-monitoring techniques described in the chronic pain assessment literature are very similar to the daily activity diaries that were originally advocated by Fordyce (1976). These diaries consisted of standard forms on which outpatients recorded on an hourly basis the amount of time spent reclining, sleeping, sitting, walking or standing as well as medication intake. The amount of time recorded in each behavioral category and the amount of medication intake could be calculated at the end of an initial assessment period in order to help determine appropriate treatment plans (Keefe, 1982). The patients could also be asked to continue self-monitoring during treatment and follow-up periods to suggest modifications in treatment and to evaluate outcome (see Fig. 1).

Although early investigators tended to assume that self-monitoring would produce reliable and accurate recordings of behavior (e.g., Sternbach, 1974), the majority of recent studies have shown low levels of association between inpatients' self-monitored recordings and relatively objective measures of medication intake (e.g., Ready et al., 1982) and activity levels or social behavior (e.g., Sanders, 1983). These low correlations may have been due to

Hour Beginning	Sitting		Walking or Standing		Reclining		Medications		Absence	Pain					Unbearable
	Major Activity	Time	Major Activity	Time	Activity	Time	Type	Amount	0	1	2	3	4	5	
12:00 am	watching TV	30	in kitchen	10	in bed	20	Darvocet	2 tablets				•			
1:00					sleep	60									
2:00						60									
3:00						60									
4:00	reading	30	in bathroom	5	sleep	25	Darvocet	2 tablets			•				
5:00						60									
6:00						60									
7:00	eating/reading	40	in bathroom/kitchen	20						•					
8:00	car/desk	40	walking to work	20						•					
9:00	at desk	55	break	5			Aspirin	2 tablets			•				
10:00	at desk	60									•				
11:00	at desk/meeting	50	walking	10							•				
12:00 noon	lunch	30	walking	10	resting	20				•					
1:00	at desk	40	talking with friends	20						•					
2:00	at desk	60										•			
3:00	at desk	55	break	5			Darvocet	2 tablets				•			
4:00	at desk/car	30	grocery shopping	30							•				
5:00			" & in kitchen	60							•				
6:00	watching TV	30	in kitchen	30							•				
7:00	eating	40	cleaning up	20							•				
8:00	reading paper	20	walking	40						•					
9:00	on phone	30			resting/TV	30				•					
10:00	sewing	50	ironing	10							•				
11:00					sleep	60	Elavil	50 mg		•					

Fig. 1. Example of a daily activity diary used for self-monitoring of patient behavior.

impression management efforts by the patients as well as impaired cognitive functioning secondary to depression (Romano and Turner, 1985), narcotic medication dependency (McNairy et al., 1984) or traumatic head/neck injury (Schwartz et al., 1987). Thus, it is clear that self-monitored observations must be compared with some external criterion (e.g., direct observations of patient behavior or medication screens) before they can be accepted as reliable or valid. Furthermore, health care providers and investigators may wish to defer using self-monitoring procedures with patients suffering from even subtle cognitive impairment due to depression, head injury or narcotic medication dependence.

Self-reports of functional disability

Despite the emphasis upon reducing pain behavior and increasing healthy behavior in many pain-treatment programs (e.g., Fordyce, 1976), only recently have investigators devoted substantial atten-

tion to measurement of functional disability in activities of daily living. The Sickness Impact Profile (SIP; Bergner et al., 1981) has shown particular promise as a disability measure with chronic pain patients. For example, the SIP provides a profile of patient functioning in several areas (e.g., ambulation, mobility, body care, movement) which can provide targets for behavioral intervention (Bradley et al., 1985). In addition, research with arthritis patients has shown the measurement efficiency of the SIP to be equal or superior to that of several other instruments with respect to change in patient mobility, global functional ability and social functions (Liang et al., 1985). Follick and his colleagues have also produced positive evidence regarding the concurrent validity and sensitivity to change of the SIP scores produced by chronic back pain patients (Follick et al., 1985).

Other investigators have attempted to develop their own measures of functional disability such as the Chronic Illness Problem Inventory (Kames et al., 1984) and the West Haven–Yale Multidimensional Pain Inventory (Kerns et al., 1985). Most of these instruments evaluate variables such as stressful life events, subjective estimates of pain, mood and self-esteem as well as functional disability. Although the multidimensional character of the instruments probably makes them appealing to health care providers, it should be noted that none of the disability scale components has been validated using the SIP or other accepted devices as criterion measures. Thus, it is recommended that both health care providers and investigators use the SIP or other well-validated disability measures (e.g., Functional Status Index, Health Assessment Questionnaire, Index of Functional Impairment) to measure the functional impairments of chronic pain patients.

Summary

The measurement of overt motor behaviors is a challenging endeavor. There are unique advantages and limitations associated with the use of direct behavioral observations, self-monitored observations and self-reports of functional disability. Moreover, the low to moderate correlations among these measures indicate that each assesses a relatively distinct aspect of patient behavior. It is recommended, therefore, that health care providers and investigators use at least two measures of overt motor behaviors for patient evaluation.

Measurement of cognitive-verbal responses

The major portion of the cognitive-verbal assessment literature has been devoted to studies of patients' affective responses and perceptions of pain. However, some attention also has been devoted to assessment of patients' coping strategies and cognitive distortions as well as to their interactions with family members. The following discussion examines the current literature concerning each of these topics with the exception of family interactions. Roy (1987) discusses this topic in detail in Chapter 30.

Affective responses

MMPI. The MMPI is the most commonly used instrument for the assessment of patients' affective responses (Bradley et al., 1981). It has been argued, however, that clinical interpretation of chronic pain patients' MMPI profiles is made difficult by the content of the MMPI items. Naliboff and his colleagues (Naliboff et al., 1982, 1983), for example, have demonstrated that chronic pain patients produce MMPI profiles which are quite similar to those produced by patients with chronic illnesses such as hypertension and diabetes. These investigators have also shown that between 20% and 31% of the variance in patients' *Hypochondriasis*, *Depression*, and *Hysteria* scale scores was determined by self-reports of functional disability. Pincus and his colleagues (Pincus et al., 1986) have reported similar findings in a study of rheumatoid arthritis patients.

There has recently been an effort to develop novel approaches to the interpretation of chronic pain patients' MMPI profiles. For example, Prokop (1986) and Moore and colleagues (Moore et al., 1988) have shown that interpretation of chronic pain patients' scores on the *Hysteria* and *Schizophrenia* scales is aided by examining the Harris and Lingoes subscales (described in Greene, 1980). Examining the patients' subscale responses revealed that their scores on the *Hysteria* and *Schizophrenia* scales were determined largely by complaints of physical dysfunction or depression.

Prokop and I have used hierarchical clustering methods to delineate replicable and relatively homogeneous MMPI profile subgroups among patients with chronic low back pain (Bradley et al., 1978) and multiple pain complaints (Prokop et al., 1980). We have suggested that MMPI profile interpretations would be improved by attempting to identify the behavioral correlates associated with each of the subgroups and the treatments that might be optimal for each subgroup (Bradley et al., 1981). Indeed, several investigators have replicated successfully the profile subgroups we originally derived using diverse samples of chronic pain patients

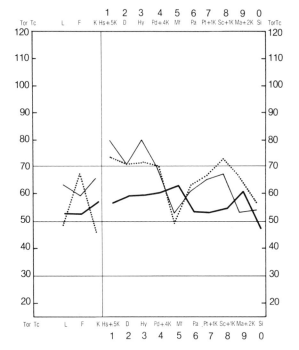

Fig. 2. Examples of mean MMPI profiles produced by three empirically derived subgroups of chronic pain patients. These profiles are based on data reported by Bradley and Van der Heide (1984).

(e.g., Armentrout et al., 1982) and headache patients (Rappaport et al., 1987). Also, several studies have demonstrated that the profile subgroups differ significantly from one another on variables such as duration of pain and number of hospitalizations (McGill et al., 1983), pain intensity ratings (Bradley and Van der Heide, 1984) and degree of physical activity restriction and deterioration in marital communication and social relationships (e.g., Armentrout et al., 1982) (see Fig. 2).

Three investigations have examined the degree to which MMPI profile subgroup membership might predict treatment outcome (McGill et al., 1983; McCreary, 1985; Moore et al., 1986). Two studies showed that profile subgroup membership did not predict outcome in multimodal pain management programs (McGill et al., 1983; Moore et al., 1986). However, McCreary (1985) reported that chronic back pain patients' responses to conservative orthopedic management could be predicted accurately by subgroup membership.

An important factor which might account for some of the predictive error associated with profile subgroup membership is excessive variability within subgroups (Henrichs, 1987). Henrichs recently replicated the MMPI profile subgroups derived both by Bradley et al. (1978) and Armentrout et al. (1982). However, a large number of patients within each subgroup were classified as outliers when a stringent (Sines, 1964) criterion for determining subgroup membership was applied. Nevertheless, application of this criterion produced subgroups which were very homogeneous with regard to behavioral correlates and responses to surgical or nonsurgical treatment. It may be possible, then, to improve the predictive power of MMPI profile subgroup membership by further refinement of the subgroups after their initial derivation by clustering methods.

Other assessment instruments. Given the problems associated with the clinical interpretation and the predictive validity of the MMPI, several alternative instruments have been developed or tested for use with chronic pain patients. These include the Illness Behavior Questionnaire (Pilowsky and Spence, 1975), Back Pain Classification Scale (Leavitt and Garron, 1979), Symptom Checklist-90 (Derogatis, 1977) and Millon Behavioral Health Inventory (MBHI; Millon et al., 1982).

Due to the absence of MBHI items concerned with physical symptoms, our research group has recently begun to study the utility of this instrument with chronic non-cardiac chest pain patients. We have shown that the Somatic Anxiety and Gastrointestinal Susceptibility scales of the MBHI reliably differentiated patients with chronic non-cardiac chest pain or the irritable bowel syndrome from patients with benign esophageal diseases and two groups of healthy control subjects (Richter et al., 1986) (see Table II). Among the chest pain patients, the prevalence rates of significant psychological disturbance identified by the MBHI and the more complex Diagnostic Interview Schedule were nearly equivalent. Other investigators have demonstrated that various MBHI scales are associated with chronic pain patients' responses to multidisciplinary pain clinic treatment (e.g., Sweet et al., 1985). Unfortunately, these studies have failed to show consistently strong relationships between the MBHI Pain Treatment Responsivity scale and patients' changes on subjective and objective outcome measures across assessment periods.

Cognitive distortion and coping strategies

There has been a great deal of recent interest in developing cognitive assessment instruments for use with chronic pain patients. This interest was originally generated by the gate-control theory's postulate that cognitive factors interact with sensory and emotional factors in perceptions of pain (Melzack and Wall, 1965). The most substantial cognitive assessment research has been devoted to measurement of (a) cognitive distortions related to depression, and (b) coping strategies among chronic pain patients.

TABLE II

Subjects' mean scores on the gastrointestinal susceptibility and somatic anxiety scales of the Millon Behavioral Health Inventory

Subject group	Millon Behavioral Health Inventory scale	
	Gastrointestinal susceptibility	Somatic anxiety
Non-cardiac chest pain	64.35 (17.87)	50.95 (28.34)
Irritable bowel syndrome	63.20 (20.56)	59.20 (26.38)
Benign esophageal disease	50.75 (17.46)	36.55 (21.57)
Healthy volunteers – hospital staff	39.00 (20.23)	30.80 (27.72)
Non-hospital healthy volunteers	48.50 (15.53)	26.20 (17.11)

These data were originally reported by Richter et al. (1986). Standard deviations are in parentheses below the mean scores.

Cognitive distortions. Depression is commonly found among chronic pain patients (Romano and Turner, 1985) although there is disagreement regarding whether depression is primary (e.g., Blumer and Heilbronn, 1982) or secondary (e.g., Ahles et al., 1987) to chronic pain. Beck's (1967) cognitive model of depression suggests that depressed individuals systematically distort the meaning of events in order to perceive themselves and their experiences in a consistently negative fashion. Accordingly, Lefebvre (1981) has developed two questionnaires which measure cognitive distortions concerning general life experiences and low back pain-related problems. It has been demonstrated that cognitive distortions are common among depressed back pain patients particularly with regard to pain-related situations. Three cognitive distortions appear to be especially salient. These are: *catastrophizing* (misinterpreting an event as a catastrophe), *overgeneralization* (assuming that the outcome of one experience applies to the same or similar future experiences) and *selective abstraction* (selectively attending to negative aspects of experiences) (Lefebvre, 1981). Smith and his colleagues (Smith et al., 1986) have recently shown that low back pain patients' cognitive distortions, especially overgeneralization, were associated with functional disability as measured by the SIP even after controlling for depression, pain severity and number of pain treatments. Thus, treatment of chronic back pain patients may be hindered by patients' erroneous beliefs that their functional disabilities will remain stable in all future situations.

Measurement of coping strategies for chronic pain.

Rosenstiel and Keefe (1983) have recently developed a questionnaire for the assessment of chronic pain patients' cognitive and behavioral coping strategies. A factor analysis of chronic low back pain patients' responses to the Coping Strategies Questionnaire produced three related underlying dimensions. These were: (a) Cognitive Coping and Suppression (e.g., reinterpreting pain sensations); (b) Helplessness (e.g., catastrophizing); and (c) Diverting Attention and Praying (e.g., praying and hoping). It also was found that patients with high scores on the Cognitive Coping and Suppression or the Diverting Attention and Praying factors tended to show high levels of functional impairment. Those who produced high Helplessness scores tended to display high levels of anxiety and depression.

Turner and Clancy (1986) have replicated the factor structure of the Coping Strategies Questionnaire among an independent sample of chronic back pain patients. These investigators have also shown that during a cognitive-behavioral or operant conditioning treatment program (a) decreased use of praying and hoping strategies was associated with decreased self-reports of pain intensity; and (b) decreased use of catastrophizing strategies was correlated with decreased pain intensity ratings and SIP functional impairment scores.

Factor analyses of Coping Strategies Questionnaire responses produced by patients with chronic osteoarthritis (OA) of the knee (Keefe et al., 1987a,b) have revealed underlying dimensions different from those found with chronic back pain patients. The majority of the variance in OA patients' questionnaire responses was accounted for by a Coping Attempts (e.g., reinterpreting pain sensations, praying and hoping, increasing activity level) and a Self-Control and Rational Thinking (e.g., low levels of catastrophizing, ability to control pain) factor. It also was found that Self-Control and Rational Thinking predicted patients' ratings of pain intensity, functional impairment and psychological distress even after controlling for the influence of demographic and medical status variables (Keefe et al., 1987a,b).

Despite the positive results described above, there are two major limitations associated with the cognitive assessment literature. First, all of the studies performed to date have been correlational. It is not known, then, to what extent patients' cognitive distortions and coping strategies actually produce psychological and functional impairments or result from these impairments. Furthermore, it is not known whether changes in patients' cognitions really generate improved coping efforts. This is a very important subject for future research given the emphasis of cognitive-behavioral therapists upon promoting adaptive cognitive activity among chronic pain patients (e.g., Turk et al., 1983).

Pain perceptions

One of the most difficult tasks facing investigators and health care providers is the measurement of patients' subjective experiences of pain (Bradley and Prokop, 1982). The most commonly used methods of subjective pain assessment include numerical or verbal category scales, visual analogue scales and the McGill Pain Questionnaire.

Category and visual analogue scales. Category scales require patients to rate the intensity of their pain along a finite numerical (e.g., 0–10) or verbal scale (e.g., 'mild, discomforting, distressing, horrible, excruciating'). Visual analogue scales, however, require patients to indicate their perceptions of pain intensity by placing a perpendicular mark along a 10 cm horizontal line labelled 'no pain' at one end and 'unbearable pain' at the other. Although both of these scales are easily administered and scored, several investigators have questioned their sensitivity to changes in the subjective pain experience (e.g., Gracely, 1979). Furthermore, it is not appropriate to treat category scales as interval scales since individuals generally do not respond to commonly used verbal categories (e.g., 'faint, weak, mild, moderate, strong, intense, severe') as if they were equally spaced (Heft and Parker, 1984). There also appear to be great differences among persons in their abilities to use visual analogue scales in a reliable manner (e.g., Carlsson, 1983). For example, it has been shown that age is positively associated with difficulty in using visual analogue scales (e.g., Kremer et al., 1981). Despite the problems associated with category and visual analogue scales, however, they continue to be employed by numerous investigators and health care providers in the evaluation of pain intensity, affect and other experiences associated with pain (e.g., stiffness, interference with work) (e.g., Million et al., 1982).

McGill Pain Questionnaire. The McGill Pain Questionnaire (MPQ; Melzack, 1975) represents the first attempt to develop an assessment device that measures a person's perceptions of the sensory (e.g., temporal, spatial), affective (e.g., tension, fear) and evaluative or intensity dimensions of the pain experience.

The MPQ has rapidly gained wide acceptance among health care providers and investigators (White et al., 1985) both in English-speaking countries and in countries in which translated versions of the measure have been produced (e.g., Radvila et al., 1987). Only two studies have examined the reliability of patients' choices of category scales (Melzack, 1975; Graham et al., 1980) but both have produced positive results. However, the validity of the MPQ has been examined by numerous investigators using a wide variety of methods. For example, a large number of investigators have examined the construct validity of the MPQ by performing factor analyses of patients' responses to the instrument. These investigators have attempted to determine whether the majority of variance in patients' MPQ responses is accounted for by the three major underlying dimensions (i.e., sensory, affective, evaluative or intensity) originally posited by Melzack and Torgerson (1971). Three studies of chronic pain patients' MPQ responses (Reading, 1979; Prieto et al., 1980; McCreary et al., 1981) have generated four-factor solutions, each of which included factors comprised solely of sensory and affective category scales. Prieto and his colleagues (1980) produced a particularly significant study in that the analysis generated three factors composed entirely of sensory, affective and evaluative descriptors, respectively, as well as a fourth factor which was defined by both sensory and affective descriptors. Byrne and her colleagues (1982) later derived three factors from the MPQ responses of an independent sample that were highly associated with the sensory, evaluative and affective-sensory factors found by Prieto's group. The affective factor, however, was not successfully cross-validated (see Table III). Turk, Rudy and Salovey (1985) recently used confirmatory factor analytic techniques to test the validity of

TABLE III

Results of two-factor analytic studies of chronic pain patients' McGill Pain Questionnaire responses

Factors	McGill Pain Questionnaire scales
Prieto et al. (1980)	
Sensory pressure	1–4, 6, 8, 18
Punishing affect	14, 20
Evaluative	16
Affective-sensory	7, 12, 15, 19
Byrne et al. (1982)	
Sensory pressure	2–4, 6–8
Sensory pressure – punishing affect	6, 12, 14, 18
Evaluative-affective – sensory	1, 11–17, 20
Sensory thermal – miscellaneous affective	15, 19

the tripartite MPQ model with the sample drawn by Byrne et al. from an orthopedic hospital and another sample drawn from a Veterans Administration hospital. The model was supported in both samples. However, the high levels of association among the sensory, affective and evaluative factors (r values 0.64–0.81) led Turk and his colleagues to suggest that it was not appropriate to compute separate scores for each MPQ dimension.

The evidence reviewed above suggests that the reliability and validity of the MPQ are acceptable. It should be noted, however, that several investigators have commented that patients who are unfamiliar with the English language or who come from low socioeconomic backgrounds have difficulty responding to the MPQ (Bradley et al., 1981). In addition, the scoring of the MPQ has been criticized on the grounds that scores are confounded by differences in the number of descriptors that comprise each of the 20 MPQ scales. Charter and Nehemkis (1983) and Melzack, Katz and Jeans (1985) have developed new scoring systems for the MPQ although these systems have been used only in a small number of studies. It is recommended that investigators and health care providers who wish to use an alternative to the current scoring methods employ the weighted-rank method devised by Melzack and his colleagues (1985). This recommendation is based upon the evidence that the sensitivity of the MPQ is increased when the weighted-rank method is used (Melzack et al., 1985).

Summary

Three very important advances have been made in the evaluation of chronic pain patients' cognitive and verbal responses. First, it has been shown consistently that there are reliable behavioral and affective differences among empirically derived MMPI profile subgroups. The second major advance has been the development of reliable and valid measures of patients' cognitive distortions and coping strategies. The third major advance has been the recognition among investigators that the use of unidimensional category or visual analogue scales is not sufficient to measure adequately patients' pain perceptions. The McGill Pain Questionnaire, however, allows investigators and health care professionals to evaluate the sensory, affective and evaluative dimensions of patients' pain experiences.

Some effort has already been devoted to determining the relationships among the various assessment devices described above (e.g., Bradley and Van der Heide, 1984). Much additional work remains to be performed. For example, it would be worthwhile to determine whether MMPI profile subgroups differ with respect to cognitive variables, overt motor behaviors and physiological responses. It would also be desirable to compare the utility of instruments such as the MMPI and MBHI with respect to prediction of treatment outcome.

Conclusions

There are clearly advantages and sources of error associated with each of the assessment methods described in this presentation. Moreover, none of the assessment methods provides a complete evaluation of patients' pain experiences or behavior. As a result, it is necessary for both health care providers and investigators to use multiple measures of overt motor behavior, cognitive-verbal responses and physiological variables to fully evaluate chronic pain patients and their treatment outcomes. For example, our research group (Bradley et al., 1987) recently completed an evaluation of the efficacy of a cognitive-behavioral treatment program for rheumatoid arthritis patients which reported changes with respect to (a) direct observations of overt motor behavior; (b) self-reports of functional disability; (c) visual analogue scale ratings of pain intensity and unpleasantness; (d) self-reports of depression and anxiety; (e) perceptions of control over general health outcomes and effects of rheumatoid arthritis (cognitive activity); and (f) peripheral skin temperature levels at the most painful joints as well as several clinical and laboratory measures of disease activity (physiological variables). As is often the case with psychological interventions, significant treatment effects were found in overt motor behavior, anxiety and several of the physiological variables but not in the other outcome measures. This example illustrates the need for comprehensive testing of chronic pain patients in order to fully assess their pain-related difficulties and the effects of treatment.

References

Ahles, T.A., Yunus, M.B. and Masi, A.T. (1987) Is chronic pain a variant of depressive disease? The case of primary fibromyalgia syndrome. Pain, 29: 105–111.

Anderson, K.O., Bradley, L.A., McDaniel, L.K., Young, L.D., Turner, R.A., Agudelo, C.A., Keefe, F.J., Pisko, E.J., Snyder, R.A. and Semble, E.L. (1987a) The assessment of pain in rheumatoid arthritis: validity of a behavioral observation method. Arthritis Rheum., 30: 36–43.

Anderson, K.O., Bradley, L.A., McDaniel, L.K., Young, L.D,

Turner, R.A., Agudelo, C.A., Gaby, N.S., Keefe, F.J., Pisko, E.J., Snyder, R.M. and Semble, E.L. (1987b) The assessment of pain in rheumatoid arthritis: disease differentiation and temporal stability of a behavioral observation method. J. Rheumatol., 14: 700–704.

Armentrout, D.P., Moore, J.E., Parker, J.C., Hewett, J.E. and Feltz, C. (1982) Pain patient MMPI subgroups: the psychological dimensions of pain. J. Behav. Med., 5: 201–211.

Beck, A.T. (1967) Depression: Clinical, Experimental and Theoretical Aspects, University of Pennsylvania Press, New York.

Bergner, M., Bobbitt, R.A., Carter, W.B. and Gibson, B.S. (1981) The Sickness Impact Profile: development and final revision of a health status measure. Med. Care, 19: 787–805.

Blumer, D. and Heilbronn, M. (1982) Chronic pain as a variant of depressive disease: the pain-prone disorder. J. Nerv. Ment. Dis., 170: 381–406.

Bradley, L.A. and Prokop, C.K. (1982) Research methods in contemporary medical psychology. In P.C. Kendall and J.N. Butcher (Eds.), Handbook of Research Methods in Clinical Psychology, John Wiley, New York, pp. 591–649.

Bradley, L.A. and Van der Heide, L.H. (1984) Pain-related correlates of MMPI profile subgroups among back pain patients. Health Psychol., 3: 157–174.

Bradley, L.A., Prokop, C.K., Margolis, R. and Gentry, W.D. (1978) Multivariate analyses of the MMPI profiles of low back pain patients. J. Behav. Med., 1: 253–272.

Bradley, L.A., Prokop, C.K., Gentry, W.D., Van der Heide, L.H. and Prieto, E.J. (1981) Assessment of chronic pain. In C.K. Prokop and L.A. Bradley (Eds.), Medical Psychology: Contributions to Behavioral Medicine, Academic Press, New York, pp. 91–117.

Bradley, L.A., Anderson, K.O., Young, L.D., McDaniel, L.K., Turner, R.A., Agudelo, C.A. and Salinger, M.C. (1985) Psychological aspects of arthritis. Bull. Rheum. Dis., 35: 1–12.

Bradley, L.A., Young, L.D., Anderson, K.O., Turner, R.A., Agudelo, C.A., McDaniel, L.K. and Pisko, E.J. (1987) Effects of cognitive-behavioral therapy on rheumatoid arthritis pain behavior: one-year follow-up. Pain, Suppl. 4: S169. (abstract)

Byrne, M., Troy, A., Bradley, L.A., Marchisello, P.J., Geisinger, K.F., Van der Heide, L.H. and Prieto, E.J. (1982) Cross-validation of the factor structure of the McGill Pain Questionnaire. Pain, 13: 193–201.

Carlsson, A.M. (1983) Assessment of chronic pain. I. Aspects of the reliability and validity of the visual analogue scale. Pain, 16: 87–101.

Charter, R.A. and Nehemkis, A.M. (1983) The language of pain intensity and complexity: new methods of scoring the McGill Pain Questionnaire. Percept. Motor Skills, 56: 519–537.

Derogatis, L.R. (1977) SCL-90 Administration and Scoring Procedures Manual, Johns Hopkins University Press, Baltimore.

Follick, M.J., Smith, T.W. and Ahern, D.K. (1985) The Sickness Impact Profile: a global measure of disability in chronic low back pain. Pain, 21: 67–76.

Fordyce, W.E. (1976) Behavioral Methods for Chronic Pain and Illness, CV Mosby, St. Louis.

Fordyce, W.E., Fowler, R.S., DeLateur, B.J., Sand, P.L. and Trieschmann, R.B. (1973) Operant conditioning in the treatment of chronic pain. Arch. Phys. Med. Rehabil., 54: 399–408.

Fordyce, W.E., Fowler, R.S., Lehmann, J.F. and DeLateur, B.J. (1968) Some implications of learning in problems of chronic pain. J. Chron. Dis., 21: 179–190.

Fordyce, W.E., Lansky, D., Calsyn, D.A., Shelton, J.L., Stolov, W.C. and Rock, D.L. (1984) Pain measurement and pain behavior. Pain, 18: 53–69.

Gracely, R.H. (1979) Psychophysical assessment of human pain. In J.J. Bonica, J.C. Liebeskind and D. Albe-Fessard (Eds.),

Advances in Pain Research and Therapy, Vol. 3, Raven Press, New York, pp. 805–824.

Graham, C., Bond, S., Gerkovich, M.N. and Cook, M.R. (1980) Use of the McGill Pain Questionnaire in the assessment of cancer pain: replicability and consistency. Pain, 8: 377–387.

Greene, R.L. (1980) The MMPI: An Interpretive Manual, Grune & Stratton, New York.

Heft, M.W. and Parker, S.R. (1984) An experimental basis for revising the graphic rating scale for pain. Pain, 19: 153–161.

Henrichs, T.F. (1987) MMPI profiles of chronic pain patients: some methodological considerations concerning clusters and descriptors. J. Clin. Psychol., 43: 650–660.

IASP Subcommittee on Taxonomy (1979) Pain terms: a list with definitions and notes on usage. Pain, 6: 249–252.

Kames, L.D., Naliboff, B.D., Heinrich, R.L. and Coscarelli-Schag, C. (1984) The Chronic Illness Problem Inventory: problem-oriented psychosocial assessment of patients with chronic illness. Int. J. Psychiat. Med., 14: 65–75.

Keefe, F.J. (1982) Behavioral assessment and treatment of chronic pain: current status and future directions. J. Consult. Clin. Psychol., 50: 896–911.

Keefe, F.J. and Block, A.R. (1982) Development of an observation method for assessing pain behavior in chronic low back pain patients. Behav. Ther., 13: 363–375.

Keefe, F.J., Brantley, A., Manuel, G. and Crisson, J.E. (1985) Behavioral assessment of head and neck cancer pain. Pain, 23: 327–336.

Keefe, F.J., Crisson, J.E., Maltbie, A., Bradley, L. and Gil, K.M. (1986) Illness behavior as a predictor of pain and overt behavior patterns in chronic low back pain patients. J. Psychosom. Res., 30: 543–551.

Keefe, F.J., Caldwell, D.S., Queen, K., Gil, K.M., Martinez, S., Crisson, J.E., Ogden, W. and Nunley, J. (1987a) Osteoarthritis knee pain: a behavioral analysis. Pain, 28: 309–321.

Keefe, F.J., Caldwell, D.S., Queen, K.T., Gil, K.M., Martinez, S., Crisson, J.E., Ogden, W. and Nunley, J. (1987b) Pain coping strategies in osteoarthritis patients. J. Consult. Clin. Psychol., 55: 208–212.

Kerns, R.D., Turk, D.C. and Rudy, T.E. (1985) The West Haven–Yale Multidimensional Pain Inventory (WHYMPI). Pain, 23: 345–356.

Kremer, E.F., Block, A. and Gaylor, M.S. (1981) Behavioral approaches to treatment of chronic pain: the inaccuracy of patient self-report measures. Arch. Phys. Med. Rehabil., 61: 188–191.

Leavitt, F. and Garron, D.C. (1979) Validity of a back pain classification scale among patients with low back pain not associated with demonstrable organic disease. J. Psychosom. Res., 23: 301–306.

Lefebvre, M.F. (1981) Cognitive distortion and cognitive errors in depressed psychiatric and low back pain patients. J. Consult. Clin. Psychol., 49: 517–525.

Liang, M.H., Larson, M.G., Cullen, K.E. and Schwartz, J.A. (1985) Comparative measurement efficiency and sensitivity of five health status instruments for arthritis research. Arthritis Rheum., 28: 542–547.

McCreary, C. (1985) Empirically derived MMPI profile clusters and characteristics of low back pain patients. J. Consult. Clin. Psychol., 53: 558–560.

McCreary, C., Turner, J. and Dawson, E. (1981) Principal dimensions of the pain experience and psychological disturbance in chronic low back pain patients. Pain, 11: 85–92.

McDaniel, L.K., Anderson, K.O., Bradley, L.A., Young, L.D., Turner, R.A., Agudelo, C.A. and Keefe, F.J. (1986) Development of an observation method for assessing pain behavior in rheumatoid arthritis patients. Pain, 24: 165–184.

McGill, J.C., Lawlis, G.F., Selby, D., Mooney, V. and McCoy, C.E. (1983) The relationship of Minnesota Multiphasic Personality Inventory (MMPI) profile clusters to pain behaviors. J. Behav. Med., 6: 77–92.

McNairy, S.L., Maruta, T., Ivnik, R.J., Swanson, D.W. and Ilstrup, D.M. (1984) Prescription medication dependence and neuropsychologic function. Pain, 18: 169–177.

Melzack, R. (1975) The McGill Pain Questionnaire: major properties and scoring methods. Pain, 1: 277–299.

Melzack, R., Katz, J. and Jeans, M.E. (1985) The role of compensation in chronic pain: analysis using a new method of scoring the McGill Pain Questionnaire. Pain, 23: 101–112.

Melzack, R. and Torgerson, W.S. (1971) The language of pain. Anesthesiology, 34: 50–59.

Melzack, R. and Wall, P.D. (1965) Pain mechanisms: a new theory. Science, 50: 971–979.

Million, R., Hall, W., Nilsen, K.H., Baker, R.D. and Jayson, I.V. (1982) Assessment of the progress of the back-pain patient. Spine, 7: 204–212.

Millon, T., Green, C. and Meagher, R. (1982) Millon Behavioral Health Inventory Manual, 3rd edn., National Computer Systems, Minneapolis.

Moore, J.E., Armentrout, D.P., Parker, J.C. and Kivlahan, D.R. (1986) Empirically derived pain-patient MMPI subgroups: prediction of treatment outcome. J. Behav. Med., 9: 51–63.

Moore, J.E., McFall, M.E., Kivlahan, D.R. and Capestany, F. (1988) Risk of misinterpretation of MMPI Schizophrenia scale elevations in chronic pain patients. Pain, 32: 207–213.

Naliboff, B.D., Cohen, M.J. and Yellin, A.N. (1983) Frequency of MMPI profile types in three chronic illness populations. J. Clin. Psychol., 39: 843–847.

Naliboff, B.D., Cohen, M.J. and Yellin, A.N. (1982) Does the MMPI differentiate chronic illness from chronic pain? Pain, 13: 333–341.

Pilowsky, I. and Spence, N.D. (1975) Patterns of illness behavior in patients with intractable pain. J. Psychosom. Res., 19: 279–287.

Pincus, T., Callahan, L.F., Bradley, L.A., Vaughn, W.K. and Wolfe, F. (1986) Elevated MMPI scores for hypochondriasis, depression, and hysteria in patients with rheumatoid arthritis reflect disease rather than psychological status. Arthritis

Rheum., 29: 1456–1466.

Prieto, E.J., Hopson, L., Bradley, L.A., Byrne, M., Geisinger, K.F., Midax, D. and Marchisello, P.J. (1980) The language of low back pain: factor structure of the McGill Pain Questionnaire. Pain, 8: 11–19.

Prokop, C.K. (1986) Hysteria scale elevations in low back pain patients: a risk factor for misdiagnosis? J. Consult. Clin. Psychol., 54: 558–562.

Prokop, C.K., Bradley, L.A., Margolis, R. and Gentry, W.D. (1980) Multivariate analyses of the MMPI profiles of multiple pain patients. J. Personal Assess., 44: 246–252.

Radvila, A., Adler, R.H., Galeazzi, R.L. and Vorkauf, H. (1987) The development of a German language (Berne) pain questionnaire and its application in a situation causing acute pain. Pain, 28: 185–195.

Rappaport, N.B., McAnulty, D.P., Waggoner, C.D. and Brantley, P.J. (1987) Cluster analysis of Minnesota Multiphasic Personality Inventory (MMPI) profiles in a chronic headache population. J. Behav. Med., 10: 49–60.

Reading, A.E. (1979) The internal structure of the McGill Pain Questionnaire in dysmenorrhea patients. Pain, 7: 353–358.

Ready, L.B., Sarkis, E. and Turner, J.A. (1982) Self-reported vs. actual use of medications in chronic pain patients. Pain, 12: 285–294.

Richter, J.E., Obrecht, W.F., Bradley, L.A., Young, L.D., Anderson, K.O. and Castell, D.O. (1986) Psychological profiles of patients with the nutcracker esophagus. Dig. Dis. Sci., 31: 131–138.

Romano, J.M. and Turner, J.A. (1985) Chronic pain and depression: does the evidence support a relationship? Psychol. Bull., 97: 18–34.

Rosenstiel, A.K. and Keefe, F.J. (1983) The use of coping strategies in chronic low back pain patients: relationship to patient characteristics and current adjustment. Pain, 17: 33–44.

Roy, R. (1987) Impact of chronic pain on family system. Pain, Suppl. 4: S214. (abstract)

Sanders, S.H. (1983) Automated versus self-monitoring of 'uptime' in chronic low-back pain patients: a comparative study. Pain, 15: 399–405.

Schwartz, D.P., Barth, J.T., Dane, J.R., Drenan, S.E., DeGood, D.E. and Rowlingson, J.C. (1987) Cognitive deficits in chronic pain patients with or without history of head/neck injury: development of a brief screening battery. Clin. J. Pain, 3: 94–101.

Sines, J.O. (1964) Actuarial methods as appropriate strategy for the validation of diagnostic tests. Psychol. Rev., 71: 517–523.

Smith, T.W., Follick, M.J., Ahern, D.K. and Adams, A. (1986) Cognitive distortion and disability in chronic low back pain. Cog. Ther. Res., 10: 201–210.

Sternbach, R.A. (1974) Pain Patients: Traits and Treatments, Academic Press, New York.

Sweet, J.J., Brewer, S.R., Hazlewood, L.A., Toye, R. and Pawl, R.P. (1985) The Millon Behavioral Health Inventory: concurrent and predictive validity in a pain treatment center. J. Behav. Med., 8: 215–226.

Turk, D.C., Meichenbaum, D.H. and Genest, M. (1983) Pain and Behavioral Medicine: A Cognitive-Behavioral Perspective, Guilford Press, New York.

Turk, D.C., Rudy, T.E. and Salovey, P. (1985) The McGill Pain Questionnaire reconsidered: confirming the factor structure and examining appropriate uses. Pain, 21: 385–397.

Turner, J.A. and Clancy, S. (1986) Strategies for coping with chronic low back pain: relationship to pain and disability. Pain, 24: 355–364.

von Knorring, L. (1987) Affect and pain: neurochemical mediators and therapeutic approaches. Pain, Suppl: 4, S215 (abstract).

White, M.C., Bradley, L.A. and Prokop, C.K. (1985) Behavioral assessment of chronic pain. In W.W. Tryon (Ed.), Behavioral Assessment in Behavioral Medicine, Springer, New York, pp. 166–199.

R. Dubner, G.F. Gebhart & M.R. Bond (Eds.)
Proceedings of the Vth World Congress on Pain
© 1988 Elsevier Science Publishers BV (Biomedical Division)

CHAPTER 29

Affective disorders and pain

Issy Pilowsky

The University of Adelaide, Department of Psychiatry, Adelaide, South Australia, 5000, Australia

Summary

The relationship between pain and depression may be elucidated in a number of ways. Thus the two states may be compared in terms of the clinical picture, associated personality characteristics, psychological and psychodynamic features, neurochemical and other biological correlates, and finally the response to treatment.

This paper focuses particularly on clinical aspects, and the need for clearly stated definitions is emphasized.

Since the advent of the Diagnostic and Statistical Manual, 3rd edition (DSM-III), of the American Psychiatric Association, it has become more feasible to compare findings from a variety of studies. These indicate a significant overlap between chronic pain syndromes and the affective disorders, but not to the point where they can be regarded as equivalent. It is possible that pain and depression share some biological and psychological correlates. It also appears that antidepressants may play a role in the treatment of chronic pain, but their general use does not seem indicated by the evidence currently available.

Introduction

Any consideration of the relationship between two conditions must begin with a definition of each. In the case of pain and depression the task is far from simple. Indeed the earliest observations on the relationship did not attempt definitions but simply used the words 'pain' and 'depression' as if their meanings were generally understood and agreed upon.

These early writings emanated in the main from psychiatrists who wished to draw attention to the fact that the complaint of pain could mask a depressive disorder. For example Bradley (1963) described a group of patients with severe pain, who on closer examination were found to suffer from a depressive illness, and Delaney (1976) described facial pain as a defence against psychosis.

Probably the first psychiatrist to formulate a definition of pain was Harold Merskey (Merskey and Spear, 1967), who described it as "an unpleasant experience which we primarily associate with tissue damage, or describe in terms of tissue damage or both". This definition formed the basis for that later accepted by the International Association for the Study of Pain: "Pain is an unpleasant sensory and emotional experience associated with actual or potential tissue damage or described in terms of such damage".

Using his definition Merskey investigated pain in patients referred for psychiatric treatment to the University of Sheffield Department of Psychiatry, headed by Professor Erwin Stengel, himself a graduate of the University of Vienna Medical School and much influenced in his psychobiological approach by his early association with Paul Schilder. Merskey found that in psychiatric patients pain was most often associated with anxiety and depression and commonly attacted a diagnosis of 'hysteria' when it presented as a chronic problem.

Merskey's studies were carried out at a time when the reliability of psychiatric diagnoses was very much in question and there was considerable controversy over the classification of depression.

As is well known, depression can be regarded as an affect, a mood or symptom or a syndrome. As an affect depression is one of many feeling tones which are "the pain-pleasure accompaniments of an idea or mental representation" (Kolb, 1977). A mood, however, is a "sustained affective state of considerable duration" (Kolb, 1977). When depression is of a particular quality it may represent a symptom of an illness which on occasion may constitute a psychiatric syndrome and a nosological entity. In the early sixties a long-standing controversy existed as to whether depressive syndromes should be classified into two distinct types, i.e neurotic (reactive, exogenous) and psychotic (endogenous). The major differences between these two types was believed to be that neurotic depressions were clearly precipitated by an external stress, did not show 'vegetative' symptoms such as early morning wakening, loss of appetite, diurnal variation of mood (worse in the morning), loss of libido or depressive delusions and did not respond to pharmacological treatments or electroconvulsive therapy, all of which were features of 'endogenous' or 'psychotic' depression. Along with this approach to classification was the underlying assumption that biological factors played a particularly important aetiological role in the endogenous depressions.

This debate was difficult to resolve, with some writers offering evidence to support the existence of two distinct forms of depression while others preferred to regard depressive illnesses as lying on a continuum with the two forms at extreme ends of a normally distributed phenomenon. This was not, of course, a purely academic debate, since choice of treatment was to a considerable degree dependent on the diagnostic decision, especially when this involved the giving or withholding of electroconvulsive therapy (ECT). However, with the advent of the monoamine oxidase inhibitor and tricyclic antide-

pressants in the late 1950s the issue of precise diagnosis and classification receded into the background at first, since a trial of an antidepressant in cases of doubt was obviously more practicable and acceptable than a trial of ECT. However, as the number of antidepressants began to multiply in the 60s and 70s and careful drug trials were necessary to choose between them, once again the need to diagnose patients accurately became important.

The response to this need took a number of forms with the development of rating scales (Hamilton, 1960), questionnaires (Zung, 1965; Beck et al., 1961; Pilowsky et al., 1969) standardized interviews and eventually Research Diagnostic Criteria (Feighner, 1972; Spitzer et al., 1975) and the Diagnostic and Statistical Manual of the American Psychiatric Association (DSM-III). DSM-III, which first appeared in 1980, was of particular importance because it was based on a phenomenological-descriptive approach to the illness, and provided criteria for diagnosis.

Since the DSM-III is a widely used diagnostic system, particularly in North America but also in Australia and New Zealand, it is interesting to consider in some detail the criteria it lays down for diagnosing depressive disorders. The conditions regarded as depressive include 'Major Depressive Episode' which may or may not be associated with psychotic features or with 'melancholia'. A major depressive episode involves essentially "a dysphoric mood, usually depression or loss of interest in all or almost all usual activities and pastimes". This is associated with other features of what is referred to as a 'depressive syndrome', viz. appetite disturbance, change in weight, disturbed sleep, psychomotor agitation or retardation, decreased energy, difficulties in concentration, feelings of worthlessness, guilt and suicidal thoughts.

Although such a depressive syndrome may be secondary to a number of other conditions such as an organic affective syndrome due to hypothyroidism or drugs such as reserpine, as well as dementia and schizophrenia, it may be present as a condition in its own right. For the purpose of diagnosis the dysphoric mood must be present and at least four of the other symptoms which go to make up the syndrome must be present nearly every day for at least two weeks.

The two syndromes which are of particular importance to treatment decision-making are 'major depression with mood congruent psychotic features' and 'major depression with melancholia'. These are closest to what would be described in the International Classification of Disorders (ICD-9) as 'psychotic' or 'endogenous' depression.

It may be said at the outset that psychotic depression with depressive delusions is very rarely seen in patients referred to pain clinics, which is the setting in which most attempts to establish the relationship between pain and depression are made.

On the other hand the diagnostic criteria for 'melancholia' are particularly relevant to our discussion because they form the essential basis for deciding whether patients with chronic 'benign' pain suffer from a depressive syndrome. These criteria are

(a) Distinct quality of depressed mood which is different from the feeling experienced in a bereavement;

(b) The depression is consistently worse in the morning (diurnal variation);

(c) Early morning awakening (at least 2 hours before usual time of awakening);

(d) Marked psychomotor retardation or agitation;

(e) Significant anorexia or weight loss;

(f) Excessive or inappropriate guilt.

For melancholia to be diagnosed, at least three of these features must be present.

The other depressive syndrome, so often contrasted with 'endogenous', was 'neurotic depression', also known as depressive neurosis and in DSM-III as 'dysthymic disorder'. In DSM-III it is characterized essentially as a chronic but less severe form of major depressive disorder. For the diagnosis to be made the disturbance of mood must be present for at least two years. During this time there may be normal periods lasting a few days to a few weeks.

As mentioned earlier the term reactive depression was previously used synonymously with neurotic

depression. The approach taken by the authors of DSM-III seems to accord with clinical experience in that it described separate criteria for an 'Adjustment Disorder with Depressed Mood', which is described as a maladaptive reaction to an identifiable psychosocial stressor, occurring within three months of the onset of the stressor and whose maladaptive nature is indicated either by impairment in social or occupational functioning or by symptoms that are in excess of a normal and expectable reaction to the stressor. It is assumed that the disturbance will remit when the stressor ceases or a new level of adaptation is achieved. In this disorder the predominant manifestation involves depressed mood, tearfulness and hopelessness.

The prevalence of depressive disorders in pain clinic patients

Virtually all prevalence studies have been carried out in patients referred to pain clinics of one sort or another. It will be seen that the findings vary widely and depend to a considerable extent on the nature of the patient population, the diagnostic criteria being used, whether it is being surveyed in an out-patient or in-patient setting and, presumably, whether or not the diagnosis is being made by a psychiatrist (Tables I-III).

Pilowsky et al. (1977) surveyed a series of 100 patients referred to the University of Washington Hospital Pain Clinic in Seattle. They were administered the Illness Behaviour Questionnaire (Pilowsky and Spence, 1975) and the Levine-Pilowsky Depression (LPD) Questionniare. The LPD is a 57-item self-report questionnaire which was constructed (Pilowsky et al., 1964) in order to study the classification issue. The LPD was originally administered to 200 patients referred to a psychiatric service in Sheffield, England. The responses were analysed by a statistical technique known as numerical taxonomy, in a form based on information theory. This resulted in the patients being ordered into three groups or classes: I, non-endogenous; II, endogenous; and III, non-depressive. The classes were

TABLE I

Major depression in intractable pain patients

Authors	n	Setting	Criteria	% Major depression
Maruta et al., 1976	26	Mayo	?ICD-9 DSM-II	0
Schaffer et al., 1980	20	Davis, California Pain Board	Feighner	50
Reich et al., 1983	43	Davis, Pain Board	DSM-III	23
Kramlinger et al., 1983	100	Mayo, Inpatients	RDC	25
Katon et al., 1985	37	Seattle, Inpatients	DSM-III	13.5
Krishnan et al., 1985	71	Duke, Inpatients	RDC	43.7
Haley et al., 1985	63	Seattle, Pain Centre	DSM-III	49
Fishbain et al., 1986	283	Miami, Pain Centre	DSM-III	4.6
Large, 1986	50	Auckland, Pain Clinic	DSM-III	8
France et al., 1987	73	Duke	DSM-III	43
				$\bar{x} = 26$

named on the basis of the items which distinguished them and decision rules were generated which allowed new patients to be categorized (Pilowsky and Boulton, 1970). The LPD also provides a measure of depressive severity with a possible range of scores from 1 to 20 (Pilowsky and Spalding, 1972).

In the Pilowsky et al. (1977) study the patients achieved a mean depression score of 6.25, which, compared to the norms for psychiatric patients (Pilowsky and Spalding, 1972), indicates a minor degree of depression.

Of the 100 patients (73 women, 27 men), ten were classified as having a depressive syndrome; four in the 'neurotic-reactive' or non-endogenous group and six in the 'endogenous' category. None of the male patients was in the non-endogenous group.

Schaffer et al. (1980) addressed the issue of whether the pain in patients with chronic 'non-organic' pain represented the outward sign of an atypical or 'masked' depression, by investigating the frequency of 'depressive spectrum disorders' (depression, alcoholism, sociopathy) in the first-degree relatives of chronic pain patients. The sample studied comprised 20 consecutive chronic pain patients referred by their community physicians to the Pain Board (a multi-specialty evaluation unit) at the medical Centre of the University of California at Davis. Each patient experienced chronic pain for at least 6 months and posed a diagnostic problem, a treatment problem or both. Patients and spouses (or close relatives) were interviewed by a psychiatrist, the former being evaluated for clinical depres-

TABLE II

Endogenous depression in intractable pain patients

Authors	Year	n	Setting	%Endogenous
Pilowsky et al.	1977	100	Seatlle, Pain Clinic referrals	6
Kramlinger et al.	1983	100	Mayo, Inpatients	5
Krishnan et al.	1985	71	Duke, Inpatients	14
Large	1986	50	Auckland, referrals	2
Pilowsky	1987	394	Adelaide, Pain Clinic referrals.	6.4
				$\bar{x} = 6.8$

TABLE III

Non-endogenous depression in intractable pain patients

Author	Year	n	Setting	Criteria	%
Maruta et al.	1976	26	Mayo	ICD-9	38
Pilowsky et al.	1977	100	Seattle	LPD	4
Reich et al.	1983	43	Davis	DSM-III	12
Krishnan et al.	1985	71	Duke	RDC	11
Fishbain et al.	1986	283	Miami	DSM-III	51
France et al.	1987	73	Duke	DSM-III	7
Large	1986	50	Auckland	DSM-III	28
Pilowsky	1987	394	Adelaide	LPD	27
					$\bar{x}=21.6$

sion using Research Diagnostic Criteria (Feighner et al., 1972). A control group matched for sex, age, race, socioeconomic background and education, drawn from the Family Practice Outpatient Clinic, was evaluated in the same way. They were being seen in the clinic for a routine medical evaluation.

The results of this study indicated that the pain patients were more often clinically depressed when there was no significant medical pathology contributing to the pain. In this group of 13 patients, 7 scored in an arbitrarily chosen depressive range on the MMPI depression scale and were also rated as showing clinically significant depression by the interviewer. Of the 20 pain patients, 10 were regarded as clinically depressed by the interviewer. Six of the 7 patients with depression and no medical pathology had a positive family history of depressive spectrum disorders.

A second study conducted in the same clinical setting was reported in 1983 by Reich et al., who applied DSM-III criteria to a sample of 43 patients. All data were reviewed by a senior psychiatrist for diagnostic impressions.

Forty-two of the 43 patients had at least one Axis I diagnosis. According to the text, most patients had a somatoform disorder (30%), while 15% had an affective disorder. The table provided lists 3 patients (7%) with a dysthymic disorder, one with major depression with psychotic features (2%) and 4 with recurrent major depression.

Kramlinger et al. (1983) pose the question "are patients with chronic pain depressed". They surveyed 100 patients treated in the Mayo Clinic in-patient pain management programme for chronic pain. Patients selected for the programme had to meet a number of criteria including a pain problem for 6 months or longer, no related malignant disease, no specific medical or surgical treatment applicable, no litigation and acceptance of the programme by the patient. An extensive history and personal data were recorded. A diagnosis was made using Research Diagnostic Criteria and scores were obtained on the MMPI, Shipley-Hartford Scale and the Hamilton Rating Scale for Depression.

In the 100 patients studied, it was possible to make a 'definite' diagnosis of major depression in 25%. Only 5% were given a diagnosis of endogenous depression. It was their opinion that reactive depression predominated in patients with chronic pain and they also made the important observation that, in almost 90% of the definitely depressed patients, a resolution of the depression occurred without the use of antidepressants.

Katon et al. (1985) also studied patients admitted to an in-patient pain programme, in this instance at the University of Washington Pain Center. The sample comprised 37 patients with chronic pain for at least one year and no evidence of organic pathology. Chronic back pain was the commonest complaint. The NIMH Diagnostic Interview Schedule was used as a standardized basis for arriving at a DSM-III diagnosis.

Of the 37 patients, 5 (13.5%) were found to have a current major depression. Nine (24.3%) patients had a history of a past episode.

Another study carried out in a similar population and setting is that of Krishnan et al. (1985). These workers studied 71 consecutive low back pain patients admitted to an in-patient treatment programme at Duke University Hospital in Durham, North Carolina. The low back pain was present for more than 6 months and pain was the major complaint. On the basis of a semi-structured interview Research Diagnostic Criteria diagnoses were made for various subtypes of depression. It was found that 31 (43.7%) of patients had a major depression and 8 (11.3%) a minor depression. Of the 31 patients with major depression, 20 had organic findings, in all cases described as 'failed disc syndrome'. Ten of the patients had a definite endogenous depression and seventeen a 'probable' endogenous depression.

In a further study from the University of Washington Pain Center, aimed at relating depression in chronic pain patients to pain, activity and sex differences, 63 patients were studied and DSM-III diagnoses of major depression were made in 49% of the sample (Haley et al., 1985).

Probably the largest published series of patients examined in a study of this type is that reported by Fishbain et al. (1986), who categorized 283 patients according to DSM-III criteria. The patients were investigated during a 3-day evaluation period following referral to the Comprehensive Pain Center at the University of Miami School of Medicine. All patients had pain for longer than 2 years and a poor response to conventional treatment. The primary location of the pain was in the low back in 73.1%.

An independent organic diagnosis was made by a neurosurgeon and a physiotherapist, who agreed in over 95% of cases. Special care was taken to detect the presence of myofascial syndromes, which were found in 85% of patients. A two-hour semi-structured interview was carried out with each patient, based on DSM-III flowsheets. A major depression was diagnosed in 4.6% of patients. A dysthymic disorder was found in 23.3%. An adjustment disorder with depressed mood was noted in 28.3% of patients.

In a recent unpublished study (Pilowsky, 1987) conducted in the Royal Adelaide Hospital in South Australia, the Levine-Pilowsky Depression Questionnaire was administered to 394 patients referred to the Pain Clinic, in none of whom organic factors played a significant role. The percentages in each category were: 6.4% endogenous, 27.2% non-endogenous and 66.5% non-depressive.

Clinical studies on the relationship between pain and depression

Maruta et al. (1976) at the Mayo Clinic compared age- and sex-matched patients admitted to the psychiatric ward of a general hospital with a complaint of back pain to those admitted with a primary complaint of depression. Twenty-six pain patients were thus compared to 26 with depression matched for age and sex. The pain patients were more likely to have reached only high school while the depressed patients comprised more college graduates (42% as opposed to 12%). Academic maladjustment was commoner in the pain group and 88% had started work at 18 years or earlier, compared to 58% in the depression group. A diagnosis of neurotic depression was made in 38% of the pain patients and 80% of the depressed patients. Endogenous depression occurred in 8% of the depressed and none of the pain patients.

Blumer and Heilbronn (1982) carried out a major study on the relationship between pain and depression and concluded that chronic pain of uncertain origin should be regarded as "the prime expression of a muted depressive state" – a form of masked depression which they term 'the pain-prone disorder', following a suggestion of George Engel, who wrote the now classic paper ' "Psychogenic pain" and the pain-prone patient' (1959). Blumer and Heilbronn base their conclusion on the findings of two studies. The first involved 900 patients with chronic pain of obscure origin who were referred to Dr. Blumer in his capacity as a psychiatric consultant to the Division of Neurosurgery at the Johns Hopkins Hospital (Baltimore), and to the Neurosurgical Division at the Massachusetts General Hospital and finally as Director of the Henry Ford Hospital (Detroit) Pain Clinic, at which over 300 of the patients were treated by the authors.

Blumer and Heilbronn report a striking homogeneity of clinical characteristics in these patients. These include continuous pain of obscure origin, hypochondrial preoccupation and a desire for surgery; a view of oneself as a 'solid citizen' with a denial of conflicts and idealization of self and family relationships together with a tendency to industriousness and 'workaholism' before the onset of the pain.

The depressive component of the syndrome is characterized by a lack of energy and inability to enjoy social life, leisure time and sexual relations. Appetite is usually normal, insomnia often develops. Although these symptoms may be regarded as typical of depression they are attributed by the patient to the pain and it is for this reason that the depression remains obscured. It is noteworthy that blind diagnosis of the MMPI profiles of 76 chronic pain patients showed that the two main groups were either depressed or defending against depression.

From a psychodynamic perspective the patients showed a rigidly maintained ego ideal characterized by a need to be independent, active and to care for others, with powerful underlying needs to depend on others, to be passive and to be cared for. These latter needs are concealed and denied, and overcompensated for by excessive activity and hard work. Once the pain syndrome begins it serves to rationalize the need for the passive-dependent role and the self-ideal can be preserved. Overcontrol or anger is often seen, together with masochism. Although compensation is often a significant issue, the constellation of clinical features described is also seen in patients where compensation is not an issue.

The second clinical study reported by Blumer and Heilbronn involved a comparison of 129 con-secutive patients admitted to the Henry Ford Hospital Pain Clinic with 36 patients with classical rheumatoid arthritis, receiving gold therapy in the same hospital. There were a number of significant differences between the two groups. The rheumatoid group had suffered pain for longer than the pain group, whose pain was more often continuous and began following trauma. The pain group reported more insomnia, interference with sexual life and depression. Overall the investigators felt that the differences which emerged supported Engel's (1959) Pain-Prone Disorder as a nosological entity and a variant of depressive disease.

In a similar study Pilowsky and Bassett (1982) compared 114 patients with chronic pain referred to the Pain Clinic of the Royal Adelaide Hospital with 53 patients treated for depression in the psychiatric service of the same hospital. The pain patients were found to be significantly older, likely to be married and to have larger families. While the distribution of occupations was similar in the two groups, the spouses of those in the pain group were more likely to be in skilled or professional occupations. The quality of sleep was equally poor in both groups but this was more often attributed to pain in the pain clinic group. Similarly both groups spent substantial periods asleep or reclining during the day but this was more often attributed to pain by the pain patients. As far as perceived needs were concerned, the pain patients placed a lower priority on help for emotional and inter-personal problems and high priorities on help with problems of pain and activity. Impairment was measured using the Sickness Impact Profile (Gilson et al., 1975). This revealed that pain patients reported less impairment in areas of emotional behaviour, home management, alertness behaviour and communication than depressed patients. However, they reported greater degrees of impairment in areas of body care and motivation and ambulation.

On psychometric tests the pain patients showed lower scores on the Levine-Pilowsky Depression Questionnaire (Pilowsky et al., 1969), the Zung Depression Scale (Zung, 1965) and the Spielberger State-Trait Anxiety Inventory (1970). On the Illness

Behaviour Questionnaire (Pilowsky and Spence, 1972, 1981), the pain patients scored lower on General (Phobic) hypochondriasis, affective inhibition and affective disturbance, and irritability; but higher on disease conviction, somatic focusing, denial and hypochondriasis.

The findings with regard to recent life experiences measured by the Modified Schedule of Recent Experience (Tennant and Andrews, 1976) were of some interest in that the depressed patients were more likely to have experienced stress in the previous year while the pain patients reported more stress nine and ten years before.

Pilowsky and Bassett concluded on the basis of their findings that chronic pain patients referred to a pain clinic were not suffering from a depressive illness but rather from a form of 'abnormal illness behaviour' characterized by hypochondriasis, disturbed sleep, and a degree of depression milder than that encountered in depressed psychiatric patients. They speculated that stress and disturbed sleep might contribute to the development of what Moldofsky (1976) has described as 'psychogenic rheumatism'. He proposes that traumatic life situations may trigger a non-REM sleep disturbance which leads to fatigue, irritability, depression, anxiety and musculo-skeletal aching and stiffness. It may well be that such a mechanism contributes to the clinical picture in chronic pain patients and this may be particularly the case in those whose illness follows an accident whose traumatic nature is not clearly revealed (Pilowsky, 1986). On the other hand Ahles et al. (1987), who administered The Zung Depression Scale to 45 'primary fibromyalgia syndrome' patients and 29 rheumatoid arthritis patients, found no difference between the two groups. Just as relevant is the finding of Pilowsky et al. (1983-4) that although pain clinic patients report as much depression and anxiety as patients attending a rheumatology clinic, the latter were significantly more likely to attribute their dysphoria to non-somatic problems, i.e. to psychosocial stressors rather than to physical symptoms such as pain. In other words patients referred to pain clinics with an 'idiopathic' or 'psychogenic' pain are more likely to manifest somatization or indeed a 'somatoform disorder' (DSM-III).

Personality in chronic pain and depression

A number of authors have compared chronic pain and depressed patients to determine whether common personality characteristics exist. Maruta et al. (1976) found personality differences using MMPI profiles. The pain group showed higher hypochondriasis scores, while the other two scales of the neurotic triad (depression and hysteria) were similar in the two groups. In addition the depression group had a higher score on the psychopathic deviate scale, indicating greater interpersonal difficulty and family concerns. The depression group was also more obsessive-compulsive and anxious.

Von Knorring and his coworkers (1983) studied the personality correlates of pain occurring as a symptom in depressive disorders. They administered the Karolinska Scales of Personality (The KSP) to 140 in-patients in the Department of Psychiatry, Umea University. The KSP has 135 questions grouped into 15 subscales.

46% of the patients had pain as a symptom. Patients with pain were found to have significantly more somatic anxiety, muscle tension, psychaesthenia and inhibition of aggression. The authors point out that inner-directed hostility is believed to play a part in the genesis of both depression and chronic pain and this may account for the frequent coexistence of these two syndromes.

The Karolinska Scales of Personality were also used by Carlsson (1986) to compare chronic pain patients, normal controls and depressed patients. The pain patients comprised 31 individuals with chronic non-malignant pain. All had an established somatic diagnosis (e.g. peripheral neuropathy in twenty cases and 'lumbosacral rhizopathy' in seven cases). They were compared to von Knorring et al.'s (1983) groups of depressed patients with and without pain and normal controls of 200 males and 200 females randomly selected from the Stockholm area. The data were age- and sex-standardized. It was found that compared to normal controls the pain patients showed more negative childhood experiences and less inhibition of aggression. On the other hand when compared to the depressed groups (with and without pain) the pain patients had significantly lower scores for the Aggression factor. In addition the pain patients had significantly less Muscular Tension, Detachment and Guilt than the depressed patients with pain and higher scores on Verbal Aggression.

The significance of anger and its expression in pain clinic patients was also investigated by Pilowsky and Spence (1976). Using the Illness Behaviour Questionnaire (IBQ), they compared 100 patients referred to a pain clinic to 40 patients attending various hospital clinics (rheumatology, radiotherapy, pulmonary and physiotherapy) who also reported pain as a prominent symptom. The pain clinic group reported becoming angry as often as the hospital group but inhibited anger more often. The pain clinic patients who inhibited anger were also more likely to have a 'psychological' view of their illness and to be affectively disturbed. Those who angered easily were more likely to be hypochondriacal and affectively disturbed.

The various studies on the question of personality suggest that the handling of anger is important in certain cases and point to a constellation of clinical features much as described by Engel (1959): pain, guilt, introputiveness and depression.

Psychobiological markers

A number of authors (Ward et al., 1982; Sylvalahti et al., 1985; Magni et al., 1986; France et al., 1987; Almay, 1987) have employed putative biological markers such as the Dexamethasone Suppression Test to explore the relationship between pain and depression based on the accumulated evidence that depression is associated with low brain turnover of serotonin and noradrenaline, while the endogenous pain suppression system is also dependent on the activity of these two monoamines.

These studies will not be surveyed in detail, but

in summary it may be said that since at the present time there exists no entirely satisfactory biological marker for depression, it is not surprising that the use of techniques such as the DST has not provided clear-cut answers.

Antidepressants and chronic pain

The widespread use of antidepressants in the treatment of chronic intractable pain is a consequence of the belief that these syndromes represent a form of depression. Furthermore, antidepressants have been used to seek support for the proposition that chronic pain may be a 'depressive-equivalent'. However, this support has not been forthcoming.

It is probably true to say that from a clinical point of view most psychiatrists would not expect the vast majority of those referred to a pain clinic to respond dramatically to a tricyclic antidepressant, since they rarely encounter patients who seem to show the clinical features predictive of such a response. This has led to emphasis on the idea that the tricyclics may have a direct effect on the pain by virtue of their influence on noradrenaline and serotonin (Feinmann, 1985). In the last analysis, however, this issue needs to be resolved by carefully conducted controlled trials, of which there has thus far been a relative dearth.

In an excellent review of psychopharmacological agents in the treatment of pain Atkinson et al. (1985) concluded that the heterogeneous nature of patients with the chronic pain syndrome made careful studies difficult. They highlight a number of shortcomings in the treatment of such patients. The first is the lack of clinical or biological markers to predict drug response; they note secondly that the high drop-out rate indicates that antidepressants on their own are insufficient and a more comprehensive approach is required, and thirdly that the role played by depression is unclear. This is consonant with the view of Williams (1986), who believes that the tricyclic depressants are most effective in the treatment of pain when there is an associated depressive illness.

Our own experience in a double-blind placebo-controlled cross-over trial of amitriptyline in chronic non-organic pain patients who were not selected for the presence of a depressive syndrome suggests that tricyclic antidepressants are not particularly effective in the treatment of this group, and responses are not related to improvement of depression (Pilowsky et al., 1982).

By contrast, Hameroff et al. (1985) showed that the tricyclic doxepin was significantly more effective than placebo in the treatment of a sample of 60 patients. It is important to note, however, that these were patients with 'coexisting clinical depression'.

In summary we may conclude that the role of antidepressants in treating chronic pain does not support the assertion that these syndromes are depressive equivalents. Experience in the clinic with which I am associated at The Royal Adelaide Hospital suggests that the evidence for the value of trycyclics in treated chronic 'benign' pain is not compelling. As France et al. (1984) have pointed out, there have been very few placebo-controlled studies on patients of this sort, and far more needs to be done.

Psychological and psychodynamic aspects

As already mentioned, the similarity between the dynamics discernible in chronic pain patients and depressed patients has been adduced as evidence for considering the two syndromes in some way equivalent. The similarity consists of a tendency to inhibit anger, turning it against the self and assuming a masochistic posture. Engel (1959), Blumer and Heilbronn (1982) and Beutler et al. (1986) have proposed that difficulties in expressing anger and controlling intense emotions are predisposing factors which link pain and depression. Their views are extremely interesting and space does not permit more than a brief mention of this theory, which leads to the suggestion that therapy aimed at allowing the patient to express the anger in an imaginary dialogue with the feared interpersonal target may contribute to the relief of chronic pain and depression

in patients who overcontrol and constrain emotional expression.

It is well known that cognitive factors play a significant role in chronic pain. Indeed, their modification is a central ingredient of cognitive-behavioural therapy. It has also been observed that the negative cognitions which are regarded as a central feature of depressive illnesses by Beck (1967) also occur in chronic pain states. These cognitive distortions were measured by Lefebvre (1981) in four groups: depressed psychiatric patients, depressed low back pain (LBP) patients, non-depressed LBP patients and non-depressed without LBP. He measured catastrophizing, overgeneralization, personalization and selective abstraction. He found that cognitive distortion was greater in depression with or without LBP. He concludes that depression in LBP patients is a function of both cognitive errors and LBP.

Stein and Fruchter (1983) examined the relationship between depression and illness behaviour in 37 chronic pain patients, using the IBQ and measures of depression. What emerged was a significant association between depression scores and hypochondriasis, disease conviction, somatic focusing, dysphoria and irritability. They concluded that disturbance in illness behaviour was related to the current level of depression and depressive experiences associated with self-criticism. They emphasize the "need for caution in extrapolating from syndromes of clinical depression and illness behaviour in patients with chronic pain."

Overview

In considering the relationship between the experiences of pain and affects such as depression, anger and anxiety, it seems useful to conceptualize it as one which moves from an intermingling of half-formed and vaguely sensed 'protoaffects' and 'protocognitions' to states in which the various affects and cognitions are experienced in increasingly sharp and delimited forms. Such a model would be in keeping with the writings of Zajonc (1980), who advances the view that affects "can occur without extensive perceptual and cognitive encoding, are made with greater confidence than cognitive judgements, and can be made sooner". This approach favours a model of pain in which 'fuzzy' affective and cognitive responses are generated within milliseconds to become one or other variety of pain experience and indeed pain syndrome. The factors shaping the experience range from the biological to the cultural and will vary from context to context.

A model for the link between pain and emotion has been described by Leventhal and Everhart (1979), whose ideas are deserving of more attention from pain researchers than they have thus far been accorded. Their model assumes the parallel processing of information, pain and distress from the observed stimulus, through preconscious and conscious phases to observed behaviour. They postulate a sensory-perceptual or informational path that creates the experience of location, duration intensity and attributes of the stimulus, and an emotion path that generates the perceptual experience of distress. This brief reference to their work does it no justice at all, since the full model is sophisticated and appealing to the clinician and based on a great deal of empirical research. It is a model which helps us to comprehend why there might be a greater than coincidental association between pain and depression and why the multidisciplinary approach will continue to be essential to its elucidation. Such a model would also be compatible with David Swanson's (1984) persuasive suggestion that chronic benign pain be considered as a third pathologic emotion alongside anxiety and depression. As Swanson points out, anxiety, depression and chronic pain often occur in various combinations, and that this is to be expected if they are "similar emotional states, with phenomenologic and neurochemical overlap". However, it seems reasonable to extend this overlap to pain in general whether acute or chronic. As indicated in Fig. 1, we may expect a combination of depression and pain in chronic pain states, anxiety and pain in acute pain states and dysphoric disorders when anxiety and depression overlap in situations where a bodily threat is not perceived. Where anxiety, depression and pain

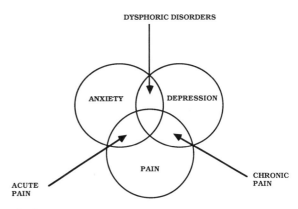

Fig. 1.

without an obvious somatic input occur in combination, we may refer to 'dysthymic pain disorder' as suggested by Blumer and Heilbronn (1987).

It is somewhat ironic that our journey through the uncertainties surrounding the relationship between chronic pain and depression leads us inexorably to the question of the relationship between somatoform disorders, such as hypochondriasis, and depression – long a controversial issue in psychiatry and as yet unresolved. As clinicians, we may need to accept that constellations of symptoms and signs which are relevant to aetiology may not be the same as those relevant to treatment and prognosis. From a practical point of view, both lines of research need to be pursued, and clearly much more needs to be done. For the time being we are led back to the conclusion that many patients with chronic intractable pain may be usefully regarded as suffering from a form of abnormal or discordant illness behaviour of a somatoform type which can only be managed by a long-standing supportive relationship with a physician who is prepared to call upon and collaborate with a range of professional colleagues, and to treat patients and their suffering with the respect and professional concern they deserve. Such a treatment approach is more likely to be successful if backed up by the resources of a multidisciplinary pain clinic.

References

Ahles, T.A., Yanus, M.B. and Masi, A.T. (1987) Is chronic pain a variant of depressive disease? The case of primary fibromyalgia syndrome. Pain, 29: 105–111.

Almay, B.G.L. (1987) Patients with idiopathic pain syndromes. Umea University Medical Dissertations, No. 191, Umea, Sweden.

Atkinson, J.H., Kremer, E.F. and Garfin, S.R. (1985) Psychopharmacological agents in the treatment of pain. J. Bone Joint Surg. 67A: 337–342.

Beck, A.T. (1969) Depression: Clinical, Experimental and Theoretical Aspects, Harper and Row, New York.

Beck, A.T., Ward, C.H., Mendelson, M., Mock, J. and Erbaugh, J. (1961) An inventory for measuring depression, Arch. Gen. Psychiatry, 4: 561–571.

Beutler, L.E., Engle, D., Oro'-Beutler, M.E., Daldrup, R. and Meredith, K. (1986) Inability to express intense affect: a common link between depression and pain? J. Consul. Clin. Psychol., 54: 752–759.

Blumer, D. and Heilbronn, M. (1982) Chronic pain as a variant of depressive disease. The pain-prone disorder. J. Nerv. Mental Dis., 170: 381–406.

Blumer, D. and Heilbronn, M. (1987) Depression and chronic pain. In O. Cameron (Ed.), Presentation of Depression, Wiley, New York, quoted in Almay (1987).

Bradley, J.J. (1963) Severe localized pain associated with the depressive syndrome. Br. J. Psychiatry, 109: 741–745.

Diagnostic and Statistical Manual of the American Psychiatric Association (1980), Washington D.C.: A.P.A.

Delaney, J.F. (1976) Atypical facial pain as a defense against psychosis. Am. J. Psychiatry, 133: 1151–1154.

Engel, G.L., (1959) 'Psychogenic' pain and the pain-prone patient. Am. J. Med., 26: 899–918.

Feighner, J.P., Robins, E. and Guze, S.B. (1972) Diagnostic criteria for use in psychiatric research. Arch. Gen. Psychiatry, 26: 57–63.

Feinmann, C. (1985) Pain relief by antidepressants: possible modes of action, Pain, 23: 1–8.

Fishbain, D.A., Goldberg, M., Meagher, B.R., Steele, R. and Rosomoff, H. (1986) Male and female chronic pain patients categorized by DSM-III psychiatric diagnostic criteria. Pain, 26: 181–197.

France, R.D., Houpt, J.L. and Ellinswood, E.H. (1984) Therapeutic effects of antidepressants in chronic pain, Gen. Hosp. Psychiatry, 6: 55–63.

France, R.D., Krishnan, K.R.R., Trainor, M. and Pelton, S. (1987) Chronic pain and depression IV. DST as a discriminator between chronic pain and depression. Pain, 28: 39–44.

Gilson, B.S., Gilson, J.S. Bergner, M., Bobbitt, R., Kresse, I.S., Pollar, W. and Vesselaso, M. (1975) The sickness impact profile. Am. J. Publ. Health, 65: 1304–1310.

Haley, W.E., Turner, J.A. and Romano, J.M. (1985) Depression in chronic pain patients: Relation to pain, activity and sex dif-

ferences. Pain, 23: 337–343.

Hameroff, S.R., Cork, R.C., Weiss, J.L., Crago, B.R. and Davis, T.P., (1985) Doxepin effects on chronic pain and depression: a controlled study. Clin. J. Pain, 1: 171–176.

Hamilton, M. (1960) A Rating Scale for depression. J. Neurol. Neurosurg. Psychiatry, 23: 53–62.

Katon, W., Egan, K. and Miller, D. (1985) Chronic pain: lifetime psychiatric diagnoses and family history. Am. J. Psychiatry, 142: 1156-1160.

Kolb, L. (1977) Modern Clinical Psychiatry, Saunders, London, pp. 24.

Kramlinger, K.G., Swanson, D.W. and Maruta, T., (1983) Are patients with chronic pain depressed? Am. J. Psychiatry, 140: 747–749.

Krishnan, K.R.R., France, R.D., Pelton, S., McCann, U.D., Davidson, J. and Urban, B.J., (1985) Chronic pain and depression. 1. Classification of depression in chronic low back pain patients. Pain, 22: 279–287.

Lefebre, M.R., (1981) Cognitive distortion in psychiatric and low back pain patients. J. Consult. Clin. Psychol., 49: 517–525.

Leventhal, H. and Everhart, D. (1979) Emotion, pain and physical illness. In C.E. Izard (Ed.), Emotions and Personality in Psychopathology, Plenum Press, New York.

Maruta, T., Swanson, D.W. and Swenson, W.M. (1976) Pain as a psychiatric symptom: comparison between low back pain and depression. Psychosomatics, 17: 123–127.

Merskey, H. and Spear, F.G. (1967): Pain: Psychological and Psychiatric Aspects, Balliere Tindall and Carsell, London.

Moldofsky, H. (1976) Psychogenic rheumatism or the fibrositic syndrome. In O. Hill (Ed.), Modern Trends in Psychosomatic Medicine, vol. 3, Butterworth, London.

Pilowsky, I. and Bassett, D.L. (1982) Pain and depression. Br. J. Psychiatry, 141: 30–36.

Pilowsky, I. (1986) Cryptotrauma and 'accident neurosis'. Br. J. Psychiatry, 147: 310–311.

Pilowsky, I. and Spence, N. (1986) Manual of the Illness Behaviour Questionnaire, Department of Psychiatry, University of Adelaide.

Pilowsky, I. and Boulton, D.M. (1970) Development of a questionnaire based decision rule for classifying depressed patients. Br. J. Psychiatry, 16: 647–650.

Pilowsky, I. and Spalding, D. (1972) A method for measuring depression. Br. J. Psychiatr, 121: 411–416.

Pilowsky, I. and Spence, N. (1975) Patterns of illness behaviour in patients with intractable pain. J. Psychosomat. Res., 19: 279–287.

Pilowsky, I., Levine, S. and Boulton, D.M., (1969) The classification of depression by numerical taxonomy. Br. J. Psychiatry, 115: 937–945.

Pilowsky, I., Chapman, C.R. and Bonica, J.J. (1977) Pain, depression and illness behaviour in a pain clinic population.

Pain, 4: 183–192.

Pilowsky, I., Bassett, D., Barrett, R., Petrovic, L. and Minniti, R. (1983-84) The illness behavior assessment schedule: reliability and validity. Int. J. Psychiatry Med., 131: 11–28.

Reich, J., Tupin, J.P. and Abramowitz, S.I. (1983) Psychiatric diagnosis of chronic pain patients. Am. J. Psychiatry, 140: 1495–1498.

Schaffer, C.B., Donlon, P.T. and Bittle, R.M. (1980) Chronic pain and depression: a clinical and family history survey. Am. J. Psychiatry, 137: 118–120.

Spielberger, C.D. (1975) The measurement of state and trait anxiety. In L. Levi (Ed.), Emotions, Raven Press, New York.

Spitzer, R.L., Endicott, T. and Robins, E. (1975) Research Diagnostic Criteria, Biometric Research, New York.

Stein, N., Fruchter, H.J. and Trief, P. (1983) Experiences of depression and illness behaviour in patients with intractable chronic pain. J. Clin. Psychol., 39: 31–33.

Swanson, D.W. (1982) Chronic pain as a third pathologic emotion. Am. J. Psychiatry, 141: 210-214.

Tennant, C. and Andrews, G. (1976) A scale to measure the stress of life events. Aust. NZ J. Psychiatry, 10: 27-32.

Williams, N.E. (1986) Current views on the pharmacological management of pain. In M. Swerdlow (Ed.), The Therapy of Pain, M.T.P. Press, Lancaster.

Zajonc, R.B. (1980) Feeling and thinking. Am. Psychol., 35: 151-175.

Zung, W.W.K. (1965) A self-rating depression scale. Arch. Gen. Psychiatry, 12: 63–70.

R. Dubner, G.F. Gebhart & M.R. Bond (Eds.)
Proceedings of the Vth World Congress on Pain
© 1988 Elsevier Science Publishers BV (Biomedical Division)

CHAPTER 30

Affect and pain: neurochemical mediators and therapeutic approaches

Lars von Knorring

Department of Psychiatry, Umeå University, Umeå, Sweden

Summary

Acute pain may promote survival and restitution and the clinical characteristics are similar to those seen in anxiety states. Chronic pain is usually destructive and the clinical symptoms and signs are similar to those seen in depressive disorders.

In idiopathic pain syndromes, no organic pathology or pathophysiological mechanism can be found to account for the pain.

In patients with idiopathic pain syndromes, as in patients with depressive disorders, the levels of the pineal hormone melatonin tend to be low in both serum and urine, the concentrations of the serotonin metabolite 5-HIAA in CSF are often low, the activity of the enzyme monoamine oxidase (MAO) in platelets tends to be low and there are often hypersecretion of cortisol and reduced suppression of cortisol in plasma after pretreatment with dexamethasone.

Although none of these biochemical or neuroendocrinological deviations is specific to the depressive syndrome, the results indicate that the idiopathic pain syndrome and the depressive syndrome at least share a common pathogenetic mechanism.

In patients with idiopathic pain syndromes, normal or high concentrations of endorphins, Fraction 1, have been demonstrated in CSF, as in patients with depressive disorders, while patients with chronic neurogenic pain syndromes tend to have low concentrations.

In extended studies, patients with idiopathic pain syndromes have been found to have low concentrations of substance P and dynorphin in CSF while the concentrations of beta-endorphin and met-enkephalin were normal. In a stepwise multiple regression analysis, it seemed as if the pain was mostly related to the levels of substance P, met-enkephalin and beta-endorphin, while sadness was related to the monoamine metabolites, 5-HIAA and HVA and to the levels of substance P in CSF.

If the idiopathic pain syndromes at least share a common pathogenetic mechanism with the depressive syndromes, it is not surprising that ECT and antidepressants have been found useful in treatment.

Acute and chronic pain

There is a very significant difference in biomedical function between the acute and the chronic pain states (Sternbach, 1981). While acute pain may promote survival and restitution, chronic pain is usually destructive – physically, psychologically and socially (Sternbach, 1974, 1984).

In acute pain the clinical symptoms and signs are

Correspondence: Lars von Knorring, M.D. Assoc. Professor, Department of Psychiatry, Umeå University, S-901 85 Umeå, Sweden.

TABLE I

A comparison of symptoms and signs seen in acute and chronic pain states (modified from Sternbach, 1981)

Acute pain	Chronic pain
Increased cardiac rate	Sleep disturbances
Increased blood pressure	Irritability
Pupillary dilatation	Appetite disturbances
Palmar sweating	Constipation
Hyperventilation	Psychomotor retardation
Hypermotility	Social withdrawal
Escape behaviour	Abnormal illness behaviour
Anxiety	Depression

similar to those seen in anxiety states, while the symptoms and signs seen in chronic pain states are similar to those seen in depressive states (Sternbach, 1981) (Table I).

Subgroups of chronic pain syndromes

There are at least four relatively separate subgroups of patients with chronic pain syndromes (Almay, 1987a).
1. Chronic pain related to non-malignant disease:
    A. Pain of predominantly nociceptive type;
    B. Pain of predominantly neurogenic type:
2. Chronic pain syndromes in malignant disease:
3. Chronic pain related to psychiatric disease (e.g., major depressive disorders or schizophrenia):
4. Idiopathic pain syndromes in which no organic pathology or pathophysiological mechanism can be found to account for the pain. An operational definition has been given by Williams and Spitzer (1982).

Furthermore, it seems reasonable to distinguish between permanent and non-permanent pain states.

As selection always takes place before a patient with a chronic pain syndrome is included in a specific research program, it is reasonable to believe that most of the contradictions that exist in the literature are due to problems related to different selection of subgroups of chronic pain patients.

In the following, the main focus will be put on

patients with chronic pain syndromes (of at least six months duration, but usually with a duration of several years) of idiopathic type, fulfilling the operational definition given by Williams and Spitzer (1982). Furthermore, most of the patients included in the series have had permanent pain, often without any interruptions.

Pain and depression

The concept depression may be used with several different meanings. Sometimes depression is used to refer to the single symptom of depressed mood. The single symptom sadness is often seen in chronic pain states (Pilowski and Basset, 1982; Almay, 1987b) in the same way as pain is often found as a symptom in patients with depressive disorders (Ward et al., 1979; von Knorring et al., 1983a).

However, the depressive syndrome is not only characterized by sadness. Anxiety, inhibition-retardation and so-called hypothalamic symptoms are also characteristic of the syndrome (APA, 1980). Thus, it is of considerable interest that anxiety, inhibition and hypothalamic symptoms such as sleep disturbances and appetite disturbances are also common symptoms in the chronic pain states (Sternbach, 1974, 1981, 1984; Almay, 1987b) (Table II).

Furthermore, depression may be used to refer to a specific disease entity, usually major depression or bipolar depressive disorders.

The exact relationship between the depressive syndrome and the chronic pain syndrome is still unclear. However, it has been suggested that the two syndromes share a common pathogenetic mechanism (Sternbach, 1974; von Knorring, 1975; Lindsay and Wycoff, 1981), that the chronic pain syndrome is a masked depression (Lopez Ibor, 1972), that the chronic pain syndrome is a special syndrome in a spectrum of depressive disorders (depressive spectrum disease) (Blumer and Heilbronn, 1981a), or that the chronic pain syndrome is in fact a variant of depressive disease (Blumer and Heilbronn, 1982).

TABLE II
Self-rating by means of a visual analogue scale in healthy volunteers ($n = 28$) and chronic pain patients with neurogenic ($n = 22$) and idiopathic pain syndromes ($n = 64$), respectively

| | Healthy volunteers | Chronic pain syndromes | | F |
		Neurogenic pain	Idiopathic pain	
Pain	2.1 ± 3.2	55.7 ± 28.8	64.1 ± 24.9	74.80
Sadness	3.8 ± 6.7	21.7 ± 22.5	32.7 ± 30.2	12.78
Inner tension	5.7 ± 8.7	32.3 ± 28.1	35.9 ± 29.0	14.16
Concentration difficulties	2.3 ± 3.8	17.5 ± 23.4	30.5 ± 25.2	16.97
Memory disturbances	1.0 ± 1.5	11.0 ± 15.3	24.1 ± 25.2	13.69

The visual analogue scales consisted of 100-mm-long horizontal lines with definitions at the ends and with no marks in between. The scores are expressed in mm, ranging from 0 to 100 mm, and are reported as $\bar{x} \pm$ S.D. The statistical analysis has been made by means of analysis of variance, one-way classification, ANOVA (data from Almay, 1987b). $P < 0.001$ in all cases.

Regardless of the exact nature of the relationship between the two syndromes, the pronounced clinical similarities make it probable that biochemical and neuroendocrinological deviations present in the depressive syndrome might also be of importance in the chronic pain syndrome.

Pathogenetic mechanisms in depressive disorders

During the last 30 years, the monoamine hypothesis has been the dominating hypothesis concerning the pathogenesis of depressive disorders (Carlsson, 1976). The hypothesis was originally formulated on the basis of knowledge about the mode of action of antidepressant drugs, both tricyclic antidepressants and MAO inhibitors, and the depressogenic action of the drug reserpine. In the last 20 years, an increasing amount of evidence has accumulated for the central role of serotonin in depressive disorders (Coppen, 1967; van Praag et al., 1973). One example is the fact that the serotonin precursor tryptophan seems to have an antidepressant effect and another is that it seems to be possible to treat depressive disorders by means of rather specific serotonin-reuptake inhibitors. Furthermore, there are studies indicating decreased concentrations of the serotonin metabolite 5-HIAA (5 hydroxyindoleacetic acid) in the cerebrospinal fluid of depressed patients, at least when careful allowance is being made for differences in age, sex and body height between the compared groups (Åsberg et al., 1984).

Apart from the central role of the monoamines, there are certain specific neuroendocrine changes described in patients with depressive disorders, including low concentrations of the pineal hormone melatonin in serum and urine (Beck Friis, 1983), hypersecretion of cortisol (Sachar, 1975) and reduced dexamethasone suppression of cortisol (Carroll et al., 1981).

Furthermore, there are results indicating a high concentration of one fraction of the endorphins (Fraction 1) as determined by means of a radio-receptor assay (RRA), in both patients with idiopathic pain syndromes and patients with depressive disorders, while patients with chronic neurogenic pain syndromes tended to have low concentrations (von Knorring et al., 1983b). All these changes may well be complementary and indicative of some basic dysfunction in the pineal-limbic-hypothalamic-pituitary system. At least the limbic and the hypothalamic areas are also under nervous control from the brain stem with the monoamines as main transmitters.

Biochemical and neuroendocrine deviations in patients with idiopathic pain syndromes

The serotonin metabolite 5-HIAA in CSF
In our studies we have been able to demonstrate low concentrations of the serotonin metabolite 5-HIAA in CSF of patients with idiopathic pain syndromes, probably indicating a low turnover rate in central serotoninergic systems (Almay et al., 1987a). At the same time, the concentrations of the dopamine metabolite HVA (homovanillic acid)

and, in earlier studies, the noradrenaline metabolite MHPG (3-methoxy-4-hydroxyphenylglycol) have been normal, indicating more normal turnover rates in central dopamine and noradrenaline systems (Table IIIa).

The determination of the serotonin metabolite 5-HIAA in CSF of depressed patients and patients with chronic pain syndromes involves several methodological problems. One problem that has often led to problems in the literature is the differences in age, sex or body height between compared groups. However, when corrections are made for age, sex and body height, there is a significantly greater frequency of subjects with low concentrations of 5-HIAA in CSF among the patients with idiopathic pain syndromes.

Thus, we have some evidence in favour of a low turnover rate in the serotoninergic systems in our patients with idiopathic pain syndromes. Such a low turnover rate in the serotoninergic systems might already have been present before the start of the chronic pain syndrome, or it may be a result of the long-standing pain syndrome.

We have approached this question in two ways. At first we looked at the possible correlation between the levels of 5-HIAA in CSF and the duration of the pain syndrome. In fact, we did find a significant positive correlation ($r = 0.31$) and thus it seems unlikely that there is a continuous decrease in 5-HIAA with time in the chronic pain syndromes (Almay et al., 1987a).

Monoamine oxidase (MAO) activity in platelets
After correction for age and sex, we found a significant overrepresentation of subjects with low platelet MAO activities among the patients with idiopathic pain syndromes (Almay et al., 1987b).

Platelet MAO activity is under strong genetic control, and it has been claimed (Oreland and Shaskan, 1983) that the activity of MAO in platelets reflects the size and/or the capacity of the central serotoninergic system, and there are experimental data in favour of such a view.

Furthermore, in healthy volunteers, there is a significant positive correlation between the activities of MAO in platelets and the levels of 5-HIAA in CSF (Oreland et al., 1981). During a depressive episode, platelet MAO activity seems to be stable, while the levels of 5-HIAA decrease. Thus, the correlation disappears. In chronic pain patients, the correlation is still present, indicating that both platelet MAO activities and the concentrations of 5-HIAA in CSF were already low before the start of the chronic pain syndrome (von Knorring et al., 1986).

Cortisol in plasma and dexamethasone non-suppression
One of the most constant findings in patients with depressive disorders is hypersecretion of cortisol (Sachar, 1975) and reduced suppression after pretreatment with dexamethasone (Carroll et al., 1981). In our patients with idiopathic pain syndromes, we also tend to find hypersecretion of cortisol, reduced diurnal variation of cortisol in plasma and a high frequency of dexamethasone non-suppression (Almay, 1987a). Abnormal dexamethasone suppression tests (DST) in patients with idiopathic pain syndromes have also been found by several other groups.

Originally, a pathological DST was claimed to be a rather specific test to identify patients with melancholic syndromes. In several studies in which pa-

TABLE IIIa
5-HIAA, HVA and substance P (determined by means of a radioimmuno assay) in CSF of patients with idiopathic pain syndromes and healthy volunteers

	5-HIAA	HVA	Substance P
Healthy volunteers ($n = 35$)	110.0 ± 25.7	207.5 ± 63.9	9.7 ± 3.2
Idiopathic pain syndromes ($n = 39$)	85.7 ± 31.4	184.6 ± 85.0	7.2 ± 5.3
	$F = 14.21$	$F = 1.70$	$F = 5.57$
	$P < 0.001$	N.S.	$P < 0.05$

The data are expressed in nmol/l and reported as $\bar{x} \pm$ S.D. The statistical analysis has been made by means of analysis of variance, one-way classification, ANOVA (data from Almay et al., 1987a,d).

tients with melancholic syndromes were compared to healthy volunteers, the specificity of the test was found to be extremely high while sensitivity was lower (Carroll et al., 1981).

Later on when patients with other psychiatric disorders were included in the studies, pathological DSTs were found also in several other diagnostic subgroups and thus the specificity of the test is not as high as has been claimed (Coppen et al., 1983). However, hypersecretion of cortisol and dexamethasone nonsuppression is most common in patients with major affective disorders. The presence in patients with idiopathic pain syndromes also indicates a certain similarity with the major affective disorders.

Melatonin in serum and urine

The functioning of the pineal gland is inversely rate-dependent on the environmental lighting. The effect is mediated by a polyneural pathway from the retina via the suprachiasmatic nuclei to the pineal gland. The final pathway is a noradrenergic neuron (Beck-Friis, 1983).

Through the excretion of melatonin, the pineal gland seems to have an extensive effect as a general tranquilizing organ on behalf of the homeostatic equilibrium in close relationship with changing environmental conditions (Romijn, 1978).

In patients with depressive disorders, melatonin has been demonstrated to be low, both in serum collected at the time of peak production at 02.00 a.m., and in urine collected during the night (Beck-Friis, 1983).

In our own studies, we have been able to demonstrate a close significant positive correlation between the values of melatonin secreted at 02.00 a.m. and the values of melatonin in urine collected during the night. In both serum and urine, patients with idiopathic pain syndromes tend to have low concentrations, as do patients with depressive disorders (Almay et al., 1987c).

Endorphins, Fraction 1, in CSF

In a long series of studies, in which the endorphins were determined by means of a radioreceptor assay

(RRA) after fractionation of the CSF, we were able to demonstrate that patients with idiopathic pain syndromes tended to have normal or high concentrations of endorphins, Fraction 1, in CSF, as do patients with depressive disorders, while patients with chronic pain syndromes of neurogenic type tended to have low concentrations (below 0.6 pmol/l) (von Knorring et al., 1983b).

Dynorphin, beta-endorphin, met-enkephalin and substance P in CSF

In a series of continuing studies, we have, by means of radioimmunoassay (RIA), determined substance P-like immunoreactivity, dynorphin, beta-endorphin and met-enkephalin in CSF of patients with idiopathic pain syndromes.

Substance P-like immunoreactivity seems to be low in both patients with idiopathic syndromes and those with chronic neurogenic pain syndromes (Almay et al., 1987d) (Table IIIa). Furthermore, there are significant negative correlations between the concentrations of substance P-like immunoreactivity in CSF and sadness, inner tension, pain, concentration difficulties and memory disturbances as determined by means of a visual analogue scale (Almay et al., 1987d). In an earlier study, we were also able to demonstrate that the low levels of sub-

TABLE IIIb

Dynorphin, beta-endorphin and met-enkephalin (determined by means of radioimmunoassay) in CSF of patients with idiopathic pain syndromes and healthy volunteers

	Dynorphin	Beta-endorphin	Met-enkephalin
Healthy volunteers (n=18)	25.9 ± 18.7	6.6 ± 2.1	82.2 ± 41.2
Idiopathic pain syndromes (n=35)	18.7 ± 9.3	6.2 ± 2.5	101.4 ± 38.1
	$F = 4.71$	$F = 0.43$	$F = 2.76$
	$P < 0.05$	N.S.	N.S.

The data are expressed in pmol/l and reported as $\bar{x} \pm$ S.D. The statistical analysis has been made by means of analysis of variance, one-way classification, ANOVA (data from von Knorring et al., 1987).

stance P-like immunoreactivity in the CSF of patients with chronic pain syndromes of neurogenic type tended to increase during treatment with transcutaneous nerve stimulation (von Knorring et al., 1985).

Dynorphin in CSF as determined by means of a RIA was also low in patients with idiopathic pain syndromes, while the levels of beta-endorphin and met-enkephalin tended to be normal (von Knorring et al., 1987) (Table IIIb).

Main biochemical basis of the experience of pain

In a multiple stepwise regression in which the pain level, as determined by means of a visual analogue scale, was included as the dependent variable and in which the concentrations of 5-HIAA, HVA, substance P, dynorphin, beta-endorphin and met-enkephalin were included as independent variables, the most significant contribution was found to come from substance P, met-enkephalin and beta-endor-

TABLE IV
Stepwise multiple regression with pain (a) and sadness (b) determined by means of a visual analogue scale as the dependent variables and 5-HIAA, HVA, substance P, dynorphin, beta-endorphin and met-enkephalin in CSF as independent variables: healthy volunteers and patients with chronic pain syndromes, $n = 63$

Step	Variable	Multiple R	Overall F	Significance
(a) Dependent variable: PAIN				
1	Substance P	0.25	4.07	$P < 0.05$
2	Met-enkephalin	0.34	4.02	$P < 0.05$
3	Beta-endorphin	0.38	3.26	$P < 0.05$
4	HVA	0.41	2.88	$P < 0.05$
5	5-HIAA	0.47	3.24	$P < 0.02$
6	Dynorphin	0.49	3.00	$P < 0.02$
(b) Dependent variable: SADNESS				
1	HVA	0.28	5.39	$P < 0.05$
2	Substance P	0.35	4.25	$P < 0.02$
3	5-HIAA	0.39	3.48	$P < 0.05$
4	Dynorphin	0.39	2.61	$P < 0.05$
5	Beta-endorphin	0.39	2.08	N.S.

phin, indicating that the peptidergic pathways are of importance for the experience of pain in chronic pain patients (von Knorring et al., 1987) (Table IVa).

It is of interest that the substance P nerve terminals are topologically associated with enkephalin nerve terminals in dorsal spinal cord as well as in brainstem and higher centers known to be involved in pain transmission and modulation (Hökfelt et al., 1977).

Main biochemical basis of the experience of sadness

In a stepwise multiple regression analysis in which sadness, as determined by means of a visual analogue scale, was included as the dependent variable and in which the concentrations of 5-HIAA, HVA, substance P, dynorphin, beta-endorphin and met-enkephalin in CSF were included as independent variables, the monoamine metabolites 5-HIAA and HVA as well as substance P were found to be of most importance for the experience of sadness (von Knorring et al., 1987) (Table IVb).

The importance of both the serotonin metabolite 5-HIAA and substance P is of interest as the coexistence of serotonin and substance P in the same nerve endings has been demonstrated (Hökfelt et al., 1978; Chan-Palay, 1979).

Therapeutic strategies

ECT and antidepressants
In early studies, it was often claimed that the experience of pain in patients with a coexisting depressive syndrome was best relieved by appropriate treatment with ECT or antidepressants (Pisetsky, 1946; Spear, 1964; Merskey, 1965). Later on it was claimed that ECT (von Hagen, 1957; Weinstein et al., 1959) or antidepressants (Webb and Lascelles, 1962; Lance and Curran, 1964) were effective in chronic pain regardless of whether a depressive syndrome was present or not.

Today, there is a very extensive literature concerning antidepressants in chronic pain syndromes. Sometimes the results are somewhat contradictory, but in the majority of studies a positive effect is claimed.

The most convincing of the studies seems to be a study performed by Blumer et al. (1980) in which consecutive patients from a pain center were included. If adequate doses of antidepressants were given and if a strict dosage regimen was followed, the effect of traditional antidepressants was as good in chronic pain as it was in depressive disorders. The results were further strengthened by means of a two-year follow up, in which the authors were able to demonstrate a long-term effect of the treatment with antidepressants (Blumer and Heilbronn, 1981b).

Selective serotonin-reuptake inhibitors

One difficult problem has been to determine whether there are pronounced differences between the different antidepressants available. Despite the fact that there are pronounced differences in biochemical profiles between the different antidepressants, some of them being almost exclusively serotonin-reuptake inhibitors, some of them almost exclusively noradrenaline-reuptake inhibitors (Maitre et al., 1980), it has been difficult to demonstrate differences in clinical profiles in the treatment of patients with depressive disorders. However, there are results indicating a better effect on anxiety by the serotonin-reuptake inhibitors, and these drugs are usually preferred in the treatment of panic disorder and obsessive-compulsive disorders.

In a double-blind, controlled study in which zimelidine, a rather specific serotonin-reuptake inhibitor, was compared to placebo (Johansson and von Knorring, 1979; Johansson et al., 1980), we have been able to demonstrate an effect on pain levels without a similar effect on the depressed mood. The selectivity of the drug was also documented through a selective effect on the serotonin metabolite 5-HIAA in CSF without any effects on dopamine or noradrenaline metabolites in CSF (Table V). Interestingly enough, there was a small change in the

TABLE V

Changes in pain levels, depression scores, 5-HIAA, HVA, MHPG and endorphins, Fraction 1, in CSF during treatment with zimelidine or placebo in a double-blind controlled study: chronic pain patients, $n = 20$

	Zimelidine ($n=9$)	Placebo ($n=11$)	Significance of the change
Baseline pain level (mm on a VAS ranging from 0 to 100)	64.0 ± 30.3	46.8 ± 18.6	$F=8.02$
Change (mm)	-16.1	$+4.1$	$P<0.05$
Baseline depression score (CPRS)	18.1 ± 2.4	19.5 ± 2.2	$F=0.47$
Change	-1.2	-0.3	N.S.
Baseline 5-HIAA/ CSF (nmol/l)	107.1 ± 35.1	113.5 ± 28.9	$F=5.54$
Change (nmol/l)	-28.6	$+1.7$	$P<0.05$
Baseline HVA/CSF (nmol/l)	201.2 ± 27.4	250.6 ± 31.5	$F=0.25$
Change (nmol/l)	$+3.7$	$+40.8$	N.S.
Baseline MHPG/ CSF (nmol/l)	36.1 ± 3.2	41.6 ± 2.8	$F=1.41$
Change (nmol/l)	-5.0	$+8.0$	N.S.
Baseline endorphin, Fract. 1/CSF (read as pmol/ml of met-enkephalin)	0.8 ± 0.3	1.4 ± 0.7	$F=5.46$
Change (pmol/ml)	-0.2	0	$P<0.05$

Analysis of covariance – initial values used as covariates. The data are reported as $\bar{x} \pm$ S.D. (data from Johansson and von Knorring, 1979; Johansson et al., 1980). VAS, visual analogue scale.

endorphins, Fraction 1, in CSF, which probably did not arise, however, through any direct effect of the drug.

Thus, it seems clear that antidepressants can have a specific effect on the pain symptomatology in patients with chronic pain syndromes without this necessarily involving an effect on a preexisting depressive syndrome. Furthermore, it is obvious that an effect can be achieved through a selective

TABLE VI

Changes in pain, sadness, inner tension, concentration difficulties and memory disturbances (determined by means of visual analogue scales) during treatment with clomipramine or maprotiline in a double-blind controlled study: Patients with idiopathic pain syndromes

	Maprotiline ($n=25$)	Clomipramine ($n=27$)
Pain	-11.8 ± 21.4[a]	-23.5 ± 29.1[c]
Sadness	-1.2 ± 22.4	-14.0 ± 27.2[a]
Inner tension	-6.1 ± 29.7	-15.0 ± 26.0[b]
Concentration difficulties	0.7 ± 18.2	-11.4 ± 25.2[a]
Memory disturbances	0.8 ± 17.7	-9.8 ± 21.4[a]

The visual analogue scales consisted of 100-mm-long horizontal lines with definitions at the ends and with no marks in between. The scores are expressed in mm, ranging from 0 to 100 mm, and are reported as $\bar{x} \pm$ S.D. The statistical analysis has been made by means of paired t-tests.
[a]$P<0.05$, [b]$P<0.01$, [c]$P<0.001$

action on the serotoninergic systems, which is to be expected from knowledge about the importance of the serotoninergic systems in chronic pain (Messing and Lytle, 1977).

However, it has also been demonstrated (Lindsay and Olsen, 1985) that chronic pain can be relieved by the rather specific noradrenaline-reuptake inhibitor maprotiline.

Thus, the situation is still somewhat unclear. It has been suggested by Lindsay and Wycoff (1981) that all the antidepressants may be effective through an induction of the endorphin-enkephalin systems. Our data are at least not contradictory to such a view.

To elucidate further the relative importance of the serotonin and noradrenaline systems, we have recently performed a double-blind, controlled study of the effects of clomipramine (a selective specific serotonin-reuptake inhibitor) and maprotiline (a selective noradrenaline-reuptake inhibitor). It is of considerable interest that the effect of the serotonin-reuptake inhibitor is much more pronounced than the effect of the noradrenaline-reuptake inhibitor (Table VI).

If the effect on serotonin reuptake is of the most importance and that on noradrenaline reuptake of less importance, some of the contradictions in the literature may be explained by the fact that the antidepressants used often have pronounced effects on both serotonin and noradrenaline reuptake and that the relative effect in a single patient may be dependent on the type of metabolites created.

However, the effect of antidepressants on chronic pain may well be transmitted through a variety of mechanisms. Most antidepressants are not specific serotonin- or noradrenaline-reuptake inhibitors but also have blocking effects on cholinergic, histaminergic, serotoninergic and adrenergic receptors.

Lithium

Apart from the beneficial effects of ECT and antidepressants, both believed to have their effect through increased transmission in serotoninergic and/or noradrenergic pathways, there are some reports from the end of the last century, when Lange (1886) treated patients with so-called masked depressions, many of them probably fulfilling the criteria of the idiopathic pain syndrome, by means of lithium salts with good effects. As later studies have indicated that lithium in long-term use seems to facilitate serotoninergic transmission, the results are of some interest and should be verified in more modern studies.

References

Almay, B.G.L. (1987a) Patients with idiopathic pain syndromes. A clinical, biochemical and neuroendocrinological study. Umeå University Medical Dissertations, New series, No. 191, Umeå University, Umeå.

Almay, B.G.L. (1987b) Clinical characteristics of patients with idiopathic pain syndromes. Depressive symptomatology and patient pain drawings. Pain, 29: 335–346.

Almay, B.G.L., Häggendal, J., von Knorring, L. and Oreland, L. (1987a) 5-HIAA and HVA in CSF in patients with idiopathic pain disorders. Biol. Psychiatry, 22: 403–412.

Almay, B.G.L., von Knorring, L. and Oreland, L. (1987b) Platelet MAO in patients with idiopathic pain disorders, J. Neural Transm., 69: 243–253.

Almay, B.G.L., von Knorring, L. and Wetterberg, J. (1987c)

Melatonin in serum and urine in patients with idiopathic pain syndromes. Psychiatr. Res., 22: 179–191.

Almay, B.G.L., Johansson, F., von Knorring, L., Le Grevés, P. and Terenius, L. (1987d) Substance P in CSF of patients with chronic pain syndromes. Pain, in press.

American Psychiatric Association (1980) DSM-III – Diagnostic and Statistic Manual of Mental Disorders, 3rd edn., Washington.

Asberg, M., Bertilsson, L., Mårtensson, B., Scalia-Tomba, G.-P., Thorén, P. and Träskman-Bendz, L. (1984) CSF monoamine metabolites in melancholia. Acta Psychiatr. Scand., 69: 201–219.

Beck-Friis, J. (1983) Melatonin in depressive disorders. A methodological and clinical study of the pineal-hypothalamic-pituitary-adrenal cortex system. Doctoral dissertation, Karolinska Institute, Stockholm.

Blumer, D. and Heilbronn, M. (1981a) The pain-prone disorder: a clinical and psychological profile. Psychosomatics, 22: 395–402.

Blumer, D. and Heilbronn, M. (1981b) Second-year-follow-up study on systematic treatment of chronic pain with antidepressants. Henry Ford Hosp. Med. J., 29: 67–68.

Blumer, D. and Heilbronn, M. (1982) Chronic pain as a variant of depressive disease. The pain-prone disorder. J. Nerv. Ment. Dis., 170: 381–406.

Blumer, D., Heilbronn, M., Pedraza, E. and Pope, G. (1980) Systematic treatment of chronic pain with antidepressants. Henry Ford Hosp. Med. J., 28: 15–21.

Carlsson, A. (1976) The contribution of drug research to investigating the nature of endogenous depression. Pharmacopsychiatry, 9: 2–10.

Carroll, B.J., Feinberg, M., Greden, F., Tarika, J., Albala, A.A., Haskett, R.F., McJames, N., Kronfol, Z., Lohr, N., Steiner, M., de Vigne, J.P. and Young, E. (1981) A specific laboratory test for the diagnosis of melancholia. Standardization, validation and clinical utility. Arch. Gen. Psychiatry, 38: 15–22.

Chan-Palay, V. (1979) Combined immunocytochemistry and autoradiography after in vivo injections of monoclonal antibody to substance P and serotonin: coexistence of two putative transmitters in single raphe cells and fiber plexus. Anat. Embryol., 156: 241–254.

Coppen, A. (1967) The biochemistry of affective disorders. Br. J. Psychiatry, 113: 1237–1264.

Coppen, A., Abou-Saleh, M., Milln, P., Metcalfe, M., Harwood, J. and Bailey, J. (1983) Dexamethasone suppression test in depression and other psychiatric illness. Br. J. Psychiatry, 142: 498–504.

Hökfelt, T., Ljungdahl, A., Terenius, L., Elde, R. and Nilsson, G. (1977) Immunohisto-chemical analysis of peptide pathways possibly related to pain and analgesia: enkephalin and substance P. Proc. Natl. Acad. Sci. USA, 74: 3081–3085.

Hökfelt, T., Ljungdahl, Å., Steinbusch, H., Verhofstad, A., Nilsson, G., Brodin, E., Pernow, B. and Goldstein, M. (1978) Immunohistochemical evidence of substance P like immuno-

reactivity in some 5-hydroxytryptamine containing neurons in the rat central nervous system. Neuroscience, 3: 517–538.

Johansson, F. and von Knorring, L. (1979) A double-blind controlled study of a serotonin uptake inhibitor (Zimelidine) versus placebo in chronic pain patients. Pain, 7: 69–78.

Johansson, F., von Knorring, L., Sedvall, G. and Terenius, L. (1980) Changes in endorphins and 5-HIAA in CSF as a result of treatment with a serotonin reuptake inhibitor (zimelidine) in chronic pain patients. Psychiatr. Res., 2: 167–172.

Lance, J.W. and Curran, D.A. (1964) Treatment of chronic tension headache. Lancet, I: 1236–1239.

Lange, C. (1886) Om periodiske depressionstilstande og deras patogenese. Jacob Lunds Forlag, Kobenhavn.

Lindsay, P.G. and Wycoff, M. (1981) The depression-pain syndrome and its response to antidepressants. Psychosomatics, 22: 571–577.

Lopez Ibor, J.J. (1972) Masked depression. Br. J. Psychiatry, 120: 245–258.

Maitre, L., Moser, P., Baumann, P.A. and Waldmeier, P.C. (1980) Amine uptake inhibitors: criteria of selectivity. Acta Psychiatr. Scand., 61: 97–110.

Merskey, H. (1965) The characteristics of persistent pain in psychological illness. J. Psychosom. Res., 9: 291–298.

Messing, R.B. and Lytle, L.D. (1977) Serotonin-containing neurons: their possible role in pain and analgesia. Pain, 4: 1–21.

Oreland, L. and Shaskan, E.G. (1983) Some rationale behind the use of monoamine oxidase activity as a biological marker. Trends Pharmacol. Sci., 4: 339–341.

Oreland, L., Wiberg, Å., Åsberg, M., Träskman, L., Sjöstrand, L., Thorén, P., Bertilsson, L. and Tybring, G. (1981) Platelet MAO activity and monoamine metabolites in cerebrospinal fluid in depressed and suicidal patients and in healthy volunteers. Psychiatr. Res., 4: 21–29.

Pilowsky, I. and Basset, D.L. (1985) Pain and depression: does the evidence support a relationship. Psychol. Bull., 97: 18–34.

Pisetsky, J.E. (1946) Disappearance of painful phantom limb after electric shock treatment. Am. J. Psychiatry, 102: 599–601.

Romijn, H.J. (1978) The pineal, a tranquilizing organ. Life Sci., 23: 2257–2274.

Sachar, E.J. (1975) Twenty-four-hour cortisol secretory patterns in depressed and manic patients. In W.H. Gipsen, T.B. van Wimersma Greidanus, B. Bohus and D. de Wied (Eds.), Hormones, Homeostasis and the Brain, Progress in Brain Research, Vol. 42, Elsevier, Amsterdam, pp. 81–91.

Spear, F.G. (1964) A study of pain as a symptom in psychiatric illness. M.D. Thesis, Bristol University.

Sternbach, R.A. (1968): Pain: A Psychological Analysis, Academic Press, New York.

Sternbach, R.A. (1974) Pain Patients. Traits and Treatment, Academic Press, London.

Sternbach, R.A. (1981) Chronic pain as a disease entity. Triangle (Sandoz), 20: 27–32.

Sternbach, R.A. (1984) Acute versus chronic pain. In P.D. Wall and R. Melzack (Eds.), Textbook of Pain, Churchill Livingstone, New York, pp. 173–177.

van Praag, H.M., Korf, J. and Schut, D. (1973) Cerebral monoamine and depression. Arch. Gen. Psychiatry, 28: 827–831.

Ward, N.G., Bloom, V.L. and Friedel, R.O. (1979) The effectiveness of tricyclic antidepressants in the treatment of coexisting pain and depression. Pain, 7: 331–341.

Webb, H.S. and Lascelles, R.G. (1962) Treatment of facial pain and head pain with depression. Lancet, i: 355–356.

Williams, J.B.W. and Spitzer, R.L. (1982) Idiopathic pain disorder: a critique of pain-prone disorder and a proposal for a revision of the DSM-III category psychogenic pain disorder. J. Nerv. Ment. Dis., 170: 415–419.

von Knorring, L. (1975) The experience of pain in patients with depressive disorders. A clinical and experimental study. Umeå University Medical Dissertations, New Series No. 2, Umeå University, Umeå.

von Knorring, L., Perris, C., Eisemann, M., Eriksson, U. and Perris, H. (1983a) Pain as a symptom in depressive disorders, I. Relationship to diagnostic subgroup and depressive symptomatology. Pain, 15: 19–26.

von Knorring, L., Terenius, L. and Wahlström, A. (1983b) Fraction 1 endorphin in CSF. Clinical studies. In J. Wood (Ed.), Neurobiology of CSF II, Plenum Press, New York, pp. 88–96.

von Knorring, L., Almay, B.G.L., Johansson, F., Schuber, G. and Terenius, L. (1985) Changes in CSF endorphins and monoamine metabolites related to treatment with high frequency transcutaneous nerve stimulation. Nord. J. Psychiatry, 39: Suppl. 11: 83–90.

von Knorring, L., Oreland, L., Häggendal, J., Magnusson, T., Almay, B. and Johansson, F. (1986) Relationship between platelet MAO activity and concentrations of 5-HIAA and HVA in cerebrospinal fluid in chronic pain patients. J. Neural Transm., 66: 37–46.

von Knorring, L., Almay, B.G.L., Ekman, R. and Widerlöv, E. (1987) Biological markers in chronic pain. Nord. J. Psychiatry, in press.

R. Dubner, G.F. Gebhart & M.R. Bond (Eds.)
Proceedings of the Vth World Congress on Pain
© 1988 Elsevier Science Publishers BV (Biomedical Division)

CHAPTER 31

Impact of chronic pain on marital partners: systems perspective

Ranjan Roy

School of Social Work and Department of Psychiatry, University of Manitoba, Winnipeg, Canada

Introduction

The impact of chronic pain on families is a topic that has received measurable attention over the past 15 years (Flor and Turk, 1985; Payne and Norfleet, 1986; Roy, 1982). Before proceeding any further, two points require immediate clarification. First, the term 'family', in contemporary society, calls for precise definition, as there are numerous types of family ranging from the traditional nuclear to the emerging reconstituted and single-parent families to more non-traditional homosexual families. Almost all family-related research with chronic illness pertains to nuclear families. Secondly, many of the research activities in the field of impact of chronic illness on families are cross-sectional and retrospective. In other words, impact is measured at a point in time and inevitably after the chronic nature of the condition or the illness itself has set in. Knowledge about the family functioning of chronic sick individuals at the pre-morbid stage is virtually unknown, and a patient's account to the research worker or clinician of trouble-free family life before the onset of illness is fraught with risks, for distortion is common.

This paper will (1) provide a detailed review of the current research literature on the impact of pain, especially on marital partners, and (2) report briefly on a clinical investigation of patients with head and back pain, and their spouses, and the consequent repercussion on the couple system from a systemic perspective. This particular perspective, which is described later, attempts to overcome the problem of measuring impact in the context of the cause-and-effect paradigm.

Chronic pain and marital dysfunction

Literature pertaining to the impact of chronic pain on marital partners falls into three broad categories. First, that dealing with spouses' health; second, sexual activities; and third, more general relationship problems such as communication, role alteration, etc.

Impact of chronic pain on the spouses health

The actual amount of research investigating the health of the spouses of chronic pain patients is surprisingly limited, given the prominence of this particular problem. Almost all studies have focused directly or indirectly on the presence of psychopathology in the spouse, except one, where the focus was on the level of distress experienced (Rowat and Knafll, 1985). An early major study to assess the impact of chronic pain on the spouse was undertaken by Mohamed et al. as recently as 1978. This seminal investigation yielded some very interesting results. Not only did the authors find that the thirteen depressed patients with pain complaints were on the whole more severely depressed than the 13 depressed patients without pain, but the spouses of depressed pain patients had a variety of pain complaints. This study established the presence of pain symptoms in the spouses of the depressed pain patient group as opposed to the depressed controls, albeit with a very small sample size. However, it left the question of the nature of the spouses' psychopathology unanswered. It merely implied that the somatic presentation in the spouse might be a manifestation of psychiatric disturbance.

Shanfield et al. (1979) in a subsequent study provided a more definitive answer to the question of spouses' mental health. The most significant finding was that the spouses of pain patients experienced a significant degree of psychiatric distress and, secondly, there appeared to be a clear relationship between the spouses' level of symptom intensity and the patients' symptom severity scores. High levels of distress in the patients were associated with elevated distress levels in their spouses. Perhaps the results of this finding should be generalized with some caution. First, it is not clear from the description of the sample the extent to which it can be generalized to the pain population at large due to the older mean age (52 years) of the sample compared to the mean age of chronic pain patients (Ahern and Follick, 1985). Secondly, the population studied was relatively small ($n = 44$). A third reason is that the comparison group was derived from national norms and it is doubtful that that population is likely to be comparable with the pain group.

Roberts and Reinhard (1980) compared 26 treated pain patients with 20 who rejected treatment. They found that the spouses of successfully treated subjects had lower scores on the hypochondriasis and hysteria scales of the MMPI than spouses of unsuccessfully treated patients. The precise implication of this finding is uncertain, other than to imply that non-participant subjects as well as their spouses are emotionally more disturbed compared with the participants and their spouses. A notable finding was that the non-participants had a higher level of depression as well as of hypochondriasis com-

pared with the participants. Indirectly, this study lends further credence to earlier studies by suggesting that there is a positive correlation between the level of distress in chronic pain patients and that in their spouses.

In a recent study, Kerns and Turk (1984) studied a sample of 30 male chronic pain patients and their wives. Sixteen of these individuals had mild to severe depression. Significantly, spouses' assessments of their own mood were positively correlated with those of the patients. An unusual finding was the lack of a significant relationship between pain intensity and depression in the patients. The mood of the spouses apparently did not correlate significantly with any of the variables assessed. Ahern et al. (1985), in their investigation of chronic low back patients, reported that 20% of the spouses were clinically depressed and found a strong association between the spouses' emotional distress and the patients' emotional distress. The patients' depression correlated significantly with the spouses' anxiety levels.

Finally, Rowat and Knafl (1985) assessed the effects of chronic pain on spouses. Eighty-three percent of the spouses reported experiencing some form of health disturbance which they attributed directly to living with partners with chronic pain. The researchers identified two extreme groups, namely high- and low-distress spouses. Twelve out of 25 spouses were found to be in the high-distress group. Distress was assessed on the basis of evidence of physical and emotional symptoms, changes that were brought about in the lives of these spouses as a result of pain in their partners. In this study, the focus was not exclusively on psychopathology, but on the overall level of functioning of the spouses.

On the basis of research to date it is clear that psychological and emotional distress in the spouses of chronic pain sufferers is not uncommon. Whether or not chronic pain patients demonstrate assortative mating behaviour which results in selection of psychologically and physiologically vulnerable mates, as claimed by Mohamed et al. (1978), or the spouses simply respond to an untenable and intractable situation by developing signs and signals of distress is not known. However, it is quite likely that the consequences of living with a chronically disabled individual, rather than some form of pre-selected mating behaviour, constitute the true basis for elevated levels of distress in spouses.

There are some obvious gaps in this body of research. First and foremost, the concept of 'depression' varies from study to study, thereby raising a fundamental question about the validity and generalizability of the disease. Second, data on the premorbid mental health of the spouses are never mentioned.

An equally critical omission is any mention of the family life stage. That tends to blur the differences of family responsibilities between, for example, a newly married couple and a middle-aged couple. To date there exists only limited information about the influence of social factors in the genesis of emotional disorders in the spouses of chronic pain patients. The value of the social factors has recently been reported by Kerns and Turk (1984), who found that the level of spouse support was an important factor in decreasing the possibility of depression in chronic pain patients. Stated another way, the better the mental health of spouses the higher the probability of better mental health in chronic pain patients. Kerns and Turk (1984) have noted that 'following the development of chronic pain problems, all aspects of the family change – social, recreational, marital, vocational and financial.' Predictably many of the spouses manifest symptoms of a psychophysiological nature in the face of such misfortune. Whether or not they become ill due to predisposition and/or as a response to a multitude of losses demands more research.

Marital difficulties

Knowledge about marital difficulties of chronic pain patients has existed for a considerable length of time. Merskey and Boyd (1978) and Swanson et al. (1978) noted that families of chronic pain patients are characterized by dissension, violence and acrimony. There is, however, a paucity of investigations focussing on the details of changes that occur in a marriage due to chronic pain in one partner.

Investigations related to marital disharmony fall into the following categories: (1) sexual difficulties; (2) problems of roles and communication; and (3) a very broad category, viz., marital dissatisfaction.

Sexual difficulties

Common sense dictates that sexual difficulties are common among chronic pain sufferers. Nevertheless, the actual amount of research conducted on this topic is remarkably small. A relatively early study by Hudgens (1979) on 24 pain patients and their families identified many areas of family dysfunction. Focussing on sexual conflicts, she reported that 11 families gave evidence of sexual problems.

Much of the more recent research in this field has been conducted by the pain clinic group at Mayo Clinic. Maruta and Osborne (1978), in a pioneering study, studied 66 married subjects referred to their pain-management centre. They found that 33% of the patients reported dysfunction in their sexual activities. Fifty-six percent of the women and 60% of the men reported deterioration in the broad category of sexual adjustment, and in the category of frequency 68% of women and 88% of men reported either elimination or reduction of sexual activities. Following the onset of the pain problem, most women had difficulties in reaching orgasm or in becoming aroused or simply lost interest in sex. Of the men studied, 44% reported deterioration in their sexual activities following the onset of pain problems. Major categories of dysfunction were difficulty either obtaining or keeping an erection and losing interest in sex. In terms of frequency, women demonstrated a lower level of reduction than their male partners.

Maruta et al. (1981), in a later study, interviewed 50 married patients and their spouses. An alarming 78% of the patients reported elimination or reduction of sexual activities and 84% of the spouses also reported similar deterioration. The patients and their spouses found that the effects of pain on the quality of sexual activity had resulted in poor quality of sexual life. Before the onset of pain 80% of both patients and spouses were satisfied with their sexual life but afterwards this figure dropped to 50% for both patients and spouses. This study, like the previous one, demonstrated a high rate of prevalence of sexual difficulties amongst chronic pain patients.

Role-related and communication problems

It is a matter of some curiosity that role-related changes associated with chronic illness have received such scanty attention from researchers. Tunks and Roy (1982) have examined the issues surrounding loss of employment for chronic pain patients. However, the impact of such a loss and other associated disabilities attributed to chronic pain has not been studied in any depth from the perspective of its consequences on family roles (Roy, 1984). Hudgens (1979), in a study of 24 pain patients and their families, noted that patients were inclined to become very dependent on their spouses. Just under one-third of them had conflicts over male/female roles but unfortunately the author failed to elaborate on what these conflicts entailed. Follick et al. (1985), in a study of 117 chronic low back pain patients, found that employment problems were highly significant in this group of patients. In addition, difficulties in home management were also present. Unfortunately their study did not include a comprehensive assessment of the impact of the role changes in the patients and/or their spouses. The inference is clear: namely that massive change in the patient's role functioning has to result in a major re-arrangement of roles between marital partners.

Rowat and Knafll (1985), who examined high-distress and low-distress spouses of chronic pain sufferers, reported that three-quarters of the highly distressed spouses experienced changes in relationships with children and marital partners in the areas of division of labour, decision-making, family activities and financial functioning. The role-related changes for the high-distress spouses were considerable.

Several authors have reported on the deterioration of communication between chronic pain sufferers and their spouses following the onset of chronic pain (Scheider and Bernstein, 1976; Hudgens, 1979; Swanson and Maruta, 1980, Roy, 1984). Hudgens (1979), for example, noted that 18 out of the 24 patients and families they studied engaged in indirect communications. In addition, 10 spouses of the same patients had difficulty expressing warmth and affection. Scheider and Bernstein (1976), in a single case study of a 52-year-old woman with low back pain, noted that communication between the patient and the husband was minimal. Part of the treatment strategy was to enable the patient to spend more time talking to her husband. Swanson and Maruta (1980), in a study of 120 pain patients and their close family members, discovered a very high level of agreement between them on matters of disability payments, amount of work missed, duration of pain, effect of pain on work, and influence of time of day on pain. The conclusion from the study was that this high level of congruency was indicative of extensive communication between family members about the pain problem. They concluded that 'disagreement about the pain problem does not necessarily work to the patient's advantage. In instances in which patient-relative congruency was greatest, the ultimate treatment outcome was the least favorable' (Swanson and Maruta, 1980). Such concerns may also be termed 'pseudo-mutuality'.

Several investigators have found a positive correlation between solicitous spouses and somewhat higher levels of pain (Block, 1981; Block et al., 1984; Block and Boyer, 1984, Ahern and Follick, 1985). In addition, those reporting higher levels of marital satisfaction also demonstrated greater increases in skin conductance to the painful displays of their spouses than the relatively unsatisfied spouses. The conclusion is that when marital satisfaction is high, spouses' heightened empathic responses to pain behaviour may dispose them to develop psychophysiological difficulties (Block, 1981; Block et al., 1984; Block and Boyer, 1984). The basis of such far-reaching consequences for solicitous behaviours by the spouses of chronic pain patients who are in conflict-free marriages is considerable. They engage in what is termed 'colluding behaviour.' Delvey and Hopkins (1982) have noted that 'collusion is apt to occur when unconscious contracts or agreements between two parties control the roles that each assumes in the relationship'. In other words, solicitousness in the spouse in response to pain behaviours in the patient serves as a powerful reinforcer for those behaviours. Solicitousness in that case is a type of communication which contributes towards the perpetuation of pain behaviours. Therefore collusion, as a psychological phenomenon, is one concept that aids the understanding of this type of communication.

In an interesting study Anderson and Rehm (1985) demonstrated that while pain intensity was significantly related to solicitous behaviours of family members, the reverse was true for arthritic and sickle-cell groups. They hypothesized that the sickle cell and the arthritic subjects were inclined to be more independent and not so prone to exhibiting the helplessness that is reinforced by sympathetic relatives. This particular observation is of interest from the point of view of communication patterns which seem to be common among chronic pain patients and their spouses. Solicitous communication on the part of the spouse is designed to promote and maintain pain behaviours in the patients and may very well be a further manifestation of the propensity of chronic pain patients and their spouses to engage in colluding behaviour. Clearly, solicitous spouses report a higher level of marital satisfaction than non-solicitous spouses. The fact remains, however, that the actual level of marital satisfaction of either group is unknown at the pre-morbid stage. Theoretically, the emergence of the pain problem may resolve long-standing marital difficulties. Solicitous communication on the part of the spouse could be a consequence of that. A few researchers, however, have reported only nominal difficulty in the communication patterns of chronic pain patients (Feurstein, et al., 1985; Follick et al., 1985). The bulk of research, however, seems to indicate that communication which results in pseudo-mutality, (Swanson and Maruta, 1980) collusion (Delvey and Hopkins, 1982) and/or re-inforcement of pain behaviours (Block, 1981) is common.

Marital dissatisfaction

Systematic investigation of marital dissatisfaction and maladjustment of chronic pain patients has a relatively recent history. Reports are quite diverse in their scope. For example, several recent studies more or less confirmed the existence of marital problems, but are ambiguous in terms of the actual nature of the marital disaffection detected (Mohamed et al., 1978, Hudgens, 1979; Shanfield et al., 1979; Blume and Heilbronn, 1982; Ahern et al., 1985). An exception to the general trend to be non-specific is a report by Hudgens (1979), who, as noted earlier, identified very clearly defined problem areas of marital difficulties in 24 pain patients. Eleven problem areas are clearly delineated.

Mohamed et al. (1978), utilizing the Locke and Wallace Short Marital Adjustment Test with a group of depressed pain patients and depressed patients without pain, found greater marital maladjustments in the depressed pain group compared to the depressed group. The actual nature of maladjustment or, more precisely, the elements of marital discord present were not made explicit. Shanfield et al. (1979), in a study of 24 pain patients and their spouses, also revealed a relationship between psychiatric distress scores in pain patients and their spouses and only indirectly inferred marital maladjustment. However, they did not use either clinical assessment or any standard instrument to directly measure marital conflicts or levels of marital maladjustment.

Common sense suggests a positive relationship between a high level of distress in the patient and marital maladjustment but this is not inevitable. Nichols (1978), in a study of marital interaction, observed that in many instances the higher the level of pain complaint, the greater was the degree of marital harmony. Kerns and Turk (1984) investigated 30 male chronic pain patients and their wives and found the presence of depression as well as marital dissatisfaction among chronic pain patients. On the other hand, pain intensity and either depression or marital satisfaction were not significantly related. A marital adjustment scale (Locke and Wallace) was used to establish levels of marital satisfaction but the study failed to provide any detailed information about the exact nature of marital conflict(s). Ahern and Follick (1985) also found that 'spouses' emotional distress levels were positively, but only weakly, related to patients' emotional distress levels'.

Contradictory findings in terms of association between patients' distress and pain level and levels of marital disharmony may be indicative of different measures being used to evaluate different factors. Perhaps the concept of marital disharmony, while in common usage in the literature, indicates different sets of problems being investigated by different investigators. Also, the age of patients and their spouses and the type of pain problems have varied from study to study. The problem of age is critical, since generally it reflects the life stage of the family. Families at different life stages encounter different sets of problems and none of the studies mentioned allow for that factor.

A small number of studies of family conflicts associated with chronic low back pain in patients are based on information provided solely by the latter, but it is doubtful that such data truly reflect the nature and extent of marital conflicts (Feurstein et al., 1985; Follick et al., 1985). In contrast, Rowat and Knafl (1985) conducted an in-depth investigation into spouses' stresses of living with chronic pain patients. They divided the spouse group into high- and low-distress groups and found that the high-distress group adopted an attitude of protectiveness towards the person in pain, whereas the low-distress spouses showed avoidance behaviours and generally ignored the sufferers' pain behaviours. Uncertainty about the problem of chronic pain

spilled over into uncertainty about family life. The authors noted that "the parameters of day-to-day living became ill-defined and indeterminate as a result of uncertainty as to when the pain might occur, its precipitating causes, and the degree of possible disruption it could create" (Rowat and Knafl, 1985). The low-distress spouses drew a picture of family life which conveyed less emotional upheaval. Also they used fewer negative descriptors to describe their family life than the high-distress spouses.

Collectively these studies provide a fragmentary picture of the disruptive effects of chronic pain on marriage and only two studies provide some detail of the nature of marital difficulties encountered by pain patients and their spouses (Hudgens, 1979; Rowat and Knafl, 1985). Several studies failed to investigate the marital difficulties from the spouses' perspective altogether (Shanfield et al., 1979; Feurstein et al., 1985; Follick et al., 1985) and none of the studies allows for the 'chronicity' factor. Therefore it is hardly surprising that many chronic pain sufferers and their spouses encounter marital difficulties. A marriage operates in many different dimensions and, without specifically addressing each of them and problems associated with them, the level of generalization made is unacceptable. A number of major studies reporting the impact of chronic pain on families are summarized in Table I.

The family systems perspective of chronic pain

A recent review of the family therapy research literature reveals that the impact of illness on the family is a subject that has been almost totally neglected (Russell et al., 1983). Family therapy research has yet to determine the etiological significance of family dynamics in relation to a variety of problems, including psychosomatic symptoms. In this regard, Liebman et al. (1976) applied Minuchin's (1975) psychosomatogenic model to conceptualize and treat psychogenic abdominal pain in children (Minuchin et al., 1975; Liebman et al., 1976). Hudgens' (1979) work was based on the systems approach and she attempted to adopt an interactional approach to the problem.

A study of the families of back pain or headache sufferers and based upon the Problem-Centered Systems Family Therapy (PCSFT), at the heart of which is the McMaster Model of Family Functioning (MMFF), is described. The MMFF was developed over a period of some 25 years by Epstein and Bishop (1981) and it is a model of family therapy viewed as an open system consisting of systems

TABLE I

A summary of studies of chronic pain and marital dissatisfaction

Investigators	Sample size	Mean age of patients (yr)	Sorts of pain	Duration of pain	Duration of marriage	Measure of marital distress	Results
Ahern et al. (1985)	117 (couples)	41.4	Low back	4.45 yr	–	Locke-Wallace	26.9% of patients and spouses respectively distressed
Feurstein et al. (1985)	33 (patients)	–	Low back	8.4 yr	–	Family environment scale	Patients scored significantly higher on conflict and control sub-scales of FES than healthy controls.
Follick et al. (1985)	107 (patients)	39.7	Low back	3.03 yr	–	Sickness Impact Profile	Problems with home management for 18.9%; social interaction 23.5%
Hudgens (1979)	24 (couples)	46	Mixed	–	–	Derived from clinical assessment of 6 areas of conflict	Problems ranged from 61 to 100%
Mohamed et al. (1978)	13 (couples)	48.4	Mixed	>3 months	–	Locke-Wallace	Mean score: pain depression = 70, depression = 98.2 (score below 100 suggests marital disharmony)
Rowat and Knafll (1985)	40 (couples)	spouses 55.4; patients 52.2	Mixed	Ranged from 12.3 yr for misc. pain; 9.7 yr for back pain	–	Clinical interview with spouse	25% spouses housebound; 12 spouses highly distressed
Shanfield et al. (1979)	36 (couples)	52.3	Mixed	>6 months	–	No direct measure of marital distress	↑ psychological symptoms in patients ↑ distress level in spouses
Kerns and Turk (1984)	30 (couples)	52.1	Mixed	10.6 yr	24.9 yr	Locke-Wallace	Mean score: patients = 95.3; wives = 91.9

within systems, for example, individual and marital systems which are related to other systems, such as extended family, schools, industry and religion systems. Families cannot be simply reduced to the characteristics of the individual or interaction between pairs of members but rather there are explicit or implicit rules, plus action by members, which govern and monitor behaviour (Epstein and Bishop, 1981). PCSFT, like all other family therapy models, is predicated on systems theory and is based on the following assumptions:

(a) The parts of the family are interrelated;
(b) One part of the family cannot be understood in isolation from the rest of the system;
(c) Family functioning cannot be fully understood by simply understanding each of its parts;
(d) The family structure and organization are important factors determining the behaviour of family members;
(e) Transactional patterns of the family system shape the behaviour of the family members.

Overall family functioning is assessed in six dimensions:

(a) Problem-solving,
(b) Communication,
(c) Roles,
(d) Affective responsiveness,
(e) Affective involvement,
(f) Behavioural control.

Within each of these dimensions the affective and instrumental types of issue are differentiated, and criteria are established for effective family functioning for each dimension. Epstein and Bishop (1981)

TABLE II
Age and sex distribution of back pain and headache sufferers

Age (yr)	Back pain ($n = 12$)	Head pain ($n = 20$)
20–29	0	3 (15%)
30–39	1 (8.5%)	8 (40%)
40–49	3 (25%)	7 (35%)
50–59	4 (33%)	2 (10%)
60–69	3 (25%)	0
70+	1 (8.5%)	0

have developed clear guidelines for conducting clinical assessment using the MMFF. As stated, the following study is the result of systematic assessment utilizing the MMFF of patients with backache and headache and their spouses. Application of MMFF to assess and treat chronic pain sufferers and their families has been reported in detail elsewhere (Roy, 1984, 1985, 1986).

Patient characteristics

There were 12 patients with back pain and 20 with head pain, with 75% of the latter aged between 30 and 49 years, whereas 83% of the patients with back pain were between the ages of 40 and 69 years. Overall the headache patients were younger than their back pain counterparts (Table II).

There were 6 (50%) males and 6 (50%) females with back pain, and 7 (35%) males and 13 (65%) females with headache. The mean duration of pain for the back pain group was 7.08 years, with a range of between 2 and 14 years, and for head pain it was 17.1 years, with a range of less than 1 year to 30 years. The mean duration of marriage for back pain group was 25 years, with a range of 5 to 40 years, and for head pain 12.9 years, with a range of 1 to 26 years.

Problems according to MMFF

Couples were systematically evaluated for their functioning in six dimensions of the MMFF. The overall picture that emerged for couple functioning revealed measurable strife in both groups.

(a) Problem-solving. Problem-solving is defined as a family's ability to resolve problems to a level that maintains effective family functioning. Effective families solve most problems rapidly, easily and without much thought, and Epstein and Bishop (1981) have identified the steps that healthy families follow in problem-solving. Only 3 subjects (25%) with back pain and their spouses had the

TABLE III
Problem-solving

	Completion of seven steps (healthy)	Failure to complete (unhealthy)
Backpain	3 (25%)	9 (75%)
Headpain	0	20 (100%)

TABLE IV
Communication

	CD	CI	MD	MI
Back pain	1 (8%)	0	5 (42%)	6 (50%)
Head pain	0	0	5 (25%)	15 (75%)

C = clear; D = direct; M = masked; I = indirect.

ability to solve problems and all 20 subjects with head pain and their spouses found problem-solving difficult. Problems were more commonly encountered in the affective rather than the instrumental domain (Table III).

(b) Communication. Communication is defined as the way in which a family exchanges information internally. It is sub-divided into instrumental and affective areas and there are two other dimensions along which communication is assessed. They are the clear versus masked continuum, and the direct versus indirect continuum. These groupings lead to four styles of communication; the first and most desirable is the clear and direct communication, the second is the clear and indirect, the third is the masked and direct, and the fourth and the most ineffective is the masked and indirect. Fifty percent of the back pain subjects and their spouses engaged in the masked and indirect form of communication, as against 75% of headache patients. Only 1 couple in the entire sample with back pain were found to engage in the clear and direct type of communication (Table IV).

(c) Roles. Roles are defined as the repetitive patterns of behaviour by which individuals fulfill family functions. They are again divided into instrumental and affective domains. Instrumental roles consist primarily of roles relating to the provision of resources and the affective ones include such activities as nurturing and support, and sexual gratification for marital partners. Accountability is another critical dimension of role functioning and ensures that roles are carried out. 'Allocation' ensu-

res that a family member or members are responsible for allocation of tasks that need to be carried out by individual members of the family.

In relation to accountability, 42% and 60% of back and head pain subjects and their spouses respectively were found to be functioning effectively. Head pain subjects and their spouses were twice as effective (60%) as the back pain (33.3%) with regard to role allocation. In the area of nurturing and support ineffective functioning in both groups was very pervasive. All of the headache subjects and 75% of the back pain subjects demonstrated an inability to provide nurture and support in their marital relationships. Sexual gratification was also found to be a casualty of chronic pain, with 75% of back pain sufferers and 60% of the head pain sufferers and their spouses reporting lack of sexual gratification in their marriage. Examination of occupational roles revealed dramatic differences between the two groups. Whereas 90% of headache subjects demon-

TABLE V
Roles

	Effective		Ineffective	
	Back pain	Head pain	Back pain	Head pain
Accountability	5 (42%)	12 (60%)	7 (48%)	8 (40%)
Allocation	4 (33.3%)	12 (60%)	8 (63.6%)	8 (40%)
Nurture and support	3 (25%)	0	9 (75%)	20 (100%)
Marital sexual gratification	3 (25%)	8 (40%)	9 (75%)	12 (60%)
Occupational roles	6 (50%)	18 (90%)	6 (50%)	2 (10%)
Household roles	6 (50%)	15 (75%)	6 (50%)	5 (25%)

strated effective functioning in their occupational roles, only 50% of the back pain patients demonstrated such effectiveness. Regarding household roles the headache patients and their spouses (75%) were more efficient than their back pain counterparts (50%). Overall the headache subjects and their spouses were more effective in fulfilling their roles than their back pain counterparts (Table V).

(d) Affective responsiveness. Affective responsiveness is defined as the ability to respond to a range of stimuli with appropriate quality and quantity of feelings. Responses are divided into two categories, namely, welfare feelings and emergency feelings. Welfare feelings consist of positive feelings such as love, happiness, joy, etc., and emergency emotions consist of sadness, disappointment, anger, depression, etc. Both the back pain and the head pain couples experienced considerable difficulty in the area of affective responsiveness; 66.6% of the back pain couples and 65% of the head pain couples were unable to express the whole range of affective responsiveness and revealed a pattern of only being able to express emergency emotions. However, 35% of headache couples and 33% of back pain couples were capable of expressing both emergency and welfare emotions (Table VI).

(e) Affective involvement. Affective involvement is defined as the extent to which the family shows interest in and values its activities and interests of family members. Six types of affective involvement are identified:

(1) Lack of involvement;
(2) Involvement devoid of feeling;
(3) Narcissistic involvement;

TABLE VI
Affective responsiveness

	Emergency and welfare emotions	Emergency emotions
Back pain	3 (33.3%)	9 (66.6%)
Head pain	7 (35%)	13 (65%)

TABLE VII
Affective involvement

	Emphatic (healthy)	Narcissistic; lack of involvement; over involvement; symbiotic (unhealthy)
Back pain	2 (17%)	10 (83%)
Head pain	8 (40%)	12 (60%)

(4) Empathic involvement;
(5) Over-involvement;
(6) Symbiotic involvement.

Only 17% of the back pain couples demonstrated an ability to engage in empathic involvement. A considerably higher percentage (40%) of head pain couples gave evidence of healthy, that is, empathic involvement. Also, 83% and 60% of back pain and head pain couples respectively gave evidence of ineffective involvement, which ranged from narcissistic to symbiotic (Table VII).

(f) Behaviour control. Behaviour control is defined as the pattern adopted by the family for handling behaviour in three specific situations:

(1) Physically dangerous situations;
(2) Situations involving the meeting and expressing of psychological needs and drives;
(3) Situations involving socializing behaviour both inside and outside the family.

Four kinds of behaviour control are identified:

(1) Rigid behaviour control;
(2) Flexible behaviour control;
(3) Laissez-faire behaviour control;
(4) Chaotic behaviour control.

Problems of behaviour control for both groups were extensive, with 93% and 80% of back pain and head pain couples respectively engaging in unhealthy behaviour control which ranged from rigid to chaotic. Only 2 (7%) of back pain and 4 (20%) of headache couples gave evidence of flexible, that is, healthy types of behaviour control (Table VIII).

TABLE VIII
Behaviour control

	Flexible (healthy)	Rigid; laissez-faire; chaotic (unhealthy)
Back pain	2 (17%)	10 (83%)
Head pain	4 (20%)	1 (80%)

Discussion

This investigation was based solely on detailed and systematic clinical interviews conducted by this author. The purpose of the project was to assess the impact of chronic pain, not on any individual member of the family but rather as it affected the spouse pair. The results are comparable with existing data and confirm what clinicians have suspected for a very long time, namely, that in the face of chronic pain, role performance in family life is likely to come under a great deal of strain. Communication and sexual problems pose difficulties for patients with chronic pain. However, there were some important differences between head pain and back pain sufferers. Headache patients by and large maintained their occupational role but back pain patients were less adept at doing so. Headache patients were less effective in the area of communication and problem-solving than the backache patients, but affective involvement and behavior control dimensions were more problematic areas for back pain than for headache couples. Difficulty with affective responsiveness was equally shared by both groups. On the basis of the study it is very difficult to speculate or offer clear reasons for the similarities and differences between the groups. Overall, the headache couples appeared to be more functional or less disabled than their back pain counterparts. This study shares one common problem with all the previous studies and that is that the health of the marriage before the onset of the pain problem was hard to ascertain. For many headache subjects the pain problem pre-dated the marriage and for others pain had existed for many years.

Russell et al. (1983) in a recent review observed that "the more researchers attempt to address the complexity of family therapy, the more difficult will be the methodological problems they confront. Family therapy outcome research involves too many variables for there ever to be a definitive study. However, much can be learned by considering the trends that appear across imperfect projects". This study must be viewed as a preliminary attempt to understand how marital partners function in terms of various measures of family functioning when they are forced to live with an intractable problem such as chronic pain. The family system must adapt to the changes introduced by illness, and the emergence of a new type of homeostasis in the family is the inevitable outcome of change. On the basis of this study, the prevailing homeostasis in the marriages of individuals with chronic pain problems appears to be predominantly maladaptive. Clinical evidence suggests that active intervention in such families will prevent the establishment of a maladaptive way of life. The dysfunctional elements that appear to be inevitable when faced with chronic pain can in fact be prevented or resolved.

Experience of systemic family therapy with chronic pain patients and their families remains extremely limited (Roy, 1985, 1986). This is surprising in view of the unanimity amongst researchers and clinicians that marital and family difficulties abound within such families. An explanation for this dichotomy has been offered by Russell et al. (1983), who note that "clinicians are operating more and more as if they believe in the assumption that individual symptoms often serve relationship functions and are (at least partially) maintained by the ways in which people interact in their intimate relationships. However, evaluation research and the agencies which fund it frequently operate under an old paradigm that predicts a one-to-one correspondence between symptom and etiology. The systemic concept of equifinality (the same end point evolving from different starting points) is inconsistent with this older, traditionally better funded, approach". Despite the recognition that chronic pain is multi-faceted and multi-dimensional, the treatment philosophy that prevails in many pain clinics in North America and Britain is still based on a disguised or not-so-disguised biomedical model. The old must give way to the new and the time-honoured approach of individually focused treatment must be considered alongside the systemic perspective.

References

Ahern, D., Adams, A. and Follick, M. (1985) Emotional and marital disturbance in spouses of chronic low back pain patients. Clin. J. Pain, 1: 69–74.

Ahern, D.K. and Follick, M.J. (1985) Distress in spouses of chronic pain patients. Int. J. Fam. Ther., 7: 247–257.

Anderson, L.P. and Rehm, L.P. (1985) The relationship between strategies of coping and perception of pain in these chronic pain groups. J. Clin. Psychol., 40: 1170–1177.

Block, A. (1981) An investigation of the response of the spouse to chronic pain behavior. Psychosom. Med., 43: 415–422.

Block, A.R., Boyer, S.L. and Shusterman, L.R. (1984) The spouses perception of the chronic pain patient: estimates of exercise tolerance. Pain, Suppl. 2.

Block, A. and Boyer, S. (1984) The spouse's adjustment to chronic pain: cognitive and emotional factors. Soc. Sci. Med., 19: 1313–1317.

Blumer, D. and Heilbronn, M. (1982) The pain-prone disorder. J. Nerv. Ment. Dis., 170: 381–406.

Delvey, J. and Hopkins, L. (1982) Pain patients and their partners. J. Marital Fam. Ther., 8: 135–142.

Epstein, N. and Bishop, D. (1981) Problem-centered systems therapy of the family. In A. Gurman and D. Kniskern (Eds.), Handbook of Family Therapy, Brunner/Mazel, New York, pp. 444–482.

Feurstein, M., Sult, S. and Houle, M. (1985) Environmental stresses and chronic low back pain: life events, family and work environment. Pain, 22: 295–307.

Flor, H. and Turk, D.C. (1985) Chronic illness in an adult family member: pain as a prototype. In D. Turk and R. Kerns (Eds.) Health, Illness Families: A Life-Span Perspective. John Wiley & Sons, New York.

Follick, M.J., Smith, T. and Ahern, D. (1985) The sickness impact profile: a global measure of health status in chronic pain patients. Pain, 21: 67–76.

Hudgens, A.J. (1979) Family-oriented treatment of chronic pain. J. Marital Fam. Ther., 5: 67–78.

Kerns, R. and Turk, D. (1984) Chronic pain and depression: mediating role of the spouse. J. Marriage Fam., 46: 845–852.

Liebman, R., Honig, P. and Berger, H. (1976) An integrated treatment program for psychogenic pain. Fam. Proc., 15: 397–405.

Maruta, T. and Osborne, D. (1978) Sexual activity in chronic pain patients. Psychosomatics, 20: 241–248.

Maruta, T., Osborne, D., Swenson, W. and Hallnig, J.M. (1981) Chronic pain patients and spouses: marital and sexual adjustment. Mayo Clin. Proc., 51: 307–310.

Merskey, H. and Boyd, D. (1978) Emotional adjustment and chronic pain. Pain, 5: 173–178.

Minuchin, S., Baker, L., Rosman, B., Liebman, R., Milman, L. and Todd, T. (1975) A conceptual model of psychosomatic illness in children: family organization and family therapy. Arch. Gen. Psychiatry, 32: 1031–1035.

Mohamed, S.N., Weisz, G.M. and Waring, E.M. (1978) The relationship of chronic pain to depression, marital and family dynamics. Pain, 5: 282–292.

Nichols, E.R. (1978) Chronic pain: a review of the intrapersonal and interpersonal factors and a study of marital interaction. Doctoral Dissertation, University of Tennessee, Knoxville, TN.

Payne, B. and Norfleet, M. (1986) Chronic pain and the family: a review. Pain, 26: 1–22.

Roberts, A. and Reinhardt, L. (1980) Behavioral management of chronic pain: long-term follow-up with comparison groups. Pain, 8: 151–162.

Rowat, K.M. and Knafll, K.A. (1985) Living with chronic pain: the spouse's perspective. Pain, 23: 259–271.

Roy, R. (1982) Marital and family issues in patients with chronic pain: a review. Psychother. Psychosom., 37: 1–12.

Roy, R. (1984) Chronic pain: a family perspective. Int. J. Fam. Ther., 6: 31–43.

Roy, R. (Ed.) (1985) The family and chronic pain. A special issue of Int. J. Fam. Ther., 7. Human Sciences Press, New York.

Roy, R. (1986) Problem-centered family systems approach in treating chronic pain. In A. Holzman and D. Turk (Eds.), Pain Management: A Handbook of Psychological Treatment Approaches, Pergamon Press, Elmsford, NJ, pp. 113–130.

Russell, C., Olson, D., Sprenkle, D. and Atilano, R. (1983) From family symptom to family system: review of family therapy research. Am. J. Fam. Ther., 11: 3–14.

Scheider, E. and Bernstein, D. (1976) A case of chronic pain and the 'unilateral' treatment of marital problems. J. Beh. Ther. Rep. Psychiatry, 7: 47–50.

Shanfield, S.B., Heiman, E.M., Cope, N. and Jones, J.R. (1979) Pain and the marital relationship: psychiatric distress. Pain, 7: 343–351.

Swanson, D.W., Swenson, W.M., Maruta, T. and Floreen, A.L. (1978) The dissatisfied patient with chronic pain. Pain, 4: 367–378.

Swanson, D.W. and Maruta, T. (1980) The family's view of chronic pain. Pain, 8: 163–166.

Tunks, E. and Roy, R. (1982) Chronic pain and the occupation role. In R. Roy and E. Tunks, (Eds.), Chronic Pain: Psychosocial Factors in Rehabilitation, Williams & Wilkins, Baltimore, MD, pp. 53–67.

R. Dubner, G.F. Gebhart & M.R. Bond (Eds.)
Proceedings of the Vth World Congress on Pain
© 1988 Elsevier Science Publishers BV (Biomedical Division)

CHAPTER 32

Behavioral interventions and their efficacy

Eldon Tunks

Chedoke-McMaster Hospitals, Box 2000, Stn. 'A', Hamilton, Ontario, L8N-3Z5, Canada

The relevance of psychological methods

From midcentury there has been growing recognition that psychological factors are important in pain. Two further developments that have significantly brought the psychological viewpoint into focus are the notion of the distinction between 'chronic and acute pain', and the application of psychological techniques on a large scale for the management particularly of chronic pain. This application was greatly stimulated by the disappointing results of traditional medical and surgical treatments for chronic pain (Spitzer et al., 1986; Flor and Turk, 1984), and the seminal work of Fordyce and his group, proving the relevance of environmental factors and showing how chronic pain disability could be improved by contingency management (Fordyce et al., 1968, 1973). The operant conditioning methods described by Fordyce form a major component in many pain clinics: however, other psychological treatment options also exist. The more behaviorally oriented treatments include operant conditioning, relaxation therapy, various types of biofeedback, assertiveness training and desensitization. Dynamic psychotherapy, family psychotherapy, group techniques and hypnosis represent 'mentalistic' or in a broad sense 'psychodynamic' approaches. Cognitive therapy and coping skills training represent something of a compromise between the behavioral and the 'psychodynamic' approaches (Sternbach, 1983, 1984).

Operant behavioral therapy

Chronic pain problems, which include both the subjective distress element and the illness behavior element, are very much subject to the problems of learning. The conceptual model which best describes this is the 'operant conditioning model' which states that behaviors are influenced by their consequences; if a behavior is followed by a certain consequence which increases the probability of that behavior being repeated, the consequence is said to be 'a reinforcer'. For example, a person who complains of pain may be given a drug which reduces anxiety, and family sympathy which was otherwise not forthcoming; this may increase the frequency of pain complaints. Avoidance learning is also an important instance of 'operant learning'; an individual with back pain may find that by going to bed and staying away from work, he or she no longer has to face a chronically unpleasant work situation or the fear of being reinjured.

In the operant conditioning model, 'respondent pain' is taken to mean the perceived discomfort that arises due to tissue damage; after injury the behavior of the injured person is governed significantly by the nociception from the injured area. For example, the person with the sprained ankle does not walk because it hurts more when he does. The illness behavior is thus initially understood in terms of the responses to nociception. However, the illness behavior is also apt to lead to certain consequences from the environment ('contingent responses'), which have the effect of either reinforcing the illness behavior, or permitting avoidance learning. As the original wound heals, the illness behavior comes progressively under the influence of environmental events. Operant behavioral treatment involves changing the environmental events which reinforce pain complaints or which permit avoidance (invalid) behavior. Much of the illness behavior can be changed by reinforcing responses that are incompatible with the pain behavior and by 'extinguishing' illness behaviors by no longer 'reinforcing them'.

'Behavioral therapies' are those which are specifically based on the premises of such behavioral learning theory. In this paper, we restrict the term 'behavioral' mostly to 'operant behavioral' concepts and methods, although the term 'behavioral' can also be used in a wider sense, to refer to other models of learning, such as the 'classical model'. One should also distinguish explicit 'operant conditioning' methods of 'behavioral therapy' from other rehabilitation methods which are compatible with the operant model, and which can be described in terms of it, but which are based on setting objective therapeutic goals, and activating the patient; in the latter category come the majority of multimodal programs, exercise and occupational therapy, and cognitive-behavioral treatment programs.

Evaluation problems

In the vigorous spread of pain clinics across North America in particular, a preference was given in most cases to multimodal methods in multidisciplinary clinics. It was soon found that outcome research was being confounded by multiple treatments and soft outcome measures (Linton, 1982; Turner and Chapman, 1982a,b; Aronoff et al., 1983; Turk et al., 1983; Roy, 1984; Turner and Romano, 1984). Although the effectiveness of these multimodal programs seemed to be accepted on the whole, it was difficult to establish the relative effectiveness of the component parts, including the behavioral methods which often acted as the core of

the treatment program (Sternbach, 1983, 1984).

Many reviews have been devoted to the problems of evaluation. Rather than depending only on relatively narrow terms, such as reduction of use of medication or health care services, increase in activity, and return to work, reviewers have called for broader and more diverse criteria by which outcome could be measured, including whether behavioral intervention led to change in pain levels, psychological factors, role-function improvement, and success of the whole rehabilitation effort. Improved experimental designs have been recommended, such as use of control groups, randomized control designs, refined patient selection, other experimental strategies, such as dismantling methods to better identify the relative efficacy of various components, the use of standardized or objective outcome measures, a uniform diagnostic system, and studies of therapies based on other models, such as classical conditioning or psychotherapy or group treatment models. They noted that future studies should make use of longer follow-ups, and should pay attention to factors such as response specificity with different sorts of intervention, the effect of concurrent medical interventions, the influence of family, the relationship between change in pain behavior and psychological and personality measures, and the credibility of and compliance with treatment regimens. It was recommended that more cost-effective methods could be studied (e.g. outpatient instead of inpatient), and most of the above reviews noted that even the most efficacious of pain-management programs have a significant failure or relapse rate, and that it would be desirable to study the characteristics of non-responders, and to mount trials on the prevention of pain. Fordyce et al. (1985), in a selective review, and Linton (1986) found that studies with more imaginative and sophisticated experimental designs had been published; these made use of matched controls, single-subject designs with varying baselines, ABAB reversals, and multiple baseline techniques. While the randomized control methods allowed for good comparison of between-group experimental effects, the use of within-group comparisons and the single-subject or multiple baseline designs permitted study of component factors and individual differences.

An important component in the refinement of clinical research has been the progressive improvement in different pain measures (Syrjala and Chapman, 1984). These include refinements of self-report questionnaires, self-reports of pain experienced (such as McGill Pain Questionnaire or Visual Analogue Scales), reliable observational methods for rating pain behavior, standardized assessments of physical function, and physiological measures. The IASP Subcommittee on Taxonomy has published a guide to pain taxonomy which will be of considerable assistance in future research (1986).

The impact of this critical thinking has been the appearance of a series of increasingly good studies. This paper undertakes a selective review of recent controlled studies of the efficacy of behavioral treatment. A few studies dealing with relaxation and biofeedback are also included for comparison purposes.

Are behavioral theories heuristic?

It would be important to know whether operant behavioral theory could be used to explain the origins and persistence of chronic pain problems. Fordyce et al. (1985) have addressed this issue in a selective review of several reports, from which the evidence is that operant conditioning can influence pain reports and pain behavior in the absence of correlated nociception, that verbal reinforcement is the most influential reinforcer affecting pain behavior, and that cues from family members affect the pain behavior of chronic pain sufferers.

The behavioral model proposes that pain which initially begins as 'respondent' can come increasingly under the influence of social contingencies. Linton and Gotestam (1985) carried out an elegant study of the effects of verbal reinforcement on the self-reports of pain. Experimental subjects were normal volunteers. The stimulus was pressure-cuff, with benchmarked pain stimulus levels. During repeated trials under baseline no-reinforcement conditions, there was good correlation with the amount of

pressure and pain reported. Some subjects were then given verbal reinforcement for increasing or decreasing their reports of pain. It was found that reinforcement for increasing pain report led to significant increases over the baseline or the 'down condition'. Reinforcement for decreasing the pain report led to significant decreases from the 'up condition'. A further group of subjects had baseline and then decreasing levels of pressure stimulus, without reinforcement; these reported decreases in pain levels which paralleled the changes in stimulation. Subjects were then reinforced for increasing pain report, even though the stimulation was being gradually reduced; reports of subjective pain increased during the reinforcement condition. This study shows that subjective reports of pain (and likely the pain experience) do not depend only on nociception but are influenced by reinforcement.

Intuitively, one might assume that pain ought to be aggravated proportionately to the degree of exercise, and relieved by rest. An operant learning model of pain would postulate the opposite; a chronic pain problem is reinforced by rest, whereas reinforcement of activity while withholding reinforcement of pain behavior leads to reduction in pain behavior, and increase in activity. Fordyce et al. (1981) reported a study in which 25 patients were observed by a physiotherapist while they were exercising to tolerance on specific exercises over a period of several sessions. Observations were made of the number of repetitions of each exercise performed in any given session and any kinds of pain behavior during the same session; verbal complaints, guarding or gestures indicating pain, moaning, or statements implying inability or difficulty to continue due to pain. With this regime, exercise steadily increased in successive sessions. There was a strikingly significant negative correlation between exercise performed per session and pain behavior in the same session.

If the behavioral model is correct, one should find that in cases of chronic pain there is a weaker association between 'pain' or 'pain complaint' and actual behavior, since it is postulated that the pain problem is no longer strictly governed by nociception, but by environmental contingencies. Fordyce et al. (1984) examined the relationship of chronic pain patients' self-ratings of pain intensity and associated impairment, and compared this to activity data gathered from diary forms, recording of medication intake, a standardized questionnaire about commonplace activity, and health care utilization questionnaire. From the self-reports, patients were divided into 'high', 'medium' and 'low' pain-rating subgroups. A positive relationship was found between pain report and the 'impairment index' (self-report of the amount of common activities limited due to pain), sleeping disturbance and limited sitting tolerance. However, no relationship was found between pain report and analgesic consumption, on measures of sitting, standing, walking or reclining from the diary. In short, the reports of pain and impairment did not match behavior.

In a similar study, Linton (1985) had 15 chronic back pain sufferers rate their pain and their ability to perform various activities of daily living; a correlation was found on these subjective measures. They kept an activity checklist of activities actually accomplished during one to three weeks; there was only a modest correlation between increased pain and increased activity in 5 of the 15 patients. Patients then rode an exercise bicycle to tolerance; there was no correlation between distance rode and 'average pain for the week', 'pain before the test', 'pain the day after the test', or inability to complete the exercise test.

To support the operant model as heuristic in the case of chronic pain, it should be possible to show that pain complaints and pain behavior of chronic pain patients are influenced by family members. Block et al. (1980) studied pain patients who had solicitous or non-solicitous spouses; when the patients who had solicitous spouses were aware that their spouses were observing, they rated their own pain higher than when the spouses were absent. When the patients with non-solicitous spouses were aware that their spouses were observing, they rated their pain as lower than when their spouses were absent. Gil et al. (1987) studied 51 chronic pain patients through the McGill Pain Questionnaire, a standardized Social Support Questionnaire, and an objective method for rating pain behavior by means of scoring videotaped segments. No correlation was found between the dimension of 'availability of social support' and either pain ratings from the McGill Questionnaire or objective pain behaviors. However, the individuals who reported a high level of 'satisfaction with social support' also demonstrated a high level of pain behavior. This was taken to support the hypothesis that chronic pain patients may be reinforced in their pain behavior by family members that they perceive to be solicitous.

Are behavioral methods efficacious?

Improving on control groups. A problem was encountered in a study by Sturgis et al. (1984), in which no statistical differences in outcome were found between a group treated in a multidisciplinary pain clinic and a control group of patients who were eligible for but who did not desire such treatment, and who were referred back to their family doctors for treatment. Those authors identified the need for a more suitable control group. Guck et al. (1985) discussed the problem of finding a suitable no-treatment control group for a multidisciplinary program. Their solution was to take those subjects who had been screened and accepted for admission who wished to participate but were unable to do so because of lack of sufficient insurance coverage; although it might be objected that there may be a hidden bias attached to the factor of having such coverage, their analysis of the demographic characteristics, which were very similar for the groups, appeared to satisfy that objection. Their study followed subjects for 1–5 years, and used the stringent outcome criteria proposed by Roberts and Reinhardt (1980). They found that 60% of treated patients satisfied the criteria for success, whereas none of the control group did so.

Ensuring compliance with experimental conditions. Kerns et al. (1986) conducted a randomized controlled comparison of operant conditioning and relaxation, cognitive-behavioral therapy and relaxation, or waiting-list control, on an outpatient basis. Dependent measures included several standardized psychological measures from which 'principal component scores' were calculated, use of the health-care system, subjective pain and objective goal achievement. Assessment was made for pretreatment comparability of subjects, and purity of treatment conditions was ensured by using standardized protocols along with randomized monitoring of taped segments of the sessions by blind raters. An assessment was made of treatment credibility. Follow-ups were conducted at 3 and 6 months. Both experimental groups demonstrated significant improvement in goal attainment, and a four-fold decrease in use of health care services on follow-up. At the end of treatment, improvement in pain severity and affective distress had occurred to a significantly greater degree in the cognitive-behavioral than in the behavioral or waiting-list groups, but the behavioral and the cognitive-behavioral groups later became similar in pain severity and affective distress by the time of the 6-month followup.

Behavioral therapy for prevention of chronic pain.
Fordyce et al. (1986) conducted a randomized controlled trial of outpatient operant behavioral therapy versus traditional management for acute back pain; for the behavioral condition, the use of analgesics, exercises and activity limits was based on quotas leading to restoration of normal activity, whereas in the traditional condition, use of these treatments was based on symptoms. Outcome measures were drawn from vocational status, health-care utilization, patient claims of impairment, extent of pain drawings, and two measures of activity level. Although there were no significant differences between groups in vocational status, pain medication intake or back examination at intake or at six weeks, at the follow-up (9–12 months) the behaviorally treated group was significantly better on the health care utilization, claimed impairment and pain drawings. In fact, the traditionally treated group had actually worsened on the claimed impairment variable.

Behavioral therapy combined with regular rehabilitation treatment. Linton et al. (1985) randomly assigned chronic pain patients to three outpatient conditions; waiting-list control, regular rehabilitation clinic treatment, or regular treatment plus operant behavior therapy and applied relaxation training. The regular treatment patients received more therapeutic contact than patients in the behavioral condition. Patients recorded their pain and medication intake, and sleep, depression, activities of daily living and activities participated in were assessed. Only the patients in the behavioral condition showed a significant reduction in pain intensity. The behavioral treatment group was significantly superior to the waiting-list control in the ADL questionnaire, and was the only condition to show significant change on the activities checklist. The behavioral treatment condition was superior to the other conditions on the measures of reduced medication intake and improved sleep and depression.

Testing various components of multimodal treatment. Sanders (1983) examined the contribution of relaxation training, assertiveness training, cognitive-behavioral training with self-monitoring, and verbal reinforcement, for increases in standing and walking, in a nonconcurrent multiple baseline design. After no-treatment baseline, four subjects received the four components in an additive and order-balanced fashion. Dependent variables included uptime (measured by a mechanical automatic timer), medication intake, and subjective pain ratings; chart data were collected by assistants who were blind to the study's intent. It was demonstrated that relaxation training produced meaningful improvements in pain ratings, medication intake and, to a lesser extent, in uptime. Verbal reinforcement induced meaningful increases in uptime, and lesser effects on medication intake.

In various age groups. Miller and LeLieuvre (1982) used a single-case design to study four geriatric patients with chronic pain. Operant behavior therapy was used plus exercise quotas. Medications decreased, and there was a decrease in pain as measured by the McGill Pain Questionnaire. Two of the patients stopped demonstrating pain behavior.

Masek et al. (1984) describe studies done by their group in headache pain management with outpatient children. They used a multiple baseline strategy to evaluate the components of operant behavioral training, meditative relaxation and EMG biofeedback. After treatment, and at 6 and 12 months follow-up, there were marked and stable reductions in headache frequency, mean intensity, mean duration, total hours of headache, medication use and headache activity. In a further study, children were assigned randomly to three conditions: (1) operant behavioral management, EMG biofeedback and meditative relaxation, (2) operant behavioral management, progressive muscle relaxation and meditative relaxation, and (3) self-monitoring waiting-list control. Both treatment groups improved significantly on all measures, with no change in the control group. They found no significant differences in any variable of outcome between the groups that did or did not have biofeedback.

Goal-setting and cognitive change. Two studies were particularly concerned with behavioral and psychological effects of setting behavioral goals. Dolce et al. (1986a) studied a patient with chronic neck pain in a single-case AB multiple baseline design. The patient was assigned two physical exercises; during baseline, she was asked to exercise to tolerance, and during the active condition quotas were set by the therapist and gradually increased daily. Measures were number of repetitions performed, 'self-efficacy beliefs' about the ability to succeed, and worry or concern about the exercise. Performance, 'self-efficacy' and worries failed to improve for either exercise during the baseline condition. After 4 days, when quotas were first set for one of the exercises, there was an immediate improvement in self-efficacy and reduction in worry regarding that exercise. This was followed by a steady daily increase in repetitions performed, a further decrease in worry and an increase in self-efficacy. On the 14th day when quotas were first set for the second exercise, there was a similar steady increase in

that exercise, improvement in self-efficacy and reduction in worry. Improvements remained stable up to 8 months follow-up. Part 2 of the experiment was to follow 14 chronic pain patients in a within-subjects repeated measures design. Patients were in a multimodal treatment program. As quotas were set, exercise tolerance increased steadily. Self-efficacy expectancies improved for 82% and worries decreased for 71% of the patients; the authors noted that a minority of the patients had failed to improve on the psychological variables despite having improved in the exercise. Dolce et al. (1986b) in a further report studied 64 college volunteers, using a cold pressor task, with measures of cold-pressor tolerance, pain intensity and beliefs about their ability to keep their hand submerged. They were divided into four groups; for the control condition, they established baseline tolerance, and were then urged to keep the hand submerged as long as possible. The quotas condition group were asked to double their baseline time. The quotas and reinforcement condition group were asked to double their time and were offered $5 if they succeeded. The placebo and quotas condition group were asked to double their time, but were given a tablet before the trial with the explanation that it was an analgesic. All three quota conditions improved their tolerance, reinforcement did not improve tolerance more than quota alone, and the placebo condition actually showed poorer tolerance than the other two quota groups. Self-efficacy increased according to the degree of performance improvement, and increased less in the placebo condition. On follow-up, the measures were repeated, showing that pain tolerance and self-efficacy were highest in the quota and quota with reinforcement groups. In the placebo group, pain rating and cold pressor tolerance were worse than in the other experimental conditions and control group.

Other behaviorally oriented therapies

Many pain clinics use a variety of treatments in addition to operant behavioral therapy. There is a logical and practical compatibility between these various behaviorally oriented therapies. For relaxation, it may be conceptualized that the condition of suffering pain is associated with an increased level of emotional and psychophysiological tension which has a bearing on the pain experienced; in relaxation, the patient is learning to identify this state of tension, and to reduce it, thereby changing the pain and the distress. In this way, the relaxation is seen as being oriented to 'respondent pain' rather than to 'operant mechanisms of pain'. One might also conceptualize relaxation as involving a classical extinction procedure in which the psychophysiological arousal of the pain experience, which has become conditioned to various psychological and situational cues, occurs in a controlled relaxation situation where it cannot be reinforced. It may also be considered within the operant learning paradigm as a situation in which the patient is apt to receive approval from the therapist for behaving in a manner which is incompatible with pain-distress – that is, the patient behaves as if he or she is unperturbed. The considerations above also apply to biofeedback, which will be briefly considered later.

Relaxation therapy

Like the lowly aspirin, this form of therapy has probably sometimes been underrated as more sophisticated therapies have made their appearances. Yet, in controlled studies and in clinical practice alike, relaxation therapy has proven to be efficacious and inexpensive. It is an important ingredient in other procedures such as biofeedback, desensitization and assertiveness training, and some kinds of cognitive-behavioral therapy, especially those which emphasize training in coping skills. Comparative studies of relaxation and other psychological therapies have found that relaxation compares very favourably with other psychological treatment methods and with biofeedback (Jessup et al., 1979; Zitman, 1983; Turner and Romano, 1984; Linton, 1986; Chapman, 1986). There is some reason to believe that whereas operant behavioral therapy is very effective in reducing illness behavior (reducing

medication intake, reducing verbal and nonverbal expressions of pain, and increasing activity), relaxation therapy may be somewhat more effective in reducing the subjective experience of pain and emotional distress. This seems to be illustrated in the studies by Sanders (1983) and Linton and Gotestam (1984). In another study, Sorbi and Tellegen (1986) studied migraine patients by randomly assigning them either to relaxation or to 'stress-coping training'. It was found that both groups improved significantly in headaches, but that the relaxation patients perceived significantly better training effects in migraine duration, drug consumption and awareness of stress, whereas the stress-coping patients more often believed that they had acquired control over stressful events. (These differences faded away during follow-up 8 months later.)

Attanasio et al. (1987) randomly assigned 25 tension headache sufferers to three conditions; combined treatment in the therapist's office using relaxation and cognitive therapy, with instructions for home practice, or combined treatment using the same elements but home-based, or relaxation only but home-based. All three groups improved, so that 71% of subjects in the combined office-based treatment, 62% of those in the combined home-based treatment, and 50% of those in the home-based relaxation group showed meaningful improvement in headache (but the differences were not considered to be statistically significant). Richter et al. (1986) randomly assigned 42 children and adolescents with migraine to three conditions; relaxation training, cognitive therapy, and attention-placebo treatment. Subjects in both treatment groups improved significantly and equally. Subjects with an initially high severity of headache showed the greatest response.

Office vs. home-based treatment. Larsson and Melin (1986) assigned adolescents with headaches to three conditions; applied relaxation, information-contact, or self-monitoring of headaches. Measures included headache diaries, psychological tests of anxiety, depression, stress and medication consumption. At the end of treatment, significant improvement in headache measures and stress experience occurred only with the relaxation group. There was no difference between the other two groups. This improvement was stable at 6 months follow-up.

How is relaxation applied? This raises the issue of relaxation training being tied in with coping skills, and not simply being a way to reduce the psychophysiological tension associated with respondent pain. Anseth et al. (1985) compared the effect of (1) a neuroleptic, flupenthixol, plus applied relaxation, (2) placebo and applied relaxation, (3) unspecific relaxation and flupenthixol, and (4) unspecific relaxation and placebo, on experimentally produced pressure pain. Patients given the unspecific relaxation were simply shown how to relax and practice imagery, whereas the applied relaxation group were shown how to use this imagery to help control the discomfort. Subjects who used the applied relaxation were more able to reduce their pain experience, regardless of whether they had the active or placebo drug, whereas there was little effect from the unspecific relaxation. (It was also noted that subjects receiving the active drug actually had more pain than those with the placebo.) Other research also confirms the requirement for relaxation (or biofeedback-assisted relaxation) to be accompanied by a cognitive coping element and for the relaxation to be actively applied to the problem (Holroyd et al., 1980; Flor and Turk, 1987).

Biofeedback

Reviews in general support the impression that biofeedback of some types and for some conditions is an efficacious treatment (Jessup et al., 1979; Cameron, 1982; Turner and Chapman, 1982a; Kerns et al., 1983; O'Brien and Weisbrot, 1983; Turk et al., 1983; Zitman, 1983; Keefe and Bradley, 1984; Trifiletti, 1984; Turk and Flor, 1984; Turner and Romano, 1984; Linton, 1986; Chapman, 1986). The reviews have stated the following conclusions. In most cases, biofeedback is about as effective as relaxation, and both are better than 'placebo' or no-treatment conditions. The physiological function that is monitored may show a training effect in the desired direction, but this is often small, and it may be difficult to establish a clear equation between the symptomatic improvement and the monitored physiological change. Other variables, especially the element of relaxation or cognitive variables, may have a critical role in the therapeutic outcome. However, there is still some biofeedback literature which suggests that there may be some specificity between training effect and therapeutic outcome which may show itself with more refined methods. For example, Wolf et al. (1982) found that back pain was not improved by either increasing or decreasing monitored muscle tension in the low back; rather pain was reduced when biofeedback was used to modify the synergistic function of the back during movement. Whether this specificity will be evident in further studies remains to be seen. The conclusions that one can draw are that biofeedback may be efficacious because of factors that are ingredients of the biofeedback procedure, such as relaxation, active use of coping skills and cognitive change.

Bell et al. (1983) randomly assigned 24 tension headache sufferers to biofeedback, brief psychotherapy, combined psychotherapy and biofeedback, or waiting-list control. Biofeedback was combined with lessons in the use of imagery, awareness of inner states, a brief relaxation technique, home practice and methods for applying the therapy to pain and stress. Brief psychotherapy consisted of the same number of hours of treatment, devoted to discussion of stressors, headache triggers, coping, dealing with unpleasant affect, some psychodynamic issues and use of imagery to deal with pain. The combined condition included both treatments. Measures were from headache diary and medication use, EMG levels, psychological measures, questions regarding treatment satisfaction and a compliance measure. All three treatment groups improved significantly with respect to control on the variables of headache symptoms, psychological improvement, medication use and decline in muscle spasms. Improvement was superior in degree for all biofeedback patients for ability to relax, need for medication, and the psychological variables of somatization, obsessive-compulsiveness, anxiety and total complaints. Patients receiving biofeedback perceived the ingredients of learning to relax, relaxing at home, avoiding stress and expecting to feel better as more helpful than did the psychotherapy patients. The psychotherapy combination with biofeedback was no more effective than biofeedback alone.

Combining treatment with rehabilitation. Lacroix et al. (1986) assigned 55 patients with back and neck pain, who also suffered tension headache, to frontalis EMG biofeedback, relaxation, combined relaxation-biofeedback or no-treatment control. Patients were all inpatients in a Worker's Compensation Hospital, and were also participating in rehabilitation aimed at increasing performance. A small but significant improvement was found for all three treatment groups, whereas the control group steadily worsened on headache frequency. Patients who received the relaxation training reported more improvement in all aspects of headache symptoms at the six month followup.

Efficacy with regard to perceived success. Biedermann et al. (1987) studied 24 back pain patients in three conditions; a high-success group who received an exaggerated EMG feedback signal, a low-success group who received a signal which changed to a lesser degree with a given amount of muscle activity, and linear feedback with a linear representation of the feedback signal. It was hypothesized that if symptomatic improvement were yoked to amount of success apparent to the patient, then the high-success group would improve the most. There were equal and significant treatment gains for all groups, for pain intensity, pain words used, consumption of medication, physical mobility, self-efficacy and measures of anxiety, depression and stress. This was maintained for 4 and 12 weeks follow-up. There was no relationship between reduction in muscle tension and post-treatment pain experiences, and all groups were comparable in actual

muscle tension reduction. From observation, the authors discovered that hand-in-hand with the therapy, the patients had been using the occasion to learn more about their problem, and had been developing coping skills. This emphasis on cognitive and coping change as a hidden ingredient in biofeedback treatment has also been discussed by other authors (Andrasik and Holroyd, 1980).

Cognitive-behavioral therapy

Cognitive therapy, or cognitive-behavioral therapy, is actually a group of therapeutic methods which may be applied in various combinations. At the core of the approach is the assumption that thoughts mediate actions, that maladaptive behaviors are often tied to problems in style of thinking or to lack of effective available cognitive coping methods, and that these problems can be corrected by an approach which combines behavioral tasks (such as self-monitoring, relaxation or biofeedback, assertiveness training, contracted goal-setting or stress inoculation) with cognitive training (reappraisal of stress, studying possible cognitive coping methods or analysis of maladaptive thoughts). What is common to all of these methods is that some objective and measurable therapeutic goals are central to the treatment process, self-measurement of progress is built into the treatment, and the patient is engaged in a structured therapeutic experience which is designed to enhance his or her sense of mastery. Often, cognitive coping methods are explicitly discussed and practised, with the assumption that the patient's strategies are absent or deficient. There are a number of detailed reviews of the cognitive-behavioral literature (Cameron, 1982; Tan, 1982; Turner and Chapman, 1982b; Kerns et al., 1983; Turk et al., 1983; Keefe and Bradley, 1984; Trifiletti, 1984; Turk and Flor, 1984; Turner and Romano, 1984; Linton, 1986).

Considering the wide variation in type of cognitive therapies, it is difficult to compare them. The most comprehensive reviews of the field note that laboratory studies of individual cognitive coping methods have often failed to demonstrate superiority, or even efficacy, of these methods in volunteers (Tan, 1982; Turk et al., 1983). The reason for this finding may be that many subjects may already have their own well-developed coping strategies which are preferable and more versatile: furthermore, laboratory studies of normal volunteers may not be comparable to clinical situations (Turk et al., 1983). Many multimodal therapies are currently based on combinations of cognitive therapy with other interventions (Khatami and Rush, 1978; Turk et al., 1983). One of the greatest reported levels of success in management of back pain was reported by Mayer et al. (1986), who used multimodal therapy built around cognitive-behavioral therapy. Cognitive therapies represent a compromise between behavior therapies which focus on overt behavior, and insight-oriented psychotherapies which concentrate on thinking and subjective states. Like other behavioral therapies, cognitive-behavioral therapy is based on structured therapeutic experiences, with objective behavioral goals around which the patient can orient his or her task of learning to cope.

The utility of a 'behavioral perspective' in other forms of therapy

Whatever the orientation of the therapy, results are optimized if there are clearly defined goals. Because the chronic pain problem involves disability, and not just subjective distress, therapeutic modalities of any sort which are used for people with chronic pain are likely to be more helpful if there is an element in the therapy which acknowledges the importance of the behavioral aspects. For example, if one were to use supportive psychotherapy or psychodynamic oriented psychotherapy, the treatment would be more palatable, apparently relevant and objectively helpful if the problems in physical functioning and requirements for realistic and progressive goals of rehabilitation were also addressed as part of the therapy. Such psychotherapy in no way contradicts the goals of other behaviorally oriented therapy or operant therapy, and, in fact, the effectiveness of psychotherapy is increased by including this element. Despite the widespread use of group, supportive, individual and family therapy in the regular operation of many pain clinics, there is, unfortunately, to date, a scant amount of literature regarding the appropriate use of psychotherapy for chronic pain patients (Pilowsky, 1978; Bellissimo and Tunks, 1984), and only a few studies have been done that might allow us to gain an impression of its efficacy (Draspa, 1959; Sarno, 1976; Bell et al., 1983; Bassett and Pilowsky, 1985).

References

Andrasik, F. and Holroyd, K.A. (1980) A test of specific and nonspecific effects in the biofeedback treatment of tension headache. J. Consult. Clin. Psychol., 48: 575–586.

Anseth, E., Berntzen, D. and Gotestam, K.G. (1985) A comparison of the effects of flupentixol and relaxation on laboratory pain: and experimental study. Acta Neurol. Scand., 71: 20–24.

Aronoff, G.M., Evans, W.O. and Enders, P.L. (1983) A review of followup studies of multidisciplinary pain units. Pain, 16: 1–11.

Attanasio, V., Andrasik, F. and Blanchard, E.B. (1987) Cognitive therapy and relaxation training in muscle contraction headache: efficacy and cost-effectiveness. Headache, 27: 254–260.

Bassett, D.L. and Pilowsky, I. (1985) A study of brief psychotherapy for chronic pain. J. Psychosom. Res., 29: 259–264.

Bellissimo, A. and Tunks, E. (1984) Chronic Pain: The Psychotherapeutic Spectrum, Praeger, New York.

Bell, N.W., Abramowitz, S.I., Folkins, C.H., Spensley, J. and Hutchinson, G.L. (1983) Biofeedback, brief psychotherapy, and tension headache. Headache, 23: 162–173.

Biedermann, H.J., McGhie, A., Monga, T.N. and Shanks, G.L. (1987) Perceived and actual control in EMG treatment of back pain. Behav. Res. Ther., 25: 137–147.

Block, A.R., Kremer, E.F. and Gaylor, M. (1980) Behavioral treatment of chronic pain: the spouse as a discriminative cue for pain behavior. Pain, 9: 243–252.

Cameron, R. (1982) Behavior and cognitive therapies. In R. Roy and E. Tunks (Eds.), Chronic Pain: Psychosocial Factors in Rehabilitation, Williams and Wilkins, Baltimore, pp. 79–103.

Chapman, S.L. (1986) A review and clinical perspective on the use of EMG and thermal biofeedback for chronic headaches. Pain, 27: 1–43.

Dolce, J.J., Crocker, M.F., Moletteire, C. and Doleys, D.M. (1986a) Exercise quotas, anticipatory concern and self-efficacy expectancies in chronic pain: a preliminary report. Pain, 24: 365–372.

Dolce, J.J., Doleys, D.M., Raczynski, J.M., Lossie, J., Poole, L. and Smith, M. (1986b) The role of self-efficacy expectancies in the prediction of pain tolerance. Pain, 27: 261–272.

Draspa, L.J. (1959) Psychological factors in muscular pain. Br. J. Med. Psychol., 32: 106–116.

Flor, H. and Turk, D.C. (1984) Etiological theories and treatments for chronic back pain. I. Somatic models and interventions. Pain, 19: 105–121.

Flor, H. and Turk, D.C. (1987) Pain-related cognitions, pain severity, and pain behaviors in chronic pain patients. Poster presented at the Vth World Congress on Pain, Hamburg, Aug. 2–7, 1987.

Fordyce, W.E., Fowler, R., Lehmann, J. and De Lateur, B. (1968) Some implications of learning in problems of chronic pain. J. Chron. Dis., 21: 179–190.

Fordyce, W.E., Fowler, R.S., Lehmann, J.F., De Lateur, B.J., Sand, P.L. and Trieschmann, R.B. (1973) Operant conditioning in the treatment of chronic pain. Arch. Phys. Med. Rehabil., 54: 399–408.

Fordyce, W.E., McMahon, R., Rainwater, G., Jackins, S., Questad, K., Murphy, T. and De Lateur, B. (1981) Pain complaint-exercise performance relationship in chronic pain. Pain, 10: 311–321.

Fordyce, W.E., Lansky, D., Calsyn, D.A., Shelton, J.L., Stolóv, W.C. and Rock, D.L. (1984) Pain measurement and pain behavior. Pain, 18: 53–69.

Fordyce, W.E., Roberts, A.H. and Sternbach, R.A. (1985) The behavioral management of chronic pain; a response to critics. Pain, 22: 113–125.

Fordyce, W.E., Brockway, J.A., Bergman, J.A. and Spengler, D. (1986) Acute back pain: a control-group comparison of behavioral vs. traditional management methods. J. Behav. Med., 9: 127–140.

Gil, K.M., Keefe, F.J., Crisson, J.E. and Van Dalfsen, P.J. (1987) Social support and pain behavior. Pain, 29: 209–217.

Guck, T.P., Skultety, F.M., Meilman, P.W. and Dowde, E.T. (1985) Multidisciplinary pain center follow-up study: evaluation with no treatment control group. Pain, 21: 295–307.

Holroyd, K.A., Andrasik, F. and Noble, J. (1980) A comparison of EMG biofeedback and a credible pseudotherapy in treating tension headache. J. Behav. Med., 3: 29–39.

I.A.S.P. Subcommittee on Taxonomy (1986) Classification of chronic pain: descriptions of chronic pain syndromes and definitions of pain terms. Pain, 3 (Suppl.).

Jessup, B.A., Neufeld, R.W.J. and Merskey, H. (1979) Biofeedback therapy for headache and other pains; an evaluative review. Pain, 7: 225–270.

Keefe, F.J. and Bradley, L.A. (1984) Behavioral and psychological approaches to the assessment and treatment of chronic pain. Gen. Hosp. Psychiatry, 6: 49–54.

Kerns, R.D., Turk, D.C. and Holzman, A.D. (1983) Psychological treatment for chronic pain: a selective review. Clin. Psychol. Rev., 3: 15–26.

Kerns, R.D., Turk, D.C., Holzman, A.D. and Rudy, T.E. (1986) Comparison of cognitive-behavioral and behavioral approaches to the outpatient treatment of chronic pain. Clin. J. Pain, 1: 195–203.

Khatami, M. and Rush, A.J. (1978) A pilot study of the treatment of outpatients with chronic pain: symptom control, stimulus control, and social system intervention. Pain, 5: 163–172.

Lacroix, J.M., Clarke, M.A., Carson Bock, J. and Doxey, N.C.S. (1986) Muscle-contraction headaches in multiple-pain patients: treatment under worsening baseline conditions. Arch. Phys. Med. Rehabil., 67: 14–18.

Larsson, B. and Melin, L. (1986) Chronic headaches in adolescents: treatment in a school setting with relaxation training as compared with information-contact and self-registration. Pain, 25: 325–336.

Linton, S.J. (1982) A critical review of behavioral treatments for chronic benign pain other than headache. Br. J. Clin. Psychol., 21: 321–337.

Linton, S.J. (1985) The relationship between activity and chronic back pain. Pain, 21: 289–294.

Linton, S.J. (1986) Behavioral remediation of chronic pain: a status report. Pain, 24: 125–141.

Linton, S.J. and Gotestam, K.G. (1984) A controlled study of the effects of applied relaxation and applied relaxation plus operant procedures in the regulation of chronic pain. Br. J. Clin. Psychol., 23 (Pt. 4): 291–299.

Linton, S.J. and Gotestam, K.G. (1985) Controlling pain reports through operant conditioning: a laboratory demonstration. Percept. Motor Skills, 60: 427–437.

Linton, S.J., Melin, L. and Stjernlof, K. (1985) The effects of applied relaxation and operant activity training on chronic pain. Behav. Psychother., 13: 87–100.

Masek, B.J., Russo, D.C. and Varni, J.W. (1984) Behavioral approaches to the management of chronic pain in children. Pediatric Clin. North America (W.B. Saunders, Philadelphia), 31: 1113–1131.

Mayer, T.G., Gatchel, R.J., Kishino, N., Keeley, J., Mayer, H., Capra, P. and Mooney, M. (1986) A prospective short-term study of chronic low back pain utilizing novel objective functional measurement. Pain, 25: 53–68.

Miller, C. and LeLieuvre, R.B. (1982) A method to reduce chronic pain in elderly nursing home residents. Gerontolologist, 22: 314–317.

O'Brien, C.P. and Weisbrot, M.M. (1983) Behavioral and psychological components of pain management. In R.M. Brown, T.M. Pinkert and J.P. Ludford (Eds.), Contemporary Research in Pain and Analgesia, 1983, NIDA Research Monograph 45, Washington, DC.

Pilowsky, I. (1978) Psychodynamic aspects of the pain experience. In R.A. Sternbach (Ed.), The Psychology of Pain, Raven Press, New York, pp. 203–217.

Richter, I.L., McGrath, P.J., Humphreys, P.J., Goodman, J.T., Firestone, P. and Keene, D. (1986) Cognitive and relaxation treatment of paediatric migraine. Pain, 25: 195–203.

Roberts, A.H. and Reinhardt, L. (1980) The behavioral management of chronic pain: longterm followup with comparison groups. Pain, 8: 151–162.

Roy, R. (1984) Pain clinics: reassessment of objectives and outcomes. Arch. Phys. Med. Rehabil., 65: 448–451.

Sanders, S.H. (1983) Component analysis of a behavioral treatment program for chronic low-back pain. Behav. Ther., 14: 697–705.

Sarno, J.E. (1976) Chronic back pain and psychic conflict. Scand. J. Rehabil. Med., 8: 143–153.

Sorbi, M. and Tellegen, B. (1986) Differential effects of training in relaxation and stress-coping in patients with migraine. Headache, 26: 473–481.

Spitzer, W.O. (1986) Rapport du groupe de travail Quebecois sur les aspects cliniques des affections vertebrales chez les travailleurs. L'Institut de Recherce en Sante et en Securite du Quebec, Montreal, Canada.

Sternbach, R.A. (1983) Fundamentals of psychological methods in chronic pain. In J.J. Bonica, U. Lindblom and A. Iggo (Eds.), Advances in Pain Research and Therapy, Vol. 5, Raven Press, New York, pp. 777–780.

Sternbach, R.A. (1984) Recent advances in psychologic pain therapy. In C. Benedetti, C.R. Chapman and G. Moricca (Eds.), Advances in Pain Research and Therapy, Vol. 7, Raven Press, New York, pp. 251–255.

Sturgis, E.T., Schaefer, C.A. and Sikora, T.L. (1984) Pain center follow-up of treated and untreated patients. Arch. Phys. Med. Rehabil., 65: 301–303.

Syrjala, K.L. and Chapman, C.R. (1984) Measurement of clinical pain: review and integration of research findings. In C. Benedetti, C.R. Chapman, and G. Moricca (Eds.), Advances in Pain Research and Therapy, Vol. 7, Raven Press, New York, pp. 71–101.

Tan, S.-Y. (1982) Cognitive and cognitive-behavioral methods for pain control: a selective review. Pain, 12: 201–228.

Trifiletti, R.J. (1984) The psychological effectiveness of pain management procedures in the context of behavioral medicine and medical psychology. Genet. Psychol. Monogr., 109: 251–278.

Turk, D.C. and Flor, H. (1984) Etiological theories and treatments for chronic back pain. II. Psychological models and interventions. Pain, 19: 209–233.

Turk, D.C., Meichenbaum, D. and Genest, M. (1983) Pain and Behavioral Medicine: a Cognitive-Behavioral Perspective, Guilford, New York.

Turner, J.A. and Chapman, C.R. (1982a) Psychological interventions for chronic pain: a critical review. I. Relaxation training and biofeedback. Pain, 12: 1–21.

Turner, J.A. and Chapman, C.R. (1982b) Psychological interventions for chronic pain: a critical review. II. Operant conditioning, hypnosis, and cognitive-behavioral therapy. Pain, 12: 23–46.

Turner, J.A., and Romano, J.M. (1984) Evaluating psychologic interventions for chronic pain: issues and recent developments. In C. Benedetti, C.R. Chapman, and G. Moricca (Eds.), Advances in Pain Research and Therapy, Vol. 7, Raven Press, New York, pp. 257–296.

Wolf, S.L., Nacht, M. and Kelly, J.L. (1982) EMG feedback training during dynamic movement for low back pain patients. Behav. Ther., 13: 395–406.

Zitman, F.G. (1983) Biofeedback and chronic pain. In J.J. Bonica, U. Lindblom and A. Iggo (Eds.), Advances in Pain Research and Therapy, Vol. 5, Raven Press, New York, pp. 795–808.

R. Dubner, G.F. Gebhart & M.R. Bond (Eds.)
Proceedings of the Vth World Congress on Pain
© 1988 Elsevier Science Publishers BV (Biomedical Division)

CHAPTER 33

Effects of cognitive-behavioral therapy on rheumatoid arthritis pain behavior: one-year follow-up

Laurence A. Bradley[1], Larry D. Young[1], Karen O. Anderson[1], Robert A. Turner[2], Carlos A. Agudelo[2], Lisa K. McDaniel[1] and Elliott L. Semble[2]

Sections of [1]*Medical Psychology and* [2]*Rheumatology, Bowman Gray School of Medicine of Wake Forest University, Winston-Salem, NC 27103, USA*

Introduction

Several recent papers have described the effects of various psychological interventions upon the pain associated with rheumatoid arthritis (RA) and other rheumatic diseases (e.g., Achterberg et al., 1981; Burke et al., 1985; Lorig et al., 1985). These investigations have generally found that thermal biofeedback or other cognitive-behavioral therapies produced significant reductions in RA patients' pain reports, functional disabilities or joint involvement. Unfortunately, all of these studies have suffered from critical methodological difficulties such as reliance upon patients' self-reports of outcome or inadequate follow-up. Therefore, we designed a study that eliminated the methodological problems associated with previous efforts (Bradley et al., 1987). Patients who agreed to serve as subjects received appropriate medical therapy and were assigned randomly to one of three adjunct treatment conditions: (a) biofeedback-assisted, cognitive-behavioral group therapy; (b) structured group social support therapy; or (c) no adjunct treatment. Outcome was assessed at posttreatment and 6-month follow-up using several behavioral, physiological and cognitive-verbal assessment measures. This article reviews the major results of the posttreatment and 6-month follow-up assessments described by Bradley et al. (1987) and reports the results of the one-year follow-up assessment.

Methods

Design

The study represents a 3×4 repeated measures design with the between-subject factor of treatment condition (cognitive-behavioral, social support, no adjunct treatment control) and the within-subject factor of assessment period (pretreatment, posttreatment, 6-month follow-up, one-year follow-up).

Subjects

One hundred and sixty-nine patients with definite or classical RA were asked to serve as subjects. Sixty-eight patients provided informed consent and were randomly assigned to one of the three treatment conditions.

Fifty-three subjects (43 females, 10 males) com-

Correspondence: Laurence A. Bradley, Ph.D., Section on Medical Psychology, Bowman Gray School of Medicine of Wake Forest University, Winston-Salem, NC 27103, U.S.A.

pleted all of the treatments as well as the pre- and posttreatment assessments associated with the investigation. These included 17 subjects in the cognitive-behavioral treatment condition, 18 subjects in the social support condition, and 18 control subjects. Five (1 cognitive-behavioral, 1 social support, 3 control) of the 53 subjects did not complete all portions of the follow-up assessment; their data were not included in the statistical analyses.

The mean age of the 53 subjects who completed all of the treatments was 50.09 years (SD = 12.44); the average duration of disease was 11.49 years (SD = 11.41). The rheumatologists classified 5 subjects as ARA Functional Class I, 28 subjects as Functional Class II, and 20 subjects as Functional Class III.

Procedure

Subjects assigned to the cognitive-behavioral treatment condition received five individual sessions of thermal biofeedback training to promote increased peripheral skin temperature at their most painful joints. They also participated in ten small group meetings with family members or close friends which included education, relaxation training and instruction in behavioral goal-setting and use of self-rewards (for a full description see Bradley et al., 1984, 1985).

Subjects assigned to the social support treatment condition received fifteen sessions of structured social support in small group meetings with their family members or close friends. These meetings consisted of education, discussion of present coping strategies and encouragement to develop improved coping methods (Bradley et al., 1984, 1985).

Subjects assigned to the no adjunct treatment control condition had no contact with the Medical Psychology staff with the exception of that received by all subjects at each assessment period.

Dependent variables

Several self-report, behavioral and physiological measures were evaluated at each assessment period. The self-report variables included the Trait form of the State-Trait Anxiety Inventory (Spielberger et al., 1970), Depression Adjective Checklist (Lubin,

1967), 10 cm visual analogue scale ratings of pain intensity, the Arthritis Helplessness Index (Nicassio et al., 1985) and a modified Health Assessment Questionnaire (Pincus et al., 1983). The latter two measures assess the extent to which persons believe they can control their arthritis symptoms and participate in activities of daily living, respectively. A 5-point scale of disease activity level was also completed both by the subjects and by their attending rheumatologists or rheumatology nurses (who were blind concerning subjects' treatment condition assignments).

The behavioral variable consisted of a frequency count of seven pain behaviors (e.g., guarding, grimacing) displayed by subjects as they performed for video recording a standardized, 10-minute sequence of sitting, standing, walking and reclining maneuvers (Anderson et al., 1987).

The physiological variables consisted of subjects' rheumatoid factor titers and Westergren sedimentation rates, as well as the attending rheumatologists' or their nurses' evaluations of subjects' grip strengths and number of tender joints (articular index). These four variables in addition to the subjects' and rheumatologists' (or nurses') ratings of subjects' disease activity levels comprised the Rheumatoid Activity Index (RAI; Davis et al., 1977).

Statistical methods

All of the outcome measures were entered in separate 3 (Treatment Condition) × 3 (Assessment Period) repeated measures analyses of covariance in which the pretreatment value of each measure served as the covariate. One-tailed t-tests were used to perform comparisons among the treatment condition means on each outcome measure at posttreatment and at each follow-up assessment.

Results

Fig. 1 shows that the cognitive-behavioral subjects displayed significantly less pain behavior than the social support and control subjects only at posttreatment (P values <0.03).

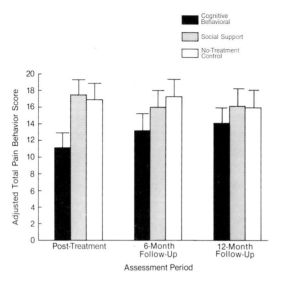

Fig. 1. Mean total pain behavior scores (± SEM) as a function of treatment condition and assessment period. Scores are adjusted to remove the effects of the pretreatment covariate.

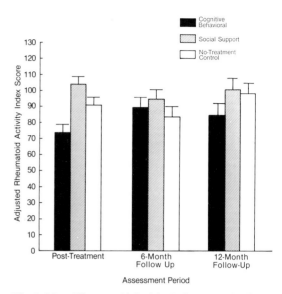

Fig. 3. Mean Rheumatoid Activity Index scores (± SEM) as a function of treatment condition and assessment period. Scores are adjusted to remove the effects of the pretreatment covariate.

Fig. 2. shows a nearly significant interaction between the independent variables ($F_{(4,90)} = 2.02$, $P < 0.10$) in which the cognitive-behavioral subjects produced significantly lower pain intensity ratings than the social support subjects at posttreat-

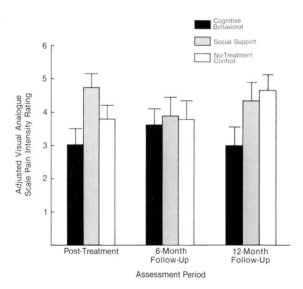

Fig. 2. Mean pain intensity ratings (± SEM) as a function of treatment condition and assessment period. Ratings are adjusted to remove the effects of the pretreatment covariate.

ment ($P < 0.005$) and the control subjects at the one-year follow-up ($P < 0.04$).

Fig. 3 illustrates a significant interaction on subjects' mean Rheumatoid Activity Index scores ($F_{(4,90)} = 5.30$, $P < 0.008$). The cognitive-behavioral subjects produced significantly lower RAI scores relative to the social support ($P < 0.001$) and control ($P < 0.02$) subjects only at posttreatment.

Fig. 4 shows that there was a nearly significant main effect of treatment condition on subjects' mean scores on the Trait Form of the State-Trait Anxiety Inventory ($F_{(2,46)} = 2.66$, $P < 0.09$). The cognitive-behavioral ($P < 0.03$) and social support ($P < 0.01$) subjects produced lower anxiety ratings than the control subjects at posttreatment. At the six-month follow-up, only the cognitive-behavioral subjects reported significantly lower anxiety levels than the controls ($P < 0.05$). However, there were no significant between-group differences at the one-year follow-up.

Fig. 5 illustrates a nearly significant main effect of treatment condition on subjects' mean Depression Adjective Checklist scores ($F_{(2,46)} = 2.80$, $P < 0.08$). The cognitive-behavioral subjects tended to report relatively low levels of depression at each assessment. However, their depression ratings were significantly lower than those of the social support ($P < 0.05$) and control ($P < 0.03$) subjects only at the one-year follow-up.

The analyses of covariance produced no significant findings on subjects' modified Health Assessment Questionnaire or Arthritis Helplessness Index scores. There were no between-group differences on these measures at any assessment period.

Discussion

The results of the present study demonstrated that a cognitive-behavioral therapy program produced significant reductions in patients' self-reports of pain intensity and depression relative to no adjunct treatment at a one-year follow-up assessment. The cognitive-behavioral subjects' significant reductions in pain behavior, disease activity and anxiety at posttreatment were not maintained at the one-year follow-up assessment. None of the reported findings was associated with systematic differences

among the treatment conditions in age, duration of disease, socioeconomic status, functional class, medication changes or initial treatment-related attitudes (Bradley et al., 1987).

The results of the present study raise three important issues. First, what factors might account for the cognitive-behavioral subjects' reductions in pain intensity and depression ratings at the one-year follow-up? Parker and his colleagues (1987) have reported findings similar to those of the current study and have attributed them to a cumulative benefit as patients consistently apply cognitive-behavioral coping strategies over time. We plan to examine this possibility by asking the cognitive-behavioral subjects to rate the degree to which they have continued to use relaxation and behavioral problem-solving strategies during the follow-up period.

The second issue concerns what factors might account for the cognitive-behavioral subjects' failure

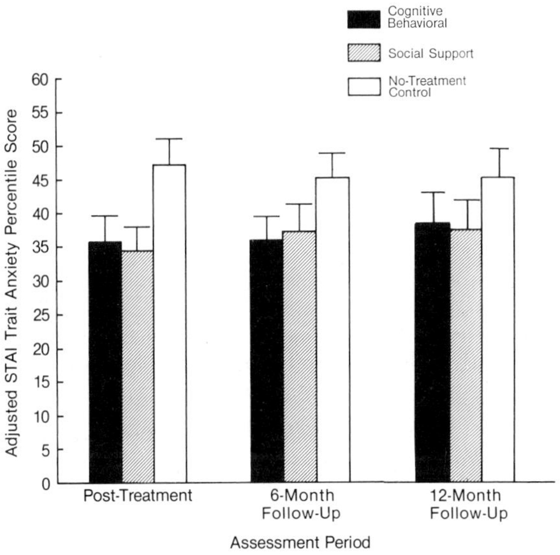

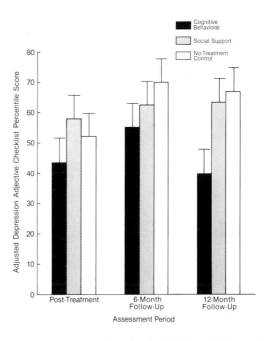

Fig. 4. Mean percentile scores ($\pm$ SEM) on the Trait form of the State-Trait Anxiety Inventory as a function of treatment condition and assessment period. Scores are adjusted to remove the effects of the pretreatment covariate.

Fig. 5. Mean percentile scores ($\pm$ SEM) on the Depression Adjective Checklist as a function of treatment condition and assessment period. Scores are adjusted to remove the effects of the pretreatment covariate.

to maintain their initial gains in pain behavior, disease activity and anxiety. Examination of the subjects' reports of their adherence with training strategies may also clarify this issue.

Finally, although the cognitive-behavioral subjects showed long-term improvements in subjective well-being, they did not show any improvement in functional disability. Future investigators should attempt to develop treatment protocols that emphasize strategies for improved functioning in activities of daily living as well as improved pain coping abilities.

In summary, this study demonstrated that cognitive-behavioral treatment produces short-term beneficial effects on patients' pain behavior, anxiety ratings and disease activity levels. It also provided the first evidence that improvements in self-reports of pain intensity and depression may be found at one year following treatment. We will attempt in future studies to identify factors associated with maintenance of treatment gains and to produce reductions in functional disability as well as in objective and subjective measures of pain.

Acknowledgement

Supported by Robert Wood Johnson Foundation Grant No. 8236 to L.A.B.

References

Achterberg, J., McGraw, P. and Lawlis, C.F. (1981) Rheumatoid arthritis: a study of relaxation and temperature biofeedback training as an adjunctive therapy. Biofeedback Self Regul., 6: 207–223.

Anderson, K.O., Bradley, L.A., McDaniel, L.K., Young, L.D., Turner, R.A., Agudelo, C.A., Keefe, F.J., Pisko, E.J., Snyder, R.M. and Semble, E.L. (1987) The assessment of pain in rheumatoid arthritis: validity of a behavioral observation method. Arthritis Rheum., 30: 36–43.

Bradley, L.A., Young, L.D., Anderson, K.O., McDaniel, L.K., Turner, R.A. and Agudelo, C.A. (1984) Psychological approaches to the management of arthritis pain. Soc. Sci. Med., 19: 1353–1360.

Bradley, L.A., Turner, R.A., Young, L.D., Agudelo, C.A., Anderson, K.O. and McDaniel, L.K. (1985) Effects of cognitive-behavioral therapy on pain behavior of rheumatoid arthritis (RA) patients: preliminary outcomes. Scand. J. Behav. Ther., 14: 51–64.

Bradley, L.A., Young, L.D., Anderson, K.O., Turner, R.A., Agudelo, C.A., McDaniel, L.K., Pisko, E.J., Semble, E.L. and Morgan, T.M. (1987) Effects of psychological therapy on pain behavior of rheumatoid arthritis patients: treatment outcome and six-month follow-up. Arthritis Rheum., 30: 1105–1114.

Burke, E.J., Hickling, E.J., Alfonso, M.-P. and Blanchard, E.B. (1985) The adjunctive use of biofeedback and relaxation training in the treatment for severe rheumatoid arthritis: a preliminary investigation. Clin. Biofeedback Health, 8: 28–36.

Davis, J.D., Turner, R.A., Collins, A., Ruchte, I.R. and Kaufman, J.S. (1977) Fenoprofen, aspirin, and gold induction in rheumatoid arthritis. Clin. Pharm. Ther., 21: 52–61.

Lorig, K., Lubeck, D., Kraines, R.G., Seleznick, M. and Holman, H.R. (1985) Outcomes of self-help education for patients with arthritis. Arthritis Rheum., 28: 680–685.

Lubin, B. (1967) Manual for the Depression Adjective Checklist, Educational and Industrial Testing Service, San Diego, CA.

Nicassio, P.M., Wallston, K.A., Callahan, L.F., Herbert, M. and Pincus, T. (1985) The measurement of helplessness in rheumatoid arthritis: the development of the Arthritis Helplessness Index. J. Rheumatol., 12: 462–467.

Parker, J.C., Frank, R.G., Beck, N.C., Smarr, K.L., Buescher, K.L., Phillips, L.R., Smith, E.I., Anderson, S.K. and Walker, S.E. (1987). Pain management in rheumatoid arthritis: a cognitive-behavioral approach. Unpublished manuscript, University of Missouri School of Medicine.

Pincus, T., Summey, J.A., Soraci, S.A., Wallston, K.A. and Hummon, N.P. (1983) Assessment of patient satisfaction in activities of daily living using a modified Stanford Health Assessment Questionnaire. Arthritis Rheum., 26: 1346–1353.

Spielberger, C.D., Gorsuch, R.L. and Lushene, R.R. (1970) Manual for the State-Trait Anxiety Inventory, Consulting Psychologists Press, Palo Alto, CA.

Wallston, B.S., Wallston, K.A., Kaplan, G.D. and Maides, S.A. (1976) Development and validation of the health locus of control scale. J. Consult. Clin. Psychol. 44: 580–585.

Pain in Children

R. Dubner, G.F. Gebhart & M.R. Bond (Eds.)
Proceedings of the Vth World Congress on Pain
© 1988 Elsevier Science Publishers BV (Biomedical Division)

CHAPTER 34

Age-related aspects of pain: pain in children

Kenneth D. Craig[1], Ruth V.E. Grunau[1,2] and Susan M. Branson[1]

[1]*Department of Psychology, University of British Columbia, and* [2]*British Columbia Children's Hospital, Vancouver, B.C.,*
Canada V6T 1Y7

Introduction

Children share the adult's capacity to experience pain and suffering, but this shared capability should not obscure qualitative differences that reflect children's biological and behavioural developmental status. When subjected to painful events, children have a considerable capacity to react with great distress which is visibly and vocally communicated to others. Nevertheless, they are biologically immature and do not have the history of accidents, diseases and pain inflicted upon them in social contexts that provide the adult with a means of interpreting what is happening to them. Our concern in this paper is with how infants and children subjectively experience and respond to noxious events in their world and the ways in which these capacities are influenced by and related to those of preceding and subsequent stages in development.

The challenge for adults is to understand just what it is that children are experiencing. Adults do not think and feel like children. We are relatively amnesic about how we experienced ourselves and the world as children. Freud coined the expression 'infantile amnesia' to characterize the almost total deficit in recall for early life experiences (Campbell and Coulter, 1976). Even when infants clearly display pain, the adult's capacity for comprehension and empathy probably does not grasp the qualities of the experience and there are risks of insensitivity and neglect. Thus, specialized training and assessment instruments are required to enable adults to discern those specific behavioural cues that signify pain in children. While there may be a generalized tendency to help children in distress, it is by no means universally displayed and it does not guarantee effective pain management. In some medical settings, it may be adaptive to suspend one's sensitivity to the distress children are experiencing in the interests of rational or mechanical delivery of care. Thus, caring for pain in children requires a special interest and effort.

Only recently has a systematic literature on pain in children become available. Clinicians and investigators have too often been misguided by beliefs that children do not experience pain as severely as adults, nor is its impact believed to persist as long as it does for adults (Eland and Anderson, 1977). These erroneous beliefs, together with an excessively conservative concern for the side-effects of analgesics, such as respiratory suppression and the potential for addiction, and another misconception that analgesics are metabolized differently in children (Schechter, et al., 1986), have led to systematic undermedication of infants and children in pain (Beyer et al., 1983; Jeans, 1983; Owens, 1984). Liebeskind and Melzack (1987) recently felt compelled

Correspondence: Dr. Kenneth D.Craig, Department of Psychology, University of British Columbia, Vancouver, B.C., Canada V6T 1Y7.

to observe: "We are appalled... by the fact that pain is most poorly managed in those most defenseless against it—the young and the elderly. Children often receive little or no treatment, even for extremely severe pain, because of the myth that they are less sensitive to pain than adults and more easily addicted to pain medication" (p. 1). There would seem to be a systematic bias toward underestimating the severity of pain children experience and acting accordingly. Recent findings (Anand et al., 1987), indicating that preterm babies given minimal anaesthesia during surgery mount much greater stress responses and have a poorer clinical outcome in terms of post-operative complications, as compared with babies given fentanyl analgesia, attest to the need to understand and recognize pain in young children.

Measurement and assessment of pain in children

Basing treatment of children on ill-founded supposition is partly a consequence of the limitations of existing measurement and assessment strategies (Beyer and Byers, 1985; Lavigne et al., 1986; McGrath, 1987; McGrath et al., 1987; Thompson and Varni, 1986). Children's capacities to introspect and to communicate qualities of subjective experiences emerge slowly, forcing clinicians and scientists to rely less on self-report and to be more dependent upon nonverbal channels of communication. Unless assessment instruments are developed which are sensitive to developmental differences, there is an increased risk of questionable inferences and unintentional mistreatment of children experiencing pain.

Indeed, one must question the conclusions of early studies, primarily because of the questionable methods used to assess pain in children. We note in particular that the distinction between acute and chronic pain is not clearly reflected in available assessment strategies for working with children. Most measures used with children have been specific to the severity of acute pain experienced during painful medical procedures. To apply the same measures to the complexities of chronic pain is particularly inadequate. This deficiency is reflected in the literature on arthritic pain in children. Physicians have reported that many children with juvenile rheumatoid arthritis (JRA) complain little of joint pain (Ansell, 1984; Cassidy, 1982). This paucity of complaint could be interpreted, mistakenly, as indicating that children actually experience little or no arthritic pain. Consistent with clinical impressions were two early studies of children with JRA that concluded that these children suffer less discomfort in affected joints than adults (Laaksonen and Laine, 1961; Scott et al., 1977). But, given limitations in the measure used (single administrations of unidimensional self-report scales that failed to consider developmental level), and the omission of statistical analyses (Laaksonen and Laine, 1961), the generalization made by these authors that children with JRA suffer minimally is overstated (Branson, 1987; Varni and Jay, 1984). Recent studies (Beales et al., 1983a,b; Thompson et al., 1987; Varni, et al., 1987) addressing methodological limitations of the earlier studies contradict the earlier reports. Beales et al. (1983a) reported that all the JRA children they studied reported uncomfortable joint sensations and endorsed the descriptor 'aching'. Older children were more likely to experience joint sensations as unpleasant and to give negatively evaluative descriptions of sensations (i.e., more likely to interpret them as pain). Varni et al. (1987) found that many of the children with JRA in their sample used descriptions such as sore, aching, uncomfortable or miserable to describe joint sensations experienced.

The criteria used to validate measures of pain must differ in children and adults. In pre-verbal children we will not be able to establish the concurrent validity of behavioural concomitants of pain as they relate to self-report of subjective experiences, as with adults, so it will be important to establish their predictive validity for unambiguously painful events. As children grow older they can provide information using self-report (e.g., free speech, facial expression matching, Visual Analogue Scales), which can be related to nonverbal expression (e.g., cry, facial activity, bodily movement), and physiological activity (e.g., autonomic activity, blood plasma levels). Systems for unobtrusive, naturalistic observation of children's verbal and nonverbal behaviour during painful events have been developed recently. We have used the approach to describe normal developmental processes (Grunau and Craig, 1987; Craig et al., 1984). Others have applied systematic behaviour-observation systems with success to the study of pediatric cancer patients who encounter painful medical procedures on a routine basis (e.g., Katz et al., 1980; Jay et al., 1983). These children regularly exhibit extreme anticipatory anxiety and behavioural distress.

Interview methods have recently demonstrated their power in the assessment and measurement of pain. Until recently, it was believed that children could not provide accurate information about their own pain experiences and coping abilities (Ross and Ross, 1984a). The interview has also allowed correction in the trend to assessing only childrens' distress reactions to pain, rather than their coping abilities (e.g., Gross et al., 1983; Jay et al., 1983). We now are becoming aware that children can exercise considerable skill in the use of behavioural and cognitive coping strategies to control distress.

There are many developmental issues requiring better measurement strategies. For example, do children engage in progressively more adaptive reactions as they grow older? Do the earlier patterns of response serve as "imperfect or nascent reflections of adult behavior" (Hall and Oppenheim, 1987)? Or, are some of the adaptations transient, serving to meet the needs of the moment and unnecessary for further development of the mature adult state, or do they always serve as building blocks for subsequent more satisfactory adaptations? For example, unchecked anger is conspicuous and commonplace in the response of young children subjected to routine, but painful, medical procedures (Izard et al., 1983). One can appreciate its functional role in restraining others, children and adults, responsible for the noxious assault. Does anger remain a universal, predominant affective response to pain in adults? If so, why is it not conspicuous? Does the mature adult no longer require anger to

control what is happening during painful events? Hall and Oppenheim (1987) conclude that of the major conceptualizations of ontogeny, the theoretical perspective "that the pathway from the embryo to the adult is seldom... straightforward" is gaining ascendancy. Thus, while there may be some continuity in development so that some patterns of atypical pain response will have their origins in childhood, certain patterns of response may be uniquely characteristic of a particular developmental level, not persisting thereafter.

The constraint of biological maturation

The experience and expression of pain in children is constrained by the organization and ontogeny of biological systems mediating the processes. One would expect a universal unfolding of specific patterns of behaviour. To capture the causal biological determinants in the broadest sense, one would have to work through numerous levels of analysis (e.g., genetic, biochemical, histological, anatomical, physiological) and understand the role of interactions of all of these with other endogenous and exogenous factors during the various stages of ontogeny. Despite the complexity of this task some insights are available.

From the broad perspective of evolutionary theory, behavioural reactions to noxious events can be constructed as adaptations with survival value. At birth, in utero protection disappears and the neonate may encounter harsh challenges, without the response repertoire that maturity will provide to meet demands. Survival depends upon utilization of those meager behavioural and physiological strategies available to immature biological systems, and the caring skills of adults. The challenge to the caretaking adult is often to decipher the significance of the child's behaviour. Success in accomplishing this would mean fulfillment of a special psychobiological interdependency between children and adults. If expressions of pain are available to children because of their communicative value, adults would also be fulfilling fundamental biological roles in serving as caretakers for children and alleviating their distress.

Attention on pain in infancy focussed initially on the possibility that infants were relatively insensitive to pain (McGraw, 1945). Sensory deficits could be the result of immaturity of the neural substrates for afferent input of noxious events, either peripheral or central, or the sensory response could be attenuated by positive inhibitory or suppressive mechanisms. A possible biological mechanism for the former exists because there continues to be myelinization of nerve fibers after birth. However, myelinization is not necessary for neural conductivity. Mechanisms for suppression of pain could be available during birth as a result of the substantial mechanical stimulation, endocrine changes and physiological demands encountered at this time. However, there are conceptual problems. It is difficult to imagine the research design necessary to demonstrate insensitivity to pain in the newborn. What are the suitable comparisons? Older children? What time frame could be selected (because biological development is dramatic at this time)? There are also some conceptual problems with the conclusion that it would be adaptive for newborns to be insensitive to pain. If the newborn child were to be seen as totally defenceless in the face of the abrupt transition of birth, or the 'birth trauma', insensitivity would be adaptive. However, would it be adaptive for the newborn to be insensitive to the striking physical demands of the extrauterine environment and not to signal their impact to caretakers at this time? In agreement with Owens (1984), we would argue that the data available from direct behavioural observation of infants exposed to noxious events directly after birth constitute ample evidence that they experience pain.

Studies in the field of developmental psychobiology (Hall and Oppenheim, 1987) of fetal sensory capabilities do not support the concept of an absence of nociceptive sensory systems at birth. Gottlieb (1976) characterizes the rate of sensory development in the human fetus as early and accelerated, relative to other species. He also notes that, in humans, all sensory systems are capable of functioning prior to birth. Cutaneous (somesthetic) sensitivities are the first among the sensory modalities to emerge in the course of fetal development (Gottlieb, 1971; Oppenheim, 1982). The evidence is largely restricted to touch and heat sensitivity, but one would expect the anatomical basis of nociception to be present. However, it seems unlikely that the intrauterine environment would provide the necessary stimulation for pain prior to birth, as would be the case for touch, or other sensory modalities, hence nociceptive systems may not become activated until birth. Demonstrating the presence of prenatal pain would be problematic, as it extends the question of whether infants experience pain to an even earlier stage of life.

Given the likelihood that sensory systems for nociception are functional at birth and infants can and do experience noxious assault, one must consider the possibility that motoric systems do not respond in a manner that would signal pain clearly to adults. While infants have a remarkably restricted response repertoire, we know that many complex motoric response systems are present prior to and at birth (Gottlieb, 1976). It is noteworthy that our appreciation of the nature of early infancy is changing. There is a growing recognition that infants display substantially greater complexity in their capacity to perceive and interact with their environment than was previously believed to be the case (Hay, 1986; Stratton, 1982). But we have only recognized these capabilities by developing measurement systems which are responsive to the limited motoric repertoire of the infant. Given the potential significance to the infant of being able to communicate threats to survival posed by injuries or the abrupt onset of disease states, one would expect activity signalling pain at this time. However, humans have been characterized as motorically immature and highly dependent upon caretaking by adults, or as displaying the altricial pattern of motor development (Gottlieb, 1971). If sensory systems are well developed in humans (as in other primates), but motoric systems are not, it may be that expressions of distress, physical and otherwise, are not well-differentiated. This is the case with cry—adults have difficulty distinguishing among hunger, fatigue, pain, and cries signalling other sources of distress, although parents seem to be astute in making distinctions. It may be that special interest and prolonged exposure do permit astute discriminations. One can conclude that it is the severely restricted response repertoire for signalling differentiated subjective states that makes it difficult for adults to recognize and understand subjective states of pain in infants. We need to develop better measures of the natural response repertoires of infants (Grunau and Craig, 1987; Johnston and Strada, 1986; Owens and Todt, 1984).

Our understanding of pain in infancy is of considerable practical importance. Recognizing pain is imperative if the physiological sequelae are to be prevented and the pain reduced or eliminated. We have encountered this most dramatically with low-birth-weight, high-risk infants whose biological immaturity and requirements for continual monitoring and health maintenance lead to frequent physically intrusive procedures. Nurses attending these tiny newborns must recognize and respond to implicit signs of pain to avoid precipitous biological collapse. In our studies (unpublished) of nurses' judgments of pain in low-birth-weight infants, they have described gross bodily movement (squirming, restlessness, agitation, irritability), body tension (arching, pushing away, pulling away, jerks, curling up), limb activity (thrashing, drawing up of the knees, clenching fists or feet, tensing the limbs), facial activity (grimaces, closing eyes tightly), crying (although difficult to recognize with respirators) and physiological signs (hypoxia, tachyapnea, respiratory changes, colour changes to duskiness, increased blood pressure, tachycardia, bradycardia, etc.) as important. These nurses are clearly sensitive to a remarkably broad range of signs of pain available in infants, but systematic development of standardized assessment systems is needed.

In our programme of research with healthy newborns (Grunau and Craig, 1987) we have considered the capacities of infants to respond to painful insult by contrasting the differing viewpoints on the one hand that newborns are capable of little more than reflexive responsivity to noxious assault, and,

on the other, that their reactions reflect complex neural organization, with variations in sleeping and waking biological rhythms modulating the impact of noxious events. The former would suggest a relatively exclusive role for spinal mechanisms, whereas the latter would implicate the participation of brain systems. We examined newborn infants' facial expressions and cries during routine heel-punctures designed to provide blood samples for the screening of metabolic diseases. If pain reactions at birth were wholly reflexive, there would be no variation in pain expression as a function of different sleep/waking states. If variations were to be observed, then the biological mechanisms that modulate pain in adults would be evident even at this earliest stage of life.

Our findings indicated that pain expression in infants did vary contingent upon the infant's sleep/waking state prior to the heel stick. Facial expressions provided the key to assessing the pain, a finding consistent with the importance of facial cues to parents. In contrast, cry did not. The infants displayed facial grimaces which differed from their reactions to having their heels cleansed and rubbed in preparation for the heel stick. The facial expressions were not dissimilar to those observed in adults (Craig and Patrick, 1984). As you would expect, infants who were awake displayed greater reactivity. However, the amount of activity was not a linear correlate of arousal. It was the infants who were awake, but inactive, and apparently attentive, who displayed the strongest pattern of reaction. This would be consistent with Brazelton's view of the alert awake state as providing optimal receptivity to environmental input (1983). The modulation of reactivity to noxious stimuli by these endogenous sleep/waking and activity states indicates the complexity and importance of the neurobiological systems regulating pain even at birth.

The similarities between the pattern of facial behaviour observed in neonates by Grunau and Craig (1987) and the facial grimaces of adults in pain (Craig and Patrick, 1984; Patrick et al., 1986) suggests that pain is organized structurally and temporally in infants in a manner strongly resembling that in adults. Thus, there appear to be stereotyped, temporally integrated patterns of response to painful assault available from birth. Other investigators have noted the potential benefits of close attention to features of facial expression during pain in infants (Owens, 1984; Johnston and Strada, 1986). We have noted that facial activity during infant pain was associated with perinatal events, including obstetric medication (Grunau and Craig, 1987). The presence of early facial behaviour patterns would have an adaptive significance. Humans at birth are motorically immature and highly dependent on maternal care for a prolonged period after birth, and thus must have effective signal systems which elicit caretaking and protection from adults (Murray, 1979).

Neurophysiological maturation and related behavioural complexity develop rapidly after birth. The patterns of pain-related activity observed above appear 'hard-wired', but solutions to the demands of a potentially harsh environment require learned adaptations and independence from succorant parents. With maturation comes the potential for more sophisticated patterns of reponse to threatening events. Social demands would begin to have an impact. Patterns of response which were once deemed satisfactory by parents would come to be seen as immature and inappropriate. Parents and other members of the family and culture would endeavour to shape the child's responses. Learned patterns of response to painful events would become superimposed on the early patterns (Craig, 1986).

In our programme of research, we have observed progressive changes as behavioural expression during noxious events transforms from global, spontaneous, nondifferentiating reaction patterns to more sophisticated behaviour disclosing anticipation, goal-directed movement and efforts to engage adult intervention. We have observed this most clearly in the transformations to be observed over the first two years of life in children's reactions to the needle stab and injection into the upper arm during routine immunization (Craig et al., 1984). Despite considerable variation in how the babies reacted, we found infants in the first year of life to cry and scream for longer periods of time, and to display a more global diffuse reaction pattern, in contrast to infants in the second year of life. The latter displayed anticipatory distress, addressed what was happening to them verbally, visually tracked the nurse who was about to hurt them, and attempted to withdraw or protect themselves. In this second year of life, children also begin to use words to describe pain.

Systematic observation of childrens's reactions to the pain inflicted by abrupt medical and dental procedures has been highly instructive about the complexity of the emotional and behavioural pain response and importance of the social context. Izard and his colleagues (Izard et al., 1983) examined infants' reactions to needle injections and demonstrated transformations in the emotional responsivity of infants as they became more socially responsive. The penetration of the needle primarily reflected pain in infants less than 4.4 months of age, but, as the children grew older, the expression of pain became less prominent, with facial expressions of anger predominating at 19 months.

Sensitivity of young children to the immediate social context has been studied by examining the effect of mother-child interactions on the behavior of children experiencing a diagnostic medical procedure (Gross et al., 1983). Mothers who become more anxious in these settings have children who display more behavioural distress (e.g., Johnson and Baldwin, 1968; Jay et al., 1983). From a behavioural perspective, the mothers' expressions of distress in that setting would serve as discriminative stimuli for the child's distress and pain behaviour, with this, in turn, serving to solicit attention, sympathy and interventions on the child's behalf. Solicitous reactions by spouses have been shown to increase pain behaviours and subjective pain intensity in adults (Turk et al., 1987). Findings on the impact of mother presence on children's distress have been equivocal (Jay et al., 1983), but in some circumstances mothers increase manifest signs of distress. The reciprocal dependence between children and their parents was apparent in our studies of children's reactions to needle injections (Craig et al., 1984), as mothers reacted in a variable manner contingent upon the child's age. While the mothers invariably comforted their children, both vocally and physically, they used verbal soothing and physical distraction sooner with the younger children. Izard et al. (1983) noted that the children who were more difficult to soothe were the ones who tended to show greater durations of anger expression.

The constraints of psychological development

Progressively more skilled patterns of interaction between the child and the social environment become apparent during the early childhood years. Children must learn to recognize potentially destructive biological events and to communicate their subjective appreciation of bodily states in a manner that will capture the attention of adults. They must do this in a manner that is socially appropriate, hence familial and cultural models for pain expression are important (Craig, 1986).

The role of psychological factors first becomes manifest when the effects of early experience persist. Learning appears to be first expressed in the form of conditioned fear. At seven or eight months, children first come to appreciate that certain settings (clinics, hospitals, etc.) and people (doctors, nurses, etc.) signal imminent pain, and react accordingly. The expression of acute distress, crying included, would be expected to have a substantial impact on adult caretakers. In this first year of life, the emotional states of both fear and anger come to coincide with pain and represent additional learned modifications of behaviour.

Behavioural changes

Developmental trends have been observed in behavioural reactions to medical and dental diagnostic and treatment procedures. In general, age has been negatively correlated with behavioural distress during medical and dental procedures (c.f., Jay et al., 1983). For example, Katz et al. (1980) examined specific behavioural reactions to bone marrow aspirations in pediatric cancer patients using a beha-

vioural observation scale. Behavioural reactions were interpreted as signifying anxiety, although they may also refect the painful impact of the procedure (Katz et al., 1981). The younger children displayed more overt signs of distress. Jay et al. (1983) similarly found the younger children to "exhibit their distress in more intense, overt, and motoric modes than older children" (p. 143). A significant drop in behavioural distress at about 7 years of age corresponds with the onset of the Piagetian stage of concrete operational thinking. These investigators believe that once children are able to understand why they have to undergo painful procedures they are more likely to cooperate, thus linking behavioural changes to cognitive changes. It would seem inappropriate to interpret these findings as indicating that the younger children were experiencing dramatically greater distress. Alternatively, it may be that older children suffer as severely, but do not display their distress in public or in the specific behaviours assessed using particular methods. LeBaron and Zeltzer (1984) adapted Katz et al.'s (1981) behavioural check list by adding 'flinching' and 'groaning' as categories for behavioural coders to note. These occurred significantly more often with adolescents than younger children, confirming that adolescents display distress differently, and that judgments as to the severity of distress experienced are subject to method errors.

Cognitive changes

The importance of cognitive processes becomes apparent as the child displays anticipation and memory of painful events and settings. Further cognitive development moves in the direction of greater cognitive complexity, allowing a more sophisticated conceptualization of illness and pain. This permits a greater ability to understand painful medical procedures and to engage in self-control (Maddux et al., 1986). Language becomes a more sophisticated tool for conceptualizing experiences and securing adult intervention. For those studying pain in childhood, it similarly provides a superior vehicle for discovering how children conceptualize and cope with pain.

Developmental trends in children's concepts and understanding of illness and pain are beginning to be understood (Lavigne et al., 1986); Thompson and Varni, 1986). Willis et al. (1982) noted that the motivational-affective, cognitive-evaluative and sensory-discriminative components of pain described by Melzack and Casey (1968) would be expected to undergo maturational change. Gaffney and Dunne (1986) documented changes which would be predicted from the multidimensional formulations. A large sample (680) of Irish schoolchildren were categorized into three age groups corresponding to the Piagetian stages of pre-operational (5–7 years), concrete operational (8 – 10 years) and formal operational thinking (11 – 14 years). Definitions of pain provided by the youngest group focussed upon perceptually dominant, physical factors. The slightly older children began to use physical analogies to describe pain, and demonstrated a developing awareness of the psychological concomitants of pain (e.g., its ability to affect the mood of the sufferer). Finally, children in the oldest age group gave definitions of pain which included both a physical and a psychological component. This latter group viewed pain more actively; they tended to define pain as something which has to be dealt with, or borne stoically.

These findings of developmental changes in definitions of pain stand in contrast to an absence of developmental trends in findings by Ross and Ross (1984), who also conducted a large-scale interview study ($n = 994$) with children aged 5 – 12 years. The different conclusion may be related to the specificity of the questions asked. Ross and Ross (1984) focussed on more concrete events and the children could respond objectively, thereby apparently eliminating the more abstract constructs cognitive maturity provides.

In a study of a clinical sample, Beales et al. (1983a) noted that in contrast to 6 – 11-year-olds, 12 – 17-year-olds with JRA universally reported negatively evaluative interpretations of joint sensations, with the sensations reminding them of their disability condition. Beales and his associates (1983) found that older children had become cap-

able of thoughts dwelling upon the unpleasant implications of their chronic arthritic disorder. For example, a 15-year-old girl with JRA stated: "I hate it when it hurts like that, because it reminds me of all the things I can't do" (p. 63). With development of an increased capacity for abstract reasoning, children become more capable of experiencing illness-related pessimistic thoughts.

One cannot consider childrens' concepts of pain in isolation from their understanding of illness in general. The Piagetian developmental sequence has provided the theoretical basis for most work in this area (Brewster, 1982; Perrin and Gerrity, 1981; Whitt et al., 1979). For example, Bibace and Walsh (1979) have proposed 6 stages in childrens' causal explanations of illness. At what were labelled the 'phenomenistic' and 'contagion' states, corresponding to preoperational thought, children were seen as giving magical explanations (e.g., "The sun made me sick") or explanations based on physical proximity. At the 'contamination' stage, that of concrete operational thought, multiple concrete, external causes were mentioned. At the 'internalization' stage, corresponding to more advanced concrete operational thought, causal explanations of illness became located inside the body. Finally, at the 'physiological' and 'psychophysiological' stages, corresponding to the attainment of formal operations, children gave multiple causal explanations of illness, both concrete and abstract, and included the role of the individual's behaviour, thoughts and feelings in contributing to health. In other words, with increasing cognitive complexity, children's understanding progressed from a view that illness is caused by external, magical factors, to a perspective that incorporated not only external factors but also personal control in determining health status.

Just as important as developmental trends in concepts of pain and illness are those relating to healing and the purposes of medical procedures. Neuhauser et al. (1978) found that personal control was increasingly prominent in causal explanations of healing as children grow older. Brewster (1982) identified three developmental stages in the thinking of chronically ill children about the intent of medical procedures. In the first, children tended to view procedures as punishment. In the second, they were correctly perceived, but the children expressed a belief that empathy from the staff depended upon the expression of pain. In the third stage, children correctly inferred both intent of the medical procedure and unconditional empathy from the medical staff. Related findings were provided by Beales et al. (1983b) to the effect that younger children (aged 7 – 11) with juvenile rheumatoid arthritis had little appreciation that painful treatments would have long-term benefits. In fact, 38% of these children believed physiotherapy made their arthritis worse, since moving inflamed joints creates discomfort. Older children (12–17) recognized the benefits, even believing that treatment needs to be unpleasant to be effective.

Recent studies examining children's coping mechanisms have attempted to describe the normal developmental process as well as the coping strategies and processes of children who do not cope well with their disorders and pain. Children report an awareness of strategies for coping with pain and willingly describe them, although direct questioning may be necessary to elicit them, a procedure that risks imposing suggestions on the children (Ross and Ross, 1984b).

In general, younger children report using behavioural strategies (Abu-Saad, 1984; Savedra et al., 1981, 1982; Tesler et al., 1981) such as information-seeking, refusal to cooperate, taking medication, attempting to relax or rest, or seeking the presence or attentions of others. Younger children tend to favour direct physical action and behavioral strategies (Jeans, 1983; Reissland, 1983; Curry and Russ, 1985). Behavioral strategies which involve seeking the intervention of others make sense for younger children because they are vulnerable; they do not have the many resources available to adults. But with increasing maturity and cognitive complexity, children seem able to add a repertoire of cognitive strategies for coping with pain and are no longer heavily dependent upon behavioural strategies (Branson, 1987). Older children appear more inclined to report cognitive strategies such as distrac-

tion, fantasy, relaxing imagery or thought-stopping (Brown et al., 1986; Curry and Russ, 1985), although as noted previously Ross and Ross (1984b) found the question format important and did not report developmental trends. Branson (1987) found that childrens's use of behavioural strategies did not decline with age, but, because there was an increase in cognitive strategies, the relative proportion of behavioural strategies children used declined with age.

As children grow older they display a greater sense of control over pain (Reissland, 1983), perhaps as a result of a greater number of coping strategies, a history of success in their application, and an increase in awareness of their own psychological processes.

Many of the strategies children use would seem to have been supplied by other people, whereas others appear to be well-ingrained and self-initiated (Jerrett, 1985; Unruh et al., 1983). Abu-Saads's (1984) observation that children's coping strategies are consistent with cultural attitudes towards illness (e.g., Asian-American children reported the use of Chinese medicine) illustrates the origins of strategies in social learning (Craig, 1986).

It would be of considerable interest to pursue exploration of the strategies children use to cope with specific painful disorders. For example, Ross and Ross (1984a) provide the interesting observation that the coping strategies of a group of children with arthritis included "knowing the physical pain-free limits, keeping within them, and refusing to allow oneself to become depressed about the limitations of activity" (p. 187).

Interesting contrasts have been made between children who have adapted well to acute or chronic pain and children who have difficulties coping with pain-producing situations (e.g., children who became more anxious during painful medical procedures or children for whom pain interferes with an excess of daily activities (Branson, 1987; Brown et al., 1986; Hunt et al., 1985)). Initial research with the latter group of children supports the view that, like adults (Reesor and Craig, 1988), they appraise somatic symptoms and pain in a manner that is self-alarming. This pattern, currently characterized as catastrophizing, includes preoccupation with pain, desperate but ineffective thoughts of escape, fear of unlikely consequences, and pessimism. It is noteworthy that Brown et al. (1986) did not find an increase in frequency of reported 'catastrophizing' thoughts with age in physically healthy children who imagined themselves undergoing dental work. Indeed, children reported relatively more coping thoughts as they grew older.

Children who could be characterized as 'catastrophizers', in terms of the self-reported thoughts dominating their reactions to stressful events, tend to differ from children who cope well, in a variety of respects. Brown et al. (1986) found the former to display greater trait anxiety. Hunt-Fitzgerald and Liddell (1985) found that children whose thoughts about dental situations were dominated by negative self-statements also self-reported higher dental anxiety. These studies were based exclusively on self-report measures so the relationships need to be confirmed with alternative methodologies.

Age-specific pain

As with adults, one can usefully discriminate among acute, recurrent and chronic pain disorders in children. Varni (1983) has provided an extensive review and description of the assessment and management of pediatric pain as it relates to specific disorders. While overlap occurs, certain commonplace adult disorders are infrequently observed in children (e.g., chronic low back pain), whereas certain complaints are associated with childhood (e.g., juvenile rheumatoid arthritis, recurrent abdominal pain, specific headache disorders, aching limbs). McGrath has recently reviewed these disorders (1987). One must also consider the diagnostic and treatment procedures for diseases unique to children which exacerbate the pain and distress inherent in the diseases themselves. Management of these painful conditions requires attention to the unique qualities of childhood, as well as the familial and social environments that are so important as determinants of illness and well behaviour.

Conclusion

While substantial progress has been achieved in our understanding of pain in children, substantial work remains to be done on the characteristics and organization of pain as it relates to other patterns of behaviour and various intrinsic and extrinsic events at various stages of development. We have only begun to systematically examine pain experiences and coping strategies characteristic of children of different ages at different levels of cognitive complexity and emotional development. The need and opportunities are there for the contributions of a broad range of scientists and professionals, ranging from ecologists and social behaviourists to geneticists and neurobiologists.

References

Abu-Saad, H. (1984) Cultural components of pain: the Asian-American child. Child. Health Care, 13: 11–14.

Anand, K.J.S., Sippell, W.G. and Aynsley-Green, A. (1987) Randomised trial of fentanyl anaesthesia in preterm babies undergoing surgery: effects of the stress response. Lancet, i: 62–66.

Ansell, B.M. (1984) Problems of assessing pain in juvenile arthritis. In R. Rizzi and M. Visentin (Eds.), Pain: Proceedings of the Joint Meeting of the European Chapters of the International Association for the Study of Pain, Abano, Terme, May, 1983, Piccin/Butterworth.

Beales, J.G., Keen, J.H. and Lennox Holt, P.J. (1983a) The child's perception of the disease and the experience of pain in juvenile chronic arthritis. Rheumatol., 10: 61–65.

Beales, J.G., Lennox Holt, P.J., Keen, J.H. and Mellor, V.P. (1983b) Children with juvenile chronic arthritis: Rheum. Dis., 42: 481–486.

Beyer, J.E. and Byers, H.L. (1985) Knowledge of pediatric pain: the state of the art. Child. Health Care, 13: 150–159.

Beyer, J.E., DeGood, D.E., Ashley, L.D. and Russell, G.A. (1983) Patterns of postoperative analgesic use with adults and children following cardiac surgery. Pain, 17: 71–811.

Bibace, R. and Walsh, M.E. (1979) Developmental stages in children's conceptions of illness. In G.C. Stone, F. Cohen and N.E. Adler (Eds.), Health Psychology, Jossey-Bass, San Francisco, pp. 285–301.

Branson, S.M. (1987) An analysis of the pain experience and spontaneous coping abilities of children and adolescents with arthritis. Unpublished Master's thesis, University of British Columbia.

Brazelton, T.B. (1983) Precursors for the development of emotions in early infancy. In R. Plutchik and H. Kellerman (Eds.), Emotion: Theory, Research and Experience, Vol. 2, Academic Press, New York, pp. 35–55.

Brewster, A.B. (1982) Chronically ill hospitalized children's concepts of their illness. Pediatrics, 69: 355–362.

Brown, J.M., O'Keefe, J., Sanders, S.H. and Baker, B. (1986) Developmental changes in children's cognition to stressful and painful situations. J. Pediatr. Psychol., 11: 343–357.

Campbell, B.A. and Coulter, X. (1976) The ontogenesis of learning and memory. In M.R. Rosenzweig and E.G. Bennett (Eds.), Neural Mechanisms of Learning and Memory, MIT Press, Cambridge, MA, pp. 209–235.

Cassidy, J.T. (1982) Juvenile rheumatoid arthritis. In J.T. Cassidy (Eds.), Textbook of Pediatric Rheumatology, Wiley, New York, pp. 169–282.

Craig, K.D. (1986) Pain in context: Social modeling influences. In R.A. Sternbach (Ed.), The Psychology of Pain, 2nd Edn., Raven Press, New York. pp. 67–96.

Craig, K.D. and Patrick, C.J. (1984) Facial expression during induced pain. J. Pers. Soc. Psychol., 48: 1089–1091.

Craig, K.D., McMahon, R.J., Morison, J.D. and Zaskow, C. (1984) Development changes in infant pain expression during immunization injections. Soc. Sci. Med., 19: 1331–1337.

Curry, S.L. and Russ, S.W. (1985) Identifying coping strategies in children. J. Clin. Child Psychol., 14: 61–69.

Eland, J.M. and Anderson, J.E. (1977) The experience of pain in children. In A. Jacox (Ed.), Pain: A Sourcebook for Nurses and Other Professionals, Little, Brown, Boston.

Gaffney, A. and Dunne, E.A. (1986) Developmental aspects of children's definitions of pain. Pain, 26: 105–117.

Gottlieb, G. (1971) Ontogenesis of sensory function in birds and mammals. In E. Tobach, L. Avonson and E. Shaw (Eds.), The Biopsychology of Development, Academic Press, New York, pp. 67–128.

Gottlieb, G. (1976) Conceptions of prenatal development. Psychol. Rev., 83: 215–234.

Gross, A.M., Stern, R.M., Levin, R.B., Dale, J. and Wojnilower, D.A. (1983) The effect of mother-child separation on the behaviour of children experiencing a diagnostic medical procedure. J. Consult. Clin. Psychol., 51: 783–785.

Grunau, R.V.E. and Craig, K.D. (1987) Pain expression in neonates: facial action and cry. Pain, 28: 395–410.

Hay, D.F. (1986) Infancy. Annu. Rev. Psychol., 37: 135–161.

Hunt-Fitzgerald, G. and Liddell, A. (1985) An analysis of children's self-talk while imagining situations related to a dental visit. Poster presented at the annual convention of the Association for the Advancement of Behavior Therapy, Houston, TX.

Hall, W.G. and Oppenheim, R.W. (1987) Developmental psychobiology: Prenatal, perinatal and early postnatal aspects of behavioral development. In M.R. Rosenzweig and L.W. Porter (Eds), Annual Review of Psychology, Vol. 38, Annual Reviews, Inc., Palo Alto, CA., pp. 91–128.

Izard, C.E., Hembree, E.A., Dougherty, L.M. and Spizzirri, C.C. (1983) Changes in facial expressions of 2 to 19 month old infants following acute pain. Dev. Psychol., 19: 418–426.

Jay, S.M., Ozolins, M., Elliott, C.H. and Caldwell, S. (1983) Assessment of children's distress during painful medical procedures. Health Psychol., 2: 133–148.

Jeans, M.E. (1983) Pain in children — a neglected area. In P. Firestone, P. McGrath and W. Feldman (Eds.), Advances in Behavioral Medicine with Children and Youth, Lawrence Erlbaum, Hillsdale, NJ.

Jerrett, M.D. (1985) Children and their pain experience. Child. Health Care, 14: 83–89.

Johnson, R. and Baldwin, D.C. (1968) Relationship of maternal anxiety to the behavior of young children undergoing dental extraction. J. Dent. Res., 47: 801–805.

Johnstone, C.C. and Strada, M.E. (1986) Acute pain response in infants: A multidimensional description. Pain, 24: 373–382.

Katz, E.R., Kellerman, J. and Siegel, D.E. (1980) Behavioral distress in children with cancer undergoing medical procedures: developmental considerations. J. Consult. Clin. Psychol., 48: 356–365.

Katz, E.R., Kellerman, J. and Siegel, D.E. (1981) Anxiety as an effective focus in the clinical study of acute behavioral distress. J. Consult. Clin. Psychol., 49: 470–471.

Laaksonen, A.L. and Laine, V. (1961) A comparative study of joint pain in adult and juvenile rheumatoid arthritis. Ann. Rheum. Dis., 20: 386–387.

Lavigne, J.V., Schulein, M.J. and Hahn, Y.S. (1986) Psychological aspects of painful medical conditions in children. I. Developmental aspects and assessment. Pain, 27: 133–146.

LeBaron, S. and Zeltzer, L. (1984) Assessment of acute pain and anxiety in children and adolescents by self-reports, observer reports, and a behavior checklist. J. Consult. Clin. Psychol., 52: 729–738.

Liebeskind, J.C. and Melzack, R. (1987) The International Pain Foundation: meeting a need for education in pain management. Pain, 30: 1.

Maddux, J.E., Roberts, M.C., Sledden, E.A. and Wright, L. (1986) Development issues in child health psychology. Am. Psychol., 41: 25–34.

McGrath, P.A. (1987) The management of chronic pain in children. In G.D. Burrows, D. Elton and G. Stanley (Eds.), Handbook of Chronic Pain Management, Elsevier, Amsterdam.

McGrath, P.A., deVeber, L.L. and Hearn, M.T. (1985) Multidimensional pain assessment in children. In H.L. Fields et al. (Eds), Advances in Pain Research and Therapy, Raven Press, New York, pp. 387–393.

McGrath, P.J., Cunningham, S.J., Goodman, J.T. and Unruh, A. (1987) The clinical measurement of pain in children: A review. Clin. J. Pain, 2: 85–90.

McGraw, M.B. (1945) The Neuromuscular Maturation of the Human Infant, Hafner, New York.

Melzack, R. and Casey, K.L. (1968) Sensory, motivational, and central control determinants of pain: A new conceptual model. In D. Kenshalo (Ed.), The Skin Senses, Thomas, Springfield, IL.

Murray, A.D. (1979) Infant crying as an elicitor of parental behavior: an examination of two models. Psychol. Bull., 86: 191–215.

Neuhauser, C., Amsterdam, B., Hines, P. and Steward, M. (1978) Children's conceptions of healing: Cognitive development and locus of control. Am. J. Orthopsychiatry, 48: 334–341.

Oppenheim, R.W. (1982) The neuroembryological study of behavior: progress, problems, perspectives. Curr. Top. Dev. Biol., 17: 257–309.

Owens, M.E. (1984) Pain in infancy: conceptual and methodological issues. Pain, 20: 213–230.

Owens, M.E. and Todt, E.H. (1984) Pain in infancy: neonatal reaction to a heel lance. Pain, 20: 77–86.

Patrick, C.J., Craig, K.D. and Prkachin, K.M. (1986) Observer judgments of acute pain: Facial action determinants. J. Pers. Soc. Psychol., 50: 1291–1298.

Perrin, E.C. and Gerrity, P.S. (1981) There's a demon in your belly: Children's understanding of illness. Pediatrics, 67: 841–849.

Reesor, K.A. and Craig, K.D. (1988) Medically incongruent chronic back pain: physical limitations, suffering, and ineffective coping. Pain, 32: 35–45.

Reissland, N. (1983) Cognitive maturity and the experience of fear and pain in hospital. Social Science and Medicine, 17: 1389–1345.

Ross, D.M. and Ross, S.A. (1984a) Childhood pain: the school-aged child's viewpoint. Pain, 20: 179–191.

Ross, D.M. and Ross, S.A. (1984b) The importance of type of question, psychological climate and subject set in interviewing children about pain. Pain, 19: 71-79.

Savedra, M., Tesler, M.D., Ward, J.A. Wegner, C. and Gibbons, P.T. (1981) Description of the pain experience: a study of school-age children. Issues Compr. Pediatr. Nurs., 5: 373–380.

Savedra, M., Gibbons, P., Tesler, M., Ward. J. and Wegner, C. (1982) How do children describe pain? Pain, 14: 95–104.

Schecter, N.L., Allen, D.A. and Hanson, K. (1986) Status of pediatric pain control: a comparison of hospital analgesic usage in children and adults. Pediatrics, 77: 11–15.

Scott, P.J., Ansell, B.M. and Huskisson, E.C. (1977) Measurement of pain in juvenile chronic polyarthritis. Ann. Rheum. Dis., 36: 186–187.

Stratton, P. (1982) Rhythmic functions in the newborn. In P. Stratton (Ed.), Psychobiology of the Human Newborn, Wiley, New York, pp. 119–141.

Tesler, M.D., Wegner, C., Savedra, M., Gibbons, P.T. and Ward, J.A. (1981) Coping strategies of children in pain. Issues Compr. Pediatr. Nurs., 5: 351–359.

Thompson, K.L. and Varni, J.W. (1986) A developmental cognitive-biobehavioral approach to pediatric pain assessment. Pain, 25: 283–296.

Thompson, K.L., Varni, J.W. and Hanson, V. (1987) Comprehensive assessment of chronic musculoskeletal pain in children with juvenile rheumatoid arthritis: An empirical model. J. Pediatr. Psychol., 12: 241–255.

Turk, D., Flor, H. and Rudy, T.E. (1987) Pain and families. I. Etiology, maintenance and psychosocial impact. Pain, 30: 3–28.

Unruh, A., McGrath, P.J., Cunningham, S.J. and Humphreys, P. (1983) Children's drawings of their pain. Pain, 17: 385–392.

Varni, J.W. (1983) Clinical Behavioral Pediatrics: An Interdisciplinary Approach, Pergamon Press, New York.

Varni, J.W. and Jay, S.M. (1984) Biobehavioral factors in juvenile rheumatoid arthritis: implications for research and practice. Clin. Psychol. Rev., 4: 543–560.

Varni, J.W., Thompson, K.L. and Hanson, V. (1987) The Varni/Thompson Pediatric Pain Questionnaire: I. Chronic musculoskeletal pain in juvenile rheumatoid arthritis. Pain, 28: 27–38.

Whitt, S.K., Dykstra, W. and Taylor, C.A. (1979) Children's conceptions of illness and cognitive development. Clin. Pediatr., 18: 327–339.

Willis, D.J., Elliott, C.H. and Jay, S. (1982) Psychological effects of physical illness and its concomitants. In J.M. Tuma (Ed.), Handbook for the Practice of Pediatric Psychology, Wiley-Interscience, New York, pp. 28–66.

R. Dubner, G.F. Gebhart & M.R. Bond (Eds.)
Proceedings of the Vth World Congress on Pain
© 1988 Elsevier Science Publishers BV (Biomedical Division)

CHAPTER 35

Does the newborn infant require potent anesthesia during surgery? Answers from a randomized trial of halothane anesthesia

Kanwal J.S. Anand[1] and A. Aynsley-Green[2]

[1]*Department of Anesthesia, Harvard Medical School, Children's Hospital, Boston, USA, and* [2]*Department of Child Health, Royal Victoria Infirmary, Newcastle-upon-Tyne, UK*

Introduction

Remarkably little is known about pain perception in the human fetus and newborn infant (Br. Med. J. Editorial, 1985). Early studies of neurological development concluded that the neonatal responses to painful stimuli were decorticate in nature and that perception or localization of pain was not present (Levy, 1960; Merskey, 1970). In addition, newborn infants were not thought capable of interpretation of pain, since they may not have a memory of painful experiences (Levy, 1960). Thus, it was concluded that preterm and term neonates do not require anesthesia during surgery or other invasive procedures and, in many centers, major surgery is frequently performed under the influence of minimal or no anesthesia (Lipman et al., 1976; Katz, 1977; Shaw, 1982; Anand and Aynsley-Green, 1985).

Although the use of halothane anesthesia has been recommended (Dierdorf and Krishna, 1981), early concerns about its margin of safety in neonates (Diaz and Lockhart, 1979; Gregory, 1982) led to the wider acceptance of anesthetic techniques using a combination of nitrous oxide and muscle relaxants or muscle relaxants alone for neonates undergoing surgery (Lipman et al., 1976; Katz, 1977; Shaw, 1982; Anand and Aynsley-Green, 1985). Subsequently, it was found that neonates have a much lower requirement of halothane than the concentrations which were used in earlier studies (Lerman et al., 1983). It was pointed out that unnecessarily high concentrations of halothane were used in earlier studies which had reported significant side-effects in newborn infants, thereby reflecting the effects of overdosage in this age group (Lerman et al., 1983).

No previous study has examined the hormonal and metabolic effects of the currently recommended doses of halothane, nor is its known whether halothane confers any advantage over the use of anesthesia with nitrous oxide and muscle relaxants. We report a randomized controlled trial designed to investigate the hypothesis that stress responses of neonates given halothane anesthesia do not differ from those given conventional anesthesia with nitrous oxide and curare.

Methods

Parental consent and approval of the Hospital Ethics Committee were obtained to study 36 neonates undergoing surgery (Table I). Food was withheld for 6 h before surgery, and an intravenous dextrose infusion was maintained at 4–6 mg/kg/min throughout the study period. Blood (1–2 ml) was

TABLE I

Patient characteristics and clinical management

	Halothane group		Non-halothane group		
Number of patients	18		18		
Age at surgery, days	24	(5)**	17	(4)	
Gestation, weeks	37	(1)	38	(1)	
Birth Weight, kg	2.8	(0.3)	2.8	(0.2)	
Weight at Surgery, kg	3.1	(0.3)	2.9	(0.2)	
Dextrose infusion, mg/kg/min	4.8	(0.4)	4.8	(0.2)	
Preoperative Starvation, h	6.0	(0.4)	6.0	(0.4)	
Temperature loss, °C	0.7	(0.2)	0.8	(0.2)	
d–Tubocurarine dose, mg/kg	0.43	(0.06)	0.66	(0.07)*	
Diagnosis					**Operation**
Pyloric stenosis	5		4		Pyloromyotomy
Inguinal hernia	3		3		Herniotomy
Abdominal wall defect	3		3		Repair
Tracheo-esophageal fistula	2		2		Repair
Diaphragmatic hernia	1		1		Repair
Imperforate anus (high)	2		2		Colostomy
Tracheo-esophageal fistula	–		1		Gastrostomy
Meningomyelocoele	–		1		Closure
Intestinal obstruction	2		1		Resection + anastomosis

**Mean (SEM)
*$P < 0.025$, Mann-Whitney U-test.

sampled just before the induction of anesthesia, at the end of surgery and at 6, 12 and 24 h after surgery. Morphine injections (i.m.) were given postoperatively by clinical personnel who were blind to the anesthetic management of the neonate; the timing of analgesia was adjusted such that an injection was not given in the 2 h before blood sampling. Urine was collected in 12-h samples during the 3 days after surgery. Blood concentrations of glucose, lactate, pyruvate, acetoacetate, 3-hydroxybutyrate, alanine, glycerol and non-esterified fatty acids (NEFA) were measured by specific enzymatic methods (Bergmeyer, 1974); plasma insulin (Albano et al., 1972); glucagon (Ghatei et al., 1983) and steroid hormones (Sippell et al., 1978) were measured by radioimmunoassay methods; plasma adrenaline and noradrenaline were measured by a double-isotope radio-enzymatic assay (Brown and

Jenner, 1981). Urine was used for measurement of 3-methylhistidine and creatinine (for 3MH/Cr ratios) by fluorimetric (Murray et al., 1981) and colorimetric methods.

Neonates undergoing surgery were randomized to two anesthesia groups, both of which were given 50% nitrous oxide and curare; one group was given halothane in addition (1–2% induction, 0.5–1% maintenance). Balanced randomization in blocks was performed by the National Perinatal Epidemiology Unit, Oxford, and the coding was retained by them until completion of the trial. Four variables were selected to test the hypothesis (plasma epinephrine, plasma norepinephrine, blood glucose, and urinary 3MH/Cr ratios), and the sample size required to give 80% power to the trial (for $\alpha = P < 0.05$) was calculated from a standard nomogram (Altman, 1982). The 'response' of each neonate was characterized by the change in each hormonal or metabolic variable from its preoperative value and non-parametric tests were used for statistical analysis.

Results

Hormonal changes

There was no significant difference between the halothane and non-halothane groups in any of the hormonal concentrations measured before surgery. In the non-halothane group, the magnitude of the plasma epinephrine response was twice ($P<0.05$) and plasma norepinephrine response was three times ($P<0.005$) that of the halothane group at the end of surgery, but no differences persisted after surgery (Fig. 1). Plasma insulin increased during surgery in both anesthesia groups; this increase was significantly greater at 6 h after surgery in the non-halothane group ($P<0.05$). Although there were no significant differences between the plasma glucagon responses of the two groups, insulin/glucagon ratios were decreased in the non-halothane group, with a significant difference ($P<0.05$) at the end of surgery (Fig. 1). Plasma cortisol increased during surgery in both groups, but this response was significantly greater in the non-halothane group at the end of surgery ($P<0.05$) and at 12 h after surgery ($P<0.05$) (Fig. 1). No diferences were observed between the two groups with regard to other steroid hormones.

Metabolic changes

Hyperglycemic responses of neonates in the non-halothane group were significantly greater than in the halothane group at the end of surgery ($P<0.025$). Total ketone bodies and plasma NEFA increased during surgery in the non-halothane group and were unchanged in the halothane group, with significant differences at the end of surgery ($P<0.02$) and 6 h after surgery ($P<0.05$) (Fig. 2). There were no significant differences between the two groups with regard to changes in blood lactate, pyruvate, glycerol and plasma triglycerides during or after surgery.

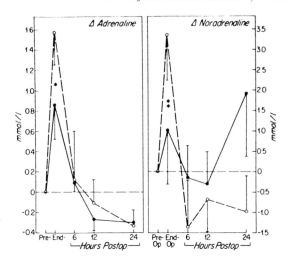

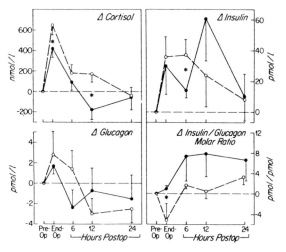

Fig. 1. Comparison of changes in plasma catecholamines, cortisol, insulin, glucagon concentrations and the insulin/glucagon molar ratios between neonates in the halothane (–, $n=18$) and non-halothane (---, $n=18$) anesthesia groups. All values are mean $\pm$ SEM. Mann-Whitney U-test: **$P<0.005$, *$P<0.05$.

Urinary nitrogenous constituents

The urinary 3-MH/Cr ratio was similar in the two groups on the day following surgery, and increased significantly in the non-halothane group on the second ($P<0.05$) and third ($P<0.01$) days after surgery, but was unchanged in the halothane group (Fig. 3).

Clinical observations

The clinical state of babies in the non-halothane

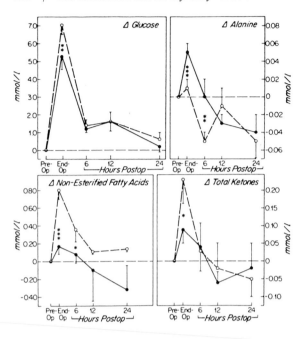

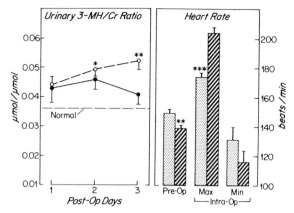

Fig. 3. Comparison of changes in the heart rate during surgery and urinary 3-methylhistidine/creatinine ratios postoperatively between neonates in the halothane (–, dotted columns, $n = 18$) and non-halothane (---, cross-hatched columns, $n = 18$) anesthesia groups. All values are mean ± SEM. Mann-Whitney U-test: ***$P < 0.005$, **$P < 0.025$, *$P < 0.05$.

Fig. 2. Comparison of changes in blood glucose, alanine, total ketone bodies, and plasma non-esterified fatty acids between neonates in the halothane (–, $n = 18$) and non-halothane (---, $n = 18$) anesthesia groups. All values are mean ± SEM. Mann-Whitney U-test: ***$P < 0.02$, **$P < 0.025$, *$P < 0.05$.

group was relatively unstable during and after surgery as compared to babies in the halothane group. Several infants in the non-halothane group had increased heart rates (Fig. 3) and muscle tone during surgery, and developed respiratory and cardiovascular instability postoperatively. Postoperative analgesia was required significantly earlier by neonates in the non-halothane group; a greater number of neonates in this group required morphine analgesia and in higher daily doses during the 3 days after surgery (Table II).

Discussion

Recent studies have suggested that the measurement of physiological stress responses can provide a reliable assessment of pain in neonates undergoing surgery (Williamson and Williamson, 1983;

Anand et al., 1985). These studies have also shown that provision of pain relief with local or opiate analgesic agents causes a decrease in the cardiovascular and hormonal-metabolic stress responses and may lead to an improved clinical outcome following surgery (Williamson and Williamson, 1983; Anand et al., 1987). This trial was designed to determine whether a similar effect can be obtained with potent inhalation anesthesia.

Hormonal changes

The hormonal responses of the two groups were strikingly different with regard to the catecholamine and cortisol responses during surgery. Neonates in the non-halothane group mounted epinephrine and norepinephrine responses that were respectively twice and three times those of the neonates in the halothane group. It is likely that potent anesthesia with halothane was responsible for decreasing the catecholamine and cortisol responses, similar to the observations from animal studies (Roizen et al., 1974) and adult patients (Roizen et al., 1981). A similar, though non-randomized study in older infants has also found that the cortisol responses were significantly greater in infants given nitrous oxide anesthesia as compared to those given halothane and nitrous oxide (Obara et al., 1984).

TABLE II

Postoperative clinical course

	Halothane group $n = 18$		Non-halothane group $n = 18$	
Perioperative complications:				
Persistent tachycardia	0		8	
Increased respiratory support	2		5	
Spontaneous bradycardias	2		6	
Poor peripheral circulation	0		2	
Gastric bleeding (stress ulcers?)	1		4	
Metabolic acidosis	0		2	
Paralytic ileus	0		2	
Postoperative oliguria	0		2	
Postoperative morphine requirements:				
First dose, hours after surgery	5.5 (1.6)		1.9 (0.03)**	
Total dose (mg/kg/day) on:	dose	no. of pts	dose	no. of pts
Postop day 1	0.23 (.06)	4	0.38 (.04)*	9
Postop day 2	0.10 (.03)	2	0.26 (.02)	7
Postop day 3	–	0	0.12 (.02)	4

All values = number of patients or mean (SEM).
Postoperative morphine injections were prescribed by clinical staff who were blind to the anesthetic management of each neonate; uniform criteria were used for giving postoperative analgesia to all neonates.
**$P < 0.001$, *$P < 0.02$, Mann-Whitney U-test.

Seven neonates were studied, although their responses were not significant due to the small number of patients and a wide variability in their data (Obara et al., 1984). In another recent study, significant cortisol responses were observed in neonates and infants undergoing various surgical procedures (Srinivasan et al., 1986).

Plasma insulin increased in response to the hyperglycemia in both groups, but the greater insulin response in the non-halothane group could have resulted either from the stimulatory effect of hyperglycemia during surgery, which was significantly greater in the non-halothane group, or from the direct inhibition of insulin secretion by halothane (Aynsley–Green et al., 1973). However, changes in the molar insulin/glucagon ratio are of greater importance than changes in the individual hormones and this ratio decreased during surgery in the non-halothane group whereas it was unchanged in the halothane group. Thus, a decrease in the insulin/

glucagon ratio, together with the increased cortisol and catecholamine responses would mediate a catabolic milieu in the non-halothane group during and after surgery (Sperling, 1982).

Metabolic changes

It is likely that surgical hyperglycemia was precipitated by the epinephrine release during surgery, and potentiated by the glucagon and cortisol responses in both groups of neonates (Bessey et al., 1984; Anand et al., 1985). Also, differences in the hyperglycemic response between the two groups may be explained by the significantly greater increases in plasma epinephrine and cortisol in the non-halothane group, together with a decrease in the insulin/glucagon ratio. A much greater suppression of the hyperglycemic response to surgery was observed in preterm babies given fentanyl anesthesia (Anand et al., 1987).

Blood lactate and pyruvate concentrations increased during surgery in both groups, probably due to epinephrine-stimulated glycogenolysis in skeletal muscle and increased glycolysis in injured tissues (Im and Hoores, 1979). Alternatively, decreased gluconeogenesis in the liver cells (Biebuyck et al, 1972) or a decreased hepatic blood flow during halothane anesthesia (Gelman et al, 1984) may contribute to this accumulation of gluconeogenic substrates. Plasma non-esterified fatty acids increased substantially during surgery in the non-halothane group and remained elevated at 6 h after surgery, whereas only a marginal response was observed in the halothane group. These responses indicate a greater degree of lipolysis, probably mediated by the marked epinephrine release and a decrease in the insulin/glucagon ratio during surgery in the non-halothane group. Total ketone bodies also increased significantly in this group, which may be related to their greater catecholamine and glucagon responses as compared to the halothane group (Williamson, 1982).

Endogenous protein breakdown was investigated by changes in the urinary 3-MH/Cr ratio, which increased significantly in the non-halothane group and was unchanged in the halothane group. Although changes in this ratio may not specifically represent skeletal muscle breakdown, increases in the urinary 3MH/Cr ratio are associated with a negative nitrogen balance, weight loss, and poor clinical condition in newborn infants (Burgoyne et al., 1982).

Clinical observations

The heart rate increased markedly during the operation in the non-halothane group, possibly due to the intraoperative release of catecholamines in this group. The increased muscle tone observed in the non-halothane group, which required extra doses of curare during surgery, may also be as a result of light anesthesia in these neonates. Other postoperative complications documented by nursing and clinical staff in the non-halothane group established a clinical pattern that was relatively unstable as compared to neonates in the halothane group (Table II). Although postoperative morphine was pre-

scribed by clinical personnel who were blind to the anesthetic group of each neonate and who used uniform criteria for giving analgesia to all neonates, it was surprising to find that neonates in the non-halothane group required postoperative analgesia earlier and more frequently during the 3 days after surgery than neonates in the halothane group.

Further clinical implications arise from this study in view of the existing notions of pain perception in the human neonate. It is believed widely that pain perception may be absent in newborn babies, due to either an immature central nervous system or an absence of the memory of previous painful experiences. The present study has confirmed that halothane obtunds the neonatal stress responses to surgery, thereby implying that painful stimuli may be perceived during surgery under unsupplemented nitrous oxide anesthesia which may be partially responsible for the marked stress responses. Also the efficacy of analgesia and anesthesia, particularly in paralysed and ventilated neonates, can be established reliably only by the measurement of physiological markers of stress. In conclusion, this randomized trial has rejected the hypothesis that halothane anesthesia does not alter the hormonal and metabolic stress responses of newborn infants subjected to surgery. We recommend that greater attention should be paid to the use of effective analgesia and anesthesia in newborn infants who are experiencing not only surgery, but other invasive medical procedures during intensive care. Clearly, the mechanisms of pain preception and the therapeutic management of painful experiences in neonates and children are important topics for future research.

Acknowledgements

Supported by the National Medical Research Fund, Oxfordshire District Research Fund and the Peel Medical Research Trust.

References

Albano, J.D.M., Ekins, R.P., Maritz, G. and Turner, R.C. (1972) A sensitive precise radioimmunoassay of serum insulin relying on charcoal separation of bound and free moieties. Acta Endocrinol., 70: 487-509.

Altman, D.G. (1982) How large a sample? In: S.M. Gore and D.G. Altman (Eds.), Statistics in Practice, British Medical Association, London, pp. 6–8.

Anand, K.J.S. and Aynsley-Green, A. (1985) Metabolic and endocrine effects of surgical ligation of patent ductus arteriosus in the human preterm neonate: are there implications for further improvement of postoperative outcome? Mod. Probl. Pediatr., 23: 143–157.

Anand, K.J.S., Brown, M.J., Bloom, S.R. and Aynsley-Green, A. (1985) Studies on the hormonal regulation of fuel metabolism in the human newborn infant undergoing anaesthesia and surgery. Hormone Res., 22: 115–128.

Anand, K.J.S., Sippell, W.G. and Aynsley-Green, A. (1987) Randomised trial of fentanyl anesthesia in preterm babies undergoing surgery: effects on the stress response. Lancet, i: 243–248.

Aynsley-Green, A., Biebuyck, J.F. and Alberti, K.G.M.M. (1973) Anaesthesia and insulin secretion: a comparative study on the effects of diethylether, halothane, sodium, pentobarbitone, and ketamine hydrochloride on blood glucose, glucose tolerance and insulin secretion in the rat. Diabetologia, 9: 274–281.

Bergmeyer, H.U. (Ed.), (1984) Methods of Enzymatic Analysis, Verlag Chemie, Weinheim, pp. 1196–1200, 1404–1414, 1446–1451, 1464–1467, 1679–1681, 1836–1843.

Bessey, P.Q., Walters, J.M., Aoki, T.T. and Wilmore, D.W. (1984) Combined hormonal infusion simulates the metabolic response to surgery. Ann. Surg. 200: 264-281.

Biebuyck, J.F., Lund, P. and Krebs, H.A. (1972) The effects of halothane on glycolysis and biosynthetic processes of the isolated perfused rat liver. Biochem. J., 128: 711–723.

Brown, M.J. and Jenner, D.A. (1981) Novel double-isotope technique for enzymatic assay of catecholamines, permitting high precision, sensitivity and plasma sample capacity. Clin. Sci., 61: 591–598.

Burgoyne, J.L., Ballard, F.J., Tomas, F.M. et al. (1982) Measurements of myofibrillar protein breakdown in newborn human infants. Clin. Sci., 63: 421–427.

Diaz, J.H. and Lockhart, C.H. (1979) Is halothane really safe in infancy? Anesthesiology, 51: S313.

Dierdorf, S.F. and Krishna, G. (1981) Anesthetic management of neonatal surgical emergencies. Anesth. Anal., 60: 204–215.

Editorial (1985) Can a fetus feel pain?, Br. Med. J., 291: 1220–1221.

Gelman, S., Fowler, K.C. and Smith, L.R. (1984) Liver circulation and function during isoflurane and halothane anesthesia. Anesthesiology, 61: 726–730.

Ghatei, M.A., Uttenthal, L.O., Bryant, M.G., Christofides, N.D., Moody, A.J. and Bloom, S.R. (1983) Molecular forms of glucagon-like immunoreactivity in porcine intestine and pancreas. Endocrinology, 112: 917–923.

Gregory, G.A. (1982) The baroresponses of preterm infants during halothane anaesthesia. Can. Anaesth. Soc. J., 29: 105–109.

Im, M.J.C. and Hoores, J.E. (1979) Energy metabolism in healing skin wounds. J. Surg. Res., 10: 459–466.

Katz, J. (1977) The question of circumcision. Int. Surg. 62: 490–492.

Lerman, J., Robinson, S., Willis, M.M. and Gregory, G.A. (1983) Anesthetic requirements for halothane in young children 0–1 month and 1-6 months of age. Anesthesiology, 59: 421–424.

Levy, D.M. (1960) The infants earliest memory of inoculation: a contribution to public health procedures. J. Genet. Psychol., 96: 3–46.

Lipman, N., Nelson, R.J. et al. (1976) Ligation of patent ductus arteriosus in premature infants. Br. J. Anaesth., 48: 365–369.

McGraw, M.D. (1943) The Neuromuscular Maturation of the Human Infant, Columbia University Press, New York.

Merskey, H. (1970) On the development of pain. Headache, 10: 116–127.

Murray, A.J., Ballard, F.J. and Tomas, F.M. (1981) A rapid method for the analysis of N-methylhistidine in human urine. Anal. Biochem., 116: 537–544.

Obara, H., Maekawa, N., Tanaka, O. and Kitamura, S. (1984) Plasma cortisol levels in paediatric anaesthesia. Can. Anaesth. Soc. J., 31:24–27.

Roizen, M.F., Moss, J., Henry, D.P. and Kopin, I.J. (1974) Effects of halothane on plasma catecholamines. Anesthesiology, (1974) 41:432–436.

Roizen, M.F., Horrigan, R.W. and Frazer, B.M. (1981) Anesthetic doses blocking adrenergic (stress) and cardiovascular responses to incision – MACBAR. Anesthesiology, 54: 390–398.

Shaw, E.A. (1982) Neonatal anaesthesia. Hosp. Update, 8: 423–434.

Sippell, W.G., Bidlingmaier, F., et al. (1978) Simultaneous radioimmunoassay of aldosterone, corticosterone, 11-deoxycorticosterone, progesterone, 17-hydroxy-progesterone, 11-deoxycortisol, cortisol and cortisone. J. Steroid Biochem. 9: 63–74.

Sperling, M.A. (1982) Integration of fuel homeostasis by insulin and glucagon in the newborn. Monogr. Paediatr., 16: 39–58.

Srinivasan, G., Jain, R., Pildes, R. and Kannan, C.R. (1986) Glucose homeostasis during anesthesia and surgery in infants. J. Pediatr. Surg., 21: 718–721.

Williamson, D.H. (1982) The production and utilization of ketone bodies in the neonate. In C.T. Jones (Ed.), Biochemical Development of the Fetus and Newborn, Elsevier Biomedical Press, Amsterdam, pp. 621–650.

Williamson, P.S. and Williamson, M.L. (1983) Physiologic stress reduction by a local anesthetic during newborn circumcision, Pediatrics, 71: 36–40.

R. Dubner, G.F. Gebhart & M.R. Bond (Eds.)
Proceedings of the Vth World Congress on Pain
© 1988 Elsevier Science Publishers BV (Biomedical Division)

CHAPTER 36

Acoustical attributes of infant pain cries: discriminating features

C.C. Johnston[1] and D. O'Shaughnessy[2]

[1]*Montreal Children's Hospital and McGill University, School of Nursing, 2300 Tupper St., Montreal, Quebec, Canada H3H 1P3, and* [2]*INRS-Télécommunications and McGill University, Dept. of Electrical Engineering, 3 Place du Commerce, Verdun, Quebec, Canada H3E 1H6*

Introduction

The human infant is extremely helpless compared to other mammalian infants and depends heavily on vocalizations for survival by signaling his state to his care-givers. In the biosocial model of crying proposed by Lester (1984), the cry signal both engages adults and reflects the biological state of the infant. Indeed, infant crying is a powerful elicitor of adult response (Lester and Boukydis, 1985) and infants that are at high risk by virtue of complicated birth histories have cries which are more arousing and urgent (Zeskind and Lester, 1978; Sirvio and Michelsson, 1976). The ability of care-givers to understand the meaning of a cry signal has been of concern to parents (Dunn, 1977). The possibility of correctly identifying the cause of the cry implies that infants have differential modes of crying related to the stressors they are experiencing.

For more than twenty-five years, the Scandinavian group has been conducting cry research (Wasz-Hockert et al., 1985) and published a monograph on healthy infant cries in four situations, pain, hunger, birth and pleasure, almost twenty years ago (Wasz-Hockert et al., 1968). They found that the initial pain cry was long, tense, high-pitched, and had a falling melody (fundamental frequency). While recent reports contain similar findings, they have elaborated various points. One fol-

lowed the entire cry episode as opposed to just the initial signal (Johnston and Strada, 1986). Another (Porter et al., 1986) examined the change in cry signals throughout varying degrees of invasiveness of newborn circumcision and found that during the most invasive part of the procedure, cries were of longer duration, higher peak fundamental frequency, more dysphonia and greater pitch variability. Technological advances have allowed more complex analyses (Rabiner and Schaffer, 1978; Golub and Corwin, 1985), so that parameters may be more precisely measured. Recently, for example, Fuller and Horii (1986) used precise measures of jitter and shimmer in an attempt to differentiate infant vocalizations in situations of pain, hunger, fussing and cooing. Although their study did not yield significant differences in the parameters of jitter and shimmer in those situations, they analysed segments of only one second's duration from each infant's vocalizations, so that differences may have been missed. In another report of their data (Fuller and Horii, 1988), they did find greater intensity in the upper spectral frequencies in the pain-induced cries.

Formants are seen as spectral resonances in cries. Tensing of the infant vocal tract as part of a physiological response to emotional state could be reflected in changes of the position in the frequency domain of the formants. Similarly, the excitation, as another physiological response to different emotional states, might be reflected in the relative intensity of the formants. Therefore, the formant parameters of frequency and intensity in a cry that was a response to acute pain might produce a cry signal which would be different from other types of infant crying. This is consistent with the stress-arousal model proposed by Fuller and Horii (1988).

Methods

Thirty-nine cry episodes were recorded from 2–6-month-old infants. The infants in this study were healthy and had no history of perinatal or postnatal complications. The cry episodes appeared to be a result of one of three stimulus situations: (1) pain/distress from routine immunization; (2) fear/startle from a jack-in-the-box; and (3) anger/frustration from head restraint. There were sixteen babies, all of whom cried from the immunization (pain) and from the head restraint (anger), but only seven cried in response to the jack-in-the-box. (These babies are a subsample of a larger study.) Recordings were analysed from the moment of the stimulus event for

60 s or until the infant had ceased crying, whichever was first. Recordings were made on a Sony TCM-500DEV cassette recorder with an omnidirectional Sennheiser MKE 2 microphone placed 10 cm from the infant's mouth. These audio tapes were then transferred to digital disc for analysis on a VAX-Venus 8600 computer. The audio signals were low-pass-filtered to 6000 Hz and sampled at 12000 samples per s with a 15-bit analogue-to-digital converter. Pitch extraction was done by the simplified inverse filter tracking (SIFT) algorithm (Markel, 1972), which was modified to accommodate high F_0 voices, that is, infant voices, which calculated an average F_0 every 10 ms of voiced segments. Thus maximum F_0 and minimum F_0 were calculated automatically. Narrow-band (filter of 50 Hz) spectrographs were visually examined to determine duration of cry episode, duration of each cry, melody, jitter, and phonation or harmonic structure (Fig. 1). Melody type was classified as falling, rising-falling or flat (Wasz-Hockert et al., 1968). Jitter, or rapid change in F_0 at least four sequential times (Fuller and Horii, 1986), was scored as either present or not present. If a cry episode had a segment of 0.5 s in which the harmonics appeared blurred, the cry

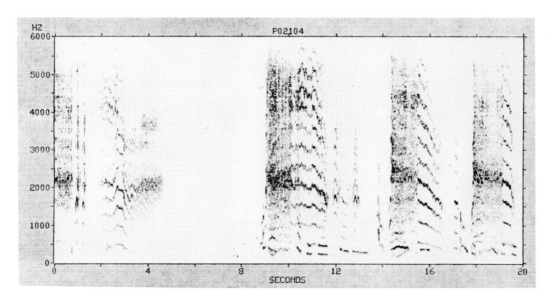

Fig. 1. Narrow-band (50 Hz filter) spectrograph of pain cry segment. Indistinct harmonics in initial part of each cry segment, jitter in latter part of each cry segment, and falling melody pattern.

was considered to have dysphonia. Formant structure was determined using a wide-band (filter of 600 Hz) spectrograph and examining a cry in the first 20 s, where formants could be clearly seen (Fig. 2).

Based on infant vocal tract size, it was expected that first formants would be around 1100 Hz and second formants around 3300 Hz (Golub and Corwin, 1985).

Results

Pain cries were different from either fear or anger cries on four parameters (Tables I and II). The frequency of the second formants in the pain cries (M = 3543.8 Hz) was higher than for either anger (M = 3150 Hz) or fear (M = 2816 Hz; F (2,37) = 4.039, P = 0.02). Also, the intensity of the second formant for pain was relatively high, -1.188 dB; for fear it was -9 dB, and for anger -4.125 dB (F (2,37) = 3.589, P = 0.05). The total time crying was longer for pain (M = 39.8 s) than for fear (M = 29.3 s) or for anger (M = 21.4 s); F (2,38) = 6.049, P = 0.005. (Although the intensity measures are affected by recording amplitude levels, an attempt was made to minimize these effects by setting the recorder levels of both the audio recorder and the computer recorder at a fixed level. Video-tape recordings of the infants show little movement during the first 20 s of the cry episodes, but the exact dis-

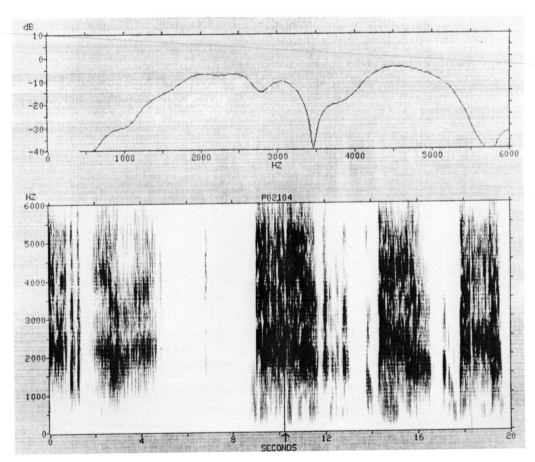

Fig. 2. Broad-band (600 Hz filter) spectrograph of pain cry. Cross-section for formant examination at 10 seconds shows first formant frequency at 2250 Hz with an intensity of -9 dB, and a second formant with a frequency of 4500 Hz and an intensity of -7.

TABLE I

Means, standard deviations and *F*-ratios for formant amplitude and cry time across conditions

Condition	Pain (n = 16)	Anger (n = 16)	Fear (n = 7)	F-ratio
2nd formant (amplitude (dB))	−1.188	−4.125	−9.000	3.59[a]
	(4.339)	(5.365)	(11.082)	
Cry duration (s)	1.656	1.188	1.857	4.396[a]
	(0.473)	(0.727)	(0.244)	
Total cry time (s)	39.8	21.4	29.3	6.049[b]

[a] $P < 0.05$; [b] $P < 0.01$.

TABLE II

Means, standard deviations and *F*-ratios for acoustical frequencies across conditions

Frequency (Hz) in condition:	Pain (n = 16)	Anger (n = 16)	Fear (n = 7)	F-ratio
F_0 maximum	679.2[a]	612	645.7	3.033[b]
	(75.3)	(88.6)	(27.0)	
F_0 minimum	384.0	342.4	364.1	2.636[b]
	(44.8)	(61.1)	(37.5)	
F_0 range	329.1	269.6	281.6	1.293
	(124.2)	(107.6)	(49.1)	
Second formant	3543.8	3150	2816.7	4.039
	(463.2)	(670.3)	(560.1)	

[a] Based on $n = 15$, one cry outside two standard deviations.
[b] $P < 0.1$; [c] $P < 0.05$.

tance between the infant's mouth and the microphone may have varied to a small extent.)

More pain cries showed dysphonation or a blurring of harmonics, χ^2 (2, $n = 39$) = 10.69, $P = 0.005$, and a greater proportion of falling melodies, χ^2 (4, $n = 39$) = 21.325, $P = 0.0001$, than either fear or anger cries.

Fear cries were more similar to pain cries than to anger cries (Table II) in the maximum pitch or F_0. Although the difference with anger cries did not reach significance, it did approach significance, F (2,37) = 3.033, $P < 0.1$, as did the minimum F_0. The fear cry duration was longer than for anger cries, F (2,38) = 4.396, $P = 0.05$. Anger cries were similar to pain cries and different from fear cries in the greater occurrence of jitter, χ^2 (2, $N = 39$) = 12.678, $P = 0.002$.

Discussion

The finding of greater intensity and higher frequency of the second formants is consistent with a stress-arousal model which proposes a tensing of muscles in the vocal tract in times of high stress or arousal. Although Fuller and Horii (1988) examined spectral energy at high frequencies, they did not examine formant frequency or intensity *per se*. The formants are a reflection of both the vocal tract shape and a result of the excitation of the vocal cords.

These results suggest that infant vocal response to pain is differentially reflected at the different levels of the physioacoustic model of infant crying proposed by Golub and Corwin (1985). The upper level processor decides whether or not the infant will respond to the stimuli; for example, there was less overt response to the jack-in-the-box than to either the head restraint or injection. This was particularly true for the 2-month-olds, for whom no rules about what events might lead to loud, unexpected noises had yet developed, and thus a loud noise from an object which had been playing music was simply not recognized as being upsetting.

The middle level of processing involves the crying as a reflexive response more than as a volitional response. The lower level involves the excitation of subglottal, glottal, supraglottal and facial movements during a cry episode. The breathing mechanisms involved at this lower level could account for the greater intensity of the second formants in the pain cries, as well as their longer vocalization. At this level as well, the changes in the vocal cord state as a result of the differential excitation are reflected in the F_0, the second formant frequency, harmonic structure and jitter differences found in these three types of cry.

Although these results appear to be consistent with a model of stress response in infant crying, caution needs to be taken in clinical use. The predictive validity of these cry parameters awaits further testing on a larger sample, particularly for the fear cries, which were few. Furthermore, inter-infant variability is great and intra-infant variability is not, which presents problems in generalizability. Cohen and Zmora (1984), however, have reported less than 5% error in correct identification of hunger and pain cries in newborns using 42 parameters, so that further work needs to be done to distinguish pain cries from other vocalizations which are similar.

Some important questions emerge from this study. Of theoretical importance is the question of distinction between arousal and pain. It is possible that a pain response, as reflected in acoustical attributes of crying which suggest greater intensity of response and tensing of the vocal tract, is simply a reflection of greater arousal, as opposed to reflecting qualitatively different responses to pain/distress, fear/startle and anger/frustration.

Of clinical interest is the question of adult listener differentiation. Pleasure vocalizations are easily distinguished from distress cries (Wasz-Hockert et al., 1968; Fuller and Horii, 1986). Studies have shown that listeners can differentiate cries of healthy newborns from high-risk newborns based on 'urgency' components, such as F_0, harmonic structure, F_0 variability and melody (Zeskind and Lester, 1978). Similarly, the cries from the most invasive part of newborn circumcisions were perceived along the same dimensions (Porter et al., 1986). No studies have investigated the effect of formant structure on listener identification. The differential formant structure of pain cries in this study suggests that this is the next step in the clinical identification of infant states of acute pain.

Acknowledgement

This project was funded by the Medical Research Council of Canada, MA-9235.

References

Cohen, A. and Zmora, E. (1984) Automatic classification of infants' hunger and pain cry. In V. Cappellini and A.G. Constantinides (Eds.), Digital Signal Processing-84, Elsevier Science Publishers, Amsterdam, pp. 667–672.

Dunn, J. (1977) Distress and Comfort, Harvard University Press, Cambridge, MA.

Fuller, B.F. and Horii, Y. (1986) Differences in fundamental frequency, jitter, and shimmer among four types of infant vocalizations. J. Commun. Disord., 19: 441–447.

Fuller, B.F. and Horii, Y. (1988) Spectral energy distribution in four types of infant vocalizations. J. Commun. Disord., in press.

Golub, H.L. and Corwin, M.J. (1985) A physioacoustic model of the infant cry. In B.M. Lester and C.F.Z. Boukydis (Eds.), Infant Crying: Theoretical and Research Perspectives, Plenum Press, New York, pp. 59–82.

Golub, H.L. and Corwin, M.J. (1982) Infant cry: a clue to diagnosis. J. Ped. Surg., 69: 197–201.

Johnston, C.C. and Strada, M.E. (1986) Acute pain response in infants: a multidimensional description. Pain, 24: 373–382.

Lester, B.M. and Boukydis, C.F.Z. (1985) Infant Crying: Theoretical and Research Perspectives, Plenum Press, New York.

Lester, B.M. (1984) A biosocial model of infant crying. In L.P. Lipsitt (Ed.), Advances in Infancy Research, Vol. 3, Ablex Publishing Corporation, Norwood, NJ, pp. 167–212.

Markel, J. (1972) The SIFT algorithm for fundamental frequency estimation. IEEE Trans. Audio Electroacoustics, AU-20: 367–377.

Porter, F.L., Miller, R.H. and Marshall, R.E. (1986) Neonatal pain cries: effect of circumcision on acoustic features and perceived urgency. Child Dev., 57: 790–802.

Rabiner, L.R. and Schafer, R.W. (1978) Digital Processing of Speech Signals, Prentice-Hall Inc., Englewood Cliffs, NJ.

Sirvio, P. and Michelsson, K. (1976) Sound-spectrographic cry analysis of normal and abnormal newborn infants. Folia Phoniat, 28: 161–173.

Wasz-Hockert, O., Lind, J., Vuorenkoski, V., Partanen, T. and Valanne, E. (1968) The infant cry: a spectrographic and auditory analysis. Clinics Developmental Medicine, Spastics International Medical Publications, London.

Wasz-Hockert, O., Michelsson, K. and Lind, J. (1985) Twenty-five years of Scandinavian cry research. In B.M. Lester and C.F.Z. Boukydis (Eds.), Infant Crying: Theoretical and Research Perspectives, Plenum Press, New York, pp. 83–104.

Zeskind, R. and Lester, B.M. (1978) Acoustic features and auditory perception of the cries of newborns with prenatal and perinatal complications. Child Dev. 49: 580–589.

R. Dubner, G.F. Gebhart & M.R. Bond (Eds.)
Proceedings of the Vth World Congress on Pain
© 1988 Elsevier Science Publishers BV (Biomedical Division)

CHAPTER 37

How children describe pain: a study of words and analogies used by 5–14-year-olds

Anne Gaffney

Department of Applied Psychology, University College, Cork, Ireland

Summary

A knowledge of children's ability to describe pain is necessary for the appropriate assessment of pain in children. This study examined developmental aspects of descriptions of pain in a sample of 680 Irish schoolchildren aged between 5 and 14 years. The results indicate developmental differences in the use of pain descriptors and in the use of analogy to describe pain. The use of pain questionnaires to assess pain in children is discussed.

Introduction

The study of pain in children has until recently been a neglected area of research. Now that attention has begun to focus on this important topic, the assessment of pain in children has been identified as a major problem for study (Jeans, 1983; McGrath and Unruh, 1987). As pain is a subjective experience not directly accessible to observers, its assessment is often difficult and depends largely on the individual's ability to describe his pain. When the sufferer is a child, the problem is compounded by limitations of verbal and communicative ability.

Correspondence: Anne Gaffney, Knockrua, Navigation Road, Mallow, Co. Cork, Ireland.

The fact that pain is a phenomenon which varies not only in intensity but also in quality and in accompanying affect adds to the complexity of its assessment.

Accurate assessment of pain in children is necessary for correct diagnosis, effective management and the evaluation of pain-relief strategies. A knowledge of children's ability to describe pain at different ages should assist in the assessment process and in the development of aids to assessment such as age-appropriate pain questionnaires.

A number of studies (Savedra et al., 1981; Abu-Saad, 1984; Ross and Ross, 1984b; Jerrett, 1985) have investigated school-aged children's ability to describe pain. While these studies concluded that these children can use a number of words and descriptive sentences to describe pain, they did not report any developmental differences between younger and older subjects in the number or type of pain descriptors used. However, a developmentally oriented study by Jeans and Gordon (1981) reported that 5-year-olds had difficulty in describing pain, and used a total of five words, in contrast with the twenty-six words used by 13-year-olds.

The study reported in this paper was aimed at further investigation of developmental aspects of children's descriptions of pain, and was part of a wider, cognitive developmental investigation of children's understanding of pain (Gaffney and Dunne, 1986, 1987). Specifically, this study examined the development of children's ability to describe pain both by the use of pain descriptors and by the use of analogy. The use of analogy to describe pain was included for study on the basis that this is a commonly used way of describing pain. Apley (1976) states "Even the most literate adult can hardly describe pain except by analogy". It was observed also that a number of the descriptive sentences used by subjects in the studies on children's descriptions of pain cited earlier were based on the use of analogy. Further, as noted by Melzack and Torgerson (1971), many single pain descriptors are used in an analogical, 'as if' sense. Thus, for example, a 'splitting' headache means that the sufferer feels as if his head is splitting.

Method

The responses of 680 Irish schoolchildren, aged 5–14 years, to two sentence completion items, 'Pain is...' and 'A pain is sometimes...', were examined for pain descriptors. These words were then listed by age of emergence in the data. Words used by both boys ($n = 341$) and girls ($n = 339$) were compared for rank order of emergence using a rank order correlation coefficient (Spearman's rho) corrected for tied ranks, as a number of words may emerge at the same age. (Note: due to the segregated Irish school system, boys and girls were tested in separate schools.)

A further sentence completion item, 'A pain can feel like...', was used to investigate the ability to describe pain by analogy. The data obtained in response to this item were analysed by dividing the 680 subjects into three age groups (5–7-year-olds, 8–10-year-olds, and 11–14-year-olds) corresponding to the Piagetian cognitive developmental stages of preoperational, concrete operational and formal operational thought. A chi-square test was then used to identify any significant differences between these age groups in the use of analogy to describe pain.

Results

The range of pain descriptors used in response to the items 'Pain is...' and 'A pain is sometimes...' increased progressively with age. Girls used more words than boys, and used more advanced words earlier than boys. As shown in Tables I and II, pain descriptors used by 5- and 6-year-olds were mainly sensory and evaluative words (hurting, sore, awful, terrible, bad). Between 8 and 10 years the range of pain descriptors broadened to include affective descriptions (annoying, irritating) and qualitative words (stinging, sharp, pricky, stabbing). Subjects in this age range also described pain in terms of fear or threat (dangerous, fatal, deadly, cruel, terrifying, frightening). The 11–14-year-olds used further qualitative words (piercing, jabbing, throbbing, sticking), complex evaluative words (uncomfortable, unpleasant, unbearable, intolerable, agonizing, acute, excruciating, overpowering), and words relating to temporal aspects of pain (persistent, prolonged, recurring). This age group also used affective words relating mainly to sadness (distressing, upsetting, worrying, depressing).

When the pain descriptors which were used by both sexes (shown in italics in Tables I and II) were listed by age of emergence in the data, and the rank order for boys was compared with the rank order for girls, significant correlations were obtained for both items. For the item 'Pain is...' $\rho = 0.76$, $P < 0.001$ (df = 15). For the item 'A pain is sometimes...' $\rho = 0.75$, $P < 0.001$, (df = 18). The frequency of use of pain descriptors used by both boys and girls was checked for the item 'A pain is sometimes...'. When pain descriptors were ranked in order of frequency of use by each sex, the rank order for boys was found to correlate significantly with the rank order for girls ($P < 0.001$). The six words used most often by boys, listed in order of use, were: sore, bad, hurting, sharp, annoying, serious. The six words used most often by girls, in order of use, were: sore, bad, hurting, annoying, sharp, serious.

TABLE I

Pain descriptors used in response to the item 'pain is...', listed by sex and age of emergence in the data: words used by both sexes are shown in italics

Age of emergence	Boys ($n = 341$)	Girls ($n = 339$)	Age of emergence	Boys ($n = 341$)	Girls ($n = 339$)
5 years	*hurting/hurtful* *sick* *sore*	*hurting/hurtful* *sick* *sore* *awful* *terrible* nervous big	11 years	*agonizing* *awful*	*agonizing* *sharp* piercing jabbing *uncomfortable* terrifying frightening
6 years	*bad* *terrible* cold *hard*	*bad* awkward	12 years	harsh unlucky	*distressing/distressful* *irritating* *unpleasant* acute miserable
7 years	nasty	tiring	13 years	frustrating *irritating* throbbing sticking	short
8 years	*annoying* horrible boring dangerous	*annoying* dreadful sickening aching desperate	14 years	*severe* *unpleasant* excruciating *uncomfortable* disturbing unwanted *distressing*	discomforting (sic)
9 years	*dreadful*	*horrible* slight *severe*			
10 years	stabbing *sharp*	troubling deadly cruel hard		Total = 30	Total = 36

Use of analogy

Chi-square analysis indicated highly significant differences ($P < 0.0001$) between the three age groups in the use of analogy in response to the item 'A pain can feel like...'. The percentage of age groups using analogies increased from 5.7% of 5–7 year-olds to 42.1% of 8–10-year-olds and to 70.1% of 11–14-year-olds. Thus the use of analogy to describe pain in response to the item 'A pain can feel like...' increased significantly with age.

When the analogies used by subjects were analysed by content, three main types emerged: 'sharp' analogies, describing a sharp object piercing the body or part of the body; 'blunt' analogies, which described pain in terms of the impact or pressure of a blunt object on the body or part of the body; and 'internal' analogies, which described pain in terms of activity within the body. 'Sharp' analogies were the most frequently used, outnumbering other types in a ratio of 3:1. All three types showed a similar pattern of increase with age. The following are some examples of analogies used by subjects:

'Sharp' analogies. A pain can feel like... a big huge long pin going through you (girl, CA 9), ...a knife in your side (boy, CA 9), ...a dog biting you (boy,

TABLE II

Pain descriptors used in response to the item 'a pain is sometimes...', listed by sex and age of emergence in the data: words used by both sexes are shown in italics

Age of emergence	Boys (*n* = 341)	Girls (*n* = 339)	Age of emergence	Boys (*n* = 341)	Girls (*n* = 339)
5 years	*hurting/hurtful* bad	*hurting/hurtful* bad sore horrible heavy *hot*	11 years	ticklish *tiring* nagging nasty	*agonizing* *aggravating* unpleasant upsetting
6 years	*sore* *awful* painful/painish	terrible awful tired	12 years	crucial *aggravating* good in ways intolerable *strong*	*unbearable* uncomfortable overpowering acute *tiring* fierce distressing throbbing sickening long persistent
7 years	hateful *cold* rough	*sharp* cold sickening *annoying* *serious*			
8 years	*serious* *irritating* *stinging* agitating *dangerous* horrible terrible	pricky *stinging* *strong* nervous	13 years	dull *depressing* horrifying troublesome	twinging worrying
9 years	*annoying* *hot* big	terrifying soft small slight little severe dreadful	14 years	*unbearable* excruciating disturbing damaging prolonged numbing	*depressing* embarrassing unexpected awkward recurring monotonous aching harsh sudden
10 years	*agonizing* deadly *sharp* rotten short long imaginary	*dangerous* frightening horrifying *irritating* funny fatal hard deep tiresome troublesome		Total = 44	Total = 61

CA 10), ...a sword gnashing into you (girl, CA 12).

'Blunt' analogies. A pain can feel like... as if a brick fell on top of you (boy, CA 9), ...a big heavy block on top of wherever the pain is (girl, CA 10), ...a hammer pounding your bones (boy, CA 13), ...a band of steel around the area (girl, CA 12).

'Internal' analogies. A pain can feel like... something tumbling in your tummy (boy, CA 10), ...a thunderstorm inside you (girl, CA 10), ...something inside you eating its way out (boy, CA 14), ...the devil inside you trying to burn your insides (girl, CA 14).

Although more girls than boys used analogies to describe pain, the difference was not significant at the 0.01 level. However, if the numbers of analogies used by each sex are compared, girls used significantly more ($p < 0.001$). Although more girls than boys used 'internal' analogies, there were no significant differences by sex in the type of analogy used.

Discussion

The aim of this study was to investigate developmental aspects of children's descriptions of pain. The finding of significant correlations between the sexes in the rank order of appearance of pain descriptors provides some evidence of a developmental pattern in the ability to describe pain. When considered in relation to the stages in cognitive development described by Piaget (Piaget and Inhelder, 1969), the data suggest that during the later part of the preoperational stage, descriptions of pain are limited to fairly basic sensory and evaluative terms. During the period of concrete operations (7–10 years) the ability to describe affective and qualitative aspects of pain appears to develop. With the acquisition of formal operations, (11–14 years) more complex words are used to describe the affective, qualitative and evaluative aspects of pain. Words beginning with 'un-' and 'dis-' were used only by this age group. While these findings need to be confirmed by further studies, they are supported by convergent findings of developmental patterns in children's definitions of pain (Gaffney and Dunne, 1986) and in children's understanding of the causality of pain (Gaffney and Dunne, 1987).

While it could be argued that the increase in range of pain descriptors with age represents only a growth in vocabulary, the finding of significant differences between age groups in the use of analogy provides stronger evidence of the effect of developmental changes in cognitive structure on the ability to describe pain. From the pattern of use of analogy in the data, it would appear that the attainment of concrete operations is necessary for the use of analogy. This finding appears to be in agreement with the literature on the relationship between cognitive stage and the use of metaphor reviewed by Kogan (1983). As noted earlier, many qualitative pain descriptors are used in an analogical sense, e.g. burning, piercing, stinging, splitting. The meaningful use of this type of word may also be linked to the development of concrete operations.

In addition to the effect of increasing age on the ability to describe pain, the data obtained in this study suggest that sex may also be a factor. Girls used more pain descriptors than boys, and tended to use more advanced words earlier than boys. Girls also used more analogies to describe pain.

Implications

The major implication of the findings of this study, which indicate that up to the age of 7 or 8 years children are limited in their ability to describe pain, is that attempts to assess parameters of pain other than the presence and intensity of pain in young children may not be productive.

The McGill Pain Questionnaire (Melzack, 1975) has proved very useful in the assessment of pain in adults, and attempts are now being made to develop pain questionnaires for use with children (Varni et al., 1987). While a checklist format is unsuitable for the investigation of developmental aspects of pain in children (Ross and Ross, 1984a), it may be useful for clinical purposes. However, the cognitive skills necessary for the meaningful completion of pain questionnaire checklists have not yet been identified. Melzack (1975) reports that adults responding to the MPQ are 'highly selective' and 'appear to feel compelled to choose only the appropriate words'. This implies that pain questionnaires may require the ability to discriminate between similar words, the introspective ability to identify appropriate words, and the self-control to limit choice to these words. At what age children might develop these skills is still uncertain. The findings of this study suggest that younger children are unlikely to be able to discriminate between various qualitative and affective words, and Piagetian theory states that up to the age of about 7 years children are not capable of introspection (Piaget, 1951). Savedra et al. (1981) reported that their sample of 9–12-year-old children concentrated seriously while selecting pain descriptors from a checklist, suggesting that the task was meaningful for them. Varni et al. (1987), using the Varni/Thompson Pediatric Pain Questionnaire on a sample of 5–15-year-old children with juvenile chronic arthritis, did not comment on any differences between younger and older children in ability to respond to the questionnaire checklist. However, Ross and Ross (1984a) noted that some children in their sample of 5–12-year-olds adopted response strategies such as avoiding words in the checklist which might result in getting an injection for pain, or checking every word in order to emphasize their pain. It is clear that the use of pain questionnaires with children is an area in which study has just begun.

The finding of a limited ability to describe pain in younger children suggests also that the reliance on spontaneous, formal complaint as a measure of pain in hospitalized children reported by Eland and Anderson (1977) is unrealistic, although the recent finding by Donovan et al. (1987) that adult patients also fail to complain adequately of their pain suggests that other factors in addition to descriptive ability may be involved.

Limitations of this study

Ross and Ross (1984a) and McGrath and Unruh (1987) have noted that children's descriptions of pain may vary with the demand characteristics of the situation. As this study examined healthy children's descriptions of pain in general, the effect of recent illness and experience of specific types of pain on children's descriptions of pain needs to be investigated. Savedra et al. (1981) have reported that hospitalized children selected an average of 13 words from a checklist of pain descriptors, compared with an average of 5 words chosen by their non-hospitalized group, and concluded that this finding reflected the recency of pain experience in the hospitalized group.

As this study examined productive rather than receptive aspects of pain descriptors, the findings may underestimate children's ability to understand and select words from a checklist.

One further point relates to cultural influences: as this study was carried out on Irish children, it is possible that some of the words used were culturally determined.

Conclusion

This study reported evidence of developmental changes in the ability to describe pain both by the use of pain descriptors and by the use of analogy.

References

Abu-Saad, H. (1984) Cultural group indicators of pain in children. Mat. Child. Nurs. J., 13: 187–196.
Apley, J. (1976) Pain in childhood, J. Psychosomat. Res., 20: 383–389.
Donovan, M., Dillon, P. and McGuire, L. (1987) Incidence and characteristics of pain in a sample of medical-surgical inpatients. Pain, 30: 69–78.
Eland, J.M. and Anderson, J.E. (1977) The experience of pain in children. In A. Jacox (Ed.), Pain: a Source Book for Nurses and other Health Professionals, Little, Brown, Boston, pp. 453–473.

Gaffney, A. and Dunne, E.A. (1986) Developmental aspects of children's definitions of pain. Pain, 26: 105–117.

Gaffney, A. and Dunne, E.A. (1987) Children's understanding of the causality of pain. Pain, 29: 91–104.

Jeans, M.E. (1983) Pain in children – a neglected area. In P. Firestone, P. McGrath and W. Feldman (Eds.), Advances in Behavioral Medicine for Children and Adolescents, Laurence Erlbaum, Hillsdale, NJ, pp. 23–27.

Jeans, M.E. and Gordon, D.J. (1981) Developmental characteristics of the concept of pain. Paper presented at the 3rd World Congress on Pain, Edinburgh, Scotland.

Jerrett, M.D. (1985) Children and their pain experience. Child. Hlth. Care, 14: 83–89.

Kogan, N. (1983) Stylistic variation in childhood and adolescence: creativity, metaphor and cognitive style. In P. Mussen (Ed.), Handbook of Child Psychology, Vol. 3, J. Flavell and E. Markman (Eds.), Wiley, New York, pp. 630–706.

McGrath, P. and Unruh, A. (1987) Pain in Children and Adolescents, Elsevier, Amsterdam, pp. 73–104.

Melzack, R. (1975) The McGill Pain Questionnaire: major properties and scoring methods. Pain, 1: 277–299.

Melzack, R. and Torgerson, W.S. (1971) On the language of pain. Anesthesiology, 34: 50–59.

Piaget, J. (1951) Judgment and Reasoning in the Child, Routledge and Kegan Paul, London, p. 147.

Piaget, J. and Inhelder, B. (1969) The Psychology of the Child, Routledge and Kegan Paul, London.

Ross, D.M. and Ross, S.A. (1984a) The importance type of question, psychological climate and subject set in interviewing children about pain. Pain, 19: 71–79.

Ross, D.M. and Ross, S.A. (1984b) Childhood pain: the school-aged child's viewpoint. Pain, 20: 179–191.

Savedra, M., Tesler, M.D., Ward, J.A., Wegner, C. and Gibbons, P.T. (1981) Description of the pain experience: a study of school-age children. Iss. Comp. Pediatr. Nurs., 5: 373–380.

Varni, J.W., Thompson, K.L. and Hanson, V. (1987) The Varni/Thompson Pediatric Pain Questionnaire: 1. Chronic musculoskeletal pain in juvenile rheumatoid arthritis. Pain, 28: 27–38.

R. Dubner, G.F. Gebhart & M.R. Bond (Eds.)
Proceedings of the Vth World Congress on Pain
© 1988 Elsevier Science Publishers BV (Biomedical Division)

CHAPTER 38

Children's language of pain

Mary Tesler, Marilyn Savedra, Judith Ann Ward, William L. Holzemer
and Diana Wilkie

School of Nursing, University of California, San Francisco, CA, USA

Summary

A sample of 958 school children, aged 8–17 years, selected from a list of 129 words those they used to describe pain and assigned intensity values to them. Fifty percent of the sample chose 67 words as useful pain descriptors.

Introduction

The value of verbal reports in the assessment and management of pain has been reported (Bailey and Davidson, 1976; Fabrega and Tyma, 1976; Craig, 1980; Gaston-Johansson, 1983). Melzack and Torgerson (1971) developed and organized a list of words to describe the sensory, affective and evaluative dimensions of pain. This work led to the McGill Pain Questionnaire, a most useful tool for assessing pain in adults. A similar tool does not exist for children. This is a report of the first stage of a program of research designed to develop and test a tool for assessing the quality, intensity and location of pain in children aged 8–17 years.

Pain words appear early in children's vocabulary. Nelson (1973) reports the use of 'hot' in a child's vocabulary as early as 13 months and 'hurt' at 24 months. Initial work of the present investigators asked children 9–12 years old (Savedra et al., 1982; Tesler et al., 1983) and in a subsequent study 13–17-year-olds (Savedra et al., 1987) to list words that described their pain experience. These words provided the basis for the present study. Ross and Ross (1984) interviewed 994 school-age children and reported that the children used colorful and discrete descriptors along with many similes to describe their pain experiences. Thompson and Varni (personal correspondence) used a word list in an instrument designed to assess pediatric pain but the source of these words was not reported. In summary, these studies provide evidence that children use words to describe pain but it is not clear whether there are sex, age, ethnic or other demographic differences in the pain descriptors used. This study identified the words children most frequently selected to describe pain. In addition, assigned intensity values and demographic differences were examined. The goal was to develop a list of words children could use to report pain quality.

Sample

The multi-ethnic sample of 958 students reflected the diverse population in the greater San Francisco Bay Area. The demographic data are presented in Table I. Twenty-six percent of the children reported that English was not their first language.

Methods

The investigators compiled a list of 129 words that

Correspondence: Mary Tesler, Clinical Professor, Department of Family Health Care Nursing N411Y, School of Nursing, University of California, San Fransisco, CA 94143, U.S.A.

children had reported using to describe pain in two previous studies (Savedra et al., 1982, 1987; Tesler et al., 1983) and from Jeans (personal correspondence). The words were printed on individual cards and randomly presented to 958 students in grades 3–12 in 5 urban and suburban high schools (grades 9–12; 14–17 yrs.), 7 middle schools (grades 6–8; 11–13 yrs.) and 5 primary schools (grades 1–5; 8–10 yrs.). The children were asked to sort the words into three categories: 'words they know and use to describe pain', 'words they do not know' and 'words they know but do not use' to describe pain. The children then assigned an intensity value to the words they use to describe pain by sorting them into categories denoting small, medium, large and worst pain.

Data analysis

Frequencies, percentages and rank orderings were tabulated for words selected, words known and not used, and words not known. The 67 words selected as known and used to describe pain by at least 50% of the sample are reported as well as the modal intensity value (most frequently occurring intensity) assigned to each word. To assess demographic differences, chi-square analyses for the variables sex, English as a first language, religion, ethnicity and grade were calculated. To allow for the effects of multiple analyses, the P value was set at 0.001.

Findings

The children sorted 129 words and at least 50% of the sample selected 67 words as those they would use to describe pain (Table II). Seventy-five percent of the sample knew 115 of the 129 words. Only three words (remorse, inhibiting and pulsating) were not known by more than 50% of the sample. Words not known were among those least frequently selected; however, children were able to discriminate among the 'known' words as pain descriptors. Fifty percent or more of the sample selected only 67

TABLE I
Sample demographic data ($n = 958$)

Variable	Categories	Frequency (%)
Sex	Boys	447 (47)
	Girls	506 (53)
English as 1st language	Yes	711 (74)
	No	244 (26)
Religion	Catholic	303 (32)
	Protestant	176 (19)
	Buddhist	31 (3)
	Jewish	31 (3)
	Others	397 (42)
Ethnicity	White	413 (43)
	Chinese	162 (17)
	Filipino	80 (8)
	Hispanic	73 (8)
	Black	69 (7)
	Others	159 (17)
Grades (ages in years)	3–4 (8– 9)	248 (26)
	5–6 (10–11)	233 (24)
	7–8 (12–13)	194 (20)
	9–10 (14–15)	164 (17)
	11–12 (16–17)	119 (12)

Frequencies may not total 958 due to missing data and percentages may not total 100% due to rounding.

of the 115 'known' words as useful pain descriptors. Only six words (see ranks 1–6, Table II) were selected by more than 75% of the sample as words known and used to describe pain.

The original list of 129 words included eight similes ('like a': sharp knife, bullet, pinch, scratch, ache, pin, hurt and sting). Six words from the original list corresponded to similes; for example, 'like a hurt' and 'hurting'. When the rankings of the similes were compared to their adjective counterparts, rank order differed for all except 'like a sharp knife' and 'sharp', which were ranked 6 and 7, respectively. However, when the intensity ratings of the similes were compared to their adjective counterparts, all but 'like a sharp knife' and 'sharp' were assigned the same intensity values.

Children were able to assign distinct intensity

TABLE II

Words selected by 50% or more of the sample ($n=958$), observed demographic differences, and relationship to McGill words

Word	Rank	Percent selected	Modal intensity[a]	Sex	English 1st lang.	Religion	Ethnic	Grade	Developmental[b]	McGill word	Word class[c]
Hurting	1	88.4	Med	Yes	No	No	No	No	No	Yes	S
Sore	2	83.9	Med	No	No	No	No	No	No	Yes	S
Burning	3	83.7	Wst	No	No	No	No	Yes	No	Yes	S
Stinging	4	80.1	Med	No	No	No	No	Yes	No	Yes	S
Aching	5	79.1	Med	No	No	No	No	Yes	Yes	Yes	S
Like a sharp knife	6	76.0	Wst	No	No	No	No	No	No	No	S
Sharp	7	74.0	Lg	No	Yes	No	No	Yes	Yes	Yes	S
Like a sting	8	73.5	Med	No	No	No	No	No	No	No	S
Pinching	9	73.4	Sml	No	No	No	No	Yes	No	Yes	S
Cramping	10	72.9	Med	No	Yes	Yes	Yes	Yes	Yes	Yes	S
Swollen	11	72.3	Med	No	No	No	No	Yes	No	No	S
Uncomfortable	12	71.6	Med	No	No	No	No	Yes	Yes	Yes	E
Pounding	13	71.0	Med,Lg	No	No	No	No	Yes	No	Yes	S
Awful	14	70.5	Lg	No	No	No	No	No	No	No	A
Stabbing	15	69.6	Wst	No	Yes	No	Yes	Yes	No	Yes	S
Cutting	16	69.2	Lg	No	No	No	No	Yes	No	Yes	S
Killing	17	68.6	Wst	No	No	No	No	No	No	Yes	A
Beating	18	67.3	Med	No	No	No	No	No	No	Yes	S
Terrible	19	67.2	Lg	No	No	No	No	No	No	No	E
Horrible	20	65.5	Lg	No	No	No	No	No	No	No	E
Like a pinch	21.5	65.4	Sml	No	No	No	No	No	No	No	S
Dizzy	21.5	65.4	Med	No	No	No	No	No	No	No	S
Like an ache	23.5	65.1	Med	No	No	No	No	Yes	No	No	S
Punching	23.5	65.1	Med	No	No	No	No	Yes	No	No	S
Miserable	25	64.9	Lg	Yes	No	No	No	Yes	No	Yes	E
Crushing	26	64.8	Lg	No	No	No	No	Yes	No	Yes	S
Itching	27	64.7	Sml	No	No	No	No	Yes	No	Yes	S
Biting	28	64.0	Med	No	No	No	No	Yes	No	No	S
Hot	29	63.8	Lg	No	No	No	No	Yes	Yes	Yes	S
Pressure	30	63.5	Med	No	No	No	No	Yes	No	Yes	S
Like a hurt	31	63.4	Med	Yes	No	No	No	Yes	No	No	S
Never goes away	32	63.2	Wst	No	No	No	No	No	No	No	M
Shocking	33	62.6	Lg	No	No	No	No	No	No	No	M
Scratching	34	62.1	Sml	No	No	No	No	No	No	No	S
Numb	35.5	60.7	Med	No	Yes	No	Yes	Yes	No	Yes	M
Splitting	35.5	60.7	Lg	No	No	No	No	Yes	No	Yes	S
Hitting	37	60.4	Med	No	No	No	No	No	No	No	S
Blistering	38.5	59.2	Med	No	No	No	No	Yes	No	No	S
Throbbing	38.5	59.2	Lg	No	Yes	Yes	Yes	Yes	Yes	Yes	S
Like a pin	40	59.0	Sml	No	No	No	No	No	No	No	S
Crying	41	58.7	Sml	Yes	No	No	No	No	No	No	A
Sickening	42	58.2	Med	Yes	No	No	No	Yes	No	Yes	A
Like a scratch	43	57.4	Sml	No	No	No	No	No	No	No	S
Dying	44	56.9	Wst	No	No	No	No	No	No	No	A
Bad	45	56.8	Med	No	No	No	No	No	No	No	E

Yes = significant, chi-square ($P<0.001$)

TABLE II (continued)

Words selected by 50% or more of the sample ($n = 958$), observed demographic differences, and relationship to McGill words

Word	Rank	Percent selected	Modal intensity[a]	Sex	English 1st lang.	Religion	Ethnic	Grade	Developmental[b]	McGill word	Word class[c]
Frightening	46	56.4	Lg	Yes	No	No	No	No	No	Yes	A
Tight	47	56.2	Med	No	No	No	No	Yes	No	Yes	M
Pin-like	48.5	55.7	Sml	No	No	No	No	No	No	No	S
Screaming	48.5	55.7	Wst	No	No	No	No	No	No	No	A
Suffocating	50	55.5	Wst	No	Yes	Yes	Yes	Yes	No	Yes	A
Deadly	51	55.2	Wst	No	No	No	No	No	No	No	A
Annoying	52	54.3	Med	No	Yes	Yes	Yes	Yes	Yes	Yes	E
Uncontrollable	53.5	54.0	Wst	No	No	No	No	Yes	No	No	E
Stiff	53.5	54.0	Med	No	No	No	Yes	No	No	No	S
Tearing	55	53.7	Lg	No	No	No	No	Yes	No	Yes	S
Unbearable	56	53.0	Wst	No	Yes	Yes	Yes	Yes	Yes	Yes	E
Like a bullet	57	52.8	Wst	No	No	No	No	No	No	No	S
Shooting	58	52.7	Wst	No	No	No	No	No	No	Yes	S
Paralyzing	59	52.6	Wst	No	No	Yes	No	Yes	No	No	A
Piercing	60	52.5	Lg	No	No	Yes	Yes	Yes	Yes	Yes	M
Frustrating	61	51.8	Med	Yes	No	Yes	No	Yes	No	No	E
Pricking	62	51.4	Sml	No	Yes	No	Yes	Yes	Yes	Yes	S
Terrifying	63	51.3	Wst	No	No	No	No	Yes	No	Yes	A
Dreadful	64	51.2	Wst	No	No	No	No	No	No	Yes	M
Scary	65	51.1	Med	Yes	No	No	No	No	No	No	A
Torturing	66	50.3	Wst	No	No	No	No	Yes	Yes	Yes	M
Fear	67	49.7	Med	No	No	No	No	Yes	No	Yes	A

[a]Modal intensity: Sml = small, Med = medium, Lg = large, Wst = worst.
[b]Developmental: Yes = developmental pattern observed, defined as frequency of word selection increasing with grade.
[c]Word classes: S = sensory, A = affective, E = evaluative, M = miscellaneous.

values. The 67 words known and used by more than 50% of the sample represented a wide range of intensities. The modal intensity for each word is presented in Table II. Overall, 9 (13%) words were designated as representing small, 27 (40%) medium, 15 (22%) large and 17 (25%) worst intensities of pain.

The top 67 words were analysed for potential difference in words selected by demographic variables as reported in Table II. Few differences were found and these are summarized by reporting the number (percent) of significant chi-square results for each demographic variable from the 67 comparisons. There were 8 (12%) significant differences for sex; girls selected the words more frequently than boys in all 8 cases. Nine (13%) words were different if English was not the child's first language; in all cases, when English was not the first language the word was selected less frequently. There were 8 (12%) significant differences among the five religions; no consistent pattern was observed. There were 10 (15%) significant differences for the six ethnic categories; Whites and Filipinos tended to select words more frequently than did Chinese, Blacks, Hispanics, or others. There were 38 (57%) significant differences by grade. Overall, children in grades 3–6 (ages 8–11 years) selected fewer words. Eleven (16%) words in the top 67 list exhibited a clear developmental trend with the frequency of word selection increasing with each grade category. Not reported in Table II is the finding that there were no significant differences between children previously hospitalized as compared to those with no previous hospitalization in their selection of words.

Table II shows that 31 (46%) of the 67 words correspond to words listed in the McGill Pain Questionnaire. Finally, the 67 words were classified according to the McGill Pain Questionnaire categories of sensory, affective and evaluative. The results were: 39 (58%) sensory, 13 (19%) affective and 9 (13%) evaluative: 7 (10%) miscellaneous.

Discussion

There are four major points in the findings. First, the enthusiasm of the children in participating in the word selection task was clear. They attended to the assignment eagerly and seriously and expressed their pleasure at being asked their opinion about how they described pain.

Second, the findings demonstrate that children between 8 and 17 years can select and reject words to describe their pain. The list of pain words proved to be developmentally appropriate given the high number of children who reported that they knew the words. Also, the number of words selected increased with age, reflecting cognitive development. This finding raises questions about the usefulness of a single tool for children across a broad age span.

Third, comparison of this list of words with those on the McGill Pain Questionnaire shows significant differences. An additional five words which appear in a different form from the McGill scale (e.g. McGill uses itchy, the children selected itching) were included among the 67 descriptors, totaling 36 McGill-related words. This study reports an additional 31 words not on the McGill Pain Questionnaire that 50% or more children selected to describe pain.

Fourth, the intensity values assigned to the words appear to reflect children's experiences with pain. For example, like a pin, pinching, and scratching were assigned small values, whereas burning, shooting, dying, killing, terrifying, suffocating, uncontrollable and screaming were assigned worst pain values. Most words in this category are affective words reflecting feelings associated with pain. Also, only 13% of the words from the list of 67 were assigned to the small intensity category. This suggests that children view pain experiences as having a moderate to high intensity.

Acknowledgements

This project was supported by the American Cancer Society, Northern California Division, and the National Institutes of Health, Center for Nursing Research (1 RO1 NU 01045-01). It was approved by the Committee on Human Research of UCSF.

References

Bailey, C.A. and Davidson, P.O. (1976) The language of pain: intensity. Pain, 2: 319–324.

Craig, K.D. (1980) Ontogenetic and cultural influences on the expression of pain in man. In H.W. Kosterlitz and L.Y. Terenius (Eds.), Pain and society, Dahlem Konferenzen 1980, Verlag Chemie Gmbh, Weinheim, pp. 37–52.

Fabrega, H., Jr. and Tyma, S. (1976) Language and cultural influences in the description of pain. Br. J. Med. Psychol., 49: 349–371.

Gaston-Johansson, F. (1984) Pain assessment: differences in quality and intensity of the words pain, ache and hurt. Pain, 20: 69–76.

Melzack, R. and Torgerson, W.S. (1971) On the language of pain. Anesthesiology, 34: 50–59.

Nelson, K. (1973) Learning to talk: a process model, Section 6. Monogr. Soc. Res. Child Dev., 34(149): 95–136.

Ross, D.M. and Ross, S.A. (1984) Childhood pain: the school-aged child's viewpoint. Pain, 20: 179–191.

Savedra, M., Gibbons, P., Tesler, M., Ward, J. and Wegner, C. (1982) How do children describe pain? A tentative assessment. Pain, 14: 95–104.

Savedra, M., Tesler, M., Ward, J. and Wegner, C. (1987) How adolescents describe pain. J. Adolescent Health Care, in press.

Tesler, M., Ward, J., Savedra, M., Wegner, C. and Gibbons, P. (1983) Developing an instrument for eliciting children's description of pain. Percept. Mot. Skills, 56: 315–321.

Pain Assessment

R. Dubner, G.F. Gebhart & M.R. Bond (Eds.)
Proceedings of the Vth World Congress on Pain
© 1988 Elsevier Science Publishers B.V. (Biomedical Division)

CHAPTER 39

Pain in the elderly

Stephen W. Harkins

Departments of Gerontology, Psychiatry, Psychology, and Biomedical Engineering, Medical College of Virginia, Virginia Commonwealth University, Richmond, VA, USA

Summary

This chapter discusses normal and abnormal aging in relation to pain. Experimental data are reviewed, and it is concluded that age does not have a major impact on perception of laboratory pain. This conclusion is contrasted with marked age-related changes that do occur in most sensory systems. The question of whether persistent and chronic pain perception changes with age is raised. Insufficient data are available to determine whether there are any such changes. Health problems which generally are restricted to the elderly are reviewed, and it is suggested that the older patient is at risk for considerable discomfort, pain and suffering, yet is infrequently treated at multidisciplinary pain clinics. There is need for better understanding of what constitutes normal aging versus diseased aging. Pain is certainly not a normal consequence of the aging process but because of social expectations it is perhaps too frequently accepted by both the patient and the health care system as a 'normal' part of the aging process. This chapter also addresses several myths concerning the aging process and suggests that systematic research is needed to understand better the psychological and social impact of pain problems in the old.

Correspondence: S.W. Harkins, Ph.D., Box 228, MCV Station, Medical College of Virginia, Virginia Commonwealth University, Richmond, VA 23298-0228, U.S.A.

Introduction

Gerontology is a science defined not as a unique discipline but by a concern with the many-sided problem of the nature and origin of differentiations in structure and function which occur with advanced aging in most living things. In humans, gerontology includes not only biological change but also social, economic, psychological and cultural factors influencing the aging process. Birren (1959) pointed out over 30 years ago that 'research on aging is controlled inquiry into the many differences between young and old organisms' (p. 4). Geriatrics, in turn, is a field concerned with medical treatment of the health problems which tend to accrue with advancing age. Thus, gerontology can be considered as a branch of basic science and geriatrics as a branch of the 'healing arts.'

This chapter presents a brief review of gerontological research related to pain. The fields of gerontology and algology have undergone dramatic expansion in the past thirty years. In both fields, myths have been dispelled, new facts made available, and theory has emerged to aid in organization of information, direct new research efforts, and permit rationally based clinical intervention. The purpose of this chapter is to outline issues in research on age changes in pain perception in the later years of life and particularly to address a myth. This myth is that the older individual in some way feels pain differently than the younger individual because of age per se.

Many myths exist with regard to old age, one of which is that being of old age is pitiful, because aging in the later years of life (1) causes a decrease in ability to conduct the active affairs of daily living, (2) causes a weakening of the body, (3) deprives the individual of all pleasures and (4) increases the probability of death. These four causes making the myth that old age is inherently pitiful or negative were debunked by Cicero in 44 BC during his old age (Cicero, translation 1967). The reader is encouraged to read and consider why Cicero decided that these are not factors which predispose to making old age pitiful. Pain at any time in the life of an individual leads to the potential for a pitiful existence. Overcoming pain problems is the challenge, and this challenge may be well met by the vast majority of both younger and older individuals.

The older segment of the world's population is increasing, and the old are indeed disposed to chronic disabling illnesses, many of which are associated with discomfort, pain and suffering. Some estimates are that 80 percent of the old (currently defined as those above 65 years of age; see Harkins et al., 1984, 1988) suffer from at least one chronic illness. Chronic pain, combined with the reduced physiological capacity of old age, probably has enormous impact upon ability to cope, quality of life, and mortality. Whether the actual capacity to feel pain changes in a clinically relevant degree in most elderly, however, is questionable, and, indeed, is unlikely. Nevertheless, a myth exists that age dulls the senses associated with nociception. Without question major changes do occur in most senses during the middle and later years of life. Many of these age-related differences in sensory processes are reviewed briefly in a subsequent section.

Population changes: demography

The world's population is growing older. This is true for both more developed and less developed countries. No single reason accounts for these changes in population characteristics, but decreases in infant mortality and birth rates have played a role. Sanitation, innoculations against childhood diseases, nutrition and education have also played a major role in these recent demographic changes. The number of individuals 65 years of age and older alive today is impressive, but estimates of total numbers of such individuals by 2030 are even more impressive. Not only will the more developed countries (MDC) show significant increases in number and percentage of older individuals in their populations but also the less developed countries (LDC) will show considerable increase in numbers of individuals above 65 years of age in the next 50 years (Hauser, 1986).

Compression of mortality. Fries and Crapo (1981) have described this 'graying' of the world's population as the 'compression of mortality' into the later years of life. That is, more and more people are surviving the early and middle years of life, but the maximum life-span is not changing. Thus, while mean population characteristics may be changing so that life expectancy at younger ages is increasing, there has been little or no change in the maximum human life-span. While older individuals are increasing in total number in both the LDCs and MDCs, longevity is not being added to the later years of life. That is, life expectancy at birth and in middle-age is increasing dramatically, but life expectancy at 75 or 85 is not. The upper biological limit of the human life-span, about 115 years, does not appear to be changing. While more individuals than ever before are living longer, the upper limit to human survival has not increased, resulting in this 'compression of mortality' into the later years of life.

Compression of morbidity. A major issue for the world's social planners and economists is the degree to which this population shift will result in increases in chronic health problems with accompanying increases in demand on services for the 'frail' and dependent elderly. Fries and Crapo (1981) also suggest that, like mortality, morbidity is being compressed into the later years of life.

Fries and Crapo (1981) argue that onset of chronic disability due to disease, age or natural loss of vital capacity with senescence will be increasingly delayed or compressed into the later years of life. Thus, the older population will be healthier according to this hypothesis. Whether morbidity is being compressed into the later years of life remains a question of major inquiry. Over the recent past there have been decreases in deaths due to cardiovascular disease and increases in survival rates for certain cancers. These gains, however, may be offset by increases in mortality and morbidity due to other diseases, including the dementias. It is currently estimated that senile dementia of the Alzheimer's type, for example, will affect over 20% of those above 80 years of age. Changes in disease patterns are occurring, particularly for chronic ailments of old age; whether morbidity, like mortality, is being compressed into the later years of life remains to be determined. Survival into the later and later years brings increasing frailty and morbidity from chronic health problems (Brody, 1982; Hauser, 1986). Today, in the elderly, chronic health problems may be controlled but they are seldom cured.

If, indeed, chronic ailments are decreasing in the increasing number of older individuals in the world, then it could be argued that discomfort, pain and suffering are also decreasing, and quality of life is increasing. Assessment of quality of life is a difficult undertaking (George and Bearon, 1980). Data reviewed here, however, suggest that chronic illnesses associated with discomfort, pain and suffering are frequent in the elderly. The impact of these health problems on quality of life has not been systematically evaluated. It is possible that while mortality is being compressed into the later years of the human life span, morbidity is expanding. Individuals may live longer but may suffer more. As Hippocrates suggested, 'old persons have fewer diseases than the young, but chronic diseases never leave them.'

Sensory changes with 'normal' aging

Decreases in sensory acuity for audition, vision, smell, certain skin senses and, to a degree, taste are well documented in both the experimental and the lay literature on aging. Age-related loss of hearing is termed presbycusis (presby = old; cusis = hearing) and is characterized as a progressive and irreversible decrease in pure-tone threshold that is greater for high than for low frequency tones. Presbycusis tends to be bilaterally symmetrical and is greater in individuals with long-term exposure to noise or with a familial history of similar hearing loss (Olsho et al. 1985; Corso, 1981). Presbyopia (opia = vision) is characterized by slow progressive changes in near-point vision, narrowing of the peripheral vision, decreases in accommodation and changes in static and dynamic acuity (Kline and Schieber, 1985). Loss in olfactory sensibilities also occurs with age. Recent research indicates that age is associated with an increase in threshold for the common chemical senses involving both nasal 'pungency' and odor 'quality', as well as a decrease in ability to identify odors (Doty et al., 1984; Stevens and Cain, 1985, 1987; Schemper et al. 1981; Stevens et al., 1982). Odor identification, however, may be more influenced by life history than age in individuals with intact olfactory reception (Wood and Harkins, 1988). While it is generally assumed that taste thresholds increase with age, such changes may not occur in healthy individuals and, where they do occur, increases in threshold are not related to suprathreshold taste experience (Bartoshuk et al., 1986). Elderly individuals do have a problem with identification of blended foods (Schiffman, 1977) but it is likely that this identification failure represents cognitive failure and not impaired sensory ability.

Age-related changes in the skin senses have been demonstrated for vibrotactile threshold but not suprathreshold perception. The excellent work of Verrillo (1980, 1982a) indicates selective age-dependent changes in vibrotactile thresholds for higher but not lower frequency cutaneous mechano-receptors. Also, it has been demonstrated that growth of sensation for suprathreshold vibratory stimuli, determined by magnitude estimation procedures, does not change with age beyond that due to increased threshold (Verrillo, 1982b).

In summary, the senses of sight, hearing and smell show changes with age. This is also true of cutaneous thresholds for vibrotactile stimuli above approximately 30 Hz. An age-related difference in taste threshold may occur but this elevated threshold does not seem to have a major impact upon suprathreshold taste sensibilities. It is true that ability to identify olfactory and gustatory stimuli diminishes with age (Doty et al. 1984; Schiffman, 1977) but ability to identify stimuli by endowed name involves higher-order cognitive factors as well as integrity of sensory processes (see Wood and Harkins, 1988).

Physiological changes with 'normal' aging

'The problem at once arises whether distinction can be made between what is "normal" and what is "pathological" in old age. At either extreme the differentiation is obvious, and a contrast is striking between a vigorous and active old man and the bedridden and decrepit senile patient. The intermediate stages are extremely difficult to evaluate, however' (Critchley, 1931, p. 1221). This problem so aptly addressed by Critchley in lectures delivered to the Royal College of Physicians of London in March of 1931 remains relevant to this day. The distinction between what constitutes illness and disease is a major question for basic research and every medical specialty concerned with prevention and treatment of health problems in middle and late life.

A vast number of changes in body systems and physiological processes do occur with aging in humans. Numerous reviews of biological and physiological aging exist, and it is beyond the scope of this chapter to review these in detail.

A note of caution is required with regard to the literature on both sensory and physiological changes in the elderly. With increasing age there is marked increase in variability between individuals in most bodily functions. The sources of these changes and their relation to 'normal' aging or ontogenetic development in the later years of life are not known. Thus, changes ascribed to 'aging' today

may indeed be shown to be due to disease processes tomorrow.

Age and pain

If age results in a loss of ability to sense noxious stimuli then presbyalgos (algos = pain) would be an appropriate term to denote such a phenomenon. This would also suggest that aging acts in some way as an 'analgesic'. Age may influence pain perception and pain-related behavior in different fashions. The following sections present a review of what is known concerning age in relation to laboratory pain and persistent and chronic pain.

Age could influence the sensory dimension of pain by resulting in changes in receptors and conduction properties of peripheral nerves and/or spinal cord mechanisms subserving nociceptive processes. Age could also affect centrally mediated processes involved in endogenous control of pain and affective-motivational response to painful stimuli. In addition, age could be related to differences in the meaning of pain to the individual due to either experience (i.e. personal history), birth cohort effects (i.e. psychosocial history) or both. Thus, age in the later years of life can be imagined to potentially influence, selectively or interactively, the three major recognized dimensions of human pain: (i.e. the sensory/discriminative, affective/motivational and cognitive/interpretive dimensions; Melzack, 1973). Age may also differentially affect responses for different types of pain. That is, age might not influence experimental pain in the laboratory, persistent pain or chronic pain in the same manner. Finally, the impact of persistent and chronic pain on the old may result in a different outcome and demand different treatments from that in young or middle-aged individuals.

Age and experimental pain. Changes with age in ability to perceive noxious laboratory stimuli were first systematically evaluated by Wolff and colleagues over 40 years ago. They concluded that age does not influence the pricking pain threshold for radiant heat in well-instructed, unprejudiced subjects (Hardy et al., 1943, 1952; Schumacher et al., 1940). Results since these early findings have been markedly conflicting. Recent reviews have dealt with this issue in considerable detail (Harkins, 1987; Harkins and Warner, 1980; Harkins et al., 1984; 1988; Kwentus et al., 1985).

Table I summarizes much of the extant literature on age differences in pain perception in the laboratory. As can be noted in this table, sensory threshold, pain threshold and pain tolerance may increase, decrease or remain unchanged between age groups. Such contradictory results probably reflect differences in choice of stimulus, stimulation procedures, psychological endpoints, instructions and training, subject selection criteria and investigator bias. Recent evidence based on contact-heat stimuli in the range 43–51°C and employing visual analogue scaling procedures indicated significant age differences in perception of experimental pain (Harkins et al., 1986). As in previous research (Harkins and Chapman, 1976, 1977a,b) older subjects tended to underrate low-intensity stimuli compared to younger individuals. These results are illustrated in

TABLE I

Effects of age on pain sensitivity

Investigators	Modality and method	Measurements of pain sensitivity in elderly compared to young groups				
		Pain threshold	Pain reaction threshold	Pain tolerance	Discrimination of suprathreshold painful stimuli	Response criterion for pain
Schumacher et al., 1940	Cutaneous – thermal	Similar	–	–	–	–
Hardy et al., 1943	Cutaneous – thermal	Similar	–	–	–	–
Chapman, 1944	Cutaneous – thermal	Higher	Higher	–	–	–
Chapman and Jones, 1944	Cutaneous – thermal	Higher	Higher	–	–	–
Birren et al., 1950	Cutaneous – thermal	Similar	Similar	–	–	–
Sherman and Robillard, 1964a,b	Cutaneous – thermal	Higher	Higher	–	–	–
Schluderman and Zubek, 1962	Cutaneous – thermal	Higher	Higher	–	–	–
Mumford, 1965, 1968	Tooth – shock	Similar	–	–	–	–
Collins and Stone, 1966	Cutaneous – shock	Lower	–	Lower	–	–
Procacci et al., 1970	Cutaneous – thermal	Higher	–	–	–	–
Clark and Mehl, 1971	Cutaneous – thermal	Higher[a]	–	–	♂ Similar[a,b] ♀ Poorer	Higher[a]
Woodrow et al., 1972	Achilles tendon – pressure	–	–	Lower	–	–
Harkins and Chapman, 1976, 1977	Tooth – shock	Similar	–	–	Poorer	Intensity-dependent – (see text)
Harkins et al., 1986	Cutaneous – thermal[c]	Higher[c]	–	–	Intensity dependent[c] (see Fig. 1 and text)	–

[a]Middle-aged subjects.
[b]Young and older males, no difference in discrimination; older females, lower discrimination than young.
[c]Used visual analogue sealing procedures; see Fig. 1 and text.

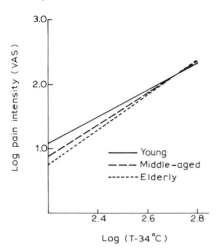

Fig. 1. Visual analogue scale (VAS) ratings of perceived pain intensity to contact heat for three age groups. Stimuli were 43°C, 45°C, 47°C, 49°C and 51°C heat pulses from an adapting temperature of 34°C. Heat pulses were 5 s delivered by a hand-held contact thermode (1 cm surface area). Stimuli were delivered to different locations on the nondominant arm. Young (n=21) mean age 25.3 (SD=4.2); middle-aged (n=10) mean age 53.4 (SD=5.7); elderly (n=13) mean age 72.5 (SD=4.6). Older groups tended to under-rate intensity of lower-intensity heat pulses compared to younger groups. (Redrawn from Harkins et al., 1986.)

Fig. 1. While a significant age effect was observed, the authors were more impressed by the similarities between the three age groups than the differences (Harkins et al., 1986).

Animal research supports the contention that normal aging has minimal effects on pain perception. The old rat, like the old human, evidences marked losses in visual and auditory acuity. But, like the old human, the old rat does not show marked loss of sensitivity to painful stimuli (Krauter et al., 1981). This finding has recently been confirmed (Hamm and Knisely, 1985). Hamm and Knisely (1985) demonstrated that, while there are no age differences in tail-flick thresholds in the rat there are differences in responses to noxious thermal stimuli as a function of age following stress-induced analgesia. These results are consistent with decreases in central control of pain (i.e. analgesia) in senescent rats due to loss, perhaps, of presynaptic modulatory process.

Over 50 years ago, Critchley (1931) asserted that 'appreciation of tactile and painful stimuli is ... impaired or even lost in a number of very aged individuals... [and] that in many cases there is a relative rise in the threshold of pain sensibility' (p. 1221). He cites a source indicating that in the elderly '... minor surgical operations and dental extractions can be carried out with but little pain and discomfort ...' (p. 1221). This assertion, that age reduces pain perception, has taken on the quality of a myth. Certainly the older diabetic may have such a significant peripheral neuropathy that pain perception is reduced to the degree that acute pain during minor surgical procedures is reduced. In turn, the patient with periodontal disease may not object to simple tooth extraction. That age alone, however, reduces pain perception to a clinically relevant degree is a myth. While further research is needed to determine the nature of age changes in nociceptive processes (particularly in systematic evaluation of age effects on so-called first or epicretic pain and second or protopathic pain), it can now be rather strongly asserted that growing older does not itself result in clinically significant changes in perception or report of laboratory pain.

Apparent stability of response to noxious laboratory-induced pain in the elderly is in direct contrast to the major losses that occur in most sensory systems. No theoretical model exists which organizes age-dependent sensory changes in later life into a meaningful whole. Perhaps a preliminary, guiding perspective is that the more complex the receptor system the greater the probability that time-dependent changes will occur. Attention to receptor complexity may well assist in a better understanding of the nature and etiology of changes in sensory processes with 'normal' aging. Currently there are no guiding principles for predicting sensory impairment or multiple sensory impairments in the later years of human life in any given individual.

Age and chronic pain. Age produces dramatic shifts in chronic illnesses likely to produce pain. For example, polymyalgia rheumatica (PMR) rarely occurs before the age of fifty and is characterized

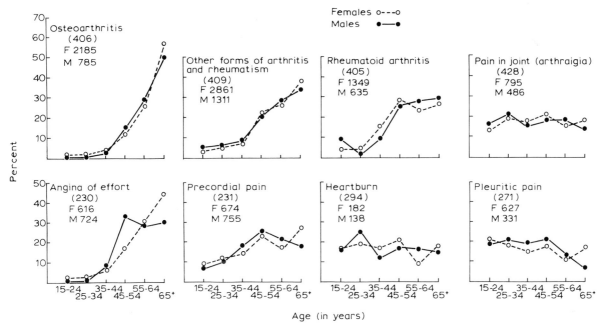

Fig. 2. Distributions by age and sex of selected reasons for visits to five family practice sites (118 family physicians) over a 2-year period in a population of 88 000 patients making over 500 000 patient problem visits. Numbers in parenthesis are Royal College of General Practitioners disease classifications. These data are substantially revised from Marsland et al., 1976, as in Harkins et al., 1988 (with permission).

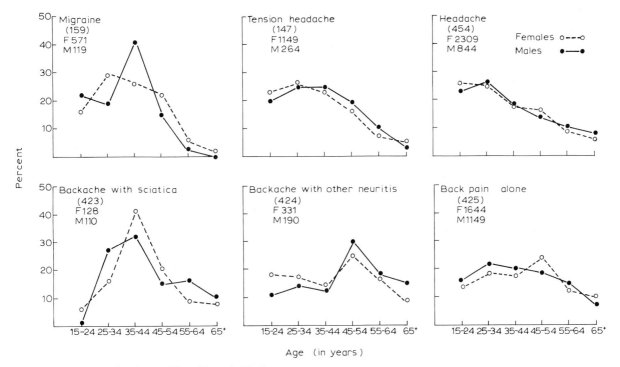

Fig. 3. Distributions of patient-problem visits as in Fig. 2.

by pain and stiffness in the hips, shoulders and neck. Untreated, PMR can lead to giant cell arteritis. Effective treatment can be achieved with low dosages of prednisone (10 mg daily) or an equivalent dosage of a similar steroid. Trigeminal neuralgia and herpes zoster occur in a higher percentage of old than of young patients (Butler and Gastel, 1980). Chronic pain problems, in general, show increases with age.

Fig. 2 presents data collected over a two-year period from a large number (over 86 000) of patients visiting family practice centers in the Commonwealth of Virginia (Marsland et al., 1976). These data are based upon over half a million patient problem visits seen at 5 family practice centers. As expected, patient problems associated with the skeletal and muscular systems and certain cardiovascular problems increase with age (see Fig. 2). In turn, patient visits associated with headaches peak in the middle years of life and subsequently decrease, as illustrated in Fig. 3. Headache (particularly apparent migraine) of recent onset in the older adult is relatively rare (Butler and Gastel, 1980) and suggests development of underlying pathology, including transient ischemic attacks or stroke (Medina et al., 1975).

Angina and precordial pain (Fig. 2) also show increasing frequency with increasing age. These contrast interestingly with the suggestion that age is associated with decreases in pain associated with myocardial infarction (MI) in the old. A recent report, designed to assess whether symptoms associated with an MI change with age evaluated 1474 MI patients admitted to a coronary care unit and diagnosed according to WHO criteria. Results indicated that pain was the major presenting symptom in 77% of the patients under 60 years of age (n = 296) and 61% of those 70 years of age or older (n = 317). The 16% difference between these two groups was significant. Nevertheless, this difference is much smaller than previously reported figures (Rodstein, 1956). Pain was, however, still the most frequent presenting symptom of acute MI in even the oldest group in this study. The results of this study, conducted by MacDonald et al. (1983), indi-

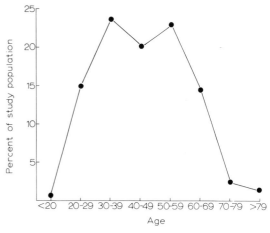

Fig. 4. Percentage of chronic pain patients as a function of age evaluated at the Medical College of Virginia Chronic Pain Clinic (n = 174). See text. (From Harkins et al., 1984; with permission.)

cate that the frequency of silent or painless MI in the old has been over-estimated. While referred pain due to MI does decrease with age, the silent MI remains atypical in the older patient. Why differences in referred pain occur with age is a question awaiting better understanding of the biological mechanisms of such pain (see Harkins et al., 1988).

Considering that up to 80% of the old have at least one chronic health problem, it is surprising that they do not constitute a larger proportion of those treated at multidisciplinary chronic pain centers. Informal inquiry of clinical directions of pain clinics conducted by the author suggests that only 7–10% of patients seen at such clinics are above 65 years of age. No systematic epidemiological data on chronic pain in the old exist. Such a study is needed and should include information regarding perceived intensity of pain, impact of pain on quality of life, causes, treatment(s) and follow-up data concerning short- and long-term outcomes. Recent, retrospective information indicates that pain and suffering are a common factor in the elderly individual during the six to twelve months immediately preceding death (Moss et al., 1986).

To a degree the data presented in Fig. 4 are surprising. These data are based upon 174 consecutive chronic pain patients evaluated and treated at a multidisciplinary pain clinic. Very few of the patients (less than 8%) were over 65 years of age. If so many of the elderly do indeed suffer from health problems associated with pain, it is noteworthy that so few are treated in state-of-the-art multidisciplinary pain clinics. From other perspectives the low utilization of these settings by the old patient is not at all surprising. First, the problems treated most frequently in the pain clinic are those which are actually less frequent in the older adult (see Fig. 3). In fact, the bimodal distribution of patients as a function of age depicted in Fig. 4 can be recreated by adding the distributions for headaches and back pain based upon primary care patients visits seen in Fig. 3. Note that migraine and backache with sciatica peak at 35–44 years and backache with other neuritis at 45–54 in Fig. 3. The primary practice setting, a major referral source for the tertiary care pain clinic, shows a decrease with patient age in

those pain problems which are indeed among the more frequent cases referred to the pain clinic. Figs. 2 and 3 also indicate that morbidity may not undergo compression in the later years of life and that the patterns of illness change with age, a not very surprising event.

Figs. 5–7 present other health problems as a function of age and sex in the primary care setting. Fig. 5 shows age – sex frequencies for selected fractures. It is well recognized that patterns of fractures and their causes change with age and that some types of fracture (e.g. hip fractures) result in considerable morbidity and mortality. There has been no systematic research on discomfort, pain and suffering related to fractures as a function of age. It is likely that considerable long-term morbidity and perhaps mortality in the old result due to the stress of pain accompanying fracture. Fig. 6 illustrates data for selected conditions which are often consid-

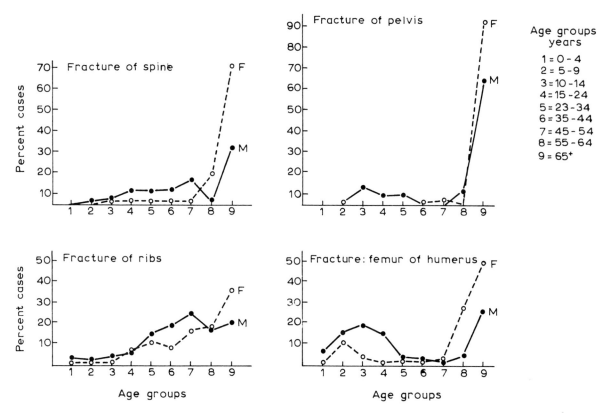

Fig. 5. Distribution by age and sex of selected fractures in family practice setting (as Fig. 1).

ered 'psychosomatic'. While the total number of patients (and relative age-dependent percentages out of the 86000 patients) is small, the increased frequency for these complaints suggests a decrease in quality of life which would be consistent with an expansion of morbidity, not a compression, in the later years of life. It is also interesting to note that a comparison of Figs. 2, 3 and 5 with Fig. 6 indicates that the greatest proportion of health visits by the elderly are related to problems with relatively easily determinable physiological and anatomical origins.

As indicated previously, the probability of dementia increases dramatically in later life. This is illustrated in Fig. 7. Senile dementia, particularly of the Alzheimer's type, represents a neurologist's diagnostic problem and a psychiatrist's or family physician's management problem. Anecdotal re-

ports suggest that patients in the early stages of some types of dementia may adopt pain complaint as a disengagement mechanism (J. Turner, personal communication). Anecdotal evidence also suggests that as the disease progresses there may be a loss of sensitivity to painful stimuli which exceeds that expected due to loss of cognitive capacity in general. For example, family members caring for such patients in the home setting have described something similar to 'la belle indifference' during and following accidental burns in such patients.

No systematic studies of age-related patterns, responses and coping mechanisms of chronic pain exist in the old. Data do exist indicating that new-pain problems are most frequent in 15–44-year-old patients (Knapp and Koch, 1984). Pain in older individuals likely has lost its newness sometime in the past (Knapp and Koch, 1984). Preliminary findings

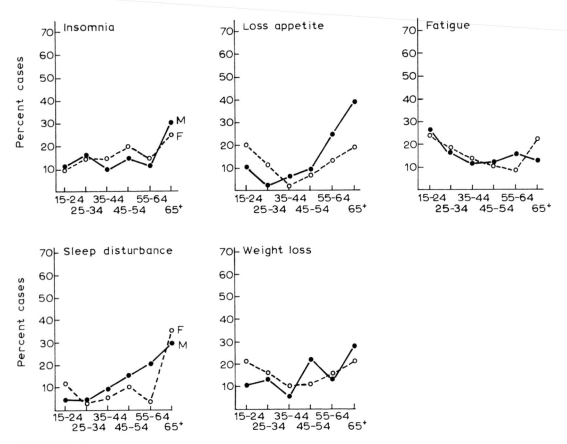

Fig. 6. As Fig. 1.

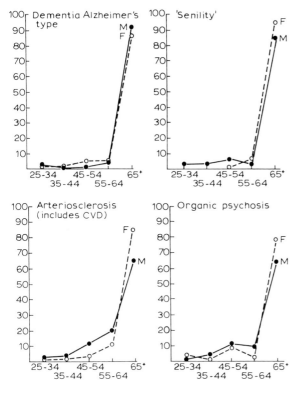

Fig. 7. As Fig. 1.

patients with persistent pain. Their findings were based on a population-based telephone survey of community-dwelling individuals. Harkins and Nowlin (1985) report a significant interaction between persistent pain and personality in volunteers in a 10-year longitudinal study of aging. Individuals who developed a persistent pain problem during the course of this study and who tended to have a more 'neurotic/anxiety'-prone personality were 3–4 times less likely to return for further study. It is probable that onset of persistent and chronic pain in the middle and later years of life is a major challenge with which many individuals are unable to cope. Further research is needed concerning the psychological impact of pain on the elderly individual and such research will need to carefully control for birth cohort effects. Because of differences in psychosocial history, birth cohort effects can influence persistent or chronic pain expressiveness, behavior, expectancies, treatment compliance and ultimate outcome. There is no necessary reason to believe that because age has minimal effects on response to experimental pain in the laboratory this would also hold true for ability to cope with pain in the real world.

In summary, pain, discomfort and suffering should not be synonymous with normal aging. Pain is not a normal consequence of being old. When present in the elderly patient it must be aggressively evaluated and treated.

are conflicting as to whether recurrent, persistent or chronic pain problems have a greater negative impact on the well-being of the elderly compared to younger patients. Crook et al. (1984) report no differential effect of age on psychological well-being in

References

Bartoshuk, L.M., Rifkin, B., Marks, L.E. and Bars, P. (1986) Taste and aging. J. of Gerontol., 41: 51–57.

Birren, J.E. (Ed.) (1959) Principles of research on aging. In Handbook of Aging and the Individual, University of Chicago Press, Chicago, pp. 3–42.

Birren, J.E., Shapiro, H.B. and Miller, J.H. (1950) The effect of salicylate upon pain sensitivity. J. Pharmacol. Exp. Ther., 100: 67–71.

Brody, J.A. (1982) Life expectancy and the health of older persons. J. of Am. Geriatr. Soc. 30: 681–683.

Butler, R.N. and Gastel, B. (1980) Care of the aged: perspectives on pain and discomfort. In L.K. Ng and J.J. Bonica (Eds.), Pain, Discomfort and Humanitarian Care, Elsevier, Amsterdam, pp. 297–312.

Chapman, W.P. and Jones, C.M. (1944) Variations in cutaneous and visceral pain sensitivity in normal subjects. J. Clin. Invest., 23: 81–91.

Cicero, M.T. Translated by H.G. Edinger (1967) On Old Age; On Friendship, Library of Liberal Arts, Vol. 213, Bobbs Merrill, Indianapolis.

Clark, W.C. and Mehl, L. (1971) Thermal pain: a sensory decision theory analysis of the effects of age and sex on various response criteria, and 50 percent pain threshold. J. Abnormal Psychol., 78: 202–212.

Collins, G. and Stone, L.A. (1966) Pain sensitivity, age and activity level in chronic schizophrenics and in normals. Br. J. Psychiatry, 112: 33–35.

Corso, J.F. (1981) Aging Sensory Systems and Perception, Praeger, New York.

Critchley, M. (1931) The neurology of old age. Lancet, i: 1221–1230.

Crook, J., Rideout, E. and Browne, G. (1984) The prevalence of pain complaints in a general population. Pain, 18: 299–314.

Doty, R.L., Shaman, P., Applebaum, S.L., Giberson, R., Sikorski, L. and Rosenberg, L. (1984) Smell identification ability: changes with age. Science, 226: 1441–1443.

Fries, J.F. and Crapo, L.M. (1981) Vitality and Aging: Implications of the Rectangular Curve, WH Freeman Co, San Francisco.

George, L.K. and Bearon, L.B. (1980) Quality of Life in Older Persons: Meaning and Measurement, Human Sciences Press, Inc., New York.

Hamm, R. and Knisely, J.S. (1985) Environmentally induced analgesia: an age-related decrease in an endogenous opioid system. J. Gerontol., 40: 268–274.

Hardy, J.D., Wolff, H.G. and Goodell, H. (1943) The pain threshold in man. Am. J. Psychiatry, 99: 744–751.

Hardy, J.D., Wolff, H.G. and Goodell, H. (1952) Pain Sensations and Reactions, Williams and Wilkins, Baltimore, MD.

Harkins, S.W. (1987) Pain. In G.L. Maddox (Ed.), The Encyclopedia of Aging, Springer, New York, pp. 509–511.

Harkins, S.W. and Chapman, C.R. (1976) Detection and decision factors in pain perception in young and elderly men. Pain, 2: 253–264.

Harkins, S.W. and Chapman, C.R. (1977a) The perception of induced dental pain perception in young and elderly women. J. Gerontol., 32: 428–435.

Harkins, S.W. and Chapman, C.R. (1977b) Age and sex differences in pain perception. In D.J. Anderson and B. Matthews (Eds), Pain in the Trigeminal Region, Elsevier, Amsterdam, pp. 435–441.

Harkins, S.W. and Nowlin, J.B. (1985) Personality factors and chronic pain complaint in community dwelling elderly persons. Paper presented at the 93rd Annual Convention of the American Psychological Association, Los Angeles, Aug. 23–27, 1985.

Harkins, S.W. and Warner, M. (1980) Age and pain. In C. Eisdorfer (Ed.), Annual Review of Gerontology and Geriatrics, Vol. 1, Springer, New York, pp. 121–131.

Harkins, S.W., Kwentus, J. and Price, D. (1984) Pain in the elderly. In C. Benedetti, C.R. Chapman and G. Moricca (Eds.), Recent Advances in Pain Research and Therapy, Vol. 7, Raven Press, New York, pp. 103–122.

Harkins, S.W., Price, D. and Martelli, M. (1986) Effects of age on pain perception: thermonociception. J. Gerontol., 41: 58–63.

Harkins, S.W., Kwentus, J. and Price, D.D. (1988) Pain, discomfort, and suffering in the elderly. In J.J. Bonica (Ed.), Clinical Management of Pain, 2nd edn., Lea and Fabiger, New York, in press.

Hauser, P.M. (1986) Aging and increasing longevity of world population. In H. Hafner and G. Moscheln (Eds.), Sartorius, Mental Health in the Elderly, Springer Verlag, Berlin, pp. 9–28.

Kline, D.W. and Schieber, F. (1985) Vision and aging. In J.E. Birren and K.W. Schaie (Eds.), Psychology of Aging, 2nd edn., Van Nostrand Reinhold, New York, pp. 296–331.

Knapp, D.A. and Koch, H. (1984) The management of new pain in office based ambulatory care: National Ambulatory Medical Care Survey, 1980 and 1981. Advance data from vital and health statistics, No. 97, DHHS Publ. No. (PHS) 84–1250, Public Health Service, Hyattsville, MD, 1.

Krauter, E.E., Wallace, J.E. and Campbell, B.A. (1981) Sensory-motor function in the aging rat. Behav. Neurol. Biol., 31: 367–392.

Kwentus, J., Harkins, Lignon, N. and Silverman, J. (1985) Current concepts of geriatric pain and its treatment. Geriatrics, 40: 48–54.

MacDonald, J.B., Baillie, J., Williams, B.O. and Ballantyne, D. (1983) Coronary care in the elderly. Age Ageing, 12: 17–20.

Marsland, D.W., Wood, M. and Mayo, F. (1976) Content of Family Practice: A Statewide Study in Virginia with its Clincial, Educational, and Research Implications, Appleton-Century-Crofts, New York.

Medina, J.L., Diamond, S. and Rubio, F.A. (1975) Headaches in patients with transcient ischemic attacks. Headache, 15: 194–197.

Melzack, R. (1973) The Puzzle of Pain, Basic Books, New York.

Moss, M.S., Lawton, M.P. and Glicksman, A. (1986) The role of pain in the last year of life of elderly persons. Gerontologist, 26: 181.

Mumford, J.M. (1965) Pain perception threshold and adaptation of normal human teeth. Arch. Oral Biol., 10: 957–968.

Mumford, J.M. (1968) Pain perception in man on electrically stimulating the teeth. In A. Soulairac, J. Cohn and J. Charpenter (Eds.), Pain, Academic Press, London, pp. 224–229.

Olsho, L.W., Harkins, S.W. and Lenhardt, M.L. (1985) Aging and the auditory system. In J.E. Birren and K.W. Schaie (Eds.), Handbook of the Psychology of Aging, 2nd Edn., Van Nostrand, New York.

Procacci, P., Bozza, G., Buzzelli, G. and Della Corte, M. (1970) The cutaneous pricking pain threshold in old age. Gerontol. Clin., 12: 213–218.

Procacci, P., Della Corte, M., Zoppi, M., Romano, S., Maresca, M. and Voegelin, M. (1974) Pain threshold measurements in man. In J.J. Bonica and P. Procacci (Eds.), Recent Advances on Pain: Pathophysiology and Clinical Aspects, Charles C. Thomas, Springfield, IL, pp. 105–147.

Rodstein, M. (1956) The characteristics of non-fatal myocardial infarction in the aged. Arch. Intern. Med., 98: 684–690.

Schemper, T., Voss, S. and Cain, W.S. (1981) Odor discrimination in young and elderly persons: sensory and cognitive limitation. J. Gerontol., 36: 446–452.

Schiffman, S. (1977) Food recognition by the elderly. J. Gerontol., 32: 586–592.

Schluderman, E. and Zubek, J.P. (1962) Effect of age on pain sensitivity. Percept. Motor Skills, 14: 295–301.

Schumacher, G.A., Goodell, H., Hardy, J.D. and Wolff, H.G. (1940) Uniformity of the pain threshold in man. Science, 92: 110–112.

Sherman, E.D. and Robillard, E. (1960) Sensitivity to pain in the aged. Canad. Med. Assoc. J., 83: 944–947.

Sherman, E.D. and Robillard, E. (1964) Sensitivity to pain in relationship to age. J. Am. Geriatr. Soc., 12: 1037–1044.

Stevens, J.C. and Cain, W.S. (1985) Age-related deficiency in the perceived strength of six odorants. Chem. Senses, 10: 517–529.

Stevens, J.C. and Cain, W.S. (1987) Old-age deficits in the sense of smell as gauged by thresholds, magnitude matching, and odor identification. Psychol. Aging, 2: 36–42.

Stevens, J.C., Bartoshuk, L.M. and Cain, W.S. (1984) Chemical senses and aging: taste versus smell. Chem. Senses, 9: 167–179.

Stevens, J.C., Plantinga, A. and Cain, W.S. (1982) Reduction of odor and nasal pungency associated with aging. Neurobiol. Aging, 3: 125–132.

Verrillo, R.T. (1980) Age related changes in the sensitivity of vibration. J. Gerontol., 35: 185–193.

Verrillo, R.T. (1982a) Effects of vibrotactile thresholds as a function of age. Sens. Processes, 3: 49–52.

Verrillo, R.T. (1982b) Effects of aging on suprathreshold response to vibrations. Percept. Psychophys., 32: 61–68.

Wood, J.B. and Harkins, S.W. (1988) Effects of age, stimulus selection, and retrieval environment on odor identification. J. Gerontol., in press.

Woodrow, K.M., Friedman, G.D., Siegalaub, A.B. and Collen, M.F. (1972) Pain tolerance: differences according to age, sex, and race. Psychosom. Med., 34: 548–556.

R. Dubner, G.F. Gebhart & M.R. Bond (Eds.)
Proceedings of the Vth World Congress on Pain
© 1988 Elsevier Science Publishers BV (Biomedical Division)

CHAPTER 40

Varieties of pain

Warren S. Torgerson, Mohammed BenDebba and Karen J. Mason

Department of Neurosurgery, The Johns Hopkins University, School of Medicine, Baltimore, MD, USA

Background

The pains of a headache, a sprained ankle, a sore throat or a bee sting differ in quality or kind, as well as in location and intensity. The term 'pain' is used to represent a broad category of perceptually different experiences or feelings. The experiences themselves, of course, cannot be directly shared with others. They can, however, be described. The words used to describe these experiences denote differences in quality, as well as differences in intensity (Melzack and Torgerson, 1971; Torgerson and BenDebba, 1983).

In 1971, Melzack and Torgerson proposed a model for specifying the relationships among the meanings of over 100 words used by patients to describe their pains. Their model represents each word by its value on a common intensity scale and its membership in one of 16 mutually exclusive classes. The classes are grouped into three major domains: sensory, affective and evaluative. The assignment of words into classes was initially based on Melzack's and Torgerson's subjective judgements, and some descriptors were reclassified to reflect the judgements of subjects who were asked to agree or disagree with the assignments. Because

words associated primarily with perceptual quality also imply different levels of severity, Melzack and Torgerson conducted several psychological scaling experiments on all the descriptors. These experiments, using Thurstone's law of categorical judgement (see Torgerson, 1958), yielded numerical values of intensity on a single scale for all descriptors, regardless of their class membership. The rank order of the descriptors on the intensity scale was essentially the same across three groups of subjects.

Melzack (1975) used this classification and intensity system to develop a tool for assessing the perceptual properties of pain. The tool, the McGill Pain Questionnaire (MPQ), has proven clinically and experimentally useful (for a summary, see Reading, 1983).

Despite the usefulness of the MPQ, the classification aspect of the system on which it is based has been questioned. Several studies have suggested that some words have not been assigned to the appropriate class (Reading et al., 1982); others have suggested that the class structure may not be optimal for specifying the relationships between the meanings of the words (Bradshaw, 1979; Torgerson and BenDebba, 1983). Melzack and Torgerson were aware of the limitation of their system; their stated aim was 'to present an approach which, hopefully, will provide some guidelines for future studies using one or another of the newer, more elaborate multidimensional scaling or classification models.'

Correspondence: Mohammed BenDebba, Ph.D., Department of Neurosurgery, The Johns Hopkins School of Medicine, 600 N. Wolfe Street, Baltimore, 21205, U.S.A.

The ideal-type model

In 1983, Torgerson and BenDebba proposed that an alternative model, an ideal-type model with a single quantitative dimension, would be more appropriate for specifying the relationships between the meanings of the words. In this model, words can vary quantitatively not only in terms of their values on an intensity dimension, but also in terms of their relationships to a set of 'ideal' pain types or qualities. Both the original class model and the newer ideal-type model represent words by values on a common intensity scale. However, the ideal-type model specifies the qualitative meaning of each word by its degree of similarity to several ideal types of pain quality, instead of by its membership in one and only one class.

The experimental and analytical procedures for determining ideal-type structures are closely related to the class of procedures known as multidimensional scaling. Multidimensional scaling procedures in general begin with observations of similarity between pairs of elements from a stimulus domain and relate the elements to points in an abstract space and their dissimilarities to distances in that space. The procedures solve for the configuration, which is specified by the projection of the points on a set of coordinate axes. Since the orientation of axes is arbitrary, these projections often cannot be directly interpreted, and additional steps are required. The most important formal feature of the configuration is its 'shape', the position of the points relative to one another in the space. Different types of underlying structure place their own restrictions on the location of points relative to one another in the spatial representation. For example, with a purely quantitative structure, the points can be located anywhere in the space, but a nominal class structure requires that the points cluster on or about the vertices of a multidimensional tetrahedron. If the class structure also includes variation along quantitative dimensions, the points must lie along the edges of a multidimensional triangular prism (Torgerson, 1965). This last is the type of structure implied by the classification and intensity system proposed by Melzack and Torgerson (1971).

Analytical procedures which can manipulate a matrix of projections to reveal the shape of an observed configuration are available (Degerman, 1970; Satalich, 1981). Studies carried out in our laboratory and elsewhere suggest that the relationships between meanings of pain descriptors are not adequately represented either in terms of quantitative dimensions or in terms of a mixture of nominal classes and quantitative dimensions (Bradshaw, 1979; Reading et al., 1982).

Our preliminary studies indicate that an ideal-type model augmented by a quantitative dimension does represent the domain of pain descriptors very well. The rationale for the purely ideal-type model leads to a spatial representation where dissimilarities are interpreted as angular distances in the positive orthant on the surface of a hypersphere: points separated by an angular distance of 90° represent stimuli that are completely dissimilar (Torgerson, 1983). Thus, all stimulus points must lie on or within the boundaries of a hyperspherical triangle. The model is formally equivalent to Thurstone's positive manifold, simple structure in factor analysis (Thurstone, 1947). Ideal types correspond mathematically to pure factors and stimuli to tests that load on several factors.

When similarity between stimuli depends not only upon the ideal-type structure but also on variation along quantitative dimensions, dissimilarities between stimuli are interpreted as distances between points in a hypercylindrical space. A hypercylindrical space combines two independent subspaces: a hyperspherical subspace and a Euclidian-dimensional subspace. When stimulus points are projected onto the hyperspherical subspace, the hyperspherical distances between them reflect stimulus variations resulting from an underlying ideal-type structure. When stimulus points are projected onto the Euclidian subspace, the distances reflect stimulus variations in continuous quantitative dimensions. This is the geometric representation of the structure of pain descriptors proposed by Torgerson and BenDebba (1983). Computer algorithms which can transform observed measures of similarity into hypercylindrical distances and solve for the projections of the stimulus points in a hypercylindrical space have been developed by Satalich (1981).

Empirical studies

A large-scale study is now being conducted to determine whether the relationships between meanings of pain descriptors can be represented by a structure resulting from a mixture of ideal types and a single quantitative dimension of intensity. The overall project involves the entire set of 102 descriptors compiled for the original paper by Melzack and Torgerson (1971). A series of interlocking studies, involving overlapping sets of 20 to 25 descriptors each, has been completed, and preliminary analyses of the data have been carried out. Since the experimental method, population and analytical procedures have been and will be essentially the same for each of the individual studies, only two studies will be described here.

The subjects for both studies were student volunteers from The Johns Hopkins University. The students either received course credit or were paid for their participation. A group of 16 students participated in one study, and a second group of 17 participated in the other.

The descriptors for the first study were drawn from Melzack's and Torgerson's sensory domain and were chosen to represent the punctate pressure, the incisive pressure, the dullness, and the miscellaneous sensory subclasses. They are listed in Table I. The descriptors for the second study, listed in Table II, were drawn from the affective domain and were chosen to represent the tension, the autonomic, the fear, and the punishment subclasses.

In both studies, the subjects' task was to rate all possible pairs of descriptors on a numerical scale of similarity from 0 (identical) to 9 (dissimilar). The subjects were asked to use the following context for their judgements: 'If the single word _____ best describes a particular pain, how close would each of the words listed below be in describing the

pain?' The blank was filled with a 'key' descriptor, and the list was composed of all the remaining words in the study. Each word served in turn as a key word for each subject, so that each subject made 380 individual judgements.

Several preliminary analyses were performed to determine the reliability of the judgements and to investigate any possible systematic differences in judgements between individuals. Since each pair of words was presented twice to each subject, the correlation between the two ratings across all pairs was used to estimate individual subject reliability. These correlations, ranging from 0.614 to 0.852 for the first study and from 0.516 to 0.808 for the second study, indicated that reliable judgements were obtained from most subjects. To determine whether or not systematic individual differences existed, the two ratings for each pair of descriptors were averaged for each subject, and an inverse principal component analysis was performed on the average ratings. No significant differences were found. The ratings for each pair were then averaged across subjects. These average ratings, with reliabilities in the nineties, were used to construct a matrix of dissimilarities for each study; these matrices were the raw input for the hypercylindrical scaling program (HYPCYL) developed by Satalich (1981).

The confirmatory option of HYPCYL was used. A single quantitative dimension was hypothesized and the intensity scale values of the stimuli, as reported in the original Melzack-Torgerson study (1971), served as the target vector for the single dimension of the quantitative subspace.

The results of the analysis for the first study showed a very close fit in a one-quantitative dimension, four ideal-type hypercylindrical space. Stress, the usual overall index of fit in multidimensional scaling, had a value of only 0.04. The projections of the stimuli on the quantitative dimension, as shown in the first column of Table I, correlated 0.93 with the original Melzack-Torgerson intensity values of the stimuli. The relationship between these values and the original Melzack-Torgerson values was linear despite the difference in the methods by which they were obtained. The projections of the descriptors in the four ideal-type hyperspherical subspace are shown in the last four data columns (these projections would all have been approximately zero or one if a class structure had been appropriate). The configuration obtained is easily interpretable. The projections of the stimuli on the first ideal-type axis can be interpreted as describing sharpness (Type I), on the second as describing dullness (Type II), on the third as describing a rasping quality (Type III), and on the fourth as describing tautness (Type IV). A surface plot illustrating the ideal-type structure obtained in this study is shown in Fig. 1. The plot gives the projections of the stimuli on the surface of the spherical subspace defined by ideal Types II, III and IV. The words lie within the boundaries of the hyperspherical triangle defined by the three Types, as required by the model. The study shows that many of the words do not closely approximate a single type of pain but tend to describe a mixture of qualities. For example, the word 'tearing' describes a pain about halfway between Types III and IV. In a like manner, tender, hurting and sore describe pains that are quite dull but tend to shade off in other directions. The plot also shows that no single descriptor uniquely describes Type IV. Taut is close but has a bit of Type II to it.

Analyses for the second study showed a very close fit in one quantitative dimension, five ideal-type hypercylindrical space. A stress value of 0.06 indicates a reasonably good fit between the data and the model. The projections of the stimuli on the quantitative dimension, as shown in column one of Table II, are linearly related to the original Melzack-Torgerson intensity value with a correlation of 0.88. The projections of the descriptors in the five ideal-type hyperspherical subspace are shown in the last five data columns. The ideal-type structure obtained is intuitively reasonable. The best single descriptors for each of the types in order are

TABLE I

Projections of descriptors on the quantitative dimension and on four orthogonal ideal-type axes for Study 1

Stimuli	Intensity	Ideal-type axes			
		I	II	III	IV
Penetrating	0.087	0.869	0.442	0.070	0.212
Piercing	0.601	0.879	0.267	0.289	0.268
Stabbing	0.489	0.936	0.130	0.232	0.229
Lancinating	0.546	0.686	0.500	0.526	0.045
Sharp	0.416	0.860	0.070	0.352	0.364
Cutting	0.408	0.697	0.025	0.379	0.609
Lacerating	0.335	0.541	−0.087	0.701	0.456
Dull	−0.592	0.282	0.952	0.037	0.116
Blurred	−0.516	0.068	0.907	0.411	0.062
Sore	−0.532	0.644	0.642	0.364	0.202
Numbing	−0.360	0.010	0.975	0.072	0.211
Hurting	−0.173	0.775	0.518	0.312	0.184
Aching	−0.375	0.634	0.729	0.133	0.223
Heavy	−0.348	0.315	0.938	−0.145	0.003
Steady	−0.324	0.420	0.782	0.085	0.453
Tender	−0.664	0.746	0.470	0.389	0.267
Taut	−0.224	0.326	0.347	0.168	0.863
Rasping	−0.009	0.312	0.150	0.937	0.055
Tearing	0.391	0.341	0.120	0.703	0.612
Splitting	0.546	0.623	0.428	0.083	0.650

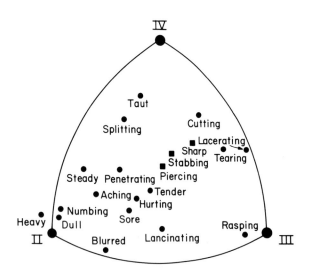

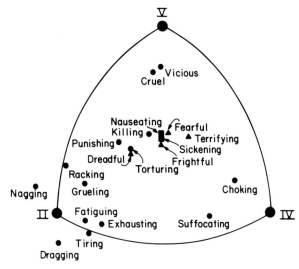

Fig. 1. Surface plot illustrating the ideal-type structure obtained for the subset of sensory words. The numbers at the vertices of the hyperspherical triangle correspond to the numbers identifying the ideal-type axes in Table I. Words identified by (■) are off the surface defined by these axes.

Fig. 2. Surface plot illustrating the ideal-type structure obtained for the subset of sensory words. The numbers at the vertices of the hyperspherical triangle correspond to the numbers identifying the ideal-type axes in Table II. Words identified by (▲ and ■) are off the surface defined by these axes.

TABLE II

Projections of descriptors on the quantitative dimension and on five orthogonal ideal-type axes for Study 2

| Stimuli | Intensity | Ideal-type axes | | | | |
		I	II	III	IV	V
Nagging	−0.635	−0.004	0.947	0.253	−0.163	0.113
Dragging	−0.676	0.078	0.956	0.223	0.127	−0.122
Tiring	−1.211	0.073	0.939	0.149	0.294	0.058
Fatiguing	−1.262	0.103	0.944	0.165	0.243	0.111
Exhausting	−0.796	0.159	0.908	0.119	0.348	0.126
Nauseating	−0.042	0.249	0.316	0.888	0.213	0.068
Choking	0.922	0.411	0.229	0.431	0.763	0.101
Sickening	0.126	0.289	0.347	0.854	0.246	0.082
Suffocating	0.528	0.360	0.429	0.297	0.773	0.023
Fearful	−0.221	0.965	0.052	0.195	0.154	0.066
Dreadful	0.150	0.894	0.300	0.317	0.100	0.029
Frightful	0.123	0.973	0.079	0.165	0.142	0.020
Terrifying	0.555	0.952	0.015	0.084	0.272	0.113
Punishing	−0.044	0.597	0.636	0.169	0.181	0.422
Gruelling	−0.473	0.429	0.841	0.158	0.140	0.255
Racking	0.499	0.452	0.830	0.137	−0.036	0.294
Cruel	0.314	0.683	0.306	0.183	0.058	0.635
Vicious	0.695	0.787	0.168	0.097	0.032	0.585
Torturing	0.381	0.667	0.578	0.235	0.224	0.339
Killing	1.065	0.721	0.457	−0.003	0.258	0.453

frightful (Type I), fatiguing (Type II), nauseating (Type III), suffocating (Type IV) and cruel (Type V). A surface plot depicting the relationships between the descriptors in the study and ideal Types II, IV and V is shown in Fig. 2. All the words tend to lie within the boundaries of a hyperspherical triangle defined by the three Types. Again, many of the words denote pains related, in different degrees, to several of the ideal pain types. There are no words that connote ideal Types III, IV or V uniquely. Nauseating and sickening, while approximating ideal Type III, shade off toward the fatiguing type of pain. Choking is close to ideal Type IV with a bit of nausea added. Suffocating is also close to ideal Type IV, but it has a little of both nausea and fatigue associated with it. Cruel and vicious approximate ideal Type V, but they also tend to denote a bit of fear.

The results of the studies reported here, along with initial results from other sets of descriptors, show that the hypercylindrical model describes the structure of the meanings of the pain descriptors very well. It appears to be an excellent structural model for representing both the quantitative and the qualitative variations in the subjective meaning of the verbal descriptors. The quantitative dimension obtained corresponds closely to independent measures of intensity of pain implied by the descriptors. Projections of the descriptors in the hyperspherical subspace do not, in general, form the tight clusters that would exist if the original Melzack-Torgerson classification structure were correct. The ideal types revealed by this completely objective procedure make very good subjective sense. Nineteen ideal types have been identified. A list of the descriptors closest to each of the types is presented in Table III.

TABLE III

Pain descriptors closest to each of the 19 idealized primary pain types

I. Sensory domain

1	2	3	4	5
Sharp	Boring	Stabbing	Dull	Rasping
Cutting	Drilling	Pricking	Numbing	Tearing
6	7	8	9	10
Taut	Tugging	Squeezing	Hot	Flickering
Splitting	Pulling	Crushing	Burning	Quivering
11	12	13	14	
Pounding	Itching	Radiating	Flashing	
Throbbing	Tickling	Spreading	Shocking	

II. Affective domain

15	16	17	18	19
Frightful	Dragging	Sickening	Choking	Cruel
Fearful	Fatiguing	Nauseating	Suffocating	Vicious

A substantial amount of work remains to be done before a complete ideal-type structure of pain descriptors is realized. However, the results obtained thus far suggest that the ideal-type structure of the descriptors may be organized into two relatively distinct subspaces: one containing the sensory types and the other the affective types. The Melzack-Torgerson evaluative domain corresponds to the intensity dimension and is shared by all descriptors whether sensory or affective.

Acknowledgement

This work was supported by the National Institutes of Health grants GM-29772 and NS-21718.

References

Bradshaw, M.H. (1979) The effect of context on the structure of pain. Doctoral dissertation. The Johns Hopkins University, Baltimore, MD.

Degerman, R. (1970) Multidimensional analysis of complex structure: Mixture of class and quantitative variation. Psychometrika, 35: 475–491.

Melzack, R. (1975) The McGill Pain Questionnaire: Major properties and scoring methods. Pain, 1: 277–299.

Melzack, R. and Torgerson, W.S. (1971) On the language of pain. Anesthesiology, 34: 50–59.

Reading, A.E. (1983) The McGill Pain Questionnaire: an appraisal. In R. Melzack (Ed.), Pain Measurement and Assessment, Raven Press, New York, pp. 55–61.

Reading, A.E., Everitt, B.S. and Sledmere, G.M. (1982) The

McGill Pain Questionnaire: a replication of its construction. Br. J. Clin. Psychol., 21: 339–349.

Satalich, T.A. (1981) Hypercylindrical multidimensional scaling: The ideal type model. Doctoral dissertation. The Johns Hopkins University, Baltimore, MD.

Thurstone, L.L. (1947) Multiple Factor Analysis, University of Chicago Press, Chicago.

Torgerson, W.S. (1958) Theory and Methods of Scaling, John Wiley & Sons, New York.

Torgerson, W.S. (1965) Multidimensional scaling of similarity. Psychometrika, 30: 379–393.

Torgerson, W.S. (1983) The Ideal type model. In H. Wainer and S. Messick (Eds.), Principals of Modern Psychological Measurement, Erlbaum, Hillsdale, New Jersey.

Torgerson, W.S. and BenDebba, M. (1983) The structure of pain descriptors. In R. Melzack (Ed.), Pain Measurement and Assessment, Raven Press, New York, pp. 49–54.

R. Dubner, G.F. Gebhart & M.R. Bond (Eds.)
Proceedings of the Vth World Congress on Pain
© 1988 Elsevier Science Publishers BV (Biomedical Division)

CHAPTER 41

Multidimensional experimental pain study in normal man: combining physiological and psychological indices

M. Luu[1], A.M. Bonnel[2] and F. Boureau[1]

[1]*Lab. Physiol. Hôpital Saint-Antoine, Paris, France, and* [2]*U.E.R., Psychol. Exp., Univ. Provence, Aix en Provence,*
France

Summary

In the same experimental session, we studied different physiological and psychological pain indices evoked by sural nerve electrical stimulation: biceps nociceptive RIII reflex (threshold and frequency of occurrence); and psychological verbal responses on sensory and affective scales of 7 categories (threshold, subjective direct estimation and Signal Detection Theory (SDT) indices for both scales). Two successive experiments were conducted to study (1) the sensitivity of the indices after morphine and naloxone i.v. administration, and (2) the intercorrelations between different indices. After morphine administration we observed a differential sensitivity of the tested indices: psychological indices were more sensitive than physiological indices; indices calculated from the affective scale were more sensitive than those calculated with the sensory scale; and attitude B SDT indices were more sensitive than discriminative P(A). We observed a good correlation but no concordance between RIII threshold and subjective sensory and affective pain thresholds. These results suggest that psychological and physiological parameters are complementary rather than equivalent. The absence of correlation between discriminative P(A) and attitude B SDT indices, the results of intercorrelation study between

these indices and the subjective thresholds and the dissociation of the sensitivity of the two rating scales may indicate that SDT parameters reflect more the discrimination and the attitude of subjects for a specific scale than sensory and affective pain dimensions per se.

Introduction

Although there is good agreement in the literature to consider pain as a complex neuropsychological phenomenon with sensory-discriminative, affective, cognitive and behavioral components (Melzack and Casey, 1968), there is still a need for valid laboratory methods permitting the discrimination and selective assessment of the above dimensions (Chapman et al., 1985).

Different methods have been proposed. Gracely et al. (1978), Tursky et al. (1982) and Price et al. (1983) have assessed sensory and affective dimensions through corresponding verbal (or visual analogue) scales. Chapman (1974) and Clark (1974), among others (for references, see Grossberg, 1976; Lloyd and Appel, 1978), suggested that Sensory Decision Theory (SDT) P(A) and B indices may reflect, respectively, sensory and affective and/or cognitive pain components. Such an interpretation of the SDT indices applied to pain evaluation is controversial, however (Rollman, 1977; Coppola and Gracely, 1983).

The aim of our experimentation was two-fold. Our purpose was firstly to combine in the same experimental session the study of different psychological and physiological indices for multidimensional experimental pain assessment; secondly, to analyse the sensitivity and the validity of the measured indices. As an objective physiological parameter, we studied the biceps nociceptive RIII reflex evoked by sural nerve electrical stimulation. The subjective verbal responses were studied with two 7-category, sensory and affective scales. The SDT indices were calculated for the two verbal scales for each consecutive intensity pair. Two successive experiments were conducted to study (1) the sensitivity of the indices after morphine and naloxone administration, and (2) the intercorrelations between different indices.

Methods

Experiment I

Subjects were two females and eight males. Age ranged from 25 to 37 years (mean = 32.5 ± 4.2 years). In the first, preliminary, session they were informed about the experimental procedures and trained in their use. During the experimental session, subjects reclined comfortably in a chair in order to produce good muscular relaxation.

Electrical stimulation and nociceptive reflex recording methodology were similar to other authors (Hugon, 1967; Willer, 1977). Electrical stimulation was delivered by a constant-intensity stimulator. The stimulus was a 20 ms train of 1 ms pulses delivered at 30 Hz to the sural nerve through surface electrodes. Time interval between two successive stimulations varied, with an approximate mean interval of 10 s. The stimulation series was composed of 5 intensity levels, ranging from 6 to 18 mA in 3 mA steps. Each intensity was delivered 10 times. The series was constructed so that sequential effects could be controlled.

Biceps femoris muscle activity was recorded with surface electrodes. Only the late component of the flexion reflex was studied. The latency of the RIII nociceptive flexion reflex ranged from 90 to 180 ms. The response was considered present when an amplitude greater than 50 μV was observed.

The experimental session was organized in the following manner. After preliminary training for 10 min, an intravenous perfusion with glucose 5% was begun. At T0, a first series of 50 stimuli was delivered during 10 min. At T10, morphine (0.14 mg/kg) was infused. The second series of 50 stimuli began five minutes later (T15). At T25, naloxone (0.01 mg/kg) was infused. Five minutes later (T30), the third series of 50 stimuli was administered. The overall duration of the experimental session lasted 40 to 60 min.

Each stimulation was judged by subjects with two ordinal scales. The sensory scale (SS) was composed of 7 categories numbered from 7 to 1: 7 = nothing; 6 = just noticeable; 5 = tactile sensation; 4 = weak pricking; 3 = moderate pricking; 2 = strong pricking; and 1 = very strong pricking.

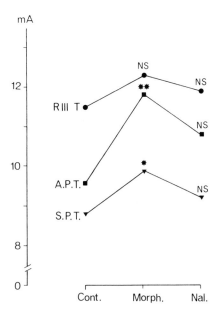

Fig. 1. Nociceptive RIII threshold (RIII T), sensory and affective pain thresholds (SPT, APT) after morphine injection (0.14 mg/kg) and naloxone (0.01 mg/kg) (paired t Student).

The affective scale (AS) was composed of 7 categories: 7 = nothing; 6 = not unpleasant; 5 = weakly unpleasant; 4 = rather unpleasant; 3 = clearly unpleasant; 2 = extremely unpleasant; and 1 = unbearable. In a preliminary study, we confirmed that these two scales were ordinal and well adapted for the phasic electrical stimulation used in the study.

Different indices were collected. We studied the RIII threshold (RIII T), defined as the intensity level which evoked 50% of the RIII response. For each intensity level, the frequency of RIII response was studied. Sensory pain threshold (SPT) was defined as the intensity level which gave 50% of 'weak pricking' response. Similarly, affective pain threshold (APT) was defined as the intensity level which gave 50% of 'weakly unpleasant' response. For each intensity level, the mean scores for sensory (SS) and affective scales (AS) were calculated. Verbal responses were also analysed with non-parametric SDT. For each intensity pair, SDT P(A) and B indices for sensory and affective scales were calculated.

Experiment II

In this experiment the subjects were five females and eleven males with ages ranging from 20 to 43 years (mean = 31.5 ± 6.5 years). This was their first experience with an experimental pain session.

Electrical stimulation, reflex response recordings, and verbal responses were similar to those in experiment I. The session was composed of preliminary training lasting 10 min followed by one stimulation series. According to the training phase, the range of the 5 stimulation levels delivered 10 times was either 3 to 15 mA or 6 to 18 mA.

The statistical tests used were paired t Student, paired T Wilcoxon for mean comparison and the non-parametric method of Spearman for the intercorrelation study.

Results

Experiment I

After morphine, RIII threshold (RIII T) was not significantly modified ($t = 1.813$, df = 9) (Fig. 1).

The mean RIII occurrence for each stimulation intensity is given in Fig. 2. At the 12 mA level, the RIII frequency decreased significantly after morphine (10 pairs, Wilcoxon $T = 0$, $P < 0.05$). This effect was not significantly modified by naloxone.

In the control session, pain thresholds for sensory and affective scales were respectively 8.8 ± 2.0 (SPT) and 9.9 ± 1.9 mA (APT). After morphine, SPT and APT increased significantly, respectively, 9.6 ± 2.7 mA ($t = 2.333$, df = 9, $P < 0.05$) and 11.8 ± 3.2 mA ($t = 3.805$, df = 9, $P < 0.001$) (Fig. 1). SPT and APT decreased after administration of naloxone, however, the reversal was not statistically significant (Fig. 1).

After morphine SS mean ratings diminished significantly at intensities 9 and 15 mA (10 pairs, respectively Wilcoxon $T = 4$ and 3, $P < 0.05$). (Fig. 3A). After naloxone a significant reversal effect was observed for these two intensities. AS mean ratings diminished for 9, 12, 15, and 18 mA intensities (Fig. 3B). These effects were significantly reversed by naloxone at 12, 15, and 18 mA intensities.

Table I presents the mean values of P(A) and B SDT indices for SS and AS for the 4 consecutive intensity pairs. For SS, P(A) indices are not statistically modified after morphine; B indices increased significantly for each intensity pair. These effects

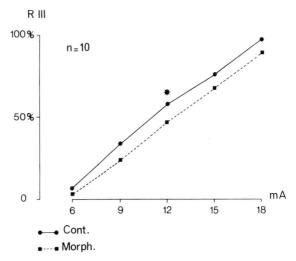

Fig. 2. Mean RIII occurrence (%) for each stimulation intensity in control condition and after morphine administration (paired T Wilcoxon, ten pairs).

TABLE I

Comparison of P(A) and B SDT indices means for Sensory Scale (SS) and Affective Scale (AS) for each intensity pair between control condition and after morphine administration (paired T Wilcoxon, ten pairs).

	Intensity pairs (mA)	9–6 mean ± SD	12–9 mean ± SD	15–12 mean ± SD	18–15 mean ± SD
S.S.					
P(A)	Control	0.74 ± 0.12	0.81 ± 0.10	0.77 ± 0.15	0.65 ± 0.20
	Morphine	0.67 ± 0.13	0.84 ± 0.12	0.76 ± 0.15	0.68 ± 0.15
		T = 12	T = 17	T = 15	T = 12
		NS	NS	NS	NS
B	Control	4.15 ± 0.46	3.51 ± 0.61	2.80 ± 0.65	2.35 ± 0.85
	Morphine	4.41 ± 0.46	3.73 ± 0.68	3.01 ± 0.65	2.54 ± 0.76
		T = 0	T = 6	T = 4	T = 2
		P < 0.01	P < 0.05	P < 0.05	P < 0.01
A.S.					
P(A)	Control	0.69 ± 0.19	0.72 ± 0.18	0.83 ± 0.08	0.67 ± 0.19
	Morphine	0.61 ± 0.15	0.72 ± 0.19	0.77 ± 0.12	0.57 ± 0.14
		T = 3	T = 13	T = 20	T = 3
		NS	NS	NS	P < 0.05
B	Control	5.20 ± 0.36	4.69 ± 0.64	4.05 ± 0.71	3.43 ± 0.78
	Morphine	5.39 ± 0.20	5.03 ± 0.48	4.51 ± 0.63	4.13 ± 0.69
		T = 0	T = 0	T = 3	T = 1
		P < 0.05	P < 0.01	P < 0.01	P < 0.01

NS, not significant.

were not significantly reversed by naloxone. For AS, P(A) dropped significantly to chance level after morphine for the 18–15 mA pair (10 pairs, Wilcoxon $T = 3$, $P < 0.05$); as for SS, B indices increased after morphine whatever the pair. These B modifications were reversed by naloxone except for the lowest 906 mA pair.

Experiment II

Sensory and affective pain thresholds (SPT, APT) were, respectively, 6.2 ± 3.1 and 5.9 ± 2.1 mA. They were not statistically different ($t = 0.468$, df = 15). They were correlated at 0.67 ($P < 0.01$). As in experiment I, RIII threshold (RII T: 12.9 ± 2.4) was statistically higher than subjective thresholds (respectively, $t = 8.774$ and $t = 15.607$, df = 15, $P < 0.001$). RIII T was correlated with SPT and APT, respectively, at 0.52 (P < 0.05) and 0.62 ($P < 0.02$).

Fig. 4 presents the frequency of RIII, 'weak pricking', 'weakly unpleasant' responses for each stimulation intensity. As is shown in this figure, an excellent superposition of sensory and affective response curves was observed. In contrast, the RIII curve was not superposed with subjective curves, confirming the non-concordance between subjective pain and RIII responses.

For each subject, SS and AS P(A) and B indices of the intensity pair which correspond to the respective thresholds were calculated. Intercorrelation study shows a correlation of 0.56 ($P < 0.05$) between the P(A) indices of the two scales, as well as between the B indices of the two scales (0.58, $P < 0.05$). For SS, neither correlation between P(A) and B were significant (0.10) nor the correlation between AS P(A) and B indices (−0.39).

The intercorrelations between thresholds and SDT indices were calculated. There was no correlation between physiological threshold (RIII T) and the SDT indices of the two scales. The correlations between P(A) and B indices and subjective thresh-

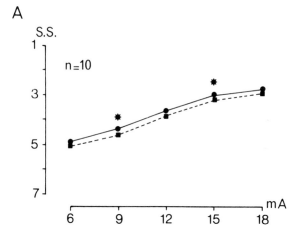

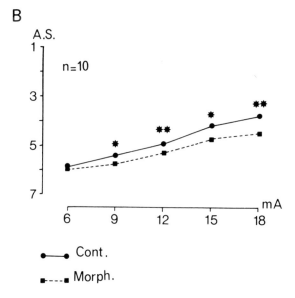

Fig. 3. Mean scores for sensory (SS) (A) and affective (AS) (B) scales for each intensity level in control condition and after morphine administration (paired *T* Wilcoxon, ten pairs).

Discussion

After morphine (0.14 mg/kg), it is interesting to observe a differential sensitivity of the tested parameters: verbal psychological indices appeared to be more sensitive than the RIII physiological indices; indices calculated from the affective scale were more sensitive than those calculated from the sensory scale; attitude B SDT indices were more sensitive than discriminative P(A). These differential effects support the use of multicriterial assessment. Since the effects of morphine were more salient with affective subjective parameters, we may have measured non-specific placebo factors. This explanation is unlikely since a previous experiment using the same assessment procedure did not show any modification of the different indices after oral administration of 10 mg morphine and a placebo. Taken together, our results suggest that low doses of morphine act mostly on the unpleasantness component of pain. However, we cannot rule out that the affective scale parameters are more sensitive than the sensory one.

The lack of effect of morphine on the RIII threshold is in agreement with Willer's data (1985) showing a clear RIII threshold increment for a higher dose of morphine (0.2 mg/kg). In our study, we did not quantify the RIII response amplitude which might be a more sensitive parameter at su-

olds were not simple. The best were between: the sensory pain threshold (SPT) and SS and AS B indices (respectively, 0.55, $P < 0.05$ and 0.85, $P < 0.01$); the affective pain threshold (APT) and SS and AS P(A) indices (respectively, -0.67, $P < 0.01$ and -0.63 $P < 0.05$). If each scale is considered, for the sensory scale SPT was correlated with B (0.55, $P < 0.05$) but not with P(A) (-0.23); for the affective scale, APT was correlated with the P(A) and B indices (respectively, 0.63 and 0.51, $P < 0.05$).

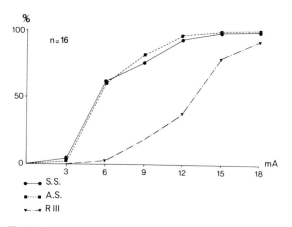

Fig. 4. Frequency (%) of RIII, 'weak pricking' (SS) and 'weakly unpleasant' (AS) responses for each stimulation intensity.

praliminar intensities. It is interesting to notice that the RIII frequency was significantly modified at a paraliminar intensity level (12 mA). These data show that the RIII frequency for each intensity value is more informative than a single index such as the statistical RIII threshold.

Furthermore, in contrast to the RIII indices, verbal indices are significantly modified after morphine. These effects are greater concerning the affective scale for pain threshold as well as direct subjective estimation. This preferential effect of morphine on the affective unpleasantness component is in agreement with the data of Price et al. (1985) showing a selective effect on this dimension with low doses of morphine IV (0.04 mg/kg). In this study, the visual analog sensory ratings were modified by a higher dose (0.08 mg/kg). Gracely et al. (1979) observed a preferential effect on the sensory intensity verbal description after fentanyl administration. However, in this experiment, fentanyl induced nausea. This unpleasantness side effect could have modified the judgement of the unpleasantness component of pain (Gracely, 1987, personal communication).

Concerning SDT indices, morphine modified attitude B indices on both verbal scales for each intensity pair. This effect was reversed by naloxone. However, discrimination P(A) indices changed only for the highest pair on the affective scale. Concerning SDT assessment of morphine analgesia, conflicting results have been reported in the literature. In normal man, Yang et al. (1979) observed modification of both SDT indices after morphine 0.14 mg/kg i.v.). However, in Buchsbaum et al.'s study (1981), the discrimination index was modified after 5 mg morphine i.m. but not the attitude index. In rhesus monkey performing a discrimination task, Lineberry and Kulics (1978), observed an opposite trend. Such conflicting results do not elicit any unambiguous interpretation of the SDT indices based on morphine analgesia.

According to the literature, SDT indices should be independent. Discriminative P(A) index would reflect the sensory dimension and attitude B index, the affective and/or cognitive dimension (Chap-

man, 1974; Clark, 1974). However, this hypothesis is not generally accepted (Rollman, 1977; Coppola and Gracely, 1983). In our study P(A) and B indices of each scale were not correlated. This is in good agreement with the independence of the two SDT indices. After morphine administration, we observed that the response criterion increased on both scales, i.e., when intensity and unpleasantness is appreciated. In contrast, P(A) was modified only on the unpleasantness scale. The non-parallel effect indicates that variations of SDT indices depend on the scale used. Thus, it seems that SDT indices may reflect discrimination and attitude for a specific scale rather than pain dimensions per se. When a global pain judgement is used, related P(A) and B indices reflect an unknown integration of the discrimination and attitude of the various sensory and affective components of pain. Our results justify the study of SDT indices for the two sensory and affective rating scales as Rollman (1983) proposed.

Yang et al. (1985) showed that subjective pain threshold was correlated with attitude B index but not with discriminative P(A) index. In our study intercorrelations between SDT indices and subjective pain thresholds are difficult to interpret. The APT was correlated with the respective P(A) and B indices but the SPT was only correlated with the respective B index and not with the respective P(A).

It is worth noting that the only modification of the P(A) index corresponds to the highest intensity pair which led to almost a 100% RIII occurrence. This result suggests that intense stimuli, instead of the usual paraliminar ones, may be investigated for the study of analgesia mechanisms on the sensitivity parameter.

The RIII flexion reflex has a protective, nociceptive function according to Sherrington's concept (1910). Willer observed the same threshold for pain sensation and RIII response (1977), and a good correlation between pain sensation and flexion reflex amplitudes for supraliminar stimulation (1985). Our results confirm a good correlation between RIII threshold and sensory or affective pain thresholds (respectively, $r = 0.53$ and 0.62). However, as is shown in Figs. 1 and 4, we have not been able to confirm a good concordance between RIII threshold and subjective threshold. In the two experiments, RIII flexion reflex threshold was higher than the sensory or affective pain threshold. Bromm and Treede (1980) also observed a discrepancy but in the opposite direction: flexion reflex threshold was smaller than pain threshold. We have no explanation for this discrepancy. A difference could be that we tested lower limb reflexes and Bromm and Treede, upper limb reflexes. Considering experiments I and II, the difference between RIII threshold and pain sensation was much less when subjects were trained. This suggests that trained subjects may learn to adjust their subjective judgement to the perceived flexion reflex.

Taken together, our results show that low doses of morphine act mostly on the unpleasantness component of pain. This result is in good agreement with empirical clinical data on morphine analgesia. This effect of morphine implicates a complex integrative mechanism. Le Bars et al. (1986) observed that analgesic low doses of morphine restore the background noise of convergent spinal neurons towards its original level through a reduction of diffuse noxious inhibitory control (DNIC) without inhibiting the spinal transmission of excitatory nociceptive messages to the higher centres. With higher doses, an inhibition of the segmental pool of active spinal neurones is superimposed on this primary mechanism. Our results with low doses of morphine are in good agreement with the observation of Le Bars et al. We observed a selective effect on the affective component without any effect on the RIII response, which reflects spinal activity. It would be interesting to study the effects of different morphine doses with our protocol. An expected result may be that higher morphine doses depress concordantly sensory verbal responses and RIII reflex.

The advantage of our assessment protocol is the combination of psychological and neurophysiological indices. These indices appear complementary rather than equivalent and reflect different integration levels in the sensory pathways. The greater sensitivity of the psychological indices after low doses of morphine reveal the complementarity of the tested indices. The measurement is not limited to the global classical subjective or RIII reflex thresholds. It permits sensory and affective subjective direct evaluation as well as the study of the frequency of occurrence of the RIII response along the stimulus continuum. Similarly, we studied the discrimination and attitude SDT indices of different intensity pairs for two scales (sensory and affective).

Multicriteria assessment increases information and this may result in greater sensitivity and better understanding of pain mechanisms.

Acknowledgements

We are grateful to R.H. Gracely for his helpful comments.

References

Bromm, B. and Treede, R.D. (1980) Withdrawal reflex, skin resistance reaction and pain ratings due to electrical stimuli in man, Pain. 9: 339–354.

Buchsbaum, M.S., Davis, G.C., Coppola, R. and Naber, D. (1981) Opiate pharmacology and individual differences I. Psychophysical pain measurements. Pain, 10: 357–366.

Chapman, C.R. (1974) An alternative threshold assessment in the study of human pain. In J.J. Bonica (Ed.), Advances in Neurology, Vol. 4, Raven Press, N.Y., pp. 115–121.

Chapman, C.R., Casey, K.L., Dubner, R., Folly, K.R., Gracely, R.H. and Reading, A.E. (1985) Pain measurement: an overview. Pain, 22: 1–33.

Clark, W.C. (1974) Pain sensitivity and the report of pain. An introduction to Sensory Decision Theory, Anesthesiology, 40: 272–287.

Coppola, R. and Gracely, R.H. (1983) Where is the noise in SDT pain assessment? Pain, 17: 257–266.

Gracely, R.H., McGrath, P. and Dubner, R. (1978) Ratio scales of sensory and affective verbal pain descriptors. Pain, 5: 5–18.

Gracely, R.H., McGrath, P. and Dubner, R. (1979) Narcotic analgesia: fentanyl reduces the intensity but not the unpleasantness of painful tooth pulp sensations. Science, 203: 1261–1263.

Grossberg, J.M. (1978) Clinical psychophysics: Applications of ratio scaling and signal detection methods to research on pain, fear, drugs, and medical decision making. Psychol. Bull. 85: 1154-1176.

Hugon, M. (1967) Reflexes polysynaptiques cutanes et commande volontaire, These Sciences, Paris.

Le Bars, D., Dickenson, A.H., Besson, J.M. and Villanueva, L. (1986) Aspects of sensory processing through convergent neurons. In T.L. Yaksh (Ed.), Spinal Afferent Processing, Plenum, New York, pp. 467–504.

Lineberry, C.G. and Kulics, A.T. (1978) The effects of diazepam, morphine and lidocaine on nociception in Rhesus monkey: a signal detection analysis. J. Pharmacol. Exp. Ther., 205: 302–310.

Lloyd, A.M. and Appel, J.B. (1976) Signal detection theory and the psychophysics of pain: an introduction and review. Psychosom. Med., 38: 79–94.

Melzack, R. and Casey, KL. (1968) Sensory, motivational and central control determinants of pain: a new conceptual model. In D. Kenshalo (Ed.), The Skin Senses, C.C. Thomas, Springfield, pp. 423–439.

Price, D.D., McGrath, P.A., Rafii, A. and Buckingham, B. (1983). The validation of visual analogue scale as ratio scale measures for chronic and experimental pain. Pain, 17: 45–56.

Price, D.D., Von der Gruen, A., Miller, J., Rafii, A. and Price, C. (1985) A psychophysical analysis of morphine analgesia. Pain, 22: 249–261.

Rollman, G.B. (1977) Signal detection theory measurement of pain. A review and critique. Pain, 3: 187–211.

Rollman, G.B. (1983) Multiple subjective representations of experimental pain. In J.J. Bonica et al. (Eds.), Advances in Pain Research and Therapy, vol. 5, Raven Press, N.Y., pp. 865–869.

Sherrington, C.S. (1910) Flexion-reflex of the limb, crossed extension-reflex and reflex stepping and standing. J. Physiol., 40: 28–121.

Tursky, B., Jammer, L.D. and Friedman, R. (1982) The pain perception profile: a psychophysical approach to the assessment of pain report. Behav. Ther., 13: 376–394.

Willer, J.C. (1977) Comparative study of perceived pain and nociceptive flexion reflex in man. Pain, 3: 69–80.

Willer, J.C. (1985) Studies on pain. Effects of morphine on a spinal nociceptive flexion reflex and related pain sensation in man. Brain Res., 331: 105–114.

Yang, J.C., Clark, W.C., Ngai, S.H., Berkowitz, B.A. and Spector, S. (1979) Analgesic action and pharmacokinetics of morphine and diazepam in man: an evaluation by sensory decision theory. Anesthesiology, 51: 495–502.

Yang, J.C., Richlin, D., Brand, L., Wagner, J. and Clark, W.C. (1985) Thermal sensory decision theory indices and pain threshold in chronic pain patients and healthy volunteers. Psychosom. Med., 47: 461–468.

R. Dubner, G.F. Gebhart & M.R. Bond (Eds.)
Proceedings of the Vth World Congress on Pain
© 1988 Elsevier Science Publishers BV (Biomedical Division)

CHAPTER 42

Use of magnitude matching for measuring group differences in pain perception

Gary H. Duncan[1,2], Jocelyn S. Feine[1,2], M. Catherine Bushnell[1,2] and Martin Boyer[1]

[1]*Faculté de Médecine Dentaire and* [2]*Centre de Recherche en Sciences Neurologiques, Université de Montréal, Montréal, Québec, Canada*

Introduction

A variety of psychophysical measures have been used to evaluate an individual's pain perception. While it is recognized that individuals and groups of individuals judge pain differently, the accurate assessment of these differences is often hindered by deficiencies inherent in the available measurement techniques. Category scales using either numbers (i.e., rating pain from 1 to 10) or words (i.e., mild = 1, moderate = 2, severe = 3, etc.) are simple to administer but restrict the precision with which the person can respond. For example, two painful stimuli could be categorized as 'moderate', although one is perceived as more painful than the other. Newer versions of these category scales, which allow better quantification of the verbal descriptors, are now available (Gracely et al., 1978; Heft and Parker, 1984); however, some of the ease and simplicity of measurement has been sacrificed for statistical sophistication, while response precision remains a practical problem.

Various cross-modality matching paradigms overcome some of the deficiencies of the category scales. In principle, cross-modality matching requires that the subject adjust the intensity of a secondary stimulus modality to match the perceptual magnitude of a primary stimulus – for example, adjusting the brightness of a light to match the painfulness of a noxious stimulus. A commonly used derivative of cross-modality matching is the visual analogue scale (VAS), which requires the subject to describe a painful stimulus by marking a position on a straight line, relative to descriptive endpoints (e.g. 'no pain' and 'intolerable pain'). Most cross-modality matching techniques allow infinitely small distinctions in responses, so that a subject can precisely indicate that two pain levels are very similar but not the same. Nevertheless, these scales are susceptible to a response artifact termed 'regression bias', in which subjects' responses are compressed near the ends of the scales (Stevens and Greenbaum, 1966). This regression effect can be particularly large whenever the response range is limited by apparatus (wattage of light stimulus, length of VAS line, strength of hand grip, etc.). For example, if a subject receives an extremely painful stimulus, he may adjust the light to its maximum intensity or mark the VAS line at the end labelled 'intolerable pain'. If he then receives another pain stimulus that is perceived as more intense than the first, he cannot indicate this, as he has already given the maximum response. Attempts to reduce such regression bias (Gracely et al., 1978) require additional experimen-

Correspondence: Gary H. Duncan, Departement de Stomatologie, Faculté de Médecine Dentaire, Université de Montréal, Case Postale 6128, Succursale A, Montréal, Québec H3C 3J7, Canada.

tal sessions and do not totally eliminate the restricted-range problems. In addition, many cross-modality matching methods are technically difficult to use with fast-adapting stimuli, such as thermal sensation (Stevens and Marks, 1980).

The method of magnitude estimation, in which the subject gives a number that indicates the perceived intensity of the stimulus, allows an unlimited range of responses, thus eliminating ceiling and floor effects. However, permitting subjects to use whatever range they prefer introduces variability which reduces the method's sensitivity in distinguishing differences between small groups of subjects.

A new method which incorporates principles of magnitude estimation and cross-modality matching seems to solve many of the practical and theoretical problems of previous scaling techniques. This method, introduced by Stevens and Marks (1980) and termed 'magnitude matching', asks the subject to make magnitude estimates of two sensory modalities, alternating from one modality to the other from trial to trial. The subject is instructed to use a common scale of magnitude estimation for both modalities. The ratings from one modality are then normalized in terms of those from the other. Individual idiosyncrasies in the use of numbers should be reflected equally in the magnitude estimates within each modality and mathematically cancel out by the normalization procedure, thus reducing the variability both between groups of subjects and within the same subject from day to day. This method has been used successfully to compare group differences for perception of odor (Stevens et al., 1982; Stevens and Cain, 1985; Cometto-Muniz and Noriega, 1985), taste (Gent and Bartoshuk, 1983; Calvino, 1986), geometric properties of visual space (Wagner, 1985) and physical exertion (Marks et al., 1983). The present study endeavours to extend the use of magnitude matching to pain measurement.

Since magnitude matching reduces variability and thus yields more consistent data with small numbers of trials and subjects (Stevens and Marks, 1980), it seems particularly suitable for the study of pain. In measuring experimental pain it is always advantageous to present the fewest painful stimuli possible to ensure subject compliance and reduce the possibility of tissue damage. Similarly, when measuring clinical pain both the number of available patients and the amount of time each patient is willing to spend are limited. The present study investigates the reliability and sensitivity of magnitude matching in measuring simulated differences in the perception of painful heat stimuli between two small groups of subjects.

Methods

Subjects. Twenty paid volunteers (13 male and 7 female) participated in these experiments. All read and signed a consent form acknowledging that the experimental procedures had been explained and that they could withdraw, without prejudice, from the experiment at any time.

Experimental design. The subjects were randomly assigned to two experiments (10 subjects each). Experiment I involved the rating of only thermal stimuli (magnitude estimation), while Experiment II required ratings of both thermal and visual stimuli (magnitude matching). To simulate a difference in pain perception between two hypothetical populations, two ranges of thermal stimuli were utilized. Half the subjects in each experiment received stimuli of 45°, 46°, 47°, 48° and 49°C, while the remaining subjects were presented a stimulus range elevated by 1°C (46° to 50°C).

Each subject participated in one experimental session, divided into three blocks of trials. In both experiments, each block contained 20 thermal stimuli (four presentations of the five stimulus levels). In Experiment II (magnitude matching), subjects also received 20 visual stimuli per block, similarly divided into four presentations of five intensity levels.

Instructions. Since a major purpose of this study was to assess the feasibility of alternately comparing noxious stimuli of one modality with innocuous stimuli from another, the subject's complete understanding of the rating methods was considered essential. Critical points were adapted from the instructions of the original magnitude matching studies (Stevens and Marks, 1980). Additionally, the standardized instructions were memorized by the experimenter and given orally to the subject, and were re-explained in paraphrased form whenever it was judged advisable (Stevens and Cain, 1985).

In brief, subjects in the magnitude matching experiment were instructed to rate pain intensity and brightness on the same scale of magnitude using whole numbers or decimals, as appropriate. Zero would indicate that the heat stimulus was not at all painful or that the visual stimulus was not detected. Subjects who were only presented with thermal stimuli were given identical instructions regarding the numerical rating of pain intensity. Both experiments were preceded by a practice set which included three examples selected from the range of relevant stimuli. Subjects could then ask additional questions or repeat the practice session if needed.

Stimulus presentation. In both experiments, the thermal stimuli were applied by the experimenter, via a hand-held contact thermode, to four spots of skin above the subject's upper lip. The order of thermal stimuli was counterbalanced across skin locations. In Experiment II, the cue light was situated 36–50 cm in front of the subject. Thermal and visual stimuli were presented on alternate trials. Neither the subject nor the experimenter knew the exact range of thermal stimuli nor the order of the intensities presented.

Following a ready signal on a computer monitor, the subject initiated a trial by pressing the 'RETURN' button on a keyboard. For the thermal trials, the temperature of the thermode increased from a baseline of 39°C to one of the five higher temperatures (45–49°C or 46–50°C). In the visual task, the cue light increased in intensity to one of five brightness levels. Following each stimulus presentation the subject typed his numerical estimate on the keyboard.

In both experiments, the intertrial intervals were adjusted to allow a minimum of one minute to elapse between presentation of consecutive thermal stimuli to the same spot of skin. We have previously shown that this period is sufficiently long to minimize response changes attributable to suppression or sensitization of nociceptive afferents (Talbot et al., 1987).

Apparatus. A minicomputer controlled all stimulus presentations, collected subjects' numerical ratings and performed statistical computations using the nonparametric Mann-Whitney test. Thermal stimuli were presented with a 1-cm diameter contact thermode which incorporated a servo-controlled heating element and active cooling via refrigerated, circulating water. The warming and cooling slopes of the thermode were approximately 6°C/s. Visual stimuli were presented through a 3-cm diameter opaque white key by a tungsten lamp whose brightness was controlled by the digital-analogue output of the computer. The luminosity of the experimental room was maintained at a constant level for all experiments.

Results

All 20 subjects completed the required tasks with little difficulty. Examination of the mean pain intensity ratings of the thermal stimuli (Table I) suggests that, in general, subjects utilized an unrestricted number range as directed by the instructions. That is, the subjects' maximum estimates do not appear to reflect an arbitrarily limited scale (0–10, 0–100, etc.). The subjects' ability to use numerical estimates to scale and, in effect, discriminate between the different levels of noxious thermal stimuli is indicated by the monotonic stimulus-response functions generated by the individual subjects (Fig. 1). Only three of the 100 mean estimates of pain intensity do not conform to the ascending order of thermal stimuli.

To assess the sensitivity of the magnitude estimation procedure in demonstrating a between-group difference in pain perception, the median pain intensity ratings estimated by the groups of subjects receiving the 45–49°C thermal stimuli were compared to those of the groups who received the higher range of temperatures (46–50°C). Fig. 2 illustrates that magnitude estimation procedures, by themselves, did not reveal group differences. The subjects rating the higher range of temperatures in Experiment I tended to produce lower, rather than higher, ratings (Fig. 2A). In Experiment II, there was a trend toward the higher temperatures receiving the higher ratings (Fig. 2B), but the overlapping distributions and small numbers of subjects do not permit a statistical difference to approach significance, either for the data collapsed across all temperatures or for any of the individual one-degree comparisons between the two groups of subjects.

The data from Experiment II, which included the ratings of visual as well as thermal stimuli, were additionally analysed in a manner similar to that described in magnitude matching paradigms utilizing two modalities of innocuous stimuli (Stevens and Cain, 1985). Specifically, all the pain intensity es-

timates of a given subject were divided by that subject's overall mean estimate of the visual stimuli. Arithmetic, rather than geometric, means were used because estimates of '0' occurred frequently for the stimuli that approximated threshold for heat pain and visual perception.

The dramatic increase in assay sensitivity permitted by the magnitude matching normalization is illustrated in Fig. 3. The median pain intensity ratings of the five subjects who received the higher range of thermal stimuli are clearly distinguished from those of the five subjects who received the lower range (Fig. 3, solid and dashed lines respectively). This difference is very robust when the data are collapsed over the entire range of temperatures ($P < 0.005$) and is also significant at each of the five individual temperature comparisons ($P < 0.05$ to $P < 0.001$).

In the light of the favourable results obtained with the magnitude-matching normalization, the data from Experiment II were further analysed to ascertain whether this procedure had sufficient sen-

TABLE I

Mean magnitude estimates of pain intensity

Subject	Thermal stimuli (°C)					Subject	Thermal stimuli (°C)				
	45	46	47	48	49		46	47	48	49	50
Experiment I:											
04	3.92	4.46	11.17	9.60	17.14	02	0.17	1.33	5.25	41.67	75.00
07	0.23	0.64	0.67	2.50	5.64	08	4.17	4.50	6.67	8.83	9.83
12	3.25	3.50	4.08	5.67	8.25	11	0.33	0.67	1.83	3.83	5.25
16	2.92	9.17	10.42	22.92	36.25	14	2.42	3.75	5.00	5.83	7.00
17	2.92	4.75	5.17	7.83	9.33	18	0.83	1.75	2.50	4.00	8.17
Means:	2.65	4.50	6.30	9.70	15.32	Means:	1.58	2.40	4.25	12.83	21.05
Medians:	2.92	4.46	5.17	7.83	9.33	Medians:	0.83	1.75	5.00	5.83	8.17
Experiment II:											
01	2.33	3.25	4.58	6.58	7.33	03	0.93	2.00	3.31	4.90	6.55
06	0.33	0.17	0.67	1.25	3.08	05	2.93	3.33	4.39	3.70	5.73
09	5.42	10.25	19.75	28.00	46.00	10	36.57	49.92	59.54	83.40	96.00
15	2.17	2.33	4.08	5.83	6.50	13	12.08	24.25	31.67	36.25	58.33
19	2.50	4.42	5.25	6.25	9.17	20	2.67	3.42	5.00	5.50	7.75
Means:	2.55	4.08	6.87	9.58	14.42	Means:	11.04	16.58	20.78	26.75	34.87
Medians:	2.33	3.25	4.58	6.25	7.33	Medians:	2.93	3.42	5.00	5.50	7.75

sitivity to distinguish group differences using smaller and smaller subsets of data. The 60 thermal and 60 visual stimuli presented to the subjects in Experiment II had initially been counterbalanced and pseudorandomized into three equivalent blocks of trials so that each of the stimulus levels would be completely represented in each block. Table II shows that, for the data collapsed over the entire range of temperatures, significant differences in the perception of pain between the two groups could be demonstrated whether the analyses were based on

Blocks A and B, or only on the data of Block A ($P < 0.005$ and $P = 0.025$, respectively). The benefit of utilizing a paradigm which includes more repetitions of the stimuli seems to be an increased sensitivity in distinguishing differences in perception at individual temperature levels. When all three blocks of trials are analysed together, all five temperature comparisons reach a significance level of 0.05, compared with only half of the comparisons based on analysis of the smaller subsets of data (Table II).

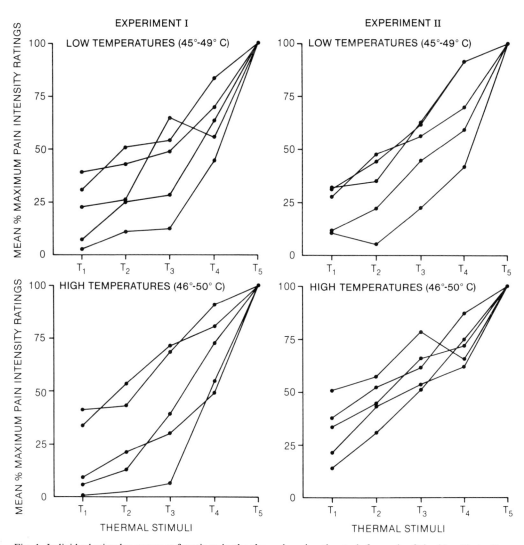

Fig. 1. Individual stimulus-response functions in the thermal nociception task for each of the 20 subjects. For each stimulus level, the subject's mean magnitude estimate of pain intensity is expressed as a percentage of his maximum estimate in that task.

Discussion

The validity and reliability of the methodological principles of magnitude matching have been demonstrated independently by several investigators (Stevens and Marks, 1980; Gent and Bartoshuk, 1983; Cometto-Muniz and Noriega, 1985; Wagner, 1985; Calvino, 1986). However, since these methods had only been applied to measuring the perception of innocuous stimuli, the question remained whether magnitude matching procedures were ap-

propriate, or even feasible, in the study of pain.

The central premise of magnitude matching requires that subjects rate their perceptions of two different types of stimulus on the same scale of magnitude. As had been shown previously for comparisons of sensory modalities such as sight and sound, and taste and smell, we now demonstrate that subjects have little or no difficulty equating the magnitude of such disparate sensations as the painfulness of thermal stimuli and the brightness of a light. In addition, comparison of the magnitude es-

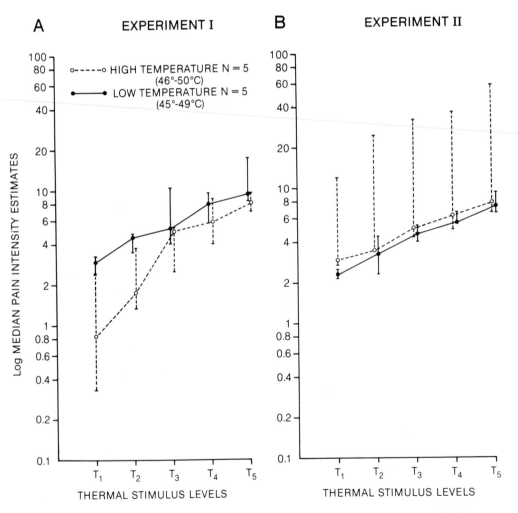

Fig. 2. Median magnitude estimates of pain intensity versus the five thermal stimulus levels. In each of the two experiments, one group of subjects ($n = 5$) rated thermal stimuli ranging from 46 to 50°C (dashed lines), while a second group ($n = 5$) rated thermal stimuli one degree cooler (45–49°C; solid lines). Variability of the numerical estimates generated by the subjects within the four groups is indicated by interquartile range.

timates of pain given by the subjects who received only thermal stimuli (Experiment I) with those who received both thermal and visual stimuli (Experiment II) gives no indication that interposing the rating of a secondary stimulus modality interferes

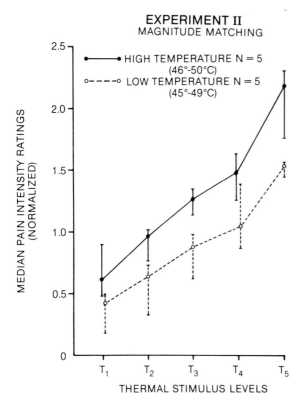

Fig. 3. Normalized median pain intensity ratings versus the five thermal stimulus levels for the two groups of subjects who received both thermal and visual stimuli. Normalized ratings were obtained by dividing each subject's mean pain intensity rating by the grand mean of his visual intensity estimates.

with one's ability to rate the magnitude of thermal pain. Moreover, the inclusion of visual ratings does not lengthen the time required for testing a subject in a paradigm using painful thermal stimuli, since the visual stimuli can be presented during the interstimulus interval that is required to prevent adaptation and sensitization. Finally, and most importantly, the data from Experiment II demonstrate the additional assay sensitivity that is gained from the normalization procedure of magnitude matching, compared with simple magnitude estimations of the single modality. Based only on an analysis of the magnitude estimates, there is no indication that the two groups of subjects in Experiment II perceived any difference in the painfulness of the thermal stimuli. However, after normalization of the thermal estimates relative to the mean visual estimates, the same statistical comparison clearly detects the difference in pain perception simulated by the 1°C disparity in thermal stimuli presented to the two groups.

The use of a magnitude matching paradigm in pain research should be most appropriate when comparisons of pain perception or analgesia must be made between different groups of subjects. The freedom to use magnitude estimates of painfulness allows the individual subjects an unrestricted range of responses (thus reducing the tendency toward regression bias, ceiling and floor effects), while the matching of the two sensory modalities mathematically cancels out the individual differences in response style (thus reducing the variability both within and between the groups of subjects). These advantages become obvious when the style of re-

TABLE II
Statistical comparisons of simulated group differences in pain perception

Blocks	Levels of significance (Mann-Whitney)					
	45–49 vs. 46–50°C	45 vs. 46°C	46 vs. 47°C	47 vs. 48°C	48 vs. 49°C	49 vs. 50°C
A B C	=0.005	=0.050	=0.010	=0.001	=0.050	=0.001
A B	=0.005	=0.100	<0.100	=0.025	=0.100	=0.005
A	=0.025	<0.050	<0.100	=0.050	=0.100	=0.025

sponding, as well as the perception of pain, may be influenced by age, gender or socio-economic background. Analysis of subsets of data from the present study revealed that the experimental design was sufficiently sensitive to detect the simulated difference in pain perception utilizing only five untrained subjects per group and requiring as little as ten minutes of the subjects' time. These results suggest that the technique of magnitude matching may be particularly applicable to scientific evaluation of patients in the clinical environment.

Acknowledgements

We wish to express our gratitude to Giovanni Filosi for graphic illustrations and to Dr. John Kalaska for his comments on earlier versions of this manuscript. G.H.D. and M.C.B. are supported in part by development grants from the Medical Research Council of Canada. M.C.B. is additionally supported by a Senior Scientist Fellowship from the Fonds de la recerche en santé du Québec. This project was funded by the Medical Research Council of Canada.

References

Calvino, A.M. (1986) Perception of sweetness: the effects of concentration and temperature. Physiol. Behav., 36: 1021–1028.

Cometto-Muniz, J.E. and Noriega, G. (1985) Gender differences in the perception of pungency. Physiol. Behav., 34: 385–389.

Gent, J.F. and Bartoshuk, L.M. (1983) Sweetness of sucrose, neohesperidin dihydrochalcone and saccharin is related to genetic ability to taste the bitter substance 6-*n*-propylthiouracil. Chem. Senses, 7: 265–272.

Gracely, R.H., McGrath, P. and Dubner, R. (1978) Ratio scales of sensory and affective verbal pain descriptors. Pain, 5: 5–18.

Heft, M.W. and Parker, S.R. (1984) An experimental basis for revising the graphic rating scale for pain. Pain, 19: 153–161.

Marks, L.E., Borg, G. and Ljunggren, G. (1983) Individual differences in perceived exertion assessed by two new methods. Percept. Psychophysics, 34: 280–288.

Stevens, J.C. and Cain, W.S. (1985) Age-related deficiency in the perceived strength of six ordorants. Chem. Senses, 10: 517–529.

Stevens, J.C. and Marks, L.E. (1980) Cross-modality matching functions generated by magnitude estimation. Percept. Psychophysics, 27: 379–389.

Stevens, J.C., Plantinga, A. and Cain, W.S. (1982) Reduction of odor and nasal pungency associated with aging. Neurobiol. Aging, 3: 125–132.

Stevens, S.S. and Greenbaum, H.B. (1966) Regression effect in psychophysical judgment. Percept. Psychophysics, 1: 439–446.

Talbot, J.D., Duncan, G.H., Bushnell, M.C. and Boyer, M. (1987) Diffuse noxious inhibitory controls (DNICs): psychophysical evidence in man for intersegmental suppression of noxious heat perception by cold pressor pain. Pain, 30: 221–232.

Wagner, M. (1985) The metric of visual space. Percept. Psychophysics, 38: 483–495.

R. Dubner, G.F. Gebhart & M.R. Bond (Eds.)
Proceedings of the Vth World Congress on Pain
© 1988 Elsevier Science Publishers BV (Biomedical Division)

CHAPTER 43

Multiple-random staircase assessment of thermal pain sensation

Richard H. Gracely

Clinical Pain Section, Neurobiology and Anesthesiology Branch, National Institute of Dental Research, NIH, Bethesda, MD 20892, USA

Two types of psychophysical procedure

Psychophysical methods of pain assessment either record the variable responses to a fixed stimulus set or determine the amount of stimulation required to evoke a predetermined response such as pain threshold. These different methods can be considered as two independent classes, distinguished by whether a psychological unit of pain magnitude or a physical unit of stimulus intensity is used as the dependent measure (Gracely, 1985, 1988; Gracely et al., 1986).

The *response-dependent* class presents a fixed set of stimulus intensities as the independent variable and records the varying responses to these stimuli as the dependent measure. This class includes almost all the suprathreshold scaling methods and also forms the basis of the Method of Constant Stimuli procedure for stimulus matching and threshold assessment. In pain assessment, several repetitions of specific stimuli (e.g. 3 each of 7 stimuli) covering the pain range are presented in random sequence. The mean response (e.g. visual analogue scale, magnitude estimation, numerical or verbal category scaling, quantified verbal descriptors) to each stimulus results in a psychophysical function relating the growth in pain magnitude to increasing stimulus intensity. Analgesia is inferred from a reduction of this function.

The other *stimulus-dependent* class performs the opposite operation. This class determines the stimulus intensity required to evoke a specific, predetermined level or quality of sensation. This stimulus intensity is the dependent variable used for subsequent data analysis. This class includes the classical methods used for threshold determination (Engen, 1971), and also contains the staircase titration method. In the simplest form of the titration method, a single stimulus staircase is used to assess threshold. Every response of 'not detected', 'nonpainful', etc., increases the intensity of the next stimulus. Every response of 'detected', 'painful', etc., lowers the intensity of the next stimulus. The result is a series of ascending and descending stimulus runs that titrate or track threshold. The method combines the up-down trials of the classical Method of Limits with the efficiency of the Method of Adjustment. It is more efficient than the classical Methods of Limits and Constant Stimuli, since more of the stimuli contribute to the assessment (Engen, 1971).

Double-random staircases

Unfortunately, this staircase method is vulnerable

Correspondence: Dr. Richard H. Gracely, Bld. 10, Rm. 3C403, NIH, Bethesda, MD 20892, U.S.A.

to bias effects, since subjects often discover that each response determines the intensity of the next stimulus. This contingency can be reduced by presenting two independent staircases and alternating randomly between them (Cornsweet, 1962). On each trial of this 'double-random staircase,' one of the two staircases is chosen and the stimulus intensity for that staircase is presented. The response determines the next stimulus presented by that staircase the next time it is randomly chosen, lowering it for a high response and increasing it for a low response. On the next trial, one of the two staircases is again randomly chosen, its stimulus is presented, and the next stimulus is determined by the response. The random choice of staircase on each trial reduces the contingency found between response and direction of stimulus change found with a single staircase. This reduction in the contingency between response and the next stimulus masks the staircase rule, reducing the possible influence of conscious or unconscious manipulation of the result.

Multiple-random staircases

Fig. 1 shows the adaptation of the double-random staircase threshold method to suprathreshold scaling of pain sensation. Three double-random staircases are used, each associated with one of the three intervals between the four response categories 'no pain', 'mild', 'moderate', and 'intense'. On each trial, one of the six staircases is randomly selected. The response to that staircase determines the intensity of the stimulus next presented by that staircase the next time it is randomly chosen. Any response above the staircase 'interval' decreases, and any response below increases stimulus intensity. Thus for the upper double-random staircase, 'intense' would decrease the intensity of the next stimulus (presented by that staircase when again selected) and either 'no pain', 'mild' or 'moderate' would increase it. For the middle pair, either 'intense' or 'moderate' would lower the next stimulus and either 'no pain' or 'mild' would increase it. 'No pain' would

increase the intensity of the next stimulus presented by the lower staircases, while either 'mild', 'moderate' or 'intense' would decrease it.

Advantages

Fig. 1 shows a single subject's data from this multiple-random staircase method. He used a four-point category scale to rate the painfulness of 3-s thermal stimuli delivered to the volar forearm at 20-s intervals by a 1-cm-diameter contact probe. This figure displays several features of this method. It graphically shows data from an individual subject, and checks for scaling consistency. The staircases within each double-random staircase pair tend to superimpose only if the subject is attending to and consistently rating the stimulus-evoked sensations. The method also makes no assumptions about psychological units of pain magnitude. Results are expressed in physical units of stimulus intensity, in

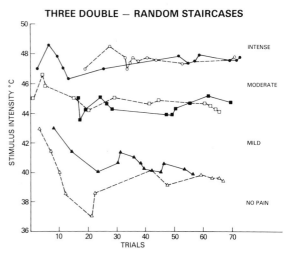

THREE DOUBLE — RANDOM STAIRCASES

Fig. 1. Multiple (three double) -random staircases. This figure shows stimulus intensity plotted against 72 stimulus trials for a single subject. On each trial, one of the six staircases is selected randomly and the stimulus temperature indicated by that staircase is presented. The subject selects one of four response categories to rate the intensity of the sensation evoked by the stimulus. Each double staircase is associated with an interval located between two response categories. Responses above the interval reduce the intensity of the next stimulus presented by that staircase. Responses below the interval increase the next stimulus.

this case, degrees Celsius. Finally, the method tracks the time course of pain sensitivity, allowing assessment of the onset, peak effect and duration of an analgesic manipulation.

Variable increment

The amount of stimulus change after each response determines sensitivity and speed of convergence. A very large change would result in rapid convergence but poor measurement. The stimulus might simply alternate between two values for the entire session. A very small increment would result in accurate measurement but slow convergence and poor temporal resolution. Thus the ideal increment size is a compromise between steps large enough to track time course and small enough to provide sensitive measurement. The present model uses a variable increment size which is adjusted throughout the session. For each staircase the algorithm attempts to maintain 3 successive stimulus changes in the same direction before the direction is reversed. If the direction is reversed before 3 successive changes, the increment is assumed to be too large and is reduced by one-half. If more than 3 changes are made in the same direction, the increment is assumed to be too small and its size is doubled.

In the present model, the increment is set initially at a maximum size of 1.6 °C and quickly reduces to 0.2–0.4 °C. Preliminary studies show that staircases assigned to the same response interval quickly converge, even when initiated at temperatures separated by 5 °C (Gracely et al., 1988).

Fentanyl analgesia

The multiple-random staircase method has been applied to several studies of thermal pain sensation. Intravenous administration of the short-acting opiate fentanyl increased staircase temperatures in both open and double-blind studies (Gracely et al., 1988). Fentanyl produced a peak increase in staircase temperature of 1–2 °C 11 min after infusion

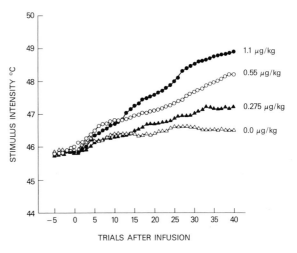

Fig. 2. Effect of fentanyl dose for the staircases titrated between 'mild' and 'moderate'. The double-random staircases titrated at this interval were combined into one mean staircase to show the results of 4 groups ($n = 16$ each) in one figure. Stimulus intensity is shown on the ordinate, and 5 trials before and 40 trials after a 2-min double-blind infusion are shown on the abcissa. This figure represents a 15 min 20 s segment of a 42 min session. Subjects received either placebo, shown by the open triangles, or 0.275, 0.55 or 1.1 µg/kg fentanyl shown respectively by the filled triangles, open circles and filled circles. Fentanyl significantly increased staircase temperatures, indicating analgesia. Both rate of onset and final temperature, which changed little for the remaining 62 trials (not shown), were significantly dose-related.

that persisted for at least 24 min. This effect appeared to be dose-related (Gracely et al., 1986).

The time course, dose relationship and effect of staircase temperature have been investigated further in a double-blind study administering 0, 0.275, 0.55 or 1.1 µg/kg fentanyl. Fig. 2 shows the mean of the two staircases titrated between 'mild' and 'moderate' for each of the four dose groups. This figure shows that fentanyl increased staircase temperatures from 46 to 47–49 °C over 40 trials (13.33 min). Both rate of onset (dose × time interaction, $F(117, 2340) = 4.27$, $P < 0.0001$) and final level (dose main effect, $F(3, 60) = 5.30$, $P < 0.005$) were significantly dose-related.

Further advantages: sensory invariance

Fig. 2 illustrates an important feature of the multiple staircase method. Following administration of an analgesic, the staircase temperatures are increased to produce the same responses, and assumed sensory magnitudes, made before administration of the drug. This increase is triggered by the use of lower response categories to describe the attenuated pain sensation. Subjects experience a slight reduction in sensory magnitude until the adjustment process is complete. In contrast, subjects in conventional response-dependent methods experience a dramatic reduction in sensory magnitude following analgesic administration.

The essentially unchanged sensory experience following analgesia with the staircase method offers several advantages over conventional scaling methods. First, the method provides minimal sensory clues of analgesia, minimizing the influence of biases mediated by knowledge that an active drug has been administered. Second, analgesia cannot be easily simulated by using higher-magnitude responses less frequently. The algorithm will simply increase the intensity of the evoked pain sensations until these responses are used. In addition, inconsistent responding can be detected by checking for similarity within a pair of double-random staircases. Finally, analgesia at intense stimulus levels can be assessed without experiencing the pain produced by these stimuli in the absence of analgesia. In a conventional response-dependent scaling

experiment analgesia to 49°C would be assessed by recording the response to this temperature before and after analgesic administration. Subjects must feel the pain evoked by 49°C. In the staircase method, subjects experience a less painful sensation before analgesia and the same sensation after analgesia. For example, the 1.1 $\mu g/kg$ group shown in Fig. 2 experienced the sensation evoked by average stimuli of 46°C from the mild-moderate staircase before analgesia and reduced sensation produced by 49°C after administration of the fentanyl.

Conclusion

The multiple-random staircase method expresses results in units of stimulus magnitude, making no assumptions about psychological units of pain magnitude, and provides a graphic check of internal consistency, identifying poor scaling performance. Preliminary results show that it can track the time course of fentanyl analgesia, showing a dose-related onset and final level. The method also produces the same subjective pain levels before and after an analgesic intervention. This feature may reduce the influence of specific biases and allow investigation of analgesic mechanisms at high stimulus intensity levels without the severe pain usually produced at these intensities.

References

Cornsweet, T.N. (1962) The staircase-method in psychophysics. Am. J. Psychol., 75: 485–491.

Engen, T. (1971) Psychophysics I. Discrimination and Detection, Psychophysics II. Scaling Methods. In J.W. Kling and L.A. Riggs (Eds.), Experimental Psychology (3rd edn.), Holt, New York, pp. 11–86.

Gracely, R.H. (1985) Pain Psychophysics. In S. Manuck (Ed.), Advances in Behavioral Medicine, JAI Press, New York, pp. 199–231.

Gracely, R.H. (1988) Methods of Pain Testing in Normal Man. In R. Melzack, and P.D. Wall (Eds.), Textbook of Pain, Vol. 2, Churchill Livingstone, London, in press.

Gracely, R.H., Lota, L., Walther, D.J. and Bernstein, S.E. (1986) Staircase assessment of thermal pain sensation: effect of fentanyl dose and staircase temperature. Am. Pain Soc. Abstr., 6.

Gracely, R.H., Lota, L., Walther, D.J. and Dubner, R. (1988) A multiple random staircase method of psychophysical pain assessment. Pain, 32: 55–63.

R. Dubner, G.F. Gebhart & M.R. Bond (Eds.)
Proceedings of the Vth World Congress on Pain
© 1988 Elsevier Science Publishers BV (Biomedical Division)

CHAPTER 44

Translated versus reconstructed McGill Pain Questionnaires: a comparative study of two French forms

F. Boureau[1] and C. Paquette[2]

[1]*Unité de Traitement de la Douleur, Laboratoire d'Explorations fonctionnelles en Neurophysiologie, Hôpital Saint-Antoine, Paris, France, and,* [2]*Faculté des Sciences Infirmières, Université de Montreal, Canada*

Introduction

Melzack's McGill Pain Questionnaire (MPQ) (Melzack, 1975) provides a quantitative and qualitative measurement of pain experience. It is a useful tool for verbal assessment of pain mechanisms and analgesia. The MPQ can be adapted from English to other languages by at least two different methodologies. The first is the MPQ translation, such as the Canadian French Viguie's Questionnaire Algie (QA) (Viguie, 1982). The second is a reconstructed questionnaire, such as the Questionnaire Douleur Saint-Antoine (QDSA), which was developed using methods similar to Melzack and Torgerson's original work (1971). The aim of this paper is to compare the two forms of pain adjective questionnaires.

Methods

One hundred consecutive chronic pain patients were administered, in a random order, the QA and QDSA as part of a larger pencil and paper assess-
ment including pain visual analogue scale (VAS), Beck Depression Inventory (BDI) (Beck et al., 1961), Spielberger State-Trait Anxiety Inventory (STAI) (Spielberger et al., 1970) and Binois-Pichot Test (BPT) (Binois and Pichot, 1968). The questionnaire session was performed after the initial consultation in an outpatient multidisciplinary university pain unit. The sample was composed of 70 females and 30 males. There were 29 patients with deafferentation pain, 27 with migraine, 11 with tension headache, 14 with idiopathic pain, 9 with neck and back pain, and 10 with miscellaneous pain.

Patients described the pain perceived during the last two weeks and not the pain present during the questionnaire session. The QDSA is a French reconstructed MPQ. The questionnaire was developed in a previous study, described elsewhere (Boureau et al., 1984a). The QDSA consists of 61 descriptors and 17 subclasses. For each pain descriptor, rank and mean values on a 5-point intensity scale have been calculated (Table I). QDSA provides quantitative numerical measures of pain. Three scores can be calculated: a sensory score (QDSA-S) (sum of values for subclasses 1 to 9), an affective score (QDSA-A) (sum of values for subclasses 10 to 16) and a total score (QDSA-T, sum of QDSA-S and QDSA-A). Three different scoring procedures can be used: (1) the sum of the rank

Correspondence: F. Boureau, Unité de Traitement de la Douleur, Hôpital St-Antoine, 184 rue du Fg. St-Antoine, Paris 75012, France.

TABLE I

Correlations between rank, mean and patient value QA-T (A) and QDSA-T (B)

	Mean	Rank
(A) QA-T		
Rank	0.97	
Patient	0.86	0.84
(B) QDSA-T		
Rank	0.96	
Patient	0.87	0.84

order value of the descriptor chosen in a subclass; (2) the sum of the mean value of the descriptor chosen in a subclass; and (3) the sum of the patient's values assigned to the descriptors chosen. We introduced this alternative scoring procedure (patient's value), in addition to the MPQ rank values and mean scoring. The patient is asked to assign each descriptor chosen to a 5-point intensity scale (0 = none, not at all; 1 = slight, a little; 2 = moderate, moderately; 3 = severe, a lot; 4 = extremely severe, extremely).

The QA is the French Canadian Viguie's MPQ translation (see Table III). The QA consists of 77 descriptors in four major classes (sensory, affective, evaluative and miscellaneous) and 20 subclasses. In a preliminary study, twenty French physicians living in France were asked to rate the intensity conveyed by the QA descriptors on a 5-point intensity scale. The mean and rank values of descriptors are given in Table III. Descriptors are well ranked for 11 subclasses out of the 20 QA subclasses. QA provides quantitative numerical measures of pain similar to those in MPQ: number of words chosen (NWC); pain rating index (PRI); present pain intensity (PPI). Only the pain rating index will be considered further in this comparative study. As with QDSA, three different scoring procedures are considered for the QA scores: (1) the sum of the rank values of descriptors for each subclass; (2) the sum of the mean values of the descriptors chosen in each subclass; and (3) the sum of the patient value of the chosen descriptor for each subclass. Five

pain ratings indices were calculated: a total score (QA-T); a sensory score (QA-S, classes 1 to 10); an affective score (QA-A, classes 11 to 15); an evaluative score (QA-E, class 16); and a miscellaneous score (QA-M, classes 17 to 20). QDSA differs from the QA in having fewer descriptors (61 vs. 77) and subclasses (17 vs. 20). Thirty-three descriptors are common to the two QA and QDSA questionnaires.

The visual analogue scale (VAS) was a 100 mm horizontal line. The extremes were defined by 'no pain' and 'maximum imaginable pain'. Depressive symptomatology was evaluated with the Beck Depression Inventory (BDI) (Beck et al., 1961). The French BDI version was validated by Delay et al. (1963). To evaluate anxiety, we used the Spielberger State-Trait Anxiety Inventory (STAI) (Spielberger et al., 1970) in a French translation, validated by Bergeron and Landry (1974). Two scores could be calculated: a score for the anxiety state (STAI-S) and a score for the anxiety trait (STAI-T). The vocabulary aptitude was assessed with the Binois-Pichot Test (BPT) (Binois and Pichot, 1968).

A principal component analysis (PCA) with varimax rotation was applied to the intercorrelation matrix. Factors with eigenvalues greater than unity were extracted. Items with factor loadings greater than 0.50 were used to identify the factors derived.

Results

The total sample mean age was 48.9 ± 16.2 years. The average duration of pain was 8.7 ± 10.9 years. The mean VAS score was 7.31 ± 1.88 mm. The mean rank order QA-T was 28.6 ± 12.3; sensory (QA-S), affective (QA-A), evaluative (QA-E) and miscellaneous (QA-M) were respectively 15.0 ± 7.8, 5.3 ± 2.8, 2.6 ± 1.6 and 5.2 ± 3.3. Mean patient value QDSA-T was 28.5 ± 12.3.

Correlations between the three scoring procedures (patient, rank and mean values). As shown in Table I, high correlations were found between rank, mean patient values QA-T and QDSA-T. Since high correlations were observed for QA-T and

QDSA-T scores as well as for other QA or QDSA subscores, only patient score values will be considered further.

Correlations between total, sensory and affective QA and QDSA scores. The correlation between

QDSA-T and QA-T was 0.87, between QDSA-S and QA-S it was 0.83, and between QDSA-A and QA-A it was 0.81. The correlation was 0.50 between the QDSA-S and QDSA-A and it was 0.44 between QA-S and QA-A.

TABLE II

Mean value and rank order of the QDSA pain descriptors as rated by physicians

Subclass	Descriptors	Mean	(S.D.)	Rank order	Subclass	Descriptors	Mean	(S.D.)	Rank order
Temporal	Battements	1.7	(0.7)	1	Dysesthesias	Picotements	1.2	(0.4)	1
	Pulsations	1.7	(0.6)	1		Fourmillements	1.2	(0.4)	1
	Elancements	2.6	(0.7)	2		Demangeaisons	1.7	(0.7)	2
	En éclairs	3.2	(0.6)	3					
	Décharges électr.	3.3	(0.8)	4	Dullness	Engourdissement	1.5	(0.6)	1
	Coups de marteau	3.3	(0.8)	4		Lourdeur	1.6	(0.7)	2
						Sourde	1.8	(0.6)	3
Spatial	Rayonnante	2.4	(0.6)	1	Fatigue	Fatigante	1.9	(0.5)	1
	Irradiante	2.5	(0.7)	2		Epuisante	2.8	(0.6)	2
						Ereintante	3.0	(0.9)	3
Incisive pressure	Piqûre	1.7	(0.5)	1					
	Coupure	1.9	(0.7)	2	Autonomic	Nauséeuse	1.8	(0.6)	1
	Pénétrante	2.6	(0.8)	3		Suffocante	3.2	(0.7)	2
	Transpercante	3.3	(0.7)	4		Syncopale	3.9	(0.3)	3
	Coups de Poignard	3.9	(0.5)	5	Anxiety	Inquiétante	2.2	(0.6)	1
						Oppressante	2.8	(0.6)	2
Constrictive pressure	Pincement	2.2	(0.6)	1		Angoissante	3.0	(0.8)	3
	Serrement	2.3	(0.7)	2					
	Compression	2.4	(0.9)	3	Punishment	Harcelante	2.8	(0.4)	1
	Ecrasement	3.3	(0.7)	4		Obsedante	3.1	(0.8)	2
	En etau	3.6	(0.5)	5		Cruelle	3.5	(0.6)	3
	Broiement	3.9	(0.4)	6		Torturante	3.8	(0.4)	4
						Suppliciante	3.9	(0.2)	5
Traction pressure	Tiraillement	1.8	(0.7)	1					
	Etirement	2.0	(0.9)	2	Evaluative	Gênante	1.3	(0.4)	1
	Distension	2.2	(0.7)	3		Désagréable	1.6	(0.5)	2
	Dechirure	3.0	(0.6)	4		Pénible	2.6	(0.6)	3
	Torsion	3.4	(0.6)	5		Insupportable	3.8	(0.6)	4
	Arrachement	3.7	(0.5)	6					
					Tension	Enervante	1.8	(0.4)	1
Thermal	Chaleur	1.6	(0.6)	1		Exasperante	2.7	(0.7)	2
	Brulure	3.2	(0.5)	2		Horripilante	3.0	(0.8)	3
Thermal	Froid	1.8	(0.6)	1	Depression	Déprimante	2.5	(0.8)	1
	Glace	2.9	(0.7)	2		Suicidaire	3.8	(0.5)	2

TABLE III

Mean value and rank order of the French-Canadian Viguie's QA pain descriptors as rated by French physicians living in France

Subclasses	French Descriptors	Mean	(S.D.)	Rank order	Subclass	Descriptors	Mean	(S.D.)	Rank order
Temporal	Fremissement	0.8	(0.81)	1					
	Pulsation	1.6	(0.94)	3	Tension	Fatigante	1.9	(0.85)	1
	Palpitation	1.3	(0.89)	2		Epuisante	2.9	(0.60)	2
	Battement	1.8	(0.87)	4					
	Martelement	2.3	(0.98)	6	Autonomic	Ecoeurante	2.5	(1.14)	1
	Cognement	2.0	(0.88)	5		Suffocante	3.6	(0.59)	2
Spatial	Elancante	2.8	(0.52)	1	Fear	Inquiétante	2.5	(0.76)	1
	En éclair	3.2	(0.55)	3		Angoissante	3.1	(0.44)	2
	Lancinante	3.0	(0.56)	2		Terrifiante	3.9	(0.30)	3
Punctuate pressure	Fourmillante	1.4	(0.59)	1	Punishment	Eprouvante	2.8	(0.76)	2
	Percante	3.2	(0.63)	2		Pénible	2.6	(0.58)	1
	Perforante	3.5	(0.60)	4		Cruelle	3.1	(0.74)	3
	En poignard	3.4	(0.60)	3		Inhumaine	3.7	(0.73)	5
						Tuante	3.4	(0.94)	4
Incisive pressure	Coupante	2.5	(0.76)	1					
	Tranchante	3.0	(0.97)	2	Affec. evaluat. miscellaneous	Déprimante	2.6	(0.67)	1
	Lacerante	3.7	(0.44)	3		Anéantissante	3.2	(1.19)	2
Constrictive pressure	Pincement	1.7	(0.55)	2	Evaluative	Ennuyante	1.2	(0.63)	1
	Pression	1.3	(0.81)	1		Contrariante	1.2	(0.78)	1
	Crampe	2.1	(0.64)	3		Affligeante	2.2	(0.95)	2
	Rongement	2.7	(0.71)	4		Harassante	2.8	(0.74)	3
	Ecrasement	3.3	(0.67)	5		Insupportable	3.8	(0.40)	4
Traction pressure	Tiraillement	2.1	(0.71)	1	Sensory miscellaneous	Diffusante	1.8	(0.81)	1
	Traction	2.3	(0.71)	2		Irradiante	2.2	(0.95)	2
	Torsion	3.0	(0.75)	3		Pénétrante	2.9	(0.51)	3
						Transpercante	3.6	(0.48)	4
Thermal	Chaleur	1.4	(1.04)	1					
	Cuisson	2.6	(0.87)	2	Sensory miscellaneous	Engourdissement	1.2	(0.83)	1
	Brulure, eau bo.	3.3	(0.65)	3		Serrement	2.3	(0.65)	3
	Brulure, fer ch.	3.5	(0.75)	4		Etirement	1.7	(0.65)	2
Brightness	Picotement	0.9	(0.55)	1		Arrachement	3.3	(0.86)	
	Démangeaison	1.4	(0.88)	2		Déchirement	3.1	(0.74)	
	Irritation	1.7	(0.86)	3					
	Inflammation	2.4	(0.50)	4	Sensory	Froid	1.4	(0.94)	1
						Gel	2.7	(0.85)	3
Dullness	Sourde	2.1	(0.48)	4		Congélation	2.5	(1.14)	2
	Diffuse	1.8	(0.81)	3					
	Localisée	1.2	(0.76)	2	Affec. evaluat. miscellaneous	Enervante	2.1	(0.78)	1
	Claire	0.9	(0.91)	1		Décourageante	2.4	(0.94)	2
	Vive	2.9	(0.44)	5		Affreuse	2.5	(1.60)	3
						Epouvantable	3.8	(0.40)	4
Sensory miscellaneous	Sensibilité	1.0	(0.88)	1		Torturante	3.8	(0.48)	4
	Raidissement	1.6	(0.99)	3					
	Eraflement	1.4	(0.82)	2					
	Fissuration	2.2	(0.91)	4					

Correlations between total QDSA-T, QA-T scores and VAS. The correlation coefficient between VAS and QDSA-T was 0.34 and between VAS and QA-T it was 0.37.

Correlations between QDSA, QA subscores and depression anxiety scores. The correlation coefficient between BDI and QDSA-A was 0.52 and between the BDI and QA-A it was 0.45. In contrast, the correlation between BDI and QDSA-S was 0.31 and between the BDI and QA-S it was 0.28. The correlation between QDSA-A and STAI-S was 0.53 and with STAI-T it was 0.58. The correlation between QA-A and STAI-S was 0.36 and with STAI-T it was 0.51.

Correlations between QDSA-T, QA-T and BPT. The correlation between BPT and QDSA-T was 0.31 and between BPT and QA-T it was 0.28. When low-verbal-aptitude subjects ($n = 8$; BPT < 15) were not considered, correlations between PBT and QDSA-T or QA-T were not significant (respectively 0.16 and 0.14).

Principal component analysis (PCA). By PCA of the intercorrelation matrix of the 16 QDSA subclasses 5 factors accounting for 61.4% of the total variance were derived (Table IV). All extracted factors are unidimensional and reflected sensory or affective aspects of the pain experience. Factor 1 accounted for 16.3% of the total variance and showed loadings on anxiety (0.82), depression (0.80), autonomic (0.61), fatigue (0.56) and punishment (0.55) submeasures. This factor reflects the anxio-depressive component of the pain experience. Factor 2 accounted for 10.9% of the total variance and showed loadings on tension (0.73) and evaluative (0.70) subclasses. This factor reflects an affective-evaluative component of the pain experience. Factor 3 accounted for 8.9% of the total variance and showed loadings on thermal-cold and paresthesias submeasures. Factor 4 accounted for 13.9% of the total variance and showed loadings on temporal (0.70), mechanical-compression (0.60), mechanical-incisive (0.58) and dullness (0.53) submeasures.

Factor 5 accounted for 11.3% of the total variance and showed loadings on spatial (0.73) and mechanical-distension (0.68) submeasures. The last three factors are all sensory and unidimensional.

PCA of the intercorrelation matrix of the QA 20 subclasses produced 5 factors accounting for 59.9% of the total variance (Table V). All extracted factors reflected unidimensional sensory or affective component aspects of pain. Factor 1 accounted for 19.8% of the total variance and showed loadings on affective-evaluative: miscellaneous (0.79), affective-evaluative-sensory miscellaneous (0.79), punishment (0.77), fear (0.69), tension (0.73) and evaluative (0.58) submeasures. This factor reflects an affective component of the pain experience. Factor 2 accounted for 13.1% of the total variance and showed loadings on constrictive pressure (0.72), traction pressure (0.66), sensory miscellaneous 10 (0.65) and 18 (0.57) submeasures. Factor 3 accounted for 10.8% of the total variance and showed

TABLE IV

Loadings of QDSA pain subclasses on five factors accounting for 61.4% of the total variance

Factors:	1 anxiety depression:	2 affective evaluative:	3 sensory	4	5
% Variance:	16.3	10.9	8.9	13.9	11.3
Subclasses					
1	0.10	0.17	0.05	0.70	−0.04
2	0.14	0.06	−0.04	0.14	0.73
3	0.04	−0.06	0.01	0.58	0.52
4	0.28	0.13	0.00	0.60	0.30
5	0.00	0.16	0.13	0.04	0.68
6	0.01	0.23	0.23	0.42	0.31
7	0.16	−0.11	0.84	−0.04	0.00
8	−0.16	0.13	0.74	0.34	0.13
9	0.16	0.31	0.19	0.53	0.12
10	0.56	0.49	0.12	0.14	0.03
11	0.61	−0.16	−0.06	0.50	−0.02
12	0.82	0.04	0.08	0.16	0.00
13	0.55	0.35	0.06	0.01	0.43
14	0.28	0.70	−0.12	0.29	−0.01
15	0.00	0.73	0.03	0.10	0.24
16	0.80	0.17	−0.06	0.06	0.13

loadings on sensory miscellaneous 17 (0.72), dullness (0.67) and punctuate pressure (0.54) submeasures. Factor 4 accounted for 10.4% of the total variance and showed loadings on thermal (0.70), incisive pressure (0.68) and brightness (0.62) submeasures. Factor 5 accounted for 5.8% of the total variance and showed loadings on sensory 19 (0.86) submeasure. Factors 2, 3, 4 and 5 are unidimensional and reflect sensory components of pain experience.

Discussion

Our results, in a French-speaking chronic pain population, provide further evidence for the validity of pain assessment through verbal descriptor questionnaires.

The major advantage of adjective questionnaires is multidimensional assessment. The MPQ has received a great amount of attention because it provides a selective evaluation of sensory and affective dimensions for studies of pain mechanisms and analgesia. In our study factor analyses confirmed the multidimensional structure of QA and QDSA. All extracted factors were unidimensional and purely sensory or affective. Melzack originally postulated a three-dimensional model for MPQ, i.e., sensory, affective and evaluative. In the literature, MPQ factor analyses have less consistently distinguished the evaluative dimension (Reading, 1982). In our study, we did not extract a purely evaluative factor. The QA evaluative subclass was associated with affective subclasses; the QDSA evaluative subclass was associated with the tension subclass. It should be observed that both MPQ and QDSA weigh the sensory or affective aspects of pain more heavily than the evaluative, which is represented by a single subclass.

Turk et al. (1985) noted that sensory, affective and evaluative components of MPQ were highly intercorrelated, suggesting that only the total score of the PRI is appropriate. Melzack argued that high intercorrelations among psychological variables do not necessarily mean that they do not represent distinct, discriminable variables. High intercorrelations between MPQ scores have not been found in all studies (Melzack, 1975). In our study, intercorrelations between factorial scores based on the sum of patient values of the 5 factorial subclass groups ranged from 0.08 to 0.48 for QDSA and from 0.02 to 0.41 for QA. Similarly, intercorrelations between the a priori classes QDSA or QA scores were significantly, but not very highly, correlated (0.50 for QSDA, from 0.39 to 0.60 for QA).

A rank order scoring system was favored by Melzack because of its simplicity and the high correlation between rank order and mean-value PRI. In each MPQ subclass, the number of descriptors varies from two to six and therefore the rank value scoring procedure tends to under- or overestimate

TABLE V

Loadings of QA pain subclasses on five factors accounting for 59.9% of the total variance

Factors:	1 anxiety depression:	2 affective evaluative:	3 sensory	4	5
% Variance:	16.3	10.9	8.9	13.9	11.3
Subclasses					
1	0.28	0.49	−0.30	0.43	−0.34
2	0.36	0.35	0.27	0.12	0.07
3	−0.06	0.34	0.54	0.32	−0.15
4	0.00	0.12	0.16	0.68	0.00
5	0.08	0.72	0.30	−0.17	0.12
6	0.14	0.66	−0.01	0.21	−0.14
7	0.19	0.03	0.11	0.70	0.09
8	−0.03	0.36	0.21	0.62	0.19
9	0.37	0.03	0.67	0.19	−0.02
10	0.07	0.65	−0.12	0.26	0.06
11	0.73	0.11	0.34	−0.01	0.04
12	0.43	0.33	−0.03	0.29	0.17
13	0.69	0.22	−0.07	−0.03	0.16
14	0.77	0.15	0.15	0.06	−0.06
15	0.79	−0.11	0.11	0.12	0.03
16	0.58	0.15	0.43	−0.07	−0.02
17	0.30	0.17	0.72	0.19	0.00
18	0.18	0.57	0.38	0.17	0.32
19	0.04	0.06	−0.08	0.16	0.86
20	0.79	0.09	0.10	0.15	−0.09

the weight of each subclass. The rank order scoring procedure loses the precise intensity of the scale value. For example, the word 'déprimante' (wretched, QA class 15) receives a rank value of 1 but has a scale value of 2.6 in QA and 2.5 in QDSA. The loss of information may mask the sensitivity of the questionnaire and therefore we introduced a weighted-patient scoring procedure. The new scoring procedure is more complicated but practicable. Our hypothesis is that the patient-value scoring procedure could be more sensitive. Clinical practice indicates that under successful treatment, chronic pain patients can, for example, describe an extremely wretched or an extremely severe burning pain which changes to a slight wretched or a slight burning pain. Correlations between the three scoring procedures are satisfactory (Table I) but further research will be necessary to test the advantages, i.e., sensitivity, of each scoring procedure.

Correlations between the translated QA and reconstructed QDSA scores are very satisfactory. Both questionnaires correlated similarly with other variables. Correlations with the overall intensity visual analogue scale are in agreement with the correlations of 0.39 and 0.10 reported between the total rank score of the MPQ and verbal and visual analogue rating scale (Reading, 1982). Correlations between anxiety-depression data and affective QDSA and QA subscores are in good agreement with the study of Kremer and Atkinson (1981) showing that the affective dimension of the MPQ provides a good summary of the affective status of chronic pain patients.

An interesting result is the relationship between QA or QDSA scores and the BPT measure of verbal aptitude. One limitation of pain adjective questionnaires is that patients sometimes have difficulty with the complexity of the pain vocabulary. Correlations between BPT and QA or QDSA global scores support the influence of verbal limitation on pain description. It is interesting to observe that when low-BPT-score subjects (BPT < 15) are removed from the analysis, the correlation is no longer significant. This observation indicates that: (1) the use of adjective questionnaires is not valid for subjects with verbal limitations; and (2) the influence of verbal aptitude is not significant for normal-verbal-aptitude subjects. To our knowledge, this result is the first attempt to study the incidence of verbal aptitude on the verbal report of pain.

Translated and reconstructed questionnaires present respective advantages and a valid MPQ translation is useful for cross-cultural studies. However, we observed that the range in a subclass may vary after translation; for example, the mean intensity values assigned by doctors to each word modify the original translated format. In our study, only 11 of the 20 QA subclasses were correctly ranked. It is interesting to observe that for the 33 QA-QDSA common words, the mean values calculated by two different groups of physicians remained very close. With some exceptions (Maiani and Sanavio, 1985), translations into other languages often modify the original MPQ format in terms of both the number of words and the number of classes (Pontinen and Ketovuori, 1983; Radvila, et al., 1987). When the purpose is not to produce a strictly parallel version of the MPQ, we suggest that a reconstructed questionnaire may be useful. In our reconstructed questionnaire we paralleled several aspects of MPQ assessment; for example, we attempted to select words easily understood by patients, we equilibrated the number of sensory and affective classes (9 versus 7), and we reduced the number of words in the new instrument.

Acknowledgements

We are grateful to R.H. Gracely for his helpful comments.

References

Beck, A.T., Ward, C.H., Mendelson, M.D., Mock, J. and Erbaugh, M.D. (1961) An inventory for measuring depression. Arch. Gen. Psychiatry, 4: 561–571.

Bergeron, J. and Landry, M. (1974) La fidelité et la validité de l'adaptation française du questionnaire d'anxiété STAI. 18e Congrès International de Psychologie Appliquée, Montreal, Canada.

Binois, R. and Pichot, P. (1968) Test de vocabulaire, Centre de Psychologie Appliquée, Paris.

Boureau, F., Luu, M., Doubrere, J.F. and Gay, C. (1984a) Elaboration d'un questionnaire d'autoévaluation de la douleur par liste de qualificatifs. Comparaison avec le McGill Pain Questionnaire de Melzack. Therapie, 39: 119–139.

Boureau, F., Luu, M. and Doubrere, J.F. (1984b) Qualitative and quantitative study of a French pain McGill adapted questionnaire in experimental and clinical conditions. Pain, Suppl. 2: S422.

Delay, J., Pichot, P., Lemperiere, T. and Mirouze, R. (1963) La nosographie des etats depressifs. Rapports entre l'etiologie et la semiologie. 2. Resultats du Questionnaire du Beck. L'encephale, 6: 497–505.

Gracely, R.H. (1980) Pain measurement in man. In J.J. Bonica (Ed.), Pain, Discomfort and Humanitarian Care, Elsevier, Amsterdam, pp. 111–137.

Kremer, E. and Atkinson, J.H. (1981) Pain measurement: construct validity of the affective dimension of the McGill Pain Questionnaire with chronic benign pain patients. Pain, 11: 93–100.

Maiani, G. and Sanavio, E. (1985) Semantics of pain in Italy: the Italian version of the McGill Pain Questionnaire. Pain, 22: 399–405.

Melzack, R. (1975) The McGill Pain Questionnaire: major properties and scoring methods. Pain, 1: 277–299.

Melzack, R. and Torgerson, W.S. (1971) On the pain language of pain, Anesthesiology, 34: 50–59.

Melzack, R., Katz, J. and Jeans, M.E. (1985) The role of compensation in chronic pain: analysis using a new method of scoring the McGill Pain Questionnaire. Pain, 23: 101–112.

Pontinen, P.J. and Ketovuori, H. (1983) Verbal measurement in non-English language: the Finnish pain questionnaire. In R. Melzack (Ed.), Pain measurement and assessment, Raven Press, New York, pp. 85–93.

Radvila, A., Adler, R.H., Galeazzi, R.L. and Vorkauf, H. (1987) The development of a German language (Berne) pain questionnaire and its application in a situation causing acute pain. Pain, 23: 185–195.

Reading, A.E. (1982) An analysis of the language of pain in chronic and acute patient groups. Pain, 13: 185–192.

Spielberger, C.D., Gorsuch, R.L. and Luschene, R.E. (1970) Manual for the State Trait Anxiety Inventory, Consulting Psychologist Press, Palo Alto.

Turk, D.C., Rudy, T.E. and Salovey, P. (1985) The McGill Pain Questionnaire reconsidered: confirming the factor structure and examining appropriate use. Pain, 21: 385–397.

Viguie, F. (1982) Questionnaire Algie. In R. Melzack and P D. Wall (Eds.), La Defi de La Douleur, Maloine, Paris, pp. 46.

R. Dubner, G.F. Gebhart & M.R. Bond (Eds.)
Proceedings of the Vth World Congress on Pain
© 1988 Elsevier Science Publishers BV (Biomedical Division)

CHAPTER 45

Effects of controlled alfentanil concentration on pain report and dental evoked potentials

C.R. Chapman[1,2], H.F. Hill[1], L. Saeger[2] and M.H. Walter[1,2]

[1]*Pain and Toxicity Research Program, Fred Hutchinson Cancer Research Center, and* [2]*Multidisciplinary Pain Center, and Department of Anesthesiology, RN-10, University of Washington, Seattle, WA 98195, USA*

Summary

A 15 μg/kg i.v. bolus of the opioid alfentanil was administered to each of 10 subjects, and blood samples were taken over 5 h. The plasma concentration measures for each subject were fitted pharmacokinetically to a curve and the resulting constants and exponents were used to individually tailor a subsequent steady-state infusion. During the infusion, 20, 40 and 80 ng/ml target plasma concentrations were held, following a matching baseline period, for 70 min each. Normally painful, repetitive tooth pulp electrical stimulation was employed to generate pain report and evoked potential measures at each alfentanil plasma concentration. Both effect measures decreased progressively and significantly as alfentanil plasma concentration increased. Although clinical pain states are more complex than the laboratory pain model used here, the outcomes suggest that the testing model may be useful for preclinical staging trials with opioid analgesics.

Correspondence: C. Richard Chapman, Ph.D., Department of Anesthesiology, RN-10, University of Washington School of Medicine, Seattle, WA 98195, U.S.A.

Introduction

A human laboratory model for opioid analgesic states provides an opportunity to bridge progress in animal-based research to controlled clinical trials with patients. Recent gains in the study of the central nervous system mechanisms of opioid analgesia and pharmacokinetic methods for characterizing drug distribution and elimination permit human laboratory investigators to manipulate plasma concentrations of opioid drugs safely and precisely in volunteers for the purposes of experimentation.

This paper demonstrates a human laboratory testing model in which opioid analgesia is inferred from the effects of the drug on the perception of painful events. In this model subjects experience repeated trials of normally painful tooth pulp electrical stimulation. Both subjective reports of pain and pain-related evoked potentials are obtained repeatedly. The drug is delivered by computer-controlled variable-rate infusion, and measures are taken at each of several levels of steady-state plasma concentration during a single experimental session. To achieve precise control of plasma concentration, the infusion is tailored to the individual subject on the basis of pharmacokinetic parameters predetermined for him.

The study reported here was designed to evaluate the therapeutic window for the short-acting opioid alfentanil. This drug has a distributional half-life of under 5 min and an elimination half-life of approximately 70 min (Bovill et al., 1982). We have previously observed that, following a bolus dose of alfentanil, the effects of the drug on pain report and dental evoked potential are evident within 1–2 min and are maximal at about 5 min; the duration of analgesia is 10–20 min (Hill et al., 1986). Alfentanil equilibrates rapidly between brain and blood and does not exhibit the marked hysteresis which characterizes other opioids such as fentanyl (Scott et al., 1985).

Below, we offer the pain report and evoked potential data on 10 subjects as a demonstration of the model. The data reported here are a subset from a larger study which included additional measures of the effects of alfentanil infusion on ventilatory function, motor performance and subjective report of nausea, mood and alertness in addition to pain. These variables were measured prior to infusion, at each of three sequential plasma drug concentrations, and during 2-h washout phase following the infusion. The effects of these manipulations on the additional measures, a characterization of the individual differences observed in tailoring opioids to different individuals and an evaluation of the degree of accuracy of pharmacokinetic tailoring have been reported elsewhere (Hill, in press).

Methods

Subjects Ten male volunteers aged 21–35 years in good health signed informed consent as approved by the Fred Hutchinson Cancer Research Center Institutional Review Board. Each received tailoring boluses of alfentanil (15 μg/kg, i.v.) prior to the infusion session.

Drug tailoring Catheters were placed in the cephalic veins of the subjects' left arms for administration of the bolus dose and in their right arms for blood sample collection. Drug boluses were given over 60 s. Blood samples were collected immediately prior to and at 1, 2, 3, 4, 5, 7, 10, 15, 20, 30, 45, 60, 90, 120, 180, 240 and 300 min following the bo-

lus. Samples were centrifuged, frozen and later subjected to radioimmunoassay for alfentanil concentration (Michiels et al., 1983). A concentration-by-time curve was fitted to each subject using a Marquardt-Levenberg algorithm (Knott, 1979). The constants and exponents derived from this fit were used for subsequent tailoring of drug infusions to the individual subjects.

Drug infusion On another day alfentanil was continuously infused via an Ivac Model 1500 infusion pump equipped with an RS-232 interface module connected to an Epson HX-20 notebook computer. This system controlled the rate of drug infusion and permitted rapid attainment and maintenance of steady-state plasma concentration. During each experimental session, subjects were studied over five 70-min blocks, the first being a pre-infusion baseline condition. Three of the other blocks corresponded to ascending steady-state plasma concentrations of alfentanil: 20, 40 and 80 ng/ml. The remaining block, not reported here, was a randomly positioned placebo (sham) increment in plasma concentration. The 2-h washout phase which followed the infusion is not discussed here.

Experimental pain Subjects experienced repetitive electrical tooth pulp stimulation (performed exactly as described by Hill et al., 1986) with randomly ordered mean interstimulus intervals of 4 s. A single dental stimulus intensity corresponding to subjectively strong pain in pre-drug condition was used throughout the experiment. In each 70-min period before and during the infusion subjects experienced two sets of 150 dental stimuli, the first set at the beginning of the period and the second at the end. Trials were delivered in subsets of 50. All subjects were well practised in the experimental paradigm before testing, and all met our criteria for subjective report and evoked potential performance before admission to the study.

Measures The pain report was derived from a scale that we have used for over a decade. In sensory decision theory studies involving multiple dental

TABLE I

Mean plasma concentrations of alfentanil and mean scores for pain report and evoked potential amplitude (*n* = 10): standard errors of the means are in parentheses

	Infusion target levels			
	Baseline	20 ng/ml	40 ng/ml	80 ng/ml
Alfentanil plasma concentration (ng/ml)	0.0 (0.0)	18.8 (1.3)	42.4 (2.5)	90.0 (6.3)
Pain report (1–5)	4.9 (0.02)	4.5 (0.18)	3.3 (0.28)	2.2 (0.38)
Evoked potential amplitude	19.0 (2.05)	14.9 (1.47)	8.7 (0.77)	7.9 (0.67)

stimulus intensities and hundreds of trials, subjects used the categories of this scale as though they were spaced at equal intervals. In this study subjects were permitted to use either whole or half numbers (e.g., either 4, 3.5 or 3, for example) to rate pain intensity, and the report was obtained at the end of each 50-trial block. The peak-to-peak amplitude (N150–P250) of the dental evoked potential waveform, formed by averaging the blocks of 50 trials, was scored in microvolts (as described by Chapman and Jacobson, 1984).

Results

Table I summarizes the accuracy of the tailored steady-state infusions across the three target concentrations of alfentanil, the corresponding changes in pain report, and the associated changes in dental evoked potential amplitude. Fig. 1 illustrates these outcomes.

Multivariate profile analyses (Morrison, 1976) were performed on both pain report and evoked potential data. Reductions in pain report over time associated with stepwise variations in alfentanil plasma concentration were statistically significant [$F(3,7) = 15.25$, $P = .002$], as were decrements in the amplitude of the evoked potential [$F(3,7) = 11.87$, $P = .004$]. The correlations between pain report and

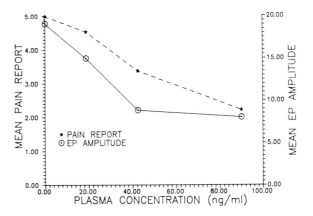

Fig. 1. The mean effects of stepwise tailored alfentanil infusions on pain report (dashed line) and dental evoked potential amplitudes (solid line) are shown for ten subjects. The target plasma concentrations of alfentanil for each of three steps in the infusions were 20, 40 and 80 ng/ml.

evoked potential were obtained at all four drug levels, subjected to a Fischer *Z* transform, averaged, and retransformed to a Pearson *r* to determine the degree of relationship between these variables across plasma concentrations. The resulting correlation coefficient was 0.07, indicating that the two variables do not yield redundant information about the effect of alfentanil on brain.

In sum, these outcomes show that alfentanil infusions were accurately tailored to the individual subjects, and this manipulation resulted in significant and progressive decreases in both reported pain and dental evoked potential. During stepwise infusions the two measures of brain effect, pain report and evoked potential, tracked the changes in plasma alfentanil concentration. The low correlation between pain report and evoked potential indicates that they provided different information about the effects of alfentanil.

Conclusions

This report demonstrates the feasibility of a human-subjects model for opioid analgesia. The use of human vs. animal subjects affords two advantages: (1) analgesia may be inferred from more sophisticated measures of pain and related variables; and (2) the results obtained can be generalized more readily to apply to the care of patients than can animal research findings. The data presented here show that individual tailoring of drug delivery allows accurate control of plasma concentration in humans and can permit intensive investigation of opioid effects under steady-state conditions.

How well results obtained with this model can predict clinical outcomes must be determined by linked laboratory and clinical trials, which we now have in progress in a bone marrow transplant unit. Initial results are promising. Other work with this model indicates that, like alfentanil, morphine administered by tailored infusion reduces laboratory pain measures only about 50% at maximal analgesic plasma concentrations and patients indicate that maximal levels of morphine infusion for oral mucositis pain result in a mean diminution from 100 on a visual analog scale to about 50 (Chapman and Hill, 1988). Clearly, clinical pain states are psychologically complex, and certain salient aspects of clinical pain cannot be modelled in normal volunteers. Moreover, the dental stimulation model is limited to pain originating in A-delta fibers, and results may differ for pain states mediated primarily by C fibers. Apart from these possible limitations in ability to mimic clinical conditions, the model provides an excellent basis for confirming predictions made from animal-model studies, regarding relative potencies of opioids in humans.

The use of human laboratory models of this type can permit preclinical staging trials of new opioid analgesics, define norms for the therapeutic windows for such drugs, and facilitate the precise evaluation of the side-effects of opioids. Such models may obviate much of the need to burden patients with analgesic drug trials.

Acknowledgements

This work was supported by program project grant CA38552 from the National Cancer Institute, training grant GM 07604 from the National Institutes of Health and by Janssen Pharmaceutica.

References

Bovill, J.G., Sebel, P.S., Blackburn, C.I. and Heykants, J. (1982) The pharmacokinetics of alfentanil (R 39209): a new opioid analgesic. Anesthesiology, 57:439–443.

Chapman, C.R. and Jacobson, R.C. (1984) Assessment of analgesic states: can evoked potentials play a role? In B. Bromm (Ed.), Pain Measurement in Man, Neurophysiological Correlates of Pain, Elsevier Science Publishers, Amsterdam.

Chapman, C.R. and Hill, H.F. (1988) Psychological perspectives in pain control: are patients at risk for addiction? Submitted.

Hill, H.F. (In press) Pharmacokinetic tailoring of computer-controlled drug infusions. In R.B. Smith, P.D. Kroboth and R.P. Juhl (Eds.), Pharmacodynamic Research: Current Problems, Potential Solutions, Harvey Whitney Books, Cincinnati.

Hill, H., Walter, M.H., Saeger, L., Sargur, M., Sizemore, W. and Chapman, C.R. (1986) Dose effects of alfentanil in human analgesia. Clin. Pharmacol. Ther., 40:178–186.

Knott, G.D. (1979) Mlab – a mathematical modeling tool. Comput. Prog. Biomed., 10:271–280.

Michiels, M., Hendricks, R. and Heykants, J. (1983) Radioimmunoassay of the new opiate analgesics alfentanil and sufentanil. Pharmacokinetic profile in man. J. Pharmacol., 35: 86–93.

Morrison, D.F. (1976) Multivariate Statistical Methods, McGraw-Hill, New York.

Scott, J.C., Ponganis, D.V. and Stanski, D.R. (1985) EEG quantitation of narcotic effect: the comparative pharmacodynamics of fentanyl and alfentanil. Anesthesiology, 62:L234–241.

R. Dubner, G.F. Gebhart & M.R. Bond (Eds.)
Proceedings of the Vth World Congress on Pain
© 1988 Elsevier Science Publishers BV (Biomedical Division)

CHAPTER 46

A pressure algometer for myofascial pain syndrome: reliability and validity testing

E. Schiffman, J. Fricton, D. Haley and D. Tylka

Department of Oral and Maxillofacial Surgery, University of Minnesota, MN, USA

Introduction

Chronic pain is a serious problem in our society to-day which costs the USA economy over sixty billion dollars per year in medications, health care and lost wages, with untold costs in human suffering (Bonica et al., 1979). Myofascial pain syndrome (MPS) is the primary diagnosis in the majority of these cases for head and neck pain (Fricton et al., 1985). Because of the lack of obvious organic findings, confusion regarding the pathophysiology and the frequent psychosocial problems associated with it, MPS is commonly misunderstood (Laskin, 1969; Sternbach, 1974; Simons, 1975; Moss et al., 1982; Travell and Simons, 1983). If misdiagnosed or inadequately treated at an early stage in development, patients with MPS may develop a complex chronic pain syndrome.

The criteria for establishing the diagnosis of MPS (Fricton et al., 1985) are based on palpation and include:

1. Localized tenderness to palpation at points in firm bands of skeletal muscle, tendons or ligaments: these are termed trigger points.
2. Pain complaints which follow consistent patterns of referral from trigger points.

3. Reproducible alteration or replication of the pain with specific palpation of the trigger point.

Assessment of severity of MPS also uses palpation to quantify the degree of tenderness found in the head and neck musculature because it is found to correlate with symptom severity and improves with treatment (Helkimo, 1974; Sharav et al., 1978; Fricton and Schiffman, 1986).

Some of the confusion in diagnosis and assessment may stem from the subjective nature and lack of reliability of this muscle palpation (Friedman and Weisberg, 1982). Although studies suggest that intra-rater reliability is improved with standardization of a palpation technique, inter-rater reliability of muscle palpation for use with epidemiological and clinical studies is still unacceptably low (Carlsson et al., 1980; Kopp and Wenneberg, 1983). The poor reliability is due to variability in the subjective experience of pain, in the exact anatomical area of palpation, in the surface area, shape and consistency of the palpating finger, and in the amount of pressure used.

In attempts to decrease this variability, the latter three factors can be made more objective through use of a palpation technique with a pressure-sensitive device. In controlling these factors, a pressure-sensitive device must provide a quantifiable pressure gradient, be agile enough to palpate specific anatomical areas, consistent in its shape, surface area and texture, simple, convenient and safe to use

Correspondence: Dr. Eric Schiffman, 7-174 Malcolm Moos Tower, 515 Delaware Street, Minneapolis, MN 55455, U.S.A.

in a clinical setting. Previous attempts to develop a device to use in palpation have shown improved reliability but lacked in clinical agility (Jaeger et al., 1984). A Pressure Algometer for Muscle Palpation (PAMP II) was designed to improve the reliability of the palpation technique and be clinically agile.

The specific aims of this study were:

1. Test the inter-rater reliability of muscle palpation with manual finger palpation and PAMP II utilizing three pairs of raters.
2. Test the validity of PAMP II by comparing the degree of tenderness in muscles in patients with MPS versus normal subjects.

Methods

The Pressure Algometer for Muscle Palpation (PAMP II) (Fig. 1) consists of two parts: the sensor and the readout apparatus. The sensor consists of a hand-held hollow aluminum tube in which is mounted an aluminum bar machined to deflect approximately 0.5 mm with a maximum pressure of 10 pounds/0.13 square inch. A Kistle-Morse strain gauge is mounted the aluminum bar to sense any deflection of the bar. A Delrin® plastic rod is attached to one end of the bar. The opposite end of the plastic rod, convex in all directions, contacts the skin and, when pressure is applied, it deflects the bar.

The readout section is a commercial box with switch, meter, batteries and a suitable amplifier for the strain gauge to provide full-scale meter deflection with application of pressure to the plastic probe tip.

In this study, inter-rater reliability was determined by having three raters (A,B,C) evaluate 45 normal subjects and 45 patients from the TMJ and Craniofacial Pain Clinic at the University of Minnesota who were diagnosed as having MPS using the previously discussed diagnostic criteria. The normal subjects had no history of MPS or TMJ problems and checked negative on all symptoms on a symptom check list. The patients and subjects were matched for sex and age. Only two raters were

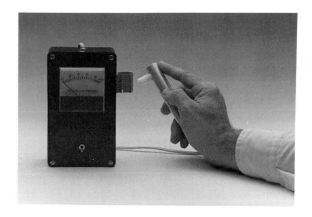

Fig. 1. Pressure algometer for muscle palpation (PAMP II). PAMP II consists of a hand-held sensor and a readout apparatus. The sensor is contained in a hollow aluminum tube in which is mounted an aluminum bar. A Delrin plastic rod is attached to one end of the bar, the other convex end contacts the skin and, when pressure is applied, the bar is deflected. A Kistler-Morse strain gauge is attached to the side of the bar to detect deflection. The readout apparatus is connected electrically to the sensor.

used to examine each patient to minimize variability due to increasing tenderness of muscles which may develop as a result of examinations. Thus, thirty patients were evaluated by each pair (A-B, A-C, B-C) to equal 90 comparisons. Each examination consisted of palpating the muscle-joint sites on the right side to determine the pain threshold with PAMP II and on the left side to determine whether tenderness existed or not with a standardized manual finger pressure technique. The exact locations of the muscle palpation sites are given in Fig. 2. The muscle and joint locations palpated include the anterior, middle and posterior temporalis, the anterior, deep and inferior masseter, posterior digastric, medial ptergyoid, vertex, superior and middle sternocleidomastoid, splenius capitis, trapezius insertion, upper trapezius and lateral aspect of the TMJ capsule.

The manual technique is performed first by locating the distinct muscle band or joint and then palpating using the sensitive spade-like pad at the end of the distal phalanx of the index finger using firm pressure. The subject/patient is asked 'does it hurt or is it just pressure?'. It is scored positive if the patient indicates that the site is clearly painful. Any equivocal response is scored as negative.

The palpation technique with PAMP II consisted of locating the distinct muscle band or part of joint with gentle index-finger pressure and then using the tip of the PAMP to place pressure on the band at the specific muscle/joint location. An 'ascending method of limits' technique was used to determine the pain threshold. The pain threshold is the first level at which the subject/patient reports even the slightest pain due to ascending pressure from palpation with PAMP II. This level was recorded and repeated in five seconds to determine mean pain

threshold for each muscle location. All the subjects/patients were given the following instructions: 'Please raise your hand when the pressure first becomes even the slightest bit painful'. If no pain was reported at the highest level, then this level was used as the pain threshold. In both cases, the second rater, blind to the first rater's determinations, repeated the evaluation after a 15-min rest to minimize aggravation of the trigger point.

The mean value at each site for the 45 comparisons for both the PAMP II technique and manual technique was then compared using the KAPPA statistic for inter-rater agreement. This statistic was

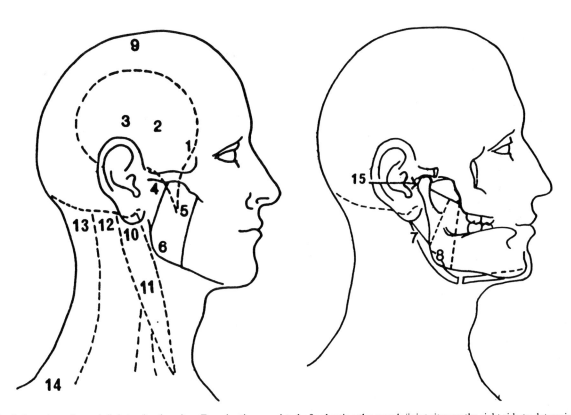

Fig. 2. Location of muscle/joint palpation sites. Examination consisted of palpating the muscle/joint sites on the right side to determine the pain threshold with PAMP II and on the left side to determine whether tenderness existed with a standardized manual finger pressure technique. The exact locations of the palpation sites are:

Muscle: extraoral
1. anterior temporalis
2. middle temporalis
3. posterior temporalis
4. deep masseter
5. anterior masseter
6. inferior masseter
7. posterior digastric
8. medial pterygoid
9. vertex
Muscle: neck
10. superior sternocleidomastoid
11. middle sternocleidomastoid
12. splenius capitus
13. insertion of trapezius
14. upper trapezius
TMJ
15. lateral capsule

used in order to provide a standardized comparison of both the PAMP II and the manual technique which considers the factor of random agreement. The PAMP II scores were converted to 0 to 1 scores by using the mean as the threshold value. In addition, for the PAMP technique, Pearson's correlation coefficient of each pair of raters (A-B, A-C, B-C) was also used to determine differences between pairs of raters and overall correlation between rating 1 and rating 2.

The mean pain thresholds for muscle palpation of the 45 MPS patients at 1st testing were compared with the mean pain threshold for muscle palpation of 45 normal subjects, matched for sex and age. Mean values for each muscle/joint palpated for the two groups were statistically compared using a paired t-test. In addition, the mean pain threshold of male subjects was compared to that of female subjects in both MPS and normal groups.

Results

Table I illustrates the mean pain threshold for palpation in MPS patients using PAMP II and the percentage of positive responses using the manual technique. Values for the first and second rating per patient are also shown and were assessed for inter-rater reliability via the Kappa Statistic (i.e. K value).

For the PAMP II technique, the reliability was at or above 0.40, demonstrating moderate to good reliability, with the exception of the posterior temporalis and deep masseter. For the manual technique, only two muscle sites, the anterior temporalis and middle sternocleidomastoid, had moderate to good reliability; that is, above 0.40. The inter-rater reliability of palpation using PAMP II was consistently higher than for manual palpation, except for the middle sternocleidomastoid.

TABLE I

Inter-rater reliability of muscle palpation was higher with PAMP II than with manual finger palpation

Muscle	MPS patients with PAMP II (mean pain threshold level)			MPS patients with manual technique (percentage positive responses)		
	Rating 1	Rating 2	K value[b]	Rating 1	Rating 2	K value[b]
Anterior temporalis	0.37	0.36	0.55*	0.46	0.47	0.51*
Middle temporalis	0.48	0.48	0.49*	0.42	0.24	0.34
Posterior temporalis	0.40	0.39	0.38	0.56	0.56	0.32
Deep masseter	0.44	0.35	0.36	0.82	0.82	0.27
Anterior masseter	0.35	0.36	0.63*	0.53	0.71	0.24
Inferior masseter	0.32	0.34	0.68*	0.67	0.73	0.24
Posterior digastric	0.26	0.26	0.40*	0.84	0.78	0.35
Medial pterygoid	0.26	0.24	0.51*	0.58	0.73	0.27
Vertex	0.67	0.58	0.69*	0.16	0.24	0.17
Superior SCM[a]	0.44	0.44	0.46*	0.27	0.27	0.02
Middle SCM[a]	0.24	0.21	0.58*	0.56	0.49	0.60*
Splenius capitis	0.47	0.48	0.68*	0.76	0.56	0.33
Trapezius insertion	0.45	0.47	0.54*	0.73	0.56	0.38
Upper trapezius	0.50	0.51	0.46*	0.64	0.73	0.37
TMJ capsule (lateral)	0.28	0.28	0.46*	0.49	0.71	0.17

Mean pain threshold and percentage of positive responses were determined from PAMP and manual finger palpation, respectively. Inter-rater reliability comparing PAMP II with the manual technique between the first and second ratings at each muscle/joint site was assessed via the Kappa Correlation Statistic. For the PAMP II technique, moderate to good reliability ($r \geq 0.4$)* was demonstrated in 13 of 15 sites. For the manual technique, only two sites had this level of reliability.
[a]Sternocleidomastoid; [b]Kappa statistic.

Table II compares each pair of raters (A-B, B-C, A-C) using the PAMP II technique: the correlations (Pearson's) involving one rater (B) were consistently lower at most sites than the other pair (A,C). This rater (B) had less experience in palpation than raters A or C; however, overall correlations were good, ranging from 0.58 to 0.82, with the exception of the posterior digastric, middle sternocleidomastoid and lateral TMJ capsule.

Validity testing is illustrated in Table III. The mean pain threshold for patients with MPS was significantly lower than in normal subjects at each muscle/joint site ($P \leq 0.001$). In addition, a comparison of mean pain thresholds in males at each site was significantly higher than that of females for the MPS patients ($P \leq 0.05$). Each of the muscle sites in normal subjects, however, had mean pain thresholds which did not differ significantly between males and females.

Discussion

The results of this study provide evidence for the adequacy of inter-rater reliability of muscle palpation of most muscle/joint sites using PAMP II. However, they also suggest that although the reliability of palpation using PAMP II is higher than with manual palpation, the latter technique can have adequate reliability when using a standardized technique with experienced raters on specific muscle/joint sites. The use of PAMP II is of questionable reliability on muscles which are difficult to palpate. The posterior digastric is small, frequently tender, and often difficult to locate. The middle sternocleidomastoid is difficult to palpate because it often rolls out from under the palpating surface. The lateral TMJ capsule can only be palpated with the mouth open a specific amount and any limitation in translation will effect palpation reliability. Also, the palpating surface is small and convex over the lateral aspect of the TMJ capsule.

In this study, one rater was less experienced than the other two raters and this affected overall reliability. This finding highlights the importance of

TABLE II

Inter-rater reliability: results are dependent on utilization of a standardized technique with experienced raters (Pearson's correlation coefficient (45 MPS patients))

Site	Raters AB	Raters AC	Raters BC	R1/R2
Anterior temporalis	0.59	0.88	0.41	0.64
Middle temporalis	0.80	0.88	0.44	0.60
Posterior temporalis	0.49	0.86	0.28	0.58
Deep masseter	0.74	0.81	0.60	0.74
Anterior masseter	0.78	0.89	0.71	0.82
Inferior masseter	0.84	0.93	0.69	0.82
Posterior digastric	0.68	0.59	0.33	0.53
Medial pterygoid	0.55	0.85	0.73	0.75
Vertex	0.80	0.76	0.69	0.70
Superior SCM[a]	0.79	0.85	0.59	0.70
Middle SCM[a]	0.49	0.88	0.61	0.53
Splenius capitis	0.55	0.77	0.79	0.70
Trapezius insertion	0.62	0.87	0.68	0.75
Upper trapezius	0.74	0.66	0.75	0.71
TMJ capsule (lateral)	0.22	0.51	0.67	0.40

Inter-rater reliability is partly dependent on the experience of the raters in performing the palpation technique. Rater B had less experience than raters A and C, which illustrates the effect of experience. However, when the results of all the raters (A,B,C) were combined (Rating 1/Rating 2, R1/R2) correlations ranging between 0.53 and 0.82 were obtained for muscle palpation, but only 0.40 for joint palpation.
[a]Sternocleidomastoid.

having experienced raters with much discussion and test comparisons of sites and techniques prior to initiating any study using palpation. The results of this study also corroborate the validity of PAMP II as an instrument which measures the pain threshold of muscle/joint sites. As hypothesized, the pain thresholds of these sites were consistently lower in patients with MPS than in normal subjects. This finding supports the trigger point theory of MPS by confirming that specific sites of muscles are more tender in patients with MPS than normal subjects. Others have confirmed that these sites are localized and more tender than adjacent sites (Jaeger et al., 1984).

Another finding of this study is that muscles/joints in females with MPS had a lower pain threshold than muscles/joints in males with MPS. This finding sheds some light on the higher prevalence of MPS in females than in males in a clinical population. A lower pain threshold in affected muscles of females suggests that smaller muscles with less bulk are more sensitive to pressure and possibly more prone to injury due to micro- or macro-trauma. This contention is also supported by the lower pain threshold found in smaller muscles such as the digastric in either sex. However, differences in care-seeking behavior, pain tolerance and hormonal balance have also been implicated.

It is hoped that the use of pressure algometry will improve the objectivity and reliability of palpation for trigger points. Past studies have suggested that the reliability of finger palpation for muscle tenderness is low (Carlsson et al., 1980; Kopp and Wenneberg, 1983). A standardized technique further im-

proves the reliability of finger palpation (Fricton and Schiffman, 1986). A pressure algometer standardizes the factors which contribute to this lower variability between raters by providing a consistent palpating surface and amount of pressure. In this way, a standardized technique utilizing an algometer produces the highest level of reliability.

In addition to confirming diagnosis, the tenderness of trigger points can also be used as an indicator of severity. This tenderness is reduced with treatment and correlated with a reduction in symptoms (Fricton and Schiffman, 1987). In most cases, though, the number of tender muscles in patients successfully treated is still higher than in a normal population. The exact nature of this localized tenderness has yet to be confirmed.

TABLE III

Validity testing: the mean pain threshold for MPS patients was significantly lower than for normal subjects: within the MPS patients, females had lower pain thresholds than males

| Sites | Mean pain threshold using PAMP II | | | | | |
| | MPS patients ($n=45$) | | | Normal subjects ($n=45$) | | |
	Male (11)	Female (34)	Combined	Male (11)	Female (34)	Combined
Anterior temporalis	0.50	0.33*	0.37	0.80	0.79	0.79**
Middle temporalis	0.66	0.43*	0.49	0.91	0.81	0.84**
Posterior temporalis	0.51	0.36*	0.40	0.86	0.79	0.81**
Deep masseter	0.63	0.32*	0.39	0.80	0.78	0.78**
Anterior masseter	0.51	0.30*	0.35	0.71	0.68	0.68**
Inferior masseter	0.51	0.27*	0.33	0.73	0.62	0.65**
Posterior digastric	0.36	0.23*	0.26	0.53	0.44	0.46**
Medial pterygoid	0.35	0.21*	0.25	0.44	0.36	0.38**
Vertex	0.68	0.61	0.63	0.83	0.85	0.84**
Superior SCM[a]	0.60	0.30*	0.43	0.78	0.75	0.76**
Middle SCM[a]	0.34	0.19*	0.23	0.52	0.48	0.49**
Splenius capitis	0.66	0.42*	0.47	0.87	0.81	0.82**
Trapezius insertion	0.64	0.40*	0.46	0.91	0.82	0.84**
Upper trapezius	0.75	0.43*	0.50	0.85	0.83	0.83**
TMJ capsule (lateral)	0.34	0.26*	0.28	0.61	0.64	0.63**

*Significance ($P \leq 0.05$) when comparing males with females in MPS group (no significance when comparing males with females in normal group).

**Significance ($P \leq 0.001$) when comparing combined (female and male) mean pain thresholds of MPS patients and normal subjects.

[a]Sternocleidomastoid

Conclusion

1. PAMP II has been shown to be more reliable for palpation of anatomical sites than a standardized finger pressure technique.
2. The mean pain threshold for MPS patients was significantly lower than for normal subjects. This validates muscle palpation tenderness as an objective sign in helping establish a diagnosis of MPS.
3. In patients with MPS, females have significantly lower mean pain thresholds upon palpation than males. This relationship was not present in the control group.
4. Neither technique eliminates the need for standardization between raters.

Acknowledgement

This research was supported by the NIDR Small Grant Program (No. 1R03DE04713-01).

References

Bonica, J.J., Liebeskind, J.C. and Albe-Fessard, D. (1979) Preface. Advances in Pain Research and Therapy, Vol. 3, Raven Press, New York, pp. v–viii.

Carlsson, G.E., Egermark-Erikson, I. and Magnusson, T. (1980) Intra- and inter-observer variation in functional examination of the masticatory system. Swed. Dent. J., 4: 187–194.

Fricton, J.R., Kroening, R., Haley, D. and Siegert, R. (1985) Myofascial pain and dysfunction of the head and neck: a review of clinical characteristics of 164 patients. Oral Surg., 60: 615–623.

Fricton, J. and Schiffman, E. (1986) Craniomandibular index: reliability. J. Dent. Res., 65: 1359–1364.

Fricton, J. and Schiffman, E. (1987) The craniomandibular index: validity. J. Prosthet. Dent., 58: 222–228.

Friedman, M.H. and Weisberg, J. (1982) Pitfalls of muscle palpation in TMJ diagnosis. J. Prosthet. Dent., 48: 331–335.

Helkimo, M. (1974) Studies on function and dysfunction of the masticatory system III. Analyses of anamnestic and clinical recordings of dysfunction with the aid of indices. Swed. Dent. J., 67: 165–182.

Jaeger, G., Reeves, J.L., Graff-Radford, S.B. and Fisher, A.A. (1984) Reliability of the pressure meter as an objective measure of myofascial trigger point sensitivity. Pain, Suppl. 2: 124.

Kopp, S. and Wenneberg, G. (1983) Intra- and inter-observer variability in the assessment of signs of disorder in the stomatognathic system. Swed. Dent. J., 7: 239–246.

Laskin, D. (1969) Etiology of pain-dysfunction syndrome. J. Am. Dent. Assoc., 79: 147.

Moss, R.A., Garrett, J. and Chiodo, J.F. (1982) Temporomandibular joint dysfunction and myofascial pain dysfunction syndromes: parameters, etiology and treatment. Psych. Bull., 92: 331–346.

Sharav, Y., Tzukert, A. and Refaeli, B. (1978) Muscle pain indices in relation to pain, dysfunction and dizziness associated with myofascial pain dysfunction syndrome. Oral Surg., 46: 742–747.

Simons, D.G. (1975) Muscle pain syndromes (Part I and II). Am. J. Phys. Med., 54: 288–311 and 55: 15–42.

Sternbach, R.A. (1974) Pain Patients: Traits and Treatment, Academic Press, New York.

Travell, J. and Simons, D.G. (1983) Myofascial Pain and Dysfunction: The Trigger Point Manual, Williams and Wilkins, Baltimore, Ch. 2–4.

The Spinal Cord and Analgesia

R. Dubner, G.F. Gebhart & M.R. Bond (Eds.)
Proceedings of the Vth World Congress on Pain
© 1988 Elsevier Science Publishers BV (Biomedical Division)

CHAPTER 47

Properties of the modulation of spinal nociceptive transmission by receptor-selective agents

Tony L. Yaksh and Craig W. Stevens

Departments of Neurosurgical Research and Pharmacology, Mayo Clinic, Rochester, Mn 55905, USA

Summary

Spinally administered agents known to act upon specific classes of pharmacologically defined receptors can produce a powerful and relatively selective alteration in spinal processing input evoked by high-intensity somatic and visceral stimuli. (1) Current evidence based on the pharmacological analysis of the effects produced by intrathecally administered drugs in a variety of animal models suggests that μ, δ and κ opioid, α_2-adrenergic, muscarinic cholinergic and to a lesser degree GABA-B and serotonin receptors can produce such selective alterations in behavior at doses which do not significantly affect motor function. (2) Chronic spinal infusion of μ, δ and α_2 receptor agonists has shown that all systems undergo a reduction in the response produced by a given concentration of the drug (tolerance). Significantly, however, such studies have shown that the tolerance is reversible and have indicated the independence of the receptor systems by demonstrating the lack of cross-tolerance between the respective class of agents. (3) Certain of these classes of receptors appear to interact in a non-linear, synergistic fashion so that small concentrations, for example, of μ and α_2 receptor agonists result in prominent physiological effects. These investigations thus provide not only an insight into the pharmacological characteristics of intrinsic receptor systems which modulate spinal nociceptive processing, but also the fundamental information

needed regarding the toxicology of these agents to permit their considered use in man. Thus, to date, based on the animal studies, it has been shown that the spinal administration of μ and δ opioid and α_2-adrenergic receptor agonists will produce a powerful analgesia in man. It appears reasonable to presume that fundamental studies on the pharmacology of the spinal cord will continue to yield fruitful information relevant to pain management in man.

Introduction

Unconditioned visceral and somatic stimuli known to activate certain populations of small afferents will evoke organized efforts to escape or will result in signs of discomfort and distress, such as vocalization or verbal report. Considerable evidence exists to suggest that the processes whereby this information is encoded, particularly those in the spinal cord, are plastic and subject to alteration by a number of intrinsic modulatory systems. Indeed, these spinal modulatory substrates themselves constitute an important element in the encoding process in that their activity can dynamically alter the meaning of the nociceptive message. Of particular importance has been the observation that these modulatory systems possess a well-defined pharmacology and that their presumed physiological effects can be mimicked by administering exogenous agents which act on the appropriate receptor postsynaptic to the modulatory terminals, e.g., by intrathecal (i.t.) or epidural injection. This approach has not only shed light on the hodology of the systems which process pain-relevant information, but in several instances it has proven to have therapeutic benefit in the treatment of pain in man.

In considering the use of spinally administered, receptor-selective agents, four points must be considered to have theoretical and therapeutic relevance:

(i) What is the receptor through which the agent mediates its effects?

(ii) What are the characteristics of the tolerance associated with the continued exposure of the receptor to the agent?

(iii) Do these receptors interact?

(iv) Are the receptors upon which the agent acts differentially associated with systems which process pain-relevant information?

Considerations of methodology

Several issues should first be considered with regard to the methods of studying spinal receptor systems which modulate pain-processing. First, from a behavioral perspective, if an agent results in an attenuation of the animal's supraspinally organized response to a strong and otherwise aversive stimulus with no detectable effect upon motor function, then this drug action, at the given dose, may be thought to reflect an antinociceptive or 'analgesic' action. However, agents may also alter motor function prominently by a receptor-selective action if the receptor is directly associated with control of motor outflow. In such cases, a drug may indeed alter sensory processing, but it cannot be thought to fit the theoretical construct of an analgetic. A variety of pain models are commonly employed which are evoked by high-threshold input and which are organized at the spinal level such as the thermally evoked tail flick (D'Amour and Smith, 1941) or skin twitch (Martin et al., 1976). Though extremely useful, caution must be taken to separate effects on motor components from those relevant to the su-

praspinal transmission of the peripheral stimulus. It follows that the characterization of the *analgesic* effects of a spinal agent absolutely depends upon the assessment of the organized behavior evoked by strong somatic/visceral stimuli in the intact and unanesthetized animal, e.g., has the spinal manipulation altered the content of the peripheral message so that there is no longer correspondence between the physical nature of the unconditioned stimulus and the evoked escape behavior? More complex measures which entail a supraspinally mediated component, and thus reflect a measure of the integrated responses of the animal evoked by strong somatic or visceral stimuli, are commonly available, ranging from those which depend upon a simple escape response such as the electrically evoked flinch jump (Evans, 1962), vocalization (Carroll and Lim, 1960) and the thermally evoked hot plate (Woolfe and MacDonald, 1944) responses, to the response to colonic distention (Ness and Gebhart, 1987), paw pressure (Randall and Selitto, 1957) or acute chemical (Dubuisson and Dennis, 1977; Hendershot and Forsyth, 1959) and chronic inflammatory (Imrie, 1976; Colpaert et al., 1980) stimuli. In addition, more complex behavioral analyses have been reported using various shock (Cooper and Vierck, 1986; Dykstra, 1979; Yaksh and Reddy, 1981) and thermal (Dubner, 1985) escape models. With few exceptions, these routine measures possess the common property that they allow the organism to rapidly escape the noxious stimuli. With the inflammatory stimuli this is not the case, but their use is predicated on presumed differences between acute and chronic pain.

Second, in attempting to define the spinal systems relevant to 'analgesia', one must administer the agents into the spinal space of the unanesthetized animal. Several such acute (Hylden and Wilcox, 1983a) and chronic (Durant and Yaksh, 1986; Yaksh and Rudy, 1976a; Yaksh and Stevens, 1986; Van de Hoogen and Colpaert, 1981) methodologies have been described.

Finally, if a given agonist produces a physiological effect after local administration, the identity of the receptor with which it interacts can be surmised on the basis of its known affinity for various classes of receptors. Given, however, that the concentration of drug at the site of action is unknown, the nature of the receptor mediating a given physiological effect must be defined by the demonstration of: (1) the appropriate agonist structure-activity relationship (SAR) posited for that receptor; (2) the SAR of the antagonists which reverse the effects of the agonist and/or the assessment of antagonist affinity (pA_2) for the site acted upon by the agonist; and (3) tolerance/cross-tolerance between agonists thought to act upon the same receptor.

Characterization of spinal receptors which alter pain processing

In the following sections we will discuss several classes of spinal receptors which have been shown to modify the organized response of the animal to strong, unconditioned somatic and visceral stimuli.

Opioid receptors

Opioid agonists administered into the vicinity of the substantia gelatinosa will suppress the discharge of spinal nociceptive neurons evoked by stimuli which activate small C–fiber afferents (Duggan et al., 1981; Fleetwood-Walker et al., 1987; Hope et al., 1987). Dorsal rhizotomy (LaMotte et al., 1976) or treatment with the small primary afferent neurotoxin capsaicin (Gamse et al., 1979) results in a significant but subtotal reduction in opioid ligand receptor binding. These observations, in conjunction with studies showing an inhibition of the release of substance P from small primary afferents in a naloxone-reversible fashion (Go and Yaksh, 1987; Jessell and Iversen, 1977; Yaksh et al., 1980), suggest a presynaptic action of spinal opiates. Alternatively, the subtotal depletion of dorsal horn opiate receptor binding produced by afferent lesions and the suppression by opioids of excitatory postsynaptic potentials evoked in dorsal horn neurons by glutamate (Zieglgansberger and Bayerl, 1976) suggest a direct postsynaptic action on a second-order neuron.

Opioids given intrathecally or epidurally will produce clear and selective changes in virtually all of the experimental and clinical pain measures employed in man (see Cousins and Mathers, 1984; Yaksh and Noueihed, 1985) and on a variety of nociceptive end-points in numerous vertebrates, including frog (Stevens et al., 1987), mouse (Hylden and Wilcox, 1983b), rabbit (Yaksh and Rudy, 1976b), rat (Tang and Schoenfeld, 1978; Tung and Yaksh, 1982; Yaksh and Rudy, 1977), cat (Yaksh, 1978a; Yaksh et al., 1986), sheep (Eisenach, 1987) and primate (Yaksh, 1983; Yaksh and Reddy, 1981). Several lines of evidence suggest that these spinal effects result from a movement of the drug into the spinal gray (Yaksh, 1981). Thus, opiates have not been shown to alter transmission through the ganglion or along primary afferents in adult in situ or ex situ models (Shefner et al., 1981; Williams and Zieglgansberger, 1981).

Current thinking suggests that there are probably several subpopulations of opioid receptors: μ = morphine, sufentanil, D-Ala^2-MePhe^4-Gly-ol^5-enkephalin (DAGO); δ = D-Ala^2-D-Leu^5-enkephalin (DADL), D-Pen^2-D-Pen^5-enkephalin (DPDPE); κ = dynorphin$_{1-13}$, U50488H; and ε = β-endorphin. Other receptor formulations suggest the likelihood of a high-affinity (μ_1-meptazinol) and low-affinity (μ_2) and δ (DPDPE) sites (Pasternak et al., 1980). The compilation of an abbreviated SAR is presented in Figs. 1 and 2 for the HP response and visceral irritant response following i.t. administration in rodents. Initial evidence of a functionally selective modulation of spinal nociceptive processing emphasized the role of μ receptor agonists (e.g., morphine, sufentanil). Animal studies have also shown that agents classified as δ (D-Pen^2-L-Pen^5-enkephalin; DPLPE) or κ (U50488H) receptor-selective are also able to alter nociceptive processing after intrathecal administration (Castillo et al., 1986; Schmauss and Yaksh, 1984; Wood et al., 1981; Yaksh, 1983). Though no single agonist is absolutely selective, several independent lines of evidence support the contention that these several classes of ligands do indeed act upon discriminable receptors:

(i) Differential structure-activity relationships for μ, δ and κ receptor agonists. Thus, as shown in Fig. 1, δ but not κ receptor agonists were very active on thermal nociceptive end-points. In contrast, as shown in Fig. 2, κ but not δ receptor agonists were active on chemical evoked responses, and μ₁ receptor agonists were equi-active on both measures (Schmauss and Yaksh, 1984). The probable role of spinal κ receptors has been proposed by several investigators (Castillo et al., 1986; Wood et al., 1981). As indicated in Fig. 1, the proposed selective μ receptor agonist (meptazinol) is without spinal effects. This differential activity of intrathecal δ and κ receptor agonists has also been confirmed on pressure tests (Millan, unpublished observations, Munich, 1987). It should be stressed that these effects do not necessarily reflect upon an absolute as-

sociation with specific stimulus modalities, rather on the intrinsic intensity of the stimuli employed. Thus, as Millan and colleagues have shown, intrathecal κ receptor ligands are in fact able to block the responses evoked by low-intensity thermal stimuli. Such results are in accord with studies examining the effects of these agents on thermally evoked ventral root reflexes (Parsons and Headley, 1987).

(ii) Distinguishable affinity of naloxone for the receptors acted upon by putative μ, δ and κ receptor agonists. Thus, where examined, the dose-response curves for these agonists are shifted to the right in a parallel fashion in the presence of increasing doses of naloxone (Yaksh and Henry, 1978; Yaksh and Rudy, 1977; Yaksh et al., 1978). However, calculation of the apparent affinity (pA₂) of naloxone for the receptor acted upon by the spinally admin-

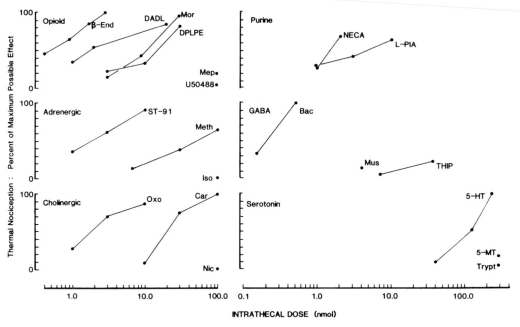

Fig. 1. Dose-response curves for the effects of intrathecally administered agents in rats (nmol/10 μl) on the hot plate response plotted in terms of percent of the maximum possible effect (baseline HP latency 10–20 s for all groups; cut-off time was 60 s). Each point shows the mean response of 4–20 rats. Drugs are: *opioid*: β–End = β-endorphin, DADL = D-Ala²-D-Leu⁵-enkephalin, Mor = morphine, DPLPE = D-Pen²-L-Pen⁵-enkephalin, Mep = meptazinol (Yaksh and Henry, 1978; Mjanger and Yaksh, unpublished observations; Schmauss et al., 1985); *adrenergic*: Meth = methoxamine, Iso = isoproterenol (Howe et al., 1983); *cholinergic*: Oxo = oxotremorine, Car = carbachol, Nic = nicotine (Yaksh et al., 1985); *purine*: NECA, 5'-N-ethylcarboxamidoadenosine (Sawynok et al., 1986); *GABA*: Bac = baclofen, Mus = muscimol (Wilson and Yaksh, 1978; Hammond and Drower, 1984); *serotonin*: 5-HT = 5-hydroxytryptamine, 5-MT = 5-methoxytryptamine, Trypt = tryptamine (Yaksh and Wilson, 1979).

istered agents differed, with naloxone showing highest affinity for μ, less for δ and least for κ receptors. This suggests distinguishable sites of action (Yaksh, 1981).

(iii) Differential antagonism by various antagonists. β-Funalnaltrexamine (β-FNA), a nonequilibrium antagonist (Ward et al., 1982) at doses which block morphine or other μ receptor agonists (DAGO, sufentanil), will not block the effects of DPLPE (Mjanger and Yaksh, unpublished observations).

(iv) Differential cross-tolerance. In a variety of studies, it has been shown that animals rendered tolerant to a μ receptor agonist (such as morphine) show relatively little loss of response to a δ-preferring ligand (see below) (Tseng, 1982; Tung and Yaksh, 1982; Yaksh, 1983; Russell et al., 1987; Stevens and Yaksh, 1986b; Yaksh, 1983).

In man, μ receptor agonists have heretofore been principally used, e.g. morphine, sufentanil, meperi-

dine, methadone. The δ-preferring peptide, DADL, has also been shown to be a powerful analgesic in man after i.t. administration (Krames et al., 1986; Moulin et al., 1985; Onofrio and Yaksh, 1983). With regard to the κ receptor, a number of the traditional partial agonists, such as nalbuphine or butorphanol, are thought to act in part at the κ site, and appear mildly effective as analgesics following epidural administration (Chu et al., 1987; Weintraub and Naulty, 1985). Whether these agents will be useful under different clinical conditions to produce adequate analgesia remains to be seen and will require systematic comparisons with full agonists such as morphine. The limited effect of these agents appears to be not because these agents are 'partial agonists', but because the receptor with which they interact (κ) may be less effectively coupled to spinal systems relevant to pain processing. β-Endorphin produces powerful analgesia when given spinally (Oyama et al., 1980). Though β-endorphin is

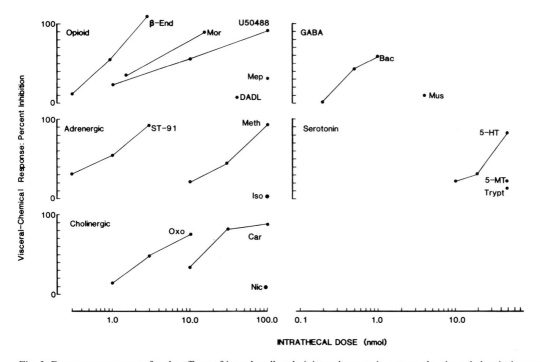

Fig. 2. Dose-response curves for the effects of intrathecally administered agents in rats on the visceral chemical response (Schmauss and Yaksh, 1984) plotted in terms of the percent inhibition. Each point presents the mean from six animals. Abbreviations are as given in Fig. 1. Opioid (Schmauss and Yaksh, 1984; Yaksh and Harty, unpublished observations); adrenergic (Yaksh, 1985); cholinergic (Yaksh et al., 1985); GABA/serotonin (Yaksh and Harty, unpublished observations).

thought to act on several sites, one of which is designated the ε receptor, systematic animal studies have suggested that its effects are mediated by a site similar to that acted upon by morphine (Tung and Yaksh, 1982; Yaksh and Henry, 1978; Yaksh et al., 1982a).

Adrenergic receptors
The role of bulbospinal adrenergic pathways in modulating spinal functions has long been appreciated. Early studies demonstrated that L-DOPA administered systemically could alter spinal activity evoked by flexor-reflex afferents (Anden et al., 1966). Activation of bulbospinal noradrenergic pathways by brainstem manipulations such as microinjection of morphine, local activation by glutamate, or electrical stimulation in the periaqueductal gray will produce a powerful descending spinal inhibition which is mediated by adrenergic receptors (see Hammond and Yaksh, 1984; Jensen and Yaksh, 1984; Yaksh, 1979, 1985; Yaksh and Rudy, 1978). Administration of norepinephrine into the dorsal horn will produce a powerful suppression of small afferent evoked activity in dorsal horn neurons (Fleetwood-Walker et al., 1985; Headley et al., 1978). By virtue of the agonists' and antagonists' SAR, this local inhibitory effect appears to be mediated by an α_2-receptor.

Intrathecal administration of adrenergic agonists in a variety of species, including mouse (Hylden and Wilcox, 1983b), rat (Kuraishi et al., 1979; Reddy and Yaksh, 1980; Reddy et al., 1980), cat (Reddy et al., 1980), sheep (Eisenach, 1987) and primate (Yaksh and Reddy, 1981), has been shown to yield a powerful analgesia.

As suggested by the data in Figs. 1 and 2, this effect, in agreement with the pharmacology of the bulbospinal inhibition discussed above, principally reflects an action mediated by an α_2-receptor. Thus, the relative activity of spinally administered adrenergic agonists is: ST-91 (α_2 = a clonidine analogue) > norepinephrine > methoxamine (α_1) >> isoproterenol (β) = 0. With regard to antagonism, the antinociceptive effects of clonidine and norepinephrine are antagonized in a dose-dependent fash-

ion by adrenergic antagonists, with the ordering of antagonist 'potency' being yohimbine (α_2) = rauwolscine (α_2) >> corynanthine (α_1) > propranolol (β) = 0 (Howe et al., 1983; Yaksh, 1985).

In man, clonidine, a α_2-agonist, has been usefully administered epidurally in cancer patients for the treatment of pain (Coombs et al., 1984; Tamsen and Gordh, 1984).

Cholinergic receptors
Cholinergic binding sites have been identified in the dorsal horn (Wamsley et al., 1981). Iontophoretic application of muscarinic agonists onto dorsal horn neurons will result in inhibition of their evoked activity (Myslinkski and Randic, 1977). Cholinergic agonists given spinally will yield an atropine-reversible antinociception (Yaksh et al., 1985). The effects of intrathecally administered acetylcholine are markedly facilitated by cholinesterase inhibition. While the mechanism of this effect is not known, the effects of spinal cholinergic agonists are not antagonized by naloxone or monoamine antagonists (Post et al., 1987).

Adenosine
Two classes of adenosine receptors (A_1, A_2) have been proposed on the basis of differential SARs (Burnstock and Buckley, 1985). The spinal application of A_1 and A_2 agents in rats will yield analgesia, as defined on several nociceptive measures (see Fig. 1). This spinal effect is stereospecific and antagonized in a dose-dependent fashion by adenosine receptor antagonists (Post, 1984; Sawynok et al., 1986). As dorsal rhizotomy does not alter A_1 or A_2 binding, this action (unlike opiates and α_2-agonists) is not likely to be mediated by a direct presynaptic effect on primary afferents (Dr. Herb Proudfit, personal communication).

GABAergic
GABA (γ-aminobutyric acid) is considered a presynaptic neurotransmitter in the spinal cord (Game and Lodge, 1975). Pharmacological studies have shown that there are probably two subclasses of GABA receptors, GABA-A (muscimol) and

GABA-B (baclofen) (Bowery, 1982). Iontophoretic administration of baclofen will result in a depression of dorsal horn neurons (Henry, 1982). Studies with i.t. injections have shown that GABA-B (Wilson and Yaksh, 1978), but not GABA-A (Hammond and Drower, 1984), receptor agonists will produce a measurable effect on thermal nociception in the rat.

Serotonin

Brainstem microinjections of morphine or stimulation with glutamate or electrodes will result in a blockade which is partially antagonized by intrathecally administered serotonin antagonists such as methysergide (Hammond and Yaksh, 1984; Jensen and Yaksh, 1984, 1986; Yaksh, 1979). Iontophoretic application of serotonin onto dorsal horn neurons will result in inhibition and excitation (Headley et al., 1978). Early studies indicated that intrathecally administered serotonin in the rat will increase hot plate and tail flick response latencies (Schmauss et al., 1985; Yaksh and Wilson, 1979). Analogues such as MK-212 and quipazine were also shown to be active. Though not strikingly potent (see Figs. 1 and 2), the effects of i.t. serotonin could be enhanced by the concurrent administration of serotonin uptake blockers such as fluoxethine or by monoamine oxidase inhibitors. Systematic studies using the more selective agonists for the several subclasses of serotonin receptors have not to our knowledge been reported yet.

Novel systems with undefined receptors

In addition to the classes of agents outlined above, a variety of agents, notably peptides, given spinally have been reported to alter nociceptive transmission. Though it is frequently assumed that these agents act at a specific receptor, the absence of selective receptor antagonists or failure to consider the SAR of the intrathecally administered agonists (in comparison to a given 'gold-standard bioassay') permits only preliminary statements as to the characteristics of the site of action. Several representative classes of agents will be discussed below.

1. Neurotensin: this 13-amino-acid peptide occurs in the dorsal horn, where it is located in local interneurons which run longitudinally within the gray matter (Yaksh et al., 1982b). Neurotensin binding has been shown to be elevated in the dorsal horn (Nincovic et al., 1981). This agent has an excitatory effect on dorsal horn neurons (Miletic and Randic, 1979); however, i.t. administration of neurotensin in rats will result in a mild, dose-dependent increase in the nociceptive threshold (Hylden and Wilcox, 1983a; Yaksh et al., 1982b). The mechanism of this effect is not known. Some evidence exists that its effects are antagonized by naloxone, suggesting that it may act to release an endogenous opioid (Yaksh et al., 1982b).

2. Somatostatin: in spinal cord, somatostatin (SST) is found in intrinsic neurons and in small primary afferents (Hokfelt et al., 1976). Given iontophoretically, SST has been shown to have excitatory and inhibitory effects on single units (Nicoll, 1978; Randic and Miletic, 1978). Recent iontophoretic studies have suggested that two subsets of somatostatin receptors may exist which may respectively augment nociceptive activity evoked by thermal nociceptive stimuli and depress nociceptive activity (Fleetwood-Walker et al., 1987). In anesthetized animals, SST given spinally can powerfully modulate spinal reflexes (Wiesenfeld-Hallin, 1985, 1986). In the unanesthetized animal, the current literature is controversial. Though spinal administration of SST has been reported to be analgesic (Ackerman et al., 1985), when assessed with regard to spinal reflexes, these effects appear to occur largely at doses which produce hindlimb dystonia (Gaumann et al., 1987).

Long-term pharmacological effects of receptor activation

One property associated with the action of receptor agonists is that continued exposure of the receptor to the agonist results in a reduction in the physiological response otherwise produced by that agonist, i.e. tolerance. Factors governing the development of tolerance are complex and involve

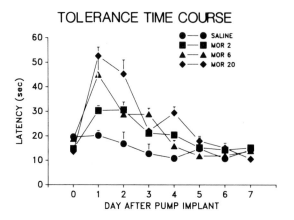

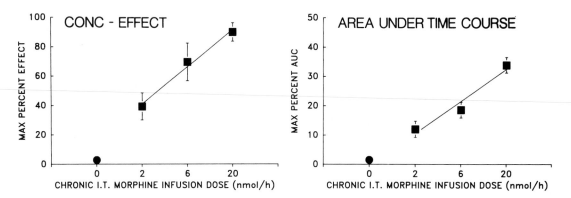

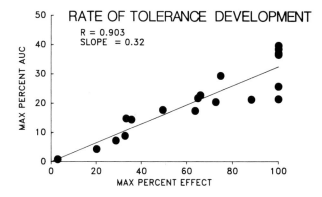

Fig. 3. (Top) Hot plate response latency assessed daily in rats receiving chronic intrathecal infusion of saline or morphine in concentrations of 2, 6 or 20 nmol/μl/h. Each line presents the mean latency from nine animals. (Middle, left) Maximum effect observed on hot plate expressed as percent of maximum possible effect versus infusion concentration. Data derived from top figure. (Middle, right) Area under the tolerance time-course curve expressed as a percent of the maximum possible area under the curve (AUC) versus infusion concentration. Data derived from top figure. (Bottom) Maximum percent AUC is plotted versus the percent of the maximum possible effect. Each point represents a single rat.

behavioral, physiological and biochemical considerations. Several issues which are intuitively relevant are the level of drug exposure and the particular agent employed.

Effects of drug concentration on tolerance development

To avoid the problems associated with periodic peak and trough levels of drug and repeated handling, chronic administration of agents into the spinal space using implantable osmotic pumps has proven of considerable benefit (Yaksh and Stevens, 1986). With this model, rats receive a constant infusion of a given concentration of agents (or vehicle) for seven days. To assess the time course of the loss of the antinociceptive action of drugs, animals are tested on a daily basis. Fig. 3 presents the time course of the changes in hot plate (HP) response latency over a 7-day period. As indicated, there was a concentration-dependent increase in the maximum HP effect (commonly observed on day 1 after implantation). Over the 7-day period, there was a progressive reduction in the antinociceptive actions until, by 3–5 days, the animals displayed baseline response latencies. The progressive decline did not arise from repeated testing, as animals infused but not tested until day 7 showed a similar baseline response latency. The area under the time-course curve (AUC) = (percent of maximum possible effect × days) was calculated and used as an index of the 'rate' of tolerance development. Plotting the maximum possible effect (MPE) vs. the maximum AUC thus permitted an assessment of the rate of tolerance development as a function of the peak effect (which was related to the log of the infusion dose). As shown in Fig. 3, the distribution of these points could be parsimoniously described by a linear function. These results thus suggest that for morphine the rate of tolerance development is independent of infusion concentration.

Experiments similar to those described above have also been employed to characterize the actions of other spinal agents known to alter nociceptive processing.

Table I summarizes the results obtained with μ, δ and α_2-preferring receptor agonists. Several points should be considered. First, the relative potency of these agents delivered by chronic i.t. infusion (as defined by the ED_{50} obtained from plotting the MPE observed on day 1) is similar to that observed following bolus intrathecal dosing. Second, as with morphine, the plots of the MPE vs. AUC curves of these several agents were described by a linear function, and third, the slopes of the MPE vs. AUC curves were identical for all agents thus far examined.

TABLE I

Summary of 'concentration-response' and 'rate of tolerance development' data for opioid and adrenergic agonists administered by chronic infusion in rats (From Stevens and Yaksh (1987)).

Infused agent	Infusion ED_{50}[a] (i.t.) (nmol/μl/rat)	Relative i.t. potency	Slope of MPE vs. AUC curve[b]
Morphine	3.4	1	0.32 (0.25–0.40)[c]
DAGO	0.3	12.1	0.48 (0.37–0.58)
Sufentanil	0.3	13.1	0.42 (0.34–0.51)
DADL	8.2	2.4	0.43 (0.29–0.57)
ST-91	13.0	0.3	0.37 (0.23–0.50)

[a]ED_{50} determined from maximum response observed after the initiation of infusion of drug (usually on 1 day). Each value is based on 3 doses with 6–12 animals/dose.
[b]Plot of MPE vs. AUC derived from infusion data of the time course as displayed in Fig. 3. All drugs showed a distribution which was significantly predicted by a linear regression.
[c]95% confidence interval.

TABLE II

ED_{50} values[a] for morphine, DADL and ST-91 assessed in rats after 7 days of intrathecal morphine infusion (from Stevens and Yaksh, (1986b), Stevens et al. (1988))

Probe drug	Morphine infusion concentration (nmol/μl/h)			
	0 (saline)	2	6	20
Morphine	0.7 (0.3–1.9)[b]	3.1 (0.4–24)	39 (20–73)	83 (49–142)
DADL	0.2 (0.1–3)	0.7 (0.2–2)	0.5 (0.1–2)	5.9 (4–8.6)
ST-91	3.0 (0.9–9.4)	27 (16–47)	39 (19–83)	81 (35–188)

[a]Each dose-response curve is constructed from results measured in 12 to 18 animals.
[b]ED_{50} value (95% confidence interval).

Evaluation of cross-tolerance between different classes of spinally administered receptor-selective agents

Given the similarity between the temporal development of spinal tolerance, it is legitimate to consider whether such receptor systems are actually independent; i.e., is there cross-tolerance? Using the chronic infusion paradigm, we devised an easily constructed 'Y'-catheter which permits external access to the IT catheter without having to expose the animal to a second surgery (Yaksh and Stevens, 1986). Dose-response curves for the selected 'probe drug' were measured 7 days after the initiation of infusion. Rats in these groups were not handled during the intervening infusion. In animals rendered tolerant to chronic infusion of vehicle, 2, 6 or 20 nmol morphine μl/h there was a parallel rightward shift in the dose-response curves for morphine. As indicated in Table II, at the highest infused concentration of morphine, this shift resulted in a 112-fold increase in the morphine ED_{50}. In contrast, at the same morphine infusion concentration, DADL (δ-preferring) and ST-91 (α_2-preferring) showed 30-fold and 27-fold increases in their ED_{50} values, respectively.

To summarize the above issues, these agents, when matched for steady-state peak effects, show the same rate of tolerance development. It thus appears likely that these particular spinal receptor systems show an alteration in function by mechanisms which have the same time courses. Though consistent with the involvement of the same processes, such observations do not prove that such is the case. Significantly, however, these agents are thought to act by suppressing the synthesis of cAMP. In spite of the similarity of the mechanisms, the apparent lack of a symmetric cross-tolerance argues not only that these agents do indeed act at discriminable receptors, but also that the coupling of each receptor to each function is independent for the sites acted upon by these three agents.

Finally, these data also point to the ultimate physiological effect and not to the native efficacy of the drug as the relevant factor. Thus, for example, morphine, DAGO and sufentanil act at the μ receptor and have potency ratios of 1:2:15, respectively, yet all show the same time course of tolerance development.

Interactions between spinal receptor systems

Given that several receptor systems exist within the spinal cord and that these several systems appear to be independent, an important issue relates to the nature of their interactions. It has been hypothesized (Yaksh and Rudy, 1978), and demonstrated (Yeung and Rudy, 1980), that the antinociceptive effects of intraventricular morphine will produce supra-additive effects when given concurrently with spinal morphine. Given the role of adrenergic systems in the bulbospinal inhibition exerted by brainstem opioid receptors, it is plausible that i.t. α receptor agonists might potentiate the effects of i.t. morphine. In rat (Monasky and Yaksh, 1986; Wilcox et al., 1987) and primate (Yaksh and Reddy, 1981) evidence of such a synergy has been demonstrated. Thus, a near maximum analgesic effect may be generated by combinations of α receptor agonists and morphine at doses which alone produce only minimal effects. This synergy reflects the fact that activation of bulbospinal adrenergic inhibition (as activated by morphine) and/or occupation of spinal opioid receptors both result in a reduction of the slope of the stimulus-response curve for dorsal horn wide-dynamic-range neurons (Gebhart et al., 1984; Yaksh, 1978a). For dorsal horn neurons, this decrease in slope would constitute a reduction in the gain of the system. The interaction between two such systems would have a net outcome which might be expressed as the product of the gain reductions and not the sum. The consequence of this would be the ability to produce an adequate physiological effect with a minimum degree of activation of the respective receptors. While the interaction between α-adrenergic and opioid drugs has been most precisely characterized, evidence exists of other spinal synergic interactions such as between baclofen and morphine (Yaksh, 1978b), leucine enkephalin and morphine (Larson et al., 1980), and serotonin and noradrenaline (Minor et al., 1985).

Functional selectivity of spinal receptor-linked systems

In the preceding sections several receptor systems have been identified which, when activated by a respective agonist, can (1) block the excitation of dorsal horn nociceptors evoked by high-threshold stimuli or small primary afferents, and (2) increase the latency of the response evoked by a given high-threshold stimulus, or increase the magnitude of the stimulus required to evoke a given response. These are minimum criteria to establish a drug having analgesic properties. Other effects, however, must be considered. From a theoretical perspective, the con-

cept of analgesia implies a specific alteration in 'pain'-related input. Thus, while an anesthetic produces analgesia, it is not classified as an analgesic. Unfortunately, there has been little systematic effort made to ascertain whether a given spinal drug alters non-nociceptive input.

A second issue of importance, particularly in the animal studies, is whether the observed changes in response latency or frequency are due to an impairment in the ability of the animal to make the response. It is particularly easy to see why absolute dependence upon, for example, the tail flick of withdrawal could lead to misleading results when employed as a single measure of analgesia. While sensitive and easily used, an increase in latency might well be obtained with no change in sensory processing (a fundamental issue in the theoretic construct of analgesia). Thus, inhibition of motor horn outflow, inhibition of interneurons which allow for inhibition between antagonistic muscle groups, and co-activation of motor horn outflow to antagonistic muscle groups could all lead to changes in latency in the absence of alterations in sensory input.

From a practical perspective, the potential clinical use of these agents requires assessment of (1) whether the receptor acted upon by the respective agents is associated with modulating substrates, the function of which is not pain processing, and (2) whether these agents, given in high concentrations in the spinal canal, have any untoward effects on other receptors or on tissue. Table III summarizes, in the rat model, the effects of the several agents on a given nociceptive end-point and the 'therapeutic' ratio with respect to other end-points. Space precludes any extensive description of this information but the following points can be emphasized.

Motor function
In animal studies, μ receptor agonists produce no detectable motor dysfunction at doses in excess of 50-times the analgesic ED_{50}. While high doses of spinal opioids can produce increased truncal rigidity (described as catalepsy), this phenomenon likely results from a supraspinal redistribution of the

agent, as it is commonly observed after intracerebral injection into mesencephalic and medullary sites (see Yaksh and Rudy, 1978). In primates, i.t. morphine or DADL has no effect on motor strength at analgesic doses (Yaksh and Reddy, 1981). U50488H, a κ-ligand, has no effect on motor

TABLE III

Therapeutic ratio intrathecally administered receptor-selective agents in rat

Receptor	ED$_{50}$ (nM)[a]	Therapeutic ratio: observed end point				References
		Motor dysfunction[b]	Bladder dysfunction[c]	Sensory disturbances[d]	Spinal tissue toxicity[e]	
Opioid						
μ: Morphine	5.4 (H)	>50	1 (I)	50 (A)	>100	Brent et al., 1983; Schmauss et al., 1985; Yaksh and Harty, 1987; Yaksh et al., 1986b
Sufentanil	0.3 (H)	>50	1 (I)	>100	>100	Yaksh et al., 1986c; Yaksh and Harty, 1987[i-h]
δ: DPLPE	15 (H)	?[f]	1 (I)	?	?	
DADL	2.3 (H)	21 (W)	1 (I)		>50	Brent et al., 1983; Schmauss et al., 1985
κ: U50488H	20 (V)	>11	>11	>11	?	Brent et al., 1983; Stevens and Yaksh, 1986a[g]
Dynorphin$_{1-13}$	>2 (V)	1 (W)	1 (I)	1 (AN)	1	Stevens and Yaksh, 1986a[g,j]
ε: β-Endorphin	0.05(H)	>5	1 (I)	?	?	Brent et al., 1983; Yaksh and Henry, 1978
Adrenergic						
α_1: Methoxamine	65 (H)	3 (W)	>2	>3	?	Durant, 1987; Howe et al., 1983
α_2: ST-91	2 (H)	48 (W)	50 (I)	>48	>48	Durant, 1987; Howe et al., 1983[i]
Cholinergic						
Carbachol	23	7 (H)	0.4 (I)	?	?	Durant, 1987; Yaksh et al., 1985
GABAergic						
Muscimol	>1 (H)	1 (W)	?	>1	?	Hammond and Drower, 1984
Baclofen	1 (H)	5 (W)	?	>5	?	Wilson and Yaksh, 1978
Purinergic						
LPIA	43 (T)	? (W)	?	?	?	Sawynok et al., 1986
NECA	2 (T)	? (W)	?	?	?	
Serotonin	120 (H)	3 (H)	>6	?	?	Yaksh and Wilson, 1978; Schmauss et al., 1985
Somatostatin	>18 (H)	1 (W)	1 (I)	1 (S,A)	1	Gaumann et al., 1987

[a](H) = hot plate; (T) = tail flick; (V) = visceral chemical response. [b](W) = hindlimb paralysis/weakness and loss of placing and stepping reflex; (H) = hypertonus. [c](I) = inhibition of volume evoked bladder contraction; (H) = hyperactivity. [d](A) = allodynia; (S) = spontaneous pain behavior; (AN) = anesthesia.

[e]Chromatolysis and/or inflammatory response. [f](?) = not examined.

[g]Yaksh, Grabow and Gaumann, unpublished observations; [h]Mjanger and Yaksh, unpublished observations; [i]Yaksh, unpublished observations; [j]Gaumann and Yaksh, in preparation.

function at elevated doses in rats. In contrast, dynorphin$_{1-13}$, a putative endogenous κ ligand, results in a hindlimb paralysis in rats. Significantly, there appears to be little dose differentiation between the putative 'analgesic' effects of dynorphin and its blockade of motor function (Herman and Goldstein, 1985; Kaneko et al., 1983; Przewlocki et al., 1983; Stevens and Yaksh, 1986a). Motor effects produced by δ receptor agonists and dynorphin, unlike the rigidity induced by high doses of μ receptor agonists, appear poorly antagonized by naloxone.

α_1 Receptor agonists result in a hypertonus and athetoid movement of the tail. High doses of α_2 receptor agonists at 50-times their analgesic ED_{50} evoke a reversible waxy paralysis. Davis and colleagues (Astrachan et al., 1983; Davis and Astrachan, 1981) have shown that i.t. α_1 receptor agonists increase while α_2 receptor agonists diminish the motor reflex component of the startle response. Spinal motor neurons are hyperpolarized and a suppression of interneurons in the vicinity of the motor neuron pool has been reported following norepinephrine (Engberg and Ryall, 1966; Jordan et al., 1977; Weight and Salmoriaghi, 1966). Excitation after focal administration has also been observed. This appears to correlate with the observations that norepinephrine, with an action in the ventral horn, can produce a facilitation of C-fiber-evoked ventral root reflexes (Bell and Matsumiya, 1981). The effect on ventral horn activity has not been fully characterized with regard to pharmacology. It appears that the suppressive effects are mediated by an α_2 receptor, whereas the facilitative effects are mediated by an α_1 site.

In man, at therapeutic doses, opiates and α_2 receptor agonists do not obtund normal sensation and do not alter tendon reflexes (Cousins and Mather, 1984; Tamsen and Gordh, 1984). In contrast, baclofen will produce a concentration-dependent flaccidity (Penn and Kroin, 1985).

For GABA receptor agonists (baclofen and muscimol) and adenosine, the analgesic versus motor effects ratio is low. Intrathecal injections of these agents produce at doses less than 5-times the ED_{50}

a prominent weakness and loss of voluntary motor movement.

Sensory disturbances

At analgesic doses, none of the opioids produces any evident effects on the behavior of the animal emitted or evoked in response to non-noxious stimuli. Primates, trained to avoid ear shock cued by a light tactile stimulus applied to the foot, showed no change in the avoidance behavior of the animal (Yaksh and Reddy, 1981). At high concentrations, drugs structurally resembling morphine, having a free 3-OH position, no ether bond and no substitutions on the N-methyl group, yield a prominent hypersensitivity (allodynia). This phenomenon is not naloxone-reversible, does not show tolerance and is produced at relatively low concentrations by 3-OH-SO_4 or 3-glucuronide conjugates of morphine. Agents lacking these structural characteristics (e.g. sufentanil, or 3-methyl morphine) do not display this phenomenon (Yaksh and Harty, 1987; Yaksh et al., 1986b). Though the mechanism is not clear, the phenomenon is not mediated by an opioid receptor and possesses many of the characteristics produced by low doses of glycine or GABA antagonist. Such a phenomenon with high doses of morphine has been reported in man (Stillman et al., 1981).

Intrathecal somatostatin (Seybold et al., 1982; Gaumann and Yaksh, in preparation), in common with a number of the peptides (such as substance P; Hylden and Wilcox, 1983b), has been shown to produce biting and scratching of the flanks and frank vocalization, suggesting a painful stimulus.

Bladder function

Considerable emphasis has been directed at the spinal pharmacology of the volume-evoked micturition reflex (VEMR). In man, spinal opiates will block the reflex in a naloxone-reversible fashion (Rawal et al., 1983). In animal models, Dray and colleagues (1985) have emphasized the role of spinal μ and δ, but not κ receptors in modulating this response. Work in our laboratory using a chronic model (Yaksh et al., 1986a) has examined other neurotransmitter systems and has similarly found that adrenergic, cholinergic and serotonergic agents will produce dose-dependent changes in the VEMR which are antagonized by the respective receptor antagonists (see Table I). Significantly, the pharmacology of the spinal substrate modulating the VEMR is similar to that related to analgesia with the therapeutic ratios frequently approaching 1. Other agents, such as SST, also block the VEMR, but this blockade is frequently irreversible (Gaumann and Yaksh, in preparation), as are the somatic motor effects.

Tissue toxicity

It is clear that receptor-selective agents may potentially exert effects directly upon neural tissue by virtue of the high concentrations achieved when agents are administered spinally. The direct activation of the respective receptor may also set in motion events such as vasoconstriction or massive depolarization which could lead to the demise of the cell. Though systematic examination of all agents has not been accomplished, examination of spinal tissue in rats after high intrathecal doses of a variety of agents such as morphine, sufentanil, DADL or ST-91 revealed that no evidence of tissue toxicity is observed even at concentrations over 50-times that required for analgesia (see Table III). Similar results have been obtained in other species at analgesic concentrations (Gordh et al., 1986; Yaksh and Reddy, 1981; Yaksh et al., 1986). In contrast, agents such as SST have been observed to produce clear evidence of chromatolysis and inflammation following doses at or near those required to produce physiological effects (Gaumann and Yaksh, in preparation). The mechanism of this toxicity is not precisely known, but severe reductions in spinal cord blood flow have been noted (Mollenholdt and Post, personal communication).

Future directions

The current burgeoning of information regarding the pharmacology of the spinal systems which process sensory information suggests major advances in the ability to modulate the encoding process which translates the physical stimulus to one we interpret as a pain event. We would like to conclude with several comments as to future considerations.

Advances in therapeutic methodology

1. Other receptor systems Currently, aside from μ and δ opioid receptors, α_2 receptor agonists have been shown to produce a powerful analgesia by mechanisms readily appreciated on the basis of physiological and pharmacological investigations. We believe that, as our understanding of other receptor systems advances, more such modulating substrates will be defined, such as those acted upon by the purines or the peptides, e.g. somatostatin. Of particular significance will be those receptor systems which do not display cross-tolerance, as they provide the potential for methodical investigation of classes of agents which have the same end-points (altering nociception), but different receptors.

2. Receptor interactions The demonstration that μ opioid and α_2-adrenergic receptors show a synergistic interaction suggests the possibility of producing major physiological consequences with a minimal level of receptor occupancy. We believe these mechanisms reflect on the nature of the physiology of the receptor coupling to the evoked discharge of the cell. This type of interaction is particularly attractive when the two agents synergize in terms of their desired end-points (analgesia) and not of their other actions (respiratory depression and cardiovascular effects). As noted, other interactions also appear probable and emphasis should be put on the systematic assessment of this interaction.

3. Tolerance Though there is controversy about the relevance of tolerance to chronic pain therapy, the phenomenon indeed represents a characteristic of most receptor-mediated agonist effects. While the mechanism of tolerance is not known, several points are evident: (1) changes in either receptor number or coupling appear likely, (2) the degree of tolerance certainly appears proportional to the time of exposure to the given agent, and (3) spinal tolerance appears reversible over time (Yaksh, 1983). Short of determining the cellular mechanisms of tolerance, practical approaches based on current understanding certainly point to the use of alternating drug therapy, using agents which do not show cross-tolerance, allowing a reversal of the tolerance process. Alternatively, with the opioid receptor, there is evidence that a rapid upregulation of opioid receptors can be achieved in the presence of an antagonist (Tempel et al., 1986). Such ploys might serve to reverse the tolerance process more rapidly, while pain management is achieved by alternate means.

4. Pharmacokinetics Single-injection regimens require a long-lasting agent and morphine has thus been eminently suitable. However, it has a relatively slow onset and a long residence time in the CSF, as expected from its hydrophilicity. The use of chronic catheters allows one to decide whether a continuous or intermittent administration protocol might be more useful given (1) that pain may vary from patient to patient and from hour to hour within a given patient and (2) that side-effects and possible tolerance depend upon the presence of drug. It is reasonable to believe that the resensitization to the receptor-selective agent begins in its absence. A regimen allowing the patient to administer drug or not depending upon his pain state would be at least theoretically advantageous. For an efficient coupling of the drug effect to the need, the agent should have a rapid onset, a reasonably fast clearance (several hours vs. 10–20 hours) and no tendency toward peripheral accumulation. Lipid-soluble agents which are rapidly metabolized in the periphery, such as alfentanil, might be considered a theoretical alternative.

Preclinical testing
While the promise of specific manipulations of spinal cord systems is significant, it must be stressed in the strongest terms that the spinal administration of these agents in man must be approached with the greatest degree of caution and concern. We have discussed elsewhere issues related to preclinical studies (Yaksh et al., 1987), but we note the following. Even 'benign' drugs such as peptides can exert potent toxicological effects on spinal tissue. Thus, as discussed above, several agents such as dynorphin and somatostatin can result in paralysis and spinal nucleolysis in rats. In recent studies, similar evidence of somatostatin toxicity has been observed in cats (Gaumann and Yaksh, unpublished observations).

Aside from tissue toxicity, the receptors upon which these agents act are never uniquely associated with pain-processing systems. As noted, many intrathecally injected agents not only affect pain transmission, but block bladder function as well. After supraspinal redistribution (which inevitably occurs, though to varying degrees), untoward effects on other respiratory or cardiovascular systems may be more likely. It is clear that adequate animal studies must be carried out in the appropriate models to determine the physiological profile of the drug effect. If a drug reaching the brainstem has no untoward physiological effects, all well and good. But, if it does, we must be able to anticipate the side-effect and have an adequate pharmacological strategy for management. Thus, while respiratory depression with opiates is an untoward clinical consequence, one can imagine the strictures against spinal opiates were it not for the ability to control opioid effects with selective receptor antagonists. In contrast, a variety of agents currently considered, such as somatostatin, may have no such antagonists.

We thus conclude this paper by pointing to the likely advances in the management of pain which will derive from fundamental studies on the pharmacology and biochemistry of the spinal cord. The local use of receptor-selective agents potentially provides the ability to discretely modulate the complex processing which occurs in the spinal cord. It should be stressed, however, that such agents are potentially as dangerous as they are beneficial and the precise characterization of their effects, both physiological and toxicological, must be achieved in the animal model prior to their use in man.

Acknowledgement

We would like to dedicate this paper to Dr. F.W.L. Kerr, who died August 28, 1983.

References

Ackerman, E., Chrubasik, J., Weinstock, M. and Wunsch, E. (1985) Effect of intrathecal somatostatin of pain threshold in rats. Schmerz Pain Douleur, 2: 41–42.

Anden, N.E., Jukes, M.G.M. and Lundberg, A. (1966) The effect of DOPA on the spinal cord. 2. A pharmacological analysis. Acta Physiol. Scand., 67: 387–397.

Astrachan, D.I., Davis, M. and Gallager, D.W. (1983) Behavior and binding: correlations between α_1-adrenergic stimulation of acoustic startle and α_1-adrenoceptor occupancy and number in rat lumbar spinal cord. Brain Res., 260: 81–90.

Bell, J.A. and Matsumiya, T. (1981) Inhibitory effects of dorsal horn and excitant effects of ventral horn intraspinal microinjections of norepinephrine and serotonin in the cat. Life Sci., 29: 1507–1514.

Bowery, N.G. (1982) Baclofen: 10 years on. Trends Pharmacol. Sci., 3: 400–403.

Brent, C.R., Harty, G. and Yaksh, T.L. (1983) The effects of spinal opiates on micturition in unanesthetized animals. Soc. Neurosci. Abstr., 9: 743.

Burnstock, G. and Buckley, N.J. (1985) The classification of receptors for adenosine and adenine nucleotides. In D.M. Paton (Ed.) Methods Used in Adenosine Research, Methods in Pharmacology, Vol. 6, Plenum Press, New york, pp. 193–212.

Carroll, M.N. and Lim, R.K.S. (1960) Observations on the neuropharmacology of morphine and morphine-like analgesia. Arch. Int. Pharmacodyn. Ther., 125: 383–403.

Castillo, R., Kissin, I. and Bradley, E.L. (1986) Selective kappa opioid agonist for spinal analgesia without the risk of respiratory depression. Anesth. Analg., 65: 350–354.

Chu, G., Cool, M. and Kurtz, N. (1987) Comparison of epidural butorphanol and morphine for control of post-cesarian section pain. Anaesthesist, 388.

Colpaert, F.C., De Witte, P., Maroli, A.N., Awonters, F., Niemegeers, C.J.E. and Janssen, P.A.J. (1980) Self-administration of the analgesic suprofen in arthritic rats: evidence for mycobacterium butyricum-induced arthritis as an experimental model of chronic pain. Life Sci., 27: 921–928.

Coombs, D.W., Saunders, R., Gaylor, M., LaChance, D. and Jensen, L. (1984) Clinical trial of intrathecal clonidine for cancer pain. J. Regional Anesth., 9: 34–35.

Cooper, B.Y. and Vierck, C.J., Jr. (1986) Measurement of pain and morphine hypalgesia in monkeys. Pain, 26: 361–392.

Cousins, M.J. and Mather, L.E. (1984) Intrathecal and epidural administration of opioids. Anesthesiology, 61: 276–310.

D'Amour, F.E. and Smith, D.L. (1941) A method for determining loss of pain sensation. J. Pharmacol. Exp. Ther., 72: 74–79.

Davis, M. and Astrachan, D.I. (1981) Spinal modulation of acoustic startle: opposite effects of clonidine and D-amphetamine. Psychopharmacology (Berlin), 75: 219–225.

Dray, A., Nunan, L. and Wire, W. (1985) Central δ-opioid receptor interactions and the inhibition of reflex urinary bladder contractions in the rat. Br. J. Pharmac., 85: 717–726.

Dubner, R. (1985) Specialization in nociceptive pathways: sensory discrimination, sensory modulation, and neural connectivity. In H.L. Fields, et al. (Eds.), Advances in Pain Research and Therapy, Vol. 9, Raven Press, New York, pp. 111–137.

Dubuisson, D. and Dennis, G. (1977) The formalin test: a quantitative study of the analgesic effects of morphine, meperidine, and brain stem stimulation in rats and cats. Pain, 4: 161–174.

Duggan, A.W., Johnson, S.M. and Morton, C.R. (1981) Differing distributions of receptors for morphine and met^5-enkephalinamide in the dorsal horn of the cat. Brain Res., 229: 379–387.

Durant, P.A.C. (1987) Central and peripheral pharmacology of the urinary bladder in unanesthetized rats. Ph.D. Thesis, Mayo Graduate School of Medicine, Rochester, MN.

Durant, P.A.C. and Yaksh, T.L. (1986) Epidural injections of bupivacaine, morphine, fentanyl, lofentanil, and DADL in chronically implanted rats: a pharmacologic and pathologic study. Anesthesiology, 64: 43–53.

Dykstra, L.A. (1979) Effects of morphine, pentazocine and cyclazocine alone and in combination with naloxone on electric shock titration in the squirrel monkey. J. Pharmacol. Exp. Ther., 211: 722–732.

Eisenach, J.C., Dewan, D.M., Rose, J.C. and Angelo, J.M. (1987) Epidural clonidine produces antinociception, but not hypotension in sheep. Anesthesiology, 66: 496–501.

Engberg, I. and Ryall, R.W. (1966) The inhibitory action of noradrenaline and other monoamines on spinal neurones. J. Physiol., 185: 298–322.

Evans, W.O. (1962) A comparison of the analgesic potency of some analgesics as measured by the 'flinch-jump' procedure. Psychopharmacology (Berlin), 3: 51–54.

Fleetwood-Walker, S.M., Mitchell, R., Hope, P.J., Molony, V. and Iggo, A. (1985) An α_2-receptor mediates the selective inhibition by noradrenaline of nociceptive responses to identified dorsal horn neurones. Brain Res., 334: 243–254.

Fleetwood-Walker, S.M., Mitchell, R., Hope, P.J., El-Yassir, N. and Molony, V. (1987) Dual regulation of spinal nociceptive processing by somatostatin. Pain, Suppl. 4: S410.

Game, C.J.A. and Lodge, D. (1975) The pharmacology of the inhibition of dorsal horn neurones by impulses in myelinated cutaneous afferents in the cat. Exp. Brain Res., 23: 75–84.

Gamse, R., Holzer, P. and Lembeck, F. (1979) Indirect evidence for presynaptic location of opiate receptors in chemosensitive primary sensory neurones. Naunyn-Schmiedberg's Arch. Pharmacol., 308: 281–285.

Gaumann, D., Yaksh, T.L. and Grabow, T. (1988) Intrathecal somatostatin in rats. No margin of safety between analgesic and toxic effects. International Anesthesia Research Society 62 Congress (Abstract), March 1988, San Diego.

Gebhart, G.F., Sandkuhler, J., Thalhammer, J.G. and Zimmerman, M. (1984) Inhibition in spinal cord of nociceptive information by electrical stimulation and morphine microinjection at identical sites in midbrain of the cat. J. Neurophysiol., 51: 75–89.

Go, V.L.W. and Yaksh, T.L. (1987) Release of substance P from the cat spinal cord. J. Physiol., 391: 141–167.

Gordh, T., Post, C. and Olsson, Y. (1986) Evaluation of the toxicity of subarachnoid clonidine, guanfacine and substance P-antagonists on rat spinal cord and nerve roots: light and electron microscopic observations after chronic intrathecal administration. Anesth. Analg., 65: 1301–1311.

Hammond, D.L. and Drower, E.J. (1984) Effects of intrathecally administered THIP, baclofen and muscimol on nociceptive threshold. Eur. J. Pharmacol., 103: 121–125.

Hammond, D.L. and Yaksh, T.L. (1984) Antagonism of stimulation-produced antinociception by intrathecal administration of methysergide or phentolamine. Brain Res., 298: 329–337.

Headley, P.M., Duggan, A.W. and Griersmith, B.T. (1978) Selective reduction by noradrenaline and 5-hydroxytryptamine of nociceptive responses of cat dorsal horn neurones. Brain Res., 145: 185–189.

Hendershot, L.C. and Forsaith, J. (1959) Antagonism of the frequency of phenylquinone-induced writhing in the mouse by weak analgesics and non-analgesics. J. Pharmacol. Exp. Ther., 125: 237–240.

Henry, J.L. (1982) Pharmacological studies on the prolonged depressant effects of baclofen on lumbar dorsal horn units in the cat. Neuropharmacology, 21: 1085–1093.

Herman, B.H. and Golstein, A. (1985) Antinociception and paralysis induced by intrathecal dynorphin A. J. Pharmacol. Exp. Ther., 232: 27–32.

Hokfelt, T., Elde, R., Johansson, O., Luft, R., Nilsson, G. and Arimura, A. (1976) Immunohistochemical evidence for separate populations of somatostatin-containing and substance P-containing primary afferent neurons in the rat. Neuroscience, 1: 131–136.

Hope, P.J., Fleetwood-Walker, S.M. and Mitchell, R. (1987) The antinociceptive actions of opioids on lamina I neurons of the dorsal horn. Pain, Suppl. 4: S409.

Howe, J.R., Wang, J.–Y. and Yaksh, T.L. (1983) Selective antagonism of the antinociceptive effect of intrathecally applied alpha-adrenergic agonists by intrathecal prazosin and intrathecal yohimbine. J. Pharmacol. Exp. Ther., 224: 552–558.

Hylden, J.L.K. and Wilcox, G.L. (1983a) Antinociceptive action of intrathecal neurotensin in mice. Peptides, 4: 517–520.

Hylden, J.L.K. and Wilcox, G.L. (1983b) Pharmacological characterization of substance P-induced nociception in mice: modulation by opioid and noradrenergic agonists at the spinal level. J. Pharmacol. Exp. Ther., 226: 398–404.

Imrie, R.C. (1976) Animal models of arthritis. Lab Anim. Sci., 26: 345–351.

Jensen, T.S. and Yaksh, T.L. (1984) Spinal monoamine and opiate system pathways mediate the antinociceptive effects produced by glutamate at brainstem sites. Brain Res., 321: 287–297.

Jensen, T.S. and Yaksh, T.L. (1986) II. Examination of spinal monoamine receptors through which brain stem opiate-sensitive systems act in the rat. Brain Res., 363: 114–127.

Jessell, T.M. and Iversen, L.L. (1977) Opiate analgesics inhibit substance P release from rat trigeminal nucleus. Nature, 268: 549–551.

Jordan, L.M., McCrea, D.A., Steeves, J.D. and Menzies, J.E. (1977) Noradrenergic synapses and effects of noradrenaline on interneurones in the ventral horn of the cat spinal cord. Can. J. Physiol. Pharmacol., 55: 399–412.

Kaneko, T., Nakazawa, M., Ikeda, M., Yamatsu, K., Iwama, T., Wada, T., Satoh, M. and Takagi, H. (1983) Sites of analgesic action of dynorphin. Life Sci. 33: 661–664.

Krames, E.S., Wilkie, D.J. and Gershow, J. (1986) Intrathecal D-Ala²-D-Leu⁵-enkephalin (DADL) restores analgesia in a patient analgetically tolerant to intrathecal morphine sulfate. Pain, 24: 205–209.

Kuraishi, Y., Harada, Y. and Takagi, H. (1979) Noradrenaline regulation of pain-transmission in the spinal cord mediated by alpha-adrenoceptors. Brain Res., 174: 333–336.

LaMotte, C., Pert, C.B. and Snyder, S.H. (1976) Opiate receptor binding in primate spinal cord: distribution and changes after dorsal root section. Brain Res., 112: 407–412.

Larson, A.A., Vaught, J.L. and Takemori, A.E. (1980) The potentiation of spinal analgesia by leucine enkephalin. Eur. J. Pharmacol., 61: 381–383.

Martin, W.R., Eades, C.G., Thompson, J.A., Huppler, R.E. and Gilbert, P.E. (1976) The effects of morphine- and nalorphine-like drugs in the nondependent and morphine-dependent chronic spinal dog. J. Pharmacol. Exp. Ther., 197: 517–532.

Miletic, V. and Randic, M. (1979) Neurotensin excites cat spinal neurones located in laminae I-III. Brain Res., 169: 600–604.

Minor, B.G., Post, C. and Archer, T. (1985) Blockade of intrathecal 5-hydroxtryptamine-induced antinociception in rats by noradrenaline depletion. Neurosci. Lett., 54: 39–44.

Monasky, M.S. and Yaksh, T.L. (1986) Synergistic interaction of intrathecal morphine and an α_2-agonist (ST-91) on antinociception in the rat. Soc. Neurosci. Abstr., 12: 1016.

Moulin, D., Max, M., Kaiko, R., Inturissi, C., Maggard, J., Yaksh, T.L. and Foley, K.M. (1985) Analgesic efficacy of IT D-Ala²-D-Leu⁵-enkephalin (DADL) in cancer patients with chronic pain. Pain, 23: 213–221.

Myslinski, N.R. and Randic, M. (1977) Responses of identified spinal neurones to acetylcholine applied by micro-electrophoresis. J. Physiol., 269: 195–219.

Ness, T.J. and Gebhart, G.F. (1987) Quantitative comparison of morphine and clonidine effects upon visceral and cutaneous spinal nociceptive transmission in the rat. Pain, Suppl. 4: S409.

Ninkovic, M., Hunt, S.P. and Kelly, J.S. (1981) Effect of dorsal root rhizotomy on the autoradiographic distribution of opiate and neurotensin-like immunoreactivity within the rat spinal cord. Brain Res., 230: 111–119.

Onofrio, B.M. and Yaksh, T.L. (1983) Intrathecal delta-receptor ligand produces analgesia in man. Lancet, i: 1386–1387.

Oyama, T., Toshiro, J.I.N. and Yamaya, R. (1980) Profound analgesic effects of beta-endorphin in man. Lancet, *i*: 122–124.

Parsons, C.G. and Headley, P.M. (1987) Have current concepts of spinal opioid receptor function been influenced by the routes of drug administration used? Pain, Suppl. 4: S397. (See Chapter 19 of this volume.)

Pasternak, G.W., Childers, S.R. and Snyder, S.H. (1980) Opiate analgesia: evidence for mediation by a subpopulation of opiate receptors. Science, 208: 514–516.

Penn, R.D. and Kroin, J.S. (1985) Continuous intrathecal baclofen for severe spasticity. Lancet, i: 125–127.

Post, C. (1984) Antinociceptive effects in mice after intrathecal injection of 5'-*N*-ethylcarboxamide adenosine. Neurosci. Lett., 51: 325–330.

Post, C., Gordh, T., Jr., Jansson, I., Hartvig, P. and Gillberg, P.-G. (1987) Interactions between spinal noradrenergic and cholinergic mechanisms for antinociception. Pain, Suppl. 4: S408.

Przewlocki, B., Shearman, G.T. and Herz, A. (1983) Mixed opioid/non-opioid effects of dynorphin related peptides after intrathecal injection in the rat. Neuropeptides, 3: 233–240.

Randall, L.O. and Selitto, J.J. (1957) A method for measurement of analgesic activity on inflamed tissue. Arch. Int. Pharmacodyn. Ther., 111: 409–419.

Rawal, N., Mollefors, K., Axelsson, K., Lingardh, G. and Widman, B. (1983) An experimental study of urodynamic effects of epidural morphine and of naloxone reversal. Anesth. Analg., 62: 641–647.

Reddy, S.V.R. and Yaksh, T.L. (1980) Spinal noradrenergic terminal system mediates antinociception. Brain Res., 189: 391–401.

Reddy, S.V.R., Maderdrut, J.L. and Yaksh, T.L. (1980) Spinal cord pharmacology of adrenergic agonist-mediated antinociception. J. Pharmacol. Exp. Ther., 213: 525–533.

Russell, R.D., Leslie, J.B., Su, Y.F., Watkins, W.D. and Chang, K.J. (1987) Continuous intrathecal opioid analgesia: tolerance and cross-tolerance of mu and delta spinal opioid receptors. J. Pharmacol. Exp. Ther., 240: 150–158.

Sawynok, J., Sweeney, M.I. and White, T.D. (1986) Classification of adenosine receptors mediating antinociception in the rat spinal cord. Br. J. Pharmac., 88: 923–930.

Schmauss, C. and Yaksh, T.L. (1984) In vivo studies on spinal opiate receptor systems mediating antinociception. II. Pharmacological profiles suggesting a differential association of mu, delta and kappa receptors with visceral chemical and cutaneous thermal stimuli in the rat. J. Pharmacol. Exp. Ther., 228: 1–12.

Schmauss, C., Shimohigashi, Y., Jensen, T.S., Rodbard, D. and Yaksh, T.L. (1985) Studies on spinal opiate receptor pharmacology. III. Analgetic effects of enkephalin dimers as measured by cutaneous thermal and visceral chemical evoked responses. Brain Res., 337: 209–215.

Seybold, V.S., Hylden, J.L.K. and Wilcox, G.L. (1982) Intrathecal substance P and somatostatin in rats: behaviors indicative of sensation. Peptides, 3: 49–54.

Shefner, S.A., North, R.A. and Zukin, R.S. (1981) Opiate effects on rabbit vagus nerve: electrophysiology and radioligand binding. Brain Res., 221: 109–116.

Stevens, C.W. and Yaksh, T.L. (1986a) Dynorphin A and related peptides administered intrathecally in the rat: a search for putative kappa opiate receptor activity. J. Pharmacol. Exp. Ther., 238: 833–838.

Stevens, C.W. and Yaksh, T.L. (1986b) Studies of opiate tolerance in spinal catheterized rats. Soc. Neurosci. Abstr. 12: 618.

Stevens, C.W. and Yaksh, T.L. (1987) Time course of tolerance development to antinociceptive agents in rat spinal cord. Soc. Neurosci. Abstr. 13: 917.

Stevens, C.W., Pezalla, P.D. and Yaksh, T.L. (1987) Spinal antinociceptive action of three representative opioid peptides in frogs. Brain Res., 402: 201–203.

Stevens, C.W., Monasky, M.S. and Yaksh, T.L. (1988) Spinal infusion of opiate and α_2-agonists in rats: tolerance and cross-tolerance studies. J. Pharmacol. Exp. Ther. 244: in press.

Tamsen, A. and Gordh, T. (1984) Epidural clonidine produces analgesia. Lancet, i: 231–232.

Tang, A.H. and Schoenfeld, M.J. (1978) Comparison of subcutaneous and spinal subarachnoid injections of morphine and naloxone in analgesic tests in the rat. Eur. J. Pharmacol., 52: 215–223.

Tempel, A., Crain, S.M., Peterson, E.R., Simon, E.J. and Zukin, R.S. (1986) Antagonist-induced opiate receptor upregulation in cultures of fetal mouse spinal cord-ganglion explants. Dev. Brain Res., 25: 287–291.

Tseng, L.-F. (1982) Tolerance and cross tolerance to morphine after chronic spinal D-Ala^2-D-Leu^5-enkephalin infusion. Life Sci., 31: 987–992.

Tung, A.S. and Yaksh, T.L. (1982) In vivo evidence for multiple opiate receptors mediating analgesia in the rat spinal cord. Brain Res., 247: 75–83.

Van de Hoogen, R.H.W.M. and Colpaert, F.C. (1981) Long term catheterization of the lumbar epidural space in rats. Pharmacol. Biochem. Behav., 15: 515–516.

Wamsley, J.K., Lewis, M.S., Young, W.S., III and Kuhar, M.J. (1981) Autoradiographic localization of muscarinic cholinergic receptors in rat brainstem. J. Neurosci., 1: 176–191.

Wang, J.J., Chan, K.H., Lee, T.Y. and Mok, M.S. (1985) Epidural nalbuphine hydrochloride in painless labour. Ma Tsui Hsueh Tsa Chi, 23: 3–11.

Ward, S.J., Portoghese, P.S. and Takemori, A.E. (1982) Pharmacological characterization in vivo of the novel opiate, β-funaltrexamine. J. Pharmacol. Exp. Ther., 220: 494–498.

Weight, F.F. and Salmoiraghi, G.C. (1966) Responses of spinal cord interneurons to acetylcholine, norepinephrine and serotonin administered by microelectrophoresis. J. Pharmacol. Exp. Ther., 153: 420–427.

Weintraub, S.J. and Naulty, J.S. (1985) Acute abstinence syndrome after epidural injection of butorphanol. Anesth. Analg., 64: 452–453.

Wiesenfeld-Hallin, Z. (1985) Intrathecal somatostatin modulates spinal sensory and reflex mechanisms: behavioral and electrophysiological studies in the rat. Neurosci. Lett., 62: 69–74.

Wiesenfeld-Hallin, Z. (1986) Substance P and somatostatin modulate spinal cord excitability via physiologically different sensory pathways. Brain Res., 372: 172–175.

Wilcox, G., Carlsson, K.H., Jochim, A. and Jurna, I. (1987) Mutual potentiation of antinociceptive effects of morphine and clonidine on motor and sensory responses in rat spinal cord. Brain Res., 405: 84–93.

Williams, J. and Zieglgansberger, W. (1981) Mature spinal ganglion cells are not sensitive to opiate-receptor mediated actions. Neurosci. Lett., 21: 211–216.

Wilson, P.R. and Yaksh, T.L. (1978) Baclofen is antinociceptive in the spinal intrathecal space of animals. Eur. J. Pharmacol., 51: 323–330.

Wood, P.L., Rackham, A. and Richard, J. (1981) Spinal analgesia: comparison of the mu agonist morphine and the kappa agonist ethylketazocine. Life Sci., 28: 2119–2125.

Woolfe, G. and MacDonald, A.D. (1944) The evaluation of the analgesic action of pethidine hydrochloride (Demerol). J. Pharmacol. Exp. Ther., 80: 300–307.

Yaksh, T.L. (1978a) Inhibition by etorphine of the discharge of dorsal horn neurons: effects upon the neuronal response to both high- and low-threshold sensory input in the decerebrate spinal cat. Exp. Neurol., 60: 23–40.

Yaksh, T.L. (1978b) The synergistic interaction of three pharmacologically distinct spinal systems mediating antinociception: the intrathecal action of morphine, serotonin and baclofen. Soc. Neurosci. Abstr. 4.

Yaksh, T.L. (1979) Direct evidence that spinal serotonin and noradrenaline terminals mediate the spinal antinociceptive effects of morphine in the periaqueductal gray. Brain Res., 160: 180–185.

Yaksh, T.L. (1981) Spinal opiate analgesia: Characteristics and principles of action. Pain, 11: 293–346.

Yaksh, T.L. (1983) In vivo studies on spinal opiate receptor systems mediating antinociception. I. Mu and delta receptor profiles in the primate. J. Pharmacol. Exp. Ther., 226: 303–316.

Yaksh, T.L. (1985) Pharmacology of spinal adrenergic systems which modulate spinal nociceptive processing. Pharmacol. Biochem. Behav., 22: 845–858.

Yaksh, T.L. and Harty, G.J. (1988) The pharmacology of the allodynia in rats evoked by high dose intrathecal morphine. J. Pharmacol. Exp. Ther., in press.

Yaksh, T.L. and Henry, J.L. (1978) Antinociceptive effects of intrathecally administered human β-endorphin in the rat and cat. Can. J. Physiol. Pharmacol., 56: 754–760.

Yaksh, T.L. and Noueihed, R. (1985) The physiology and pharmacology of spinal opiates. Annu. Rev. Pharmacol. Toxicol., 25: 433–462.

Yaksh, T.L. and Reddy, S.V.R. (1981) Studies in the primate on the analgetic effects associated with intrathecal actions of opiates, α-adrenergic agonists and baclofen. Anesthesiology, 54: 451–467.

Yaksh, T.L. and Rudy, T.A. (1976a) Chronic catheterization of the spinal subarachnoid space. Physiol. Behav., 17: 1031–1036.

Yaksh, T.L. and Rudy, T.A. (1976b) Analgesia mediated by a direct spinal action of narcotics. Science, 192: 1357–1358.

Yaksh, T.L. and Rudy, T.A. (1977) Studies on the direct spinal action of narcotics in the production of analgesia in the rat. J. Pharmacol. Exp. Ther., 202: 411–428.

Yaksh, T.L. and Rudy, T.A. (1978) Narcotic analgesics: CNS sites and mechanisms of action as revealed by intracerebral injection techniques. Pain, 4: 299–359.

Yaksh, T.L. and Stevens, C.W. (1986) Simple catheter preparation for permitting bolus intrathecal administration during chronic intrathecal infusion. Pharm. Biochem. Behav., 25: 483–485.

Yaksh, T.L. and Wilson, P.R. (1979) Spinal serotonin terminal system mediates antinociception. J. Pharmacol. Exp. Ther., 208: 446–453.

Yaksh, T.L. Frederickson, R.C.A., Huang, S.P. and Rudy, T.A. (1978) In vivo comparison of the receptor populations acted upon in the spinal cord by morphine and pentapeptides in the production of analgesia. Brain Res., 148: 516–520.

Yaksh, T.L., Jessell, T.M., Gamse, R., Mudge, A.W. and Leeman, S.E. (1980) Intrathecal morphine inhibits substance P release from mammalian spinal cord in vivo. Nature, 286: 155–156.

Yaksh, T.L., Gross, K.E. and Li, C.H. (1982a) Studies on the intrathecal effect of β-endorphin in primate. Brain Res., 241: 261–269.

Yaksh, T.L., Schmauss, C., Micevych, P.E., Abay, E.O. and Go, V.L.W. (1982b) Pharmacological studies on the application, disposition and release of neurotensin in the spinal cord. Ann. N.Y. Acad. Sci., 400: 228–242.

Yaksh, T.L., Dirksen, R. and Harty, G.J. (1985) Antinociceptive effects of intrathecally injected cholinomimetic drugs in the rat and cat. Eur. J. Pharmacol., 117: 81–88.

Yaksh, T.L., Noueihed, R.Y. and Durant, P.A.C. (1986) Studies of the pharmacology and pathology of intrathecally administered 4-anilinopiperidine analogues and morphine in rat and cat. Anesthesiology, 64: 54–66.

Yaksh, T.L., Durant, P.A.C. and Brent, C.R. (1986a) Micturition in rats: a chronic model for study of bladder function and effect of anesthetics. Am. J. Physiol., 251 (Reg. Integ. Comp. Physiol., 20): R1177–R1185.

Yaksh, T.L., Harty, G.J. and Onofrio, B.M. (1986b) High doses of spinal morphine produce a nonopiate receptor-mediated hyperesthesia: clinical and theoretic implications. Anethesiology, 64: 590–597.

Yaksh, T.L., Durant, P.A.C., Gaumann, D.M., Stevens, C.W. and Mjanger, E. (1987) The use of receptor-selective agents as analgesics in the spinal cord: trends and possibilities. J. Pain Sympt. Manag., 2: 129–138.

Yeung, J.C. and Rudy, T.A. (1980) Multiplicative interaction between narcotic agonisms expressed at spinal and supraspinal sites of antinociceptive action as revealed by concurrent intrathecal and intracerebroventricular injections of morphine. J. Pharmacol. Exp. Ther., 215: 663–642.

Zieglgansberger, W. and Bayerl, H. (1976) The mechanisms of inhibition of neuronal activity by opiates in the spinal cord of the cat. Brain Res., 115: 111–128.

R. Dubner, G.F. Gebhart & M.R. Bond (Eds.)
Proceedings of the Vth World Congress on Pain
© 1988 Elsevier Science Publishers BV (Biomedical Division)

CHAPTER 48

High-resolution autoradiography of opioid receptors and enkephalinase in the rat spinal cord

Jean-Marie Zajac[a]*, Marc Peschanski[b], Jean-Marie Besson[b] and Bernard P. Roques[a]

[a]*INSERM U 266, CNRS UA 498, 4 rue de l'Observatoire, 75006 Paris and* [b]*INSERM U 161, 2 rue d'Alésia, 75014 Paris, France*

Summary

The distribution of μ and δ opioid binding sites and of neutral endopeptidase (enkephalinase) has been studied in adjacent sections of the rat spinal cord by using highly selective ligands ([^{3}H]DAGO, [^{3}H]DTLET and [^{3}H]HACBO-Gly). Emulsion-coated coverslips were used for autoradiographic localization of the probes. All three ligands were located in the substantia gelatinosa at all levels of the spinal cord. In the medial portion of lamina V and in the motoneuronal area, only [^{3}H]DAGO binding occurred. Likewise, only [^{3}H]HACBO-Gly (an inhibitor of enkephalinase) bound to sites located in the intermediolateral column in the sacral spinal cord and in the peripheral portions of both dorsal and ventral roots. These results are discussed with regard to possible differential roles of opioids in the spinal cord.

Introduction

Numerous studies have demonstrated that opioid peptides can act on spinal sensory processing and, in particular, possess antinociceptive actions (see

Refs. in Yaksh, 1984 and Yaksh and Noueihed, 1985). Micro-iontophoretic injections of morphine into the dorsal horn as well as systemic administration of opioids significantly decrease the neuronal activity evoked in spinal dorsal horn nociceptive neurons by Aδ and C-fiber activation of peripheral nerves (see Refs. in Le Bars and Besson, 1981). This is in accordance with the presence of all three types of opioid receptors (μ, δ and κ) in the spinal cord (see Refs. in Gouarderes et al., 1985). Relevant to these findings, potent inhibitors of enkephalin-degrading enzymes such as kelatorphan produce a significant inhibition of nociceptive neurons when injected iontophoretically into the substantia gelatinosa or intrathecally (Morton et al., 1987; Dickenson et al., 1987).

It remains, however, to be determined whether opiate receptors and enkephalin-degrading enzymes are part of the same functional system. In order to provide the first clue to this problem, we have analysed the distribution of the neutral endopeptidase (enkephalinase) and opioid-binding sites in the spinal cord by using selective ligands developed for μ and δ opiate receptors and for the neutral endopeptidase (Handa et al., 1981; Zajac et al., 1983; Waksman, 1986). A high resolution autoradiographic technique, based upon the use of emulsion-coated coverslips, allowed us to compare precisely, at the light microscopic level, the distribution of all three markers within the spinal cord.

---

*To whom correspondence should be addressed.

Experimental procedures

Male Sprague-Dawley albino rats (150–200 g) were killed by decapitation and their spinal cord rapidly removed. The spinal cord was divided into several segments a few mm long and frozen in isopentane ($-40°C$). Frontal sections (10 μm thick) were cut on a cryostat ($-20°C$), thaw-mounted onto gelatinized slides and kept at $-80°C$. Three sets of adjacent sections were prepared for further incubation with one of the three ligands.

The sections were brought back to room temperature, then incubated in 50 mM Tris-HCl buffer (pH 7.4) at 25°C for 60 min with one of three ligands: DAGO, DTLET or HACBO-Gly. [³H]DAGO (Tyr-D-Ala-Gly-(Me)Phe-Gly-ol) (1.59 TBq/mmol, CEA Saclay) was used at a final concentration of 3 nM to label μ sites. [³H]DTLET (Tyr-D-Thr-Gly-Phe-Leu-Thr) (2.1 TBq/mmol, CEA Saclay) was used at a final concentration of 3 nM to label δ sites. For these two ligands, the non-specific binding was evaluated in the same conditions in the presence of 10^{-6} M levorphanol (Hoffman-LaRoche). [³H]HACBO-Gly (N-[2RS)-3-hydroxyaminocarboxyl-2-benzyl-1-oxopropyl]-glycine) (1.1 TBq/mmol, CEA Saclay) was used at a concentration of 3 nM. In this case, the non-specific binding was assessed in the presence of 10^{-6} M thiorphan.

At the end of incubation, slides were transferred sequentially through two rinses (10 min each) in the incubation buffer at 4°C and then air-dried.

Emulsion-coated coverslips were prepared by dipping into a 1:1 aqueous solution of Ilford K_5. Coverslips were allowed to dry for at least 24 h, then apposed firmly to sections, either glued at one end to the slides or left unglued. Exposure time in the dark at 4°C was 3 months. At the end of the exposure coverslips not glued to the slides were separated from the slides and the autoradiograms revealed using standard autoradiographic techniques with Kodak D 19b as a developer. Coverslips were subsequently mounted onto clean glass slides, the autoradiograms facing the slides. In parallel, sections were Nissl-stained with Cresyl violet, dehydrated and mounted with Permount. When cover-

slips had been glued to the slides, all steps (autoradiographic techniques and Nissl-staining) were performed in sequence, the unglued end of the coverslip being separated from the slide by inserting a pin between them.

For unglued coverslips, autoradiograms were observed with relatively low magnification lenses (up to 25 ×) using both bright and dark-field illuminations and the labelling was drawn using a camera lucida drawing tube and/or photographed. The labelling was subsequently compared to that of the companion Nissl-stained section, using various landmarks (blood vessels, central canal, etc.). In the cases of glued coverslips, the arrangements of silver grains with regards to neurons was studied using high magnification lenses. It should be noted, however, that this latter analysis required focussing on two different planes of section, which limited the resolution to about 10–15 μm instead of the 2–3 μm theoretically permitted by the energy of the β emission of tritium.

Results

Labelling obtained with all three ligands was visible in the substantia gelatinosa along the whole rostro-caudal extent of the spinal cord, including the spinal trigeminal subnucleus caudalis. Additional specific sites of labelling were observed with DAGO and HACBO-Gly.

Substantia gelatinosa
For all ligands the highest density of labelling was observed at the level of the superficial layer II (substantia gelatinosa) of the dorsal horn (Fig. 1). The grain density fell sharply on both sides of this layer and, in particular, the grain density in layer III did not differ significantly from that observed in the white matter. Despite the absence of a strict quantitative analysis, the autoradiograms show clearly that there are more μ than δ receptor-binding sites in this area (Fig. 2). High power photomicrographs (Fig. 3) show that the labelling by DAGO is relatively even in the substantia gelatinosa. For all li-

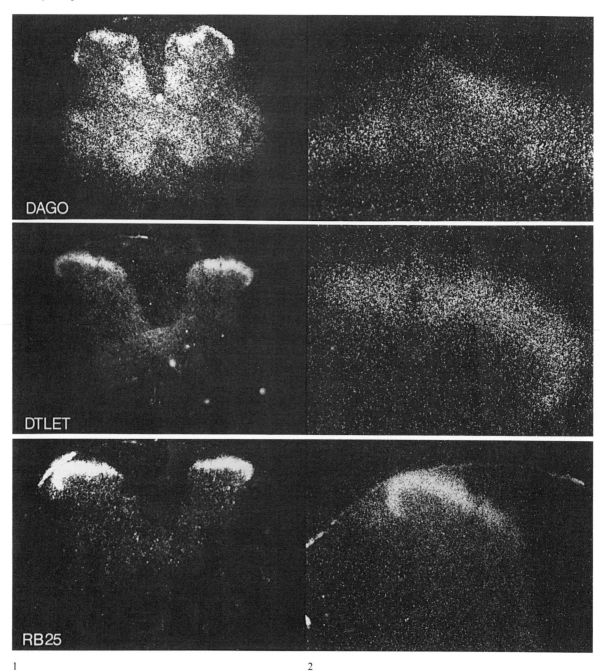

1   2

Fig. 1. Low power darkfield photomicrographs of autoradiograms from the labelling obtained at the lumbar level of the spinal cord with tritiated ligands (DAGO, μ binding sites; DTLET, δ binding sites; RB 25 (HACBO-Gly) neutral endopeptidase).

Fig. 2. Higher power darkfield photomicrographs of autoradiograms at the same level showing the labelling observed in the substantia gelatinosa.

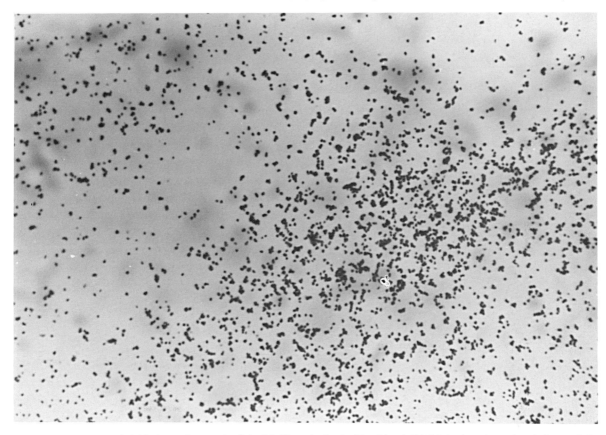

Fig. 3. High power brightfield photomicrograph of the labelling obtained with tritiated DAGO in the substantia gelatinosa of the lumbar spinal cord. The coverslip has been glued to the slide, allowing the Nissl-stained cells to appear in the background of the picture, the focus being at the level of the silver grains.

gands, there was no obvious difference between the grain density in the substantia gelatinosa along the rostro-caudal extent of the cord, including the spinal trigeminal subnucleus caudalis.

Other sites
While the labelling obtained with [³H]DTLET was essentially limited to the substantia gelatinosa, μ receptor-binding sites revealed by binding of [³H]DAGO were additionally observed in the ventromedial portion of the dorsal horn and in the medial group of motoneurons. The grain density in both of these areas was lower than in the substantia gelatinosa, but significantly higher than in the surrounding grey matter (Fig. 1). Though not directly relevant to our study, it is interesting to note that μ receptor-binding sites were also observed in the dorsal col-

umn nuclei at the level of the obex.

The neutral endopeptidase was revealed by binding of [³H]HACBO-Gly in two different zones: an area extending from the central canal to the intermediolateral cell columns in the sacral spinal cord and the peripheral portions of both ventral and dorsal roots (Fig. 4). In the latter situation, the clear-cut delineation of the labelled roots at the level of entry into the central nervous system was striking.

Discussion

The present study, performed with highly selective μ and δ receptor agonists and high resolution autoradiography, confirms the presence of opioid-bind-

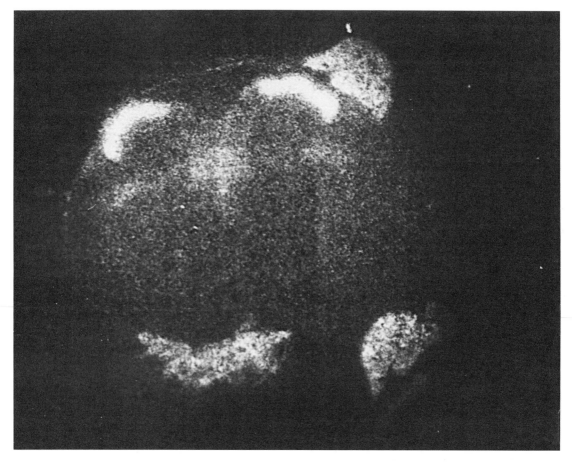

Fig. 4. Low power darkfield photomicrograph of an autoradiogram from the labelling obtained at the level of the sacral spinal cord using tritiated HACBO-Gly. In addition to the substantia gelatinosa, note the labelling in both dorsal and ventral roots and in lamina X and the intermediolateral column cell groups.

ing sites in the substantia gelatinosa (Gouarderes et al., 1985; Waksman et al., 1986). These results correspond well with those obtained in previous studies of the distribution of opioid-binding sites by using ligands which either did not discriminate between opioid receptor types (Atweh and Kuhar, 1977) or presented a relatively low selectivity for δ sites (Herkenham and Pert, 1982); moreover, the precise distribution of enkephalinase in the substantia gelatinosa reported here is in agreement with the previous mapping of neutral endopeptidase (Waksman et al., 1986; Zajac et al., 1987). Since the substantia gelatinosa is also the major spinal location of enkephalins (Hökfelt et al., 1977; Glazer and Basbaum, 1981; Ruda et al., 1984), our results

seem to indicate that the assumed endogenous opioid effector and its metabolizing enzyme are topographically associated. It is therefore very tempting to consider that they may be part of a common functional system, playing most likely a role in nociception and morphine-induced analgesia.

It should be noted, however, that the functional actions of enkephalins are classically associated with their binding to δ receptors, and this type of receptor was obviously less dense in the substantia gelatinosa than the μ type. The difference in density was not due to the difference in the occupancy of sites by the tritiated ligands (DTLET 69.7% versus DAGO 43.4%). It was not due either to the difference in specific radioactivity since [^{3}H]DTLET was more active than [³H]DAGO. It reveals, therefore, a genuine high ratio of μ/δ-binding sites in the substantia gelatinosa. The relevance of this finding for the functional role of enkephalins in pain transmission at the spinal level has yet to be demonstrated.

An interesting finding of these studies is the presence of other localizations of μ-binding sites and enkephalinase in the spinal cord. First, it was observed that μ-binding sites and enkephalinase could be observed independently in various areas of the spinal cord. The comparison of these data with those concerning the location of enkephalin-like immunoreactivity indicates some differences, but this issue is beyond the scope of this study. It is interesting to note that μ receptor-binding sites are present in two areas (lamina V and motoneurons) which contain neurons involved in various aspects of sensory-motor integration. The enkephalinase was found in areas related to vegetative functions as well as in peripheral nerves, most likely in Schwann cells as previously suggested by Matsas et al., (1986).

In conclusion, the comparison of μ and δ opioid receptor-binding sites with the distribution of a neutral endopeptidase in the spinal cord revealed that all three can be part, together with endogenous enkephalins, of a common functional system, possibly participating in nociception and opiate analgesia in the substantia gelatinosa. In parallel, μ opioid receptors on the one hand and the enkephalin-degrading enzyme on the other can be involved in other systems, possibly not directly related to pain transmission.

References

Atweh, S.F. and Kuhar, M.J. (1977) Brain Res., 124:53–67.

Dickenson, A.H. and Sullivan, A.F. (1986) Pain, 24:211–222.

Dickenson, A.H., Sullivan, A.F., Knox, R., Zajac, J.M. and Roques, B.P. (1987) Brain Res., 413:36–44.

Dickenson, A.H., Sullivan, A.F., Fournié-Zaluski, M.C. and Roques, B.P. (1987) Brain Res., 402:185–191.

Glazer, E.J. and Basbaum, A.I. (1981) J. Comp. Neurol., 196:377–389.

Gouarderes, C., Cros, J. and Quirion, R. (1985) Neuropeptides, 6:331–342.

Handa, B.K., Lane, A.C., Lord, J.A.H., Morgan, B.A., Rance, M.J. and Smith, C.F.C. (1981) Eur. J. Pharmacol., 70:531–540.

Herkenham, H. and Pert, C. (1982) Proc. Natl. Acad. Sci. USA, 77:5531–5532.

Hökfelt, T., Ljungdahl, A. Terenius, L., Elde, R. and Nilson, G. (1977) Proc. Natl. Acad. Sci. USA, 74:3031–3085.

Le Bars, D. and Besson, J.M. (1981) Trends Pharmacol. Sci., 2:323–325.

Matsas, R., Kenny, A.J. and Turner, A.J. (1986) Neuroscience, 18:991–1012.

Morton, C.R., Zhao, Z.Q. and Duggan, A.W. (1987) Eur. J. Pharmacol., 140: 195–201.

Ruda, M.A., Coffield, J. and Dubner, R. (1984) J. Neurosci., 4:2117–2132.

Waksman, G., Hamel, E., Fournié-Zaluski, M.C. and Roques, B.P. (1986) Proc. Natl. Acad. Sci. USA, 83:1523–1527.

Yaksh, T.L. (1984) Adv. Pain Res. Ther., 6:197–215.

Yaksh, T.L. and Noueihed, R. (1985) Ann. Rev. Pharmacol. Toxicol., 25:433–465.

Zajac, J.M., Charnay, Y., Soleilhac, J.M., Salès, N. and Roques, B.P. (1987) FEBS Lett., 216:118–122.

Zajac, J.M., Gacel, G., Petit, F., Dodey, P., Rossignol, P. and Roques, B.P. (1983) Biochem. Biophys. Res. Commun., 111:390–397.

R. Dubner, G.F. Gebhart & M.R. Bond (Eds.)
Proceedings of the Vth World Congress on Pain
© 1988 Elsevier Science Publishers BV (Biomedical Division)

CHAPTER 49

Inhibition of visceral and cutaneous spinal nociceptive transmission by morphine and clonidine: differential effects on intensity coding

T.J. Ness and G.F. Gebhart

Department of Pharmacology, University of Iowa College of Medicine, Iowa City, IA 52242, USA

Summary

Morphine and clonidine produced dose-dependent inhibition of spinal nociceptive transmission (both visceral and cutaneous) in spinalized rats and produced different effects upon nociceptive intensity coding. Whereas morphine produced only a small increase in the sensory threshold for neuronal response and significantly attenuated the gain of the response, clonidine had little effect upon the gain of the response, but significantly increased the threshold for neuronal response. Clonidine affected both cutaneous and visceral nociceptive transmission with roughly equal potency and was more potent than morphine. Morphine was more potent at inhibiting visceral as opposed to cutaneous nociceptive transmission. These findings indicate that clonidine and morphine, in addition to acting at different receptors, influence spinal nociceptive transmission in parametrically different ways.

Introduction

Morphine and clonidine have been increasingly employed spinally for the control of pain (Yaksh,

1981, 1986). Both opioid and α-adrenergic receptor agonists have been demonstrated electrophysiologically to produce dose-dependent inhibition of cutaneous spinal nociceptive transmission (e.g., Fleetwood-Walker et al., 1985; Wilcockson et al., 1986), but the effects of such drugs on the intensity coding of spinal nociceptive neurons have been largely ignored. Likewise, drug effects on visceral spinal nociceptive transmission have not been examined.

Distension of hollow organs such as the gall bladder or the distal colon has long been known to produce pain in man in pathological states (e.g., Bynum, 1983; Mankin and Adams, 1983) and in clinical experiments using inflatable balloons (e.g., Lipkin and Sleisinger, 1958; Ritchie, 1973). Recent work has demonstrated that balloon distension of the descending colon and rectum of the rat is a reproducible, easily controlled noxious visceral stimulus which produces avoidance behavior (i.e., is aversive; Ness and Gebhart, 1988), evokes vigorous Sherringtonian 'pseudaffective' cardiovascular and visceromotor reflexes (Ness and Gebhart, 1988) and produces stable, graded, neuronal responses in the T13–L2 and L6–S1 spinal segments (Ness and Gebhart, 1987a,c). Neurons excited by colorectal distension encode for the intensity of this noxious visceral stimulus in a monotonic, accelerating fashion that is similar to the intensity coding characteristic of spinal neurons excited by graded noxious

Correspondence: G.F. Gebhart, Dept. of Pharmacology, University of Iowa College of Medicine, Iowa City, IA 52242, U.S.A.

heating of the skin (e.g., Carstens et al., 1980; Gebhart et al., 1984; Price and Browe, 1975) and which can be described by linear stimulus-response functions (SRFs) relating the intensity of the visceral or cutaneous stimulus to the neuronal response. This coding of stimulus intensity is one of the presumed mechanisms whereby humans can perceive gradations of nociceptive stimuli. Electrical stimulation in brain sites implicated in endogenous opioid and α-adrenergic inhibition of spinal nociceptive transmission has produced differential effects upon the intensity coding of spinal nociceptive neurons (Carstens et al., 1980; Gebhart et al., 1984; Ness and Gebhart, 1987b). The two main types of inhibitory modification of the intensity coding of nociceptive neurons are: (1) a change in the minimal threshold for response demonstrable as a parallel rightward shift of characteristic SRFs; and (2) a change in the gain of the intensity coding, demonstrable as a decrease in the slope of characteristic SRFs. In the former, low-intensity stimuli are no longer effective and responses to high-intensity stimuli are also significantly reduced. In the latter, responses to low-intensity stimuli are unchanged but responses to high-intensity noxious stimuli are greatly reduced.

The present study evaluated and compared the effects of morphine and clonidine upon the intensity coding of spinal neurons excited by either graded colorectal distension (visceral nociceptive transmission) or graded radiant heating of the skin (cutaneous nociceptive transmission). In this way, similarities or differences in spinal α2-adrenergic and opioid receptor-mediated effects on the transmission of qualitatively different pains were evaluated.

Methods

Male Sprague-Dawley rats, 350–470 g, were initially anesthetized deeply with sodium pentobarbital (45–50 mg/kg i.p.). Femoral arterial and venous and tracheal cannulae were inserted and the cervical spinal cord was fully transected, followed by mechanical decerebration with forceps. The rats were artificially respired with room air for the re-

mainder of the experiment. The lower thoracic and/ or lumbar spinal cord was exposed by laminectomy and the rat was suspended from thoracic vertebral and ischial clamps. The dura mater was cut and skin flaps were arranged to form a pool for agar to stabilize the spinal cord and allow formation of a protective bath of warm paraffin oil. Rats were allowed to recover for 4–10 h after transection of the spinal cord, at which time all demonstrated reflex flexion responses. Pancuronium bromide was then administered (0.5 mg i.v. initially; 0.3 mg/h i.v. maintenance) to block reflex motor responses. Tungsten microelectrodes were used for single-unit recording of spinal neurons. Colorectal distension was produced by air inflation of a 7–8-cm-long, pressure-monitored, flexible latex balloon inserted via the anus into the descending colon and rectum. The diameter of the balloon when inflated was greater than that of the distended gut so that the air pressure within the balloon was an accurate measure of the intraluminal distending pressure. Heating of the plantar surface of the hindfoot was accomplished by a projector lamp with electronic feedback control from a thermistor placed upon the skin. To quantify neuronal responses to either colorectal distension or heating, units were discriminated conventionally from background, digitized, counted in 1 s bins and saved on computer. The total number of unit discharges during a 20 or 40 s interval starting with the onset of colorectal distension or heating was counted. Unit responses were considered reliable when control responses varied <10% on three consecutive trials. All trials were spaced 4 min apart. Graded stimuli (20–100 mmHg, 20 s colorectal distension, or 44–52°C, 15 s heating) were applied after a reliable response had been established. Cumulative doses of morphine (0.25–16.0 mg/kg i.v.) or clonidine (25–400 μg/kg i.a.), spaced 8 min apart, were administered until the neuronal response to either an 80 mmHg, 20 s colorectal distension or a 48°C, 15 s heat stimulus was inhibited to half of the control value. Graded stimuli were then again administered. Naloxone HCl (3 mg/kg i.v.), phentolamine HCl (10 mg/kg i.v.) or yohimbine HCl (2 mg/kg i.v.) were used to antagonize the ef-

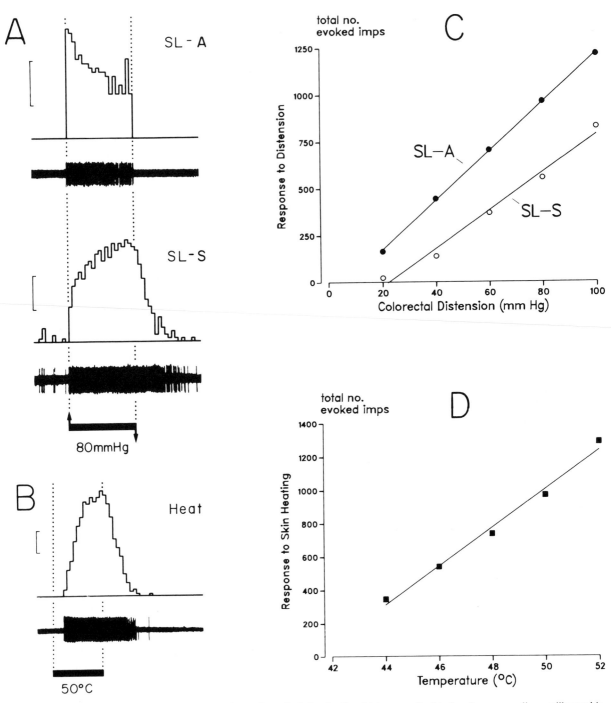

Fig. 1. Examples of neuronal responses to distension or heat. Peristimulus time histograms (1 s bins) and corresponding oscillographic tracings in A for typical SL-A and SL-S neurons excited by colorectal distension (80 mmHg, 20 s) and, in B, for a Class 3 neuron excited by heating of the plantar surface of the hindfoot (50°C, 15 s). The responses of SL-A and SL-S neurons to graded colorectal distension are characterizable by linear stimulus-response functions (SRFs, examples in C), as are the responses of neurons excited by graded heating of the hindfoot (example in D). Vertical calibrations in A and B = 20 Hz.

fects of morphine and clonidine. At the end of the experiment, rats were killed by an i.v. overdose of pentobarbital, and electrolytic lesions were made at the recording site for subsequent conventional histological localization. Data are presented as the means ± SEM. Linear regressions are least-squares-line best fits. Statistical comparisons were accomplished using two-way ANOVAs with Tukey's HSD as a post hoc test or unpaired t-tests; $P < 0.05$ was considered significant.

Results

Twenty-four dorsal horn neurons were studied. Fourteen were excited by colorectal distension and were located in the T13–L2 spinal segments; ten were excited by heating of the plantar surface of the hindfoot and were located in the L3–L5 spinal segments. Neurons excited by colorectal distension were classified according to their response to a phasic, 80 mmHg, 20 s stimulus using the terminology of a previous study (Ness and Gebhart, 1987a). Short-latency abrupt (SL-A, $n = 12$) neurons were excited at short latency (< 1 s) following the onset of the distending stimulus; following termination of the distending stimulus, SL-A neurons abruptly (< 2 s) returned to baseline (see Fig. 1A). Short-latency sustained (SL-S, $n = 2$) neurons were also excited at short latency, but had sustained (4–12 s) responses following termination of the distending stimulus (Fig. 1A). SL-A and SL-S neurons had convergent cutaneous receptive fields located on the abdomen, flank and dorsal body surface and responded to noxious pinch ($n = 14$) and light touch ($n = 12$). Neurons excited by heating of the plantar surface of the hindfoot (Fig. 1B) were classified using the schema of Menetrey et al. (1977) as either Class 2 (responsive to noxious and non-noxious cutaneous stimuli, $n = 5$) or Class 3 (responsive only to noxious cutaneous stimuli, $n = 5$).

All 24 neurons in the present study demonstrated monotonic, accelerating responses to graded stimuli characterized by linear SRFs (e.g., Fig. 1C and D) and were inhibited by morphine or clonidine in a

dose-dependent manner (e.g., Figs. 2 and 3). The responses of neurons excited by colorectal distension were inhibited to 50% of control by significantly smaller doses of morphine (visceral, 1.14 ± 0.23 mg/kg i.v.) than neurons excited by heating of the hindfoot plantar surface (cutaneous, 3.60 ± 0.40 mg/kg i.v.; $P < 0.01$, $t = 5.63$, 10 df), whereas the same was not true for clonidine (visceral, 100.0 ± 28.3 μg/kg i.a.; cutaneous, 32.5 ± 7.5 μg/kg i.a.; $P > 0.05$, $t = 1.95$, 10 df). Additionally, clonidine qualitatively appeared to have more effect on the early neuronal response (first 5 s) during either visceral or cutaneous noxious stimulation than on the late neuronal response (last 5 s), whereas the opposite was true for morphine (see Fig. 3). Quantitative analysis of this difference requires a larger neuronal sample. Morphine affected the intensity coding of both visceral and cutaneous spinal nociceptive transmission in a way which was qualitatively different from that of clonidine. Morphine produced a small increase in the threshold for neuronal response as well as a significant decrease in the gain of the neuronal response ($P < 0.05$ for the

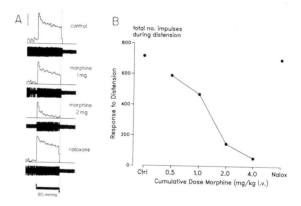

Fig. 2. Example of dose-dependent, naloxone-reversible inhibition of the neuronal response of an SL-A neuron to an 80 mmHg, 20 s distending stimulus. Peristimulus time histograms (1 s bins) and corresponding oscillographic tracings are presented in A, top to bottom, for the control response of the neuron to distension, responses of the same neuron after the administration of cumulative doses of 1 and 2 mg/kg morphine sulfate i.v., and 7 min following the i.v. administration of 3 mg/kg naloxone. Vertical calibration = 20 Hz. Data from the same neuron are presented graphically in B.

deviation from parallelism of the two lines), producing predominantly a change in the slope of the SRFs (Fig. 4A and C). Clonidine, on the other hand, produced a significant increase in the threshold of the neuronal response with no significant change in the gain of the response, thus producing a rightward parallel shift in the SRFs (Fig. 4B and D).

Discussion

The present data indicate that morphine and clonidine differentially modulate the intensity coding of

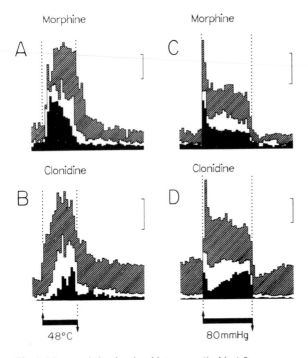

Fig. 3. Mean peristimulus time histograms (1 s bins) for neurons excited by heating of the hindfoot (A and B, $n = 5$/group) and neurons excited by colorectal distension (C and D, $n = 7$/group) which were inhibited by morphine (A and C) or clonidine (B and D). Cross-hatched histograms indicate the control responses, unfilled histograms indicate the response after administration of a dose of drug producing roughly a 50% reduction in the evoked response of a given neuron (see text), and filled histograms indicate the responses of a given neuron after administration of twice those doses. Note that morphine and clonidine apparently have differential effects upon the early and late components of the evoked neuronal responses.

spinal nociceptive transmission (both visceral and cutaneous). Morphine produces only a small change in the sensory threshold for response, but markedly attenuates the gain of intensity coding. This is in agreement with psychophysiological work in man (Willer, 1985; Willer et al., 1985) where opiates were administered spinally or systemically and it also agrees with electrophysiological and behavioral data where the effects of opiates were limited to the spinal cord (Yaksh, 1981). Opioids injected systemically or microinjected into brainstem sites have also been demonstrated to modulate similarly the intensity coding of spinal neurons (Gebhart et al., 1984). Clonidine, as opposed to morphine, produced a large increase in the sensory threshold for response with little effect upon the gain of the response. Psychophysiological work in man and experimental electrophysiological work have not, to the best of our knowledge, examined the effect of clonidine upon neuronal intensity coding, and this report is the first demonstration of such.

Morphine and clonidine have been demonstrated to act synergistically in inhibiting experimental nociceptive responses (Yaksh, 1986) and may act biochemically via the same second messenger(s) (Aghajanian and Wang, 1986). Based upon data in the present study, the receptors involved in the production of analgesia by these drugs may be located on anatomically different sites. It has been suggested previously by Carstens et al. (1980) that differential effects upon intensity coding of nociceptive transmission may be due to presynaptic vs. postsynaptic receptor sites or differential distributions of inhibitory influences on dendrites. In the spinal cord, morphine appears to be more specific than clonidine at selectively inhibiting responses to noxious levels of stimulation as opposed to responses to low-threshold noxious stimuli. Hence, morphine may act predominantly on presynaptic terminals to selectively reduce the amount of one of the excitatory neurotransmitters released from primary afferents by noxious stimuli, whereas clonidine may act presynaptically to inhibit all primary afferent terminals converging on spinal nociceptive neurons, or postsynaptically, producing a hyperpolarization of nociceptive neurons that must be overcome by a minimal level of primary afferent activity before the nociceptive neurons depolarize.

Specific dose-response relationships were not examined as part of this study. However, differences in the doses of morphine and clonidine producing inhibition to roughly 50% of control responses to colorectal distension or heating were noted. Clonidine was significantly more potent than morphine in inhibiting both cutaneous and visceral nocicepti-

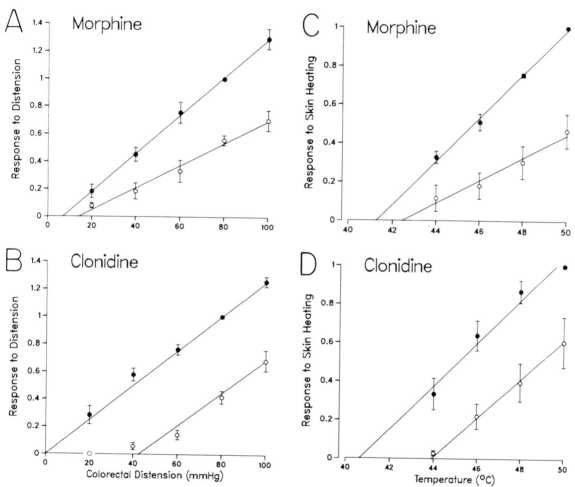

Fig. 4. Modifications of the intensity coding of neurons excited by graded colorectal distension (A and B, $n = 7$/group) and neurons excited by heating of the plantar surface of the hindfoot (C and D, $n = 5$/group) by morphine (A, 1.14 ± 0.23 mg/kg i.v.; C, 3.60 ± 0.40 mg/kg i.v.) and clonidine (B, 100.0 ± 28.3 μg/kg i.a.; D, 32.5 ± 7.5 μg/kg i.a.). Closed symbols indicate control neuronal responses to graded colorectal distension or heating; open symbols indicate neuronal responses following administration of the drug. Responses are normalized to the control neuronal response to either an 80 mmHg, 20 s colorectal distension or a 48°C, 15 s heat stimulus. Least-squares-line stimulus-response functions (SRFs) demonstrate that morphine produces a significant decrease in the gain (decrease in slope of the SRF) of the intensity coding of nociceptive neurons with only a small increase in sensory threshold (shift in ordinate intercept) whereas clonidine produces a significant increase in the sensory threshold with little effect on the gain. Data in B representing the mean neuronal response to a 40 mmHg, 20 s distending stimulus after the administration of clonidine are truncated; only 3 of the 7 neurons responded. Two of the 7 neurons responded to the 20 mmHg, 20 s distending stimulus and the linear regression did not include that point.

ve transmission and affected visceral as cutaneous nociceptive transmission similarly at comparable doses. Morphine, on the other hand, was more potent in inhibiting visceral as opposed to cutaneous nociceptive transmission. These findings are in agreement with literature demonstrating a higher potency of α-adrenergic versus opioid receptor agonists in producing inhibition of nociceptive reflexes (Yaksh, 1986) and with what is observed clinically in humans, where morphine is more efficacious for relief of poorly localized pains, such as visceral pain, than for well-localized cutaneous pains (Jaffe and Martin, 1985).

Acknowledgements

The authors would like to acknowledge the secretarial assistance of Teresa Fulton and the technical assistance of M. Burcham. This work was supported by DHHS awards NS 19912 and DA 02879. T.J.N. was supported by a Life and Health Insurance Medical Research Fellowship.

References

Aghajanian, G.K. and Wang, Y.-Y. (1986) Pertussis toxin blocks the outward currents evoked by opiate and α$_2$-agonists in locus coeruleus neurons. Brain Res., 371: 390–394.

Bynum, T.E. (1983) Abdominal Pain. In J.H. Stein (Ed.), Internal Medicine, Little, Brown and Co., Boston, pp. 85–90.

Carstens, E., Klumpp, D. and Zimmermann, M. (1980) Differential inhibitory effects of medial and lateral midbrain stimulation on spinal neuronal discharges to noxious skin heating in the cat. J. Neurophysiol., 43: 332–342.

Fleetwood-Walker, S.M., Mitchell, R., Hope, P.J., Molony, V. and Iggo, A. (1985) An α2 receptor mediates the selective inhibition by noradrenaline of nociceptive responses of identified dorsal horn neurones. Brain Res., 334: 243–254.

Gebhart, G.F., Sandkühler, J., Thalhammer, J.G. and Zimmermann, M. (1984) Inhibition in spinal cord of nociceptive information by electrical stimulation and morphine microinjection at identical sites in midbrain of the cat. J. Neurophysiol., 51: 75–89.

Jaffe, J.H. and Martin, W.R. (1985) Opioid analgesics and antagonists. In A.G. Gilman, L.S. Goodman, T.W. Rall and F. Murad (Eds.), Goodman and Gilman's Pharmacologic Basis of Therapeutics, MacMillan, New York, pp. 491–531.

Lipkin, M. and Sleisenger, M.H. (1958) Studies of visceral pain: measurements of stimulus intensity and duration associated with the onset of pain in the esophagus, ileum and colon. J. Clin. Invest., 37: 28–34.

Mankin, H.J. and Adams, R.D. (1983) Pain in the back and neck. In R.G. Petersdorf, R.D. Adams, E. Braunwald, K.J. Isselbacher, J.B. Martin and J.D. Wilson (Eds.), Harrison's Principles of Internal Medicine, McGraw-Hill, New York, pp. 35–45.

Menetrey, D., Giesler, G.J. and Besson, J.M. (1977) An analysis of response properties of spinal cord dorsal horn neurons to nonnoxious and noxious stimuli in the spinal rat. Exp. Brain Res., 27: 15–33.

Ness, T.J. and Gebhart, G.F. (1987a) Characterization of neuronal response to noxious visceral and somatic stimuli in the medial lumbosacral spinal cord of the rat. J. Neurophysiol., 57: 1867–1892.

Ness, T.J. and Gebhart, G.F. (1987b) Quantitative comparison of inhibition of visceral and cutaneous nociceptive transmission from the midbrain and medulla in the rat. J. Neurophysiol., 58: 850–865.

Ness, T.J. and Gebhart, G.F. (1987c) Characterization of T13–L2 spinal neurons responsive to noxious distension of the gut in spinalized and intact rats. Neurosci. Abstr., 13: 115.

Ness, T.J. and Gebhart, G.F. (1988) Colorectal distension as a noxious visceral stimulus: physiologic and pharmacologic characterization of pseudaffective reflexes in the rat. Brain Res., in press.

Price, D.D. and Browe, A.C. (1973) Spinal cord coding of graded nonnoxious and noxious temperature increases. Exp. Neurol., 48: 201–221.

Ritchie, J. (1973) Pain from distension of the pelvic colon by inflating a balloon in the irritable colon syndrome. Gut, 14: 125–132.

Wilcockson, W.S., Kim, J., Shin, J.M., Chung, J.M. and Willis, W.D. (1986) Actions of opioids on primate spinothalamic tract neurons. J. Neurosci., 6: 2509–2520.

Willer, J.-C. (1985) Studies on pain. Effects of morphine on a spinal nociceptive flexion reflex and related pain sensation in man. Brain Res., 331: 105–114.

Willer, J.-C., Bergeret, S. and Gaudy, J.H. (1985) Epidural morphine strongly depressed nociceptive flexion reflexes in patients with postoperative pain. Anesthesiology, 63: 675–680.

Yaksh, T.L. (1981) Spinal opiate analgesia: characteristics and principles of action. Pain, 11: 293–346.

Yaksh, T.L. (Ed.) (1986) The effects of intrathecally administered opioid and adrenergic agents on spinal function. In Spinal Afferent Processing, Plenum Press, New York, pp. 505–539.

R. Dubner, G.F. Gebhart & M.R. Bond (Eds.)
Proceedings of the Vth World Congress on Pain
© 1988 Elsevier Science Publishers BV (Biomedical Division)

CHAPTER 50

Have current concepts of spinal opioid receptor function been influenced by the routes of drug administration used?

Chris G. Parsons and P. Max Headley

Department of Physiology, The Medical School, University of Bristol, University Walk, Bristol BS8 1TD, UK

Summary

Extracellular recordings have been made from single motoneurones in ventral root filaments of α-chloralose-anaesthetized, spinalized rats. Intravenously administered opioids active at kappa (U-50,488 and tifluadom) or at mu (fentanyl and morphine) receptors were effective at reducing nociceptive reflexes to both thermal and mechanical noxious peripheral stimuli. This contrasts with the behavioural results of some, but not all, workers, who have suggested that kappa receptor agonists, whether administered systemically or intrathecally, fail to affect those nociceptive reflexes elicited by thermal stimuli, such as in the tail flick test. It seems probable that at least some of this discrepancy between our electrophysiological results and the reported behavioural data can be explained by problems associated with the routes of drug administration used. Thus, supraspinal actions will be superimposed on any direct spinal actions following systemic administration in non-spinalized preparations; following local topical application some opioids may fail to reach the appropriate opioid receptors.

Correspondence should be addressed to Dr. P.M. Headley at the above address.

Introduction

Most studies on the spinal antinociceptive actions of opioids have used behavioural models of nociception such as the tail flick, hotplate, paw pressure and writhing tests. Reports are consistent that kappa opioid receptor agonists are as effective as mu opioid receptor agonists in tests using either mechanical or visceral stimuli, whereas there is disparity on the effectiveness of kappa receptor agonists in tests using thermal stimuli. Thus, kappa receptor agonists have been reported to be ineffective in thermal tests following either systemic (Tyers, 1980, 1982; Upton et al., 1982; Ward and Takemori, 1983) or intrathecal administration (Schmauss et al., 1983; Bryant et al., 1983; Schmauss and Yaksh, 1984; see Yaksh and Noueihed, 1985). In contrast, other groups find kappa receptor agonists to be as effective as mu receptor agonists in either behavioural (Han and Xie, 1982; Kaneko et al., 1983; Przewlocki et al., 1983a,b; Vonvoigtlander et al., 1983; Herman and Goldstein, 1985) or electrophysiological (Calthrop and Hill, 1983) tests of thermal nociception.

With systemic administration in intact animals it is not possible to determine what proportion of a drug's effect is mediated at spinal rather than supraspinal sites; and following intrathecal administration, the diffusion of different drugs into the cord has been shown to vary enormously (see Durant and Yaksh, 1986; Yaksh et al., 1986). The use of systemic administration of opioids in spinally transected animals provides a means of overcoming these two problems, since any effects of spinal reflexes must be mediated caudal to the site of transection. We have therefore tested mu and kappa receptor agonists in an electrophysiological correlate of behavioural reflex experiments in an attempt to resolve some of the discrepancies referred to above.

Methods

Experimental methods have been given in detail elsewhere (see Headley et al., 1987). Briefly, the data reported here were obtained in experiments on 33 α-chloralose-anaesthetized rats which were spinalized in the lower thoracic region. Forty-four single motoneurones were recored from their axons in fine ventral root filaments, using simple silver wire electrodes. These motoneurones were activated by noxious heat and pinch of the ipsilateral hind limb alternating in a regular cycle which was electronically controlled for constancy of intensity, duration and repetition rate. Neuronal firing rates were plotted continuously on a chart recorder and great care was taken to adjust stimulus intensities so as to match neuronal firing rates elicited by the alternating heat and pinch stimuli. Counts of the spikes elicited by each stimulus were passed online to a microcomputer for the quantitative analysis reported below. Following three or more stable control cycles, the mu or kappa receptor agonist under study was given intravenously (i.v.), in a cumulative logarithmic dose progression, until responses were reduced to below 50% of control levels. With 24 of these cells, the nature of this reduction was tested with the opioid receptor antagonist naloxone (10–200 μg/kg i.v.).

Agonists tested systemically were chosen on the basis of three criteria, these being: (1) specificity for the receptor subtype under study, (2) suitability for systemic administration, and (3) half-lives that are short enough to allow multiple drug testing on any

one motoneurone; morphine has a relatively long half-life and was therefore tested as the last drug in any one experiment. The mu receptor agonists morphine and fentanyl (Sublimaze, Janssen) and the opioid receptor antagonist naloxone were obtained from commercial sources. Of the two kappa receptor agonists tested, U-50,488 (trans-3,4-dichloro-N-methyl-N-[2-(1-pyrrolidinyl)cyclohexyl]benzene-acetamide; Upjohn) was kindly provided by Dr. P.F. Vonvoigtlander, and tifluadom (1-methyl-2-(3-thienylcarbonyl)aminomethyl-5-(2-fluorophenyl)-H-2,3-dihydro-1,4-benzodiazepine; Sandoz) by Dr. D. Römer.

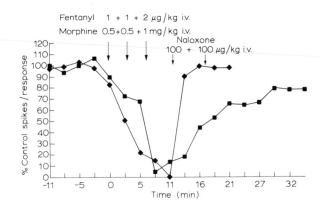

Fig. 1. Fentanyl is three orders of magnitude more potent than morphine when tested on the responses of rat motoneurones to noxious pinch stimuli. This motoneurone was activated by noxious pinching of the ipsilateral hind paw at regular 160-s intervals. The responses have been normalized as percentages of the control mean ($n = 3$) number of spikes elicited by each stimulus. Filled squares show the effect of fentanyl when administered in divided doses ($1 + 1 + 2$ μg/kg) to a cumulative dose of 4 μg/kg i.v. and the subsequent recovery from this effect over the next 30 min. Diamonds illustrate superimposed data recorded from the same cell later in the experiment and show the effect of morphine administered in divided doses ($0.5 + 0.5 + 1$ mg/kg) to a cumulative dose of 2 mg/kg i.v. This effect was rapidly and completely reversed by the subsequent administration of naloxone 100 μg/kg i.v. (an additional 100 μg/kg dose of naloxone had no further effect). U-50,488 had a similar effect on this cell when tested at 2 mg/kg i.v. Time 0 represents the administration of the first dose of agonist in both cumulative-dose regimes. Multireceptive motoneurone recorded in lumbar 5 ventral root of an α-chloralose-anaesthetized, spinalized rat.

Results

The mu receptor agonists

The mu agonist fentanyl (0.5–16 μg/kg i.v.) was tested in 21 rats on the responses of 28 motoneurones to alternating noxious heat and pinch stimuli. As expected, fentanyl reduced the nociceptive responses to thermal and mechanical stimuli equally and in a dose-dependent manner. Fentanyl was tested at 4 μg/kg i.v. on 18 of the above cells and reduced pinch responses to a mean of 30% of control (±5 SEM) whilst reducing heat responses similarly to a mean of 35% (±7). This effect was completely reversed by low i.v. doses of naloxone (20–100 μg/kg) on the 4 cells tested with this antagonist. Morphine (0.5–8 mg/kg i.v.) was equally non-selective between thermal and mechanical responses when compared with fentanyl on 5 motoneurones. Its potency was three orders of magnitude less than that of fentanyl. An example of this difference in potency is illustrated in Fig. 1, which shows that 2 mg/kg of morphine was required to produce a reduction of responses to noxious pinch similar to that produced by fentanyl at 4 μg/kg. Naloxone (10–100 μg/kg) fully reversed the depression of responses by morphine on all 5 cells.

The kappa receptor agonists

U-50,488 (0.5–16 mg/kg) was tested on 25 motoneurones in 17 rats and tifluadom (0.05–1.6 mg/kg) was tested on 16 motoneurones in 12 rats. Fig. 2 illustrates that, in common with the mu receptor agonists fentanyl and morphine, the kappa receptor agonist U-50,488 reduced thermal and mechanical nociceptive reflexes in parallel. With 15 such cells tested at 4 mg/kg i.v., responses to heat and pinch were reduced to means of 33% (±6) and 45% (±6) of control, respectively. On the 5 cells tested with both U-50,488 and morphine, the kappa and mu receptor agonists were approximately equipotent. Fig. 3 illustrates that reduction of nociceptive reflexes by U-50,488 was completely reversed by low doses of naloxone (100 μg/kg i.v.); this effect was consistent for all 8 cells tested with the opioid re-

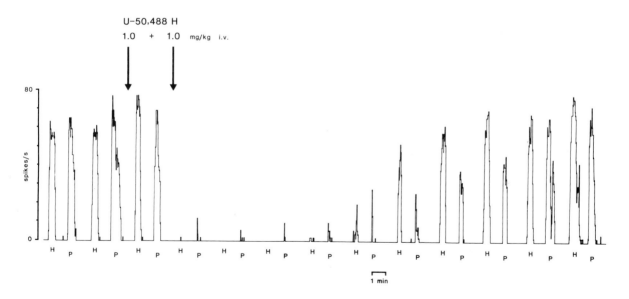

Fig. 2. Lack of selectivity of U-50,488 between the responses of a rat motoneurone to alternating thermal and mechanical noxious stimuli. The neurone was activated by noxious heat (H) of the ipsilateral plantar foot (48.5°C for 30 s) and pinch (P) of the ipsilateral hock (ankle), alternated in a regular 3-min cycle. U-50,488 was administered in divided doses (1 + 1 mg/kg) to a cumulative dose of 2 mg/kg i.v. Full recovery from the effects of U-50,488 was evident some 30 min after the second dose of this kappa receptor agonist. Multireceptive motoneurone recorded in lumbar 5 ventral root of an α-chloralose-anaesthetized, spinalized rat.

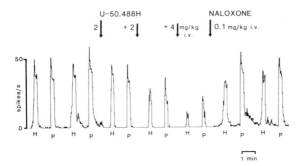

Fig. 3. Naloxone antagonized the depressant actions of U-50,488 on motoneuronal thermal and mechanical nociceptive responses. This motoneurone was activated by noxious heat (H) of the ipsilateral plantar foot (48.8°C for 30 s) and pinch (P) of the ipsilateral hock, alternated in a regular 3-min cycle. U-50,488 was administered in divided doses (2+2+4 mg/kg i.v.) to a cumulative dose of 8 mg/kg i.v. The non-selective reduction of both thermal and mechanical nociceptive responses was reversed by naloxone 0.1 mg/kg i.v. administered 3 min later. Nociceptive motoneurone recorded in lumbar 5 ventral root of an α-chloralose-anaesthetized, spinalized rat.

ceptor antagonist. Tifluadom showed a similar lack of selectivity between thermal and mechanical stimuli but was an order of magnitude more potent than both U-50,488 and morphine. Again, this effect was reversed by naloxone (100 μg/kg i.v.) on all 7 motoneurones tested.

Discussion

It is clear from these results in spinalized preparations that systemically administered kappa (U-50,488 and tifluadom) and mu (morphine and fentanyl) receptor agonists are all effective at depressing spinal reflexes to noxious heat as well as to noxious pinch stimuli. Moreover, the potency ratios for fentanyl:morphine (approximately 1000:1) and for U-50,488:morphine (approximately 1:1) are in good agreement with those found in several behavioural tests using systemic administration (e.g.

Irwin et al., 1951; Janssen et al., 1963; Römer et al., 1982; Vonvoigtlander et al., 1983). In contrast, these ratios differ markedly from those quoted for intrathecal administration, where the ratio for fentanyl:morphine is less than 20:1 and that for U-50,488:morphine is less than 0.01:1 (see Yaksh and Noueihed, 1985). This discrepancy may be explained by variable diffusion between agonists from the intrathecal space into the cord. This certainly seems to be the case for the mu receptor agonist fentanyl and the kappa receptor agonist buprenorphine, as the effective intrathecal dose can exceed the effective systemic dose (see Bryant et al., 1983; Durant and Yaksh, 1986; Yaksh et al., 1986). In the absence of specific data for the kappa receptor agonists U-50,488 and tifluadom, it is thus possible that the relative ineffectiveness of these kappa receptor agonists following intrathecal administration in behavioural tests of antinociception is due largely to inadequate penetration to the appropriate sites in the spinal cord. This problem may well be compounded by the fact that functional kappa receptors appear to be located in deeper laminae of the spinal cord than mu receptors (Fleetwood-Walker et al., 1986).

In summary, our results with systemic administration in spinalized preparations indicate that kappa receptor agonists do readily affect spinal nociceptive reflexes to thermal as well as to mechanical stimuli. Conclusions about the ineffectiveness of kappa receptor agonists in the spinal cord, when based on the relative potencies of mu and kappa agonists administered by other routes, thus need reappraisal.

Acknowledgements

Supported by the Medical Research Council and the Wellcome Trust.

References

Bryant, R.M., Olley, J.E. and Tyers, M.B. (1983) Antinociceptive actions of morphine and buprenorphine given intrathecally in the conscious rat. Br. J. Pharmacol., 78: 659–663.

Calthrop, J. and Hill, R.G. (1983) The action of κ-agonists on the nociceptive responses of neurones in the medullary dorsal horn of the anaesthetized rat. Life Sci., 33 Suppl. 1: 541–544.

Durant, P.A.C. and Yaksh, T.L. (1986) Epidural injections of bupivacaine, morphine, fentanyl, lofentanil, and DADL in chronically implanted rats: a pharmacologic and pathologic study. Anesthesiology, 64: 43–53.

Fleetwood-Walker, S.M., Hope, P.J. and Mitchell, R. (1986) Delta opioids exert antinociceptive effects in lamina I, but not lamina III-V of rat dorsal horn. J. Physiol., 382: 152P.

Han, J.S. and Xie, C.-W. (1982) Dynorphin: potent analgesic effect in spinal cord of the rat. Life Sci., 31: 1781–1784.

Headley, P.M., Parsons, C.G. and West, D.C. (1987) The role of N-methyl-aspartate receptors in mediating responses of rat and cat spinal neurones to defined sensory stimuli. J. Physiol., 385: 169–188.

Herman, B.H. and Goldstein, A. (1985) Antinociception and paralysis induced by intrathecal dynorphin A. J. Pharmacol. Exp. Ther., 232: 27–32.

Irwin, S., Houde, R.W., Bennett, D.R., Hendershot, L.C. and Seevers, M.H. (1951) The effects of morphine, methadone and meperidine on some reflex responses of spinal animals to nociceptive stimulation. J. Pharmacol. Exp. Ther., 101: 132–143.

Janssen, P.A.J., Niemegeers, C.J.E. and Dony, J.G.H. (1963) The inhibitory effect of fentanyl and other morphine-like analgesics on the warm water induced withdrawal reflex in rats. Arzneim. Forsch., 13: 502–507.

Kaneko, T., Hakazawa, T., Ikeda, M., Yamatsu, K., Iwama, T., Wada, T., Satoh, M. and Takagi, H. (1983) Sites of analgesic action of dynorphin. Life Sci., 33 Suppl. 1: 661–664.

Przewlocki, R., Stala, L., Greczek, M., Shearman, G.T., Przewlocki, B. and Herz, A. (1983a) Analgesic effects of μ-, δ- and κ-opiate agonists and, in particular, dynorphin at the spinal level. Life Sci., 33 Suppl. 1: 649–652.

Przewlocki, R., Shearman, G.T. and Herz, A. (1983b) Mixed opioid/nonopioid effects of dynorphin and dynorphin related peptides after their intrathecal injection in rats. Neuropeptides, 3: 233–240.

Römer, D., Büscher, H.H., Hill, R.C., Maurer, R., Petcher, T.J., Zeugner, H., Benson, W., Finner, E., Milkowski, W. and Thies, P.W. (1982) An opioid benzodiazepine. Nature, 298: 759–760.

Schmauss, C., Yaksh, T.L., Shimohigashi, Y., Harty, G., Jensen, T. and Rodbard, D. (1983) Differential association of spinal μ, δ and κ opioid receptors with cutaneous thermal and visceral chemical nociceptive stimuli in the rat. Life Sci., 33 Suppl. 1: 653–656.

Schmauss, C. and Yaksh, T.L. (1984) In vivo studies on spinal opiate receptor systems mediating antinociception. II. Pharmacological profiles suggesting a differential association of mu, delta and kappa receptors with visceral chemical and cutaneous thermal stimuli in the rat. J. Pharmacol. Exp. Ther., 228: 1–12.

Tyers, M.B. (1980) A classification of opiate receptors that mediate antinociception in animals. Br. J. Pharmacol., 69: 503–512.

Tyers, M.B. (1982) Studies on the antinociceptive activities of mixtures of μ- and κ-opiate receptor agonists and antagonists. Life Sci., 31: 1233–1236.

Upton, N., Sewell, R.D.E. and Spencer, P.S.J. (1982) Differentiation of potent μ- and κ-opiate agonists using heat and pressure antinociceptive profiles and combined potency analysis. Eur. J. Pharmacol., 78: 421–429.

Vonvoigtlander, P.F., Lahti, R.A. and Ludens, J.H. (1983) U-50,488, a selective and structurally novel non-mu (kappa) opioid agonist. J. Pharmacol. Exp. Ther., 224: 7–12.

Ward, S.J. and Takemori, A.E. (1983) Relative involvement of mu, kappa and delta receptor mechanisms in opiate-mediated antinociception in mice. J. Pharmacol. Exp. Ther., 224: 525–530.

Yaksh, T.L. and Noueihed, R. (1985) The physiology and pharmacology of spinal opiates. Annu. Rev. Pharmacol. Toxicol., 25: 433–462.

Yaksh, T.L., Noueihed, R.Y. and Durant, P.A.C. (1986) Studies of the pharmacology and pathology of intrathecally administered 4-anilinopiperidine analogues and morphine in the rat and cat. Anesthesiology, 64: 54–66.

R. Dubner, G.F. Gebhart & M.R. Bond (Eds.)
Proceedings of the Vth World Congress on Pain
© 1988 Elsevier Science Publishers BV (Biomedical Division)

CHAPTER 51

The spinal route of analgesia for acute and chronic pain

Michael J. Cousins*

Department of Anaesthesia and Intensive Care, The Flinders University and Flinders Medical Centre, Bedford Park, S.A., Australia

Historical perspective

A little more than one hundred years ago, in 1884, the concept of a regionalized type of pain control became a reality. When Karl Koller instilled cocaine into the eye of a patient for ophthalmological surgery, he produced blockade of axons of peripheral nerves. This was the first pharmacological attempt to aim at a relatively specific target for pain control, with the object of avoiding effects on other areas of the body, particularly the brain (Cousins et al., 1984).

The brain had been the primary target for pain control for thousands of years, with the use of agents such as plant concoctions containing belladonna, opium, hallucinogens, and other agents with an ability to produce central nervous system depression or alteration of perception of pain. Two thousand years of essentially unchanged methods of treatment of acute and chronic pain with opioids were associated with a continuing lack of fundamental information about the actions and side-effects of opioids. Spectacular progress in the past ten to fifteen years has permitted improvements in the use of opioids by all routes of administration, including the spinal route (Cousins and Phillips, 1986). Pharmacokinetic and pharmacodynamic

studies permitted a substantial increase in the efficacy of intravenous opioids and a minimization, but not complete abolition, of unwanted effects on brain, such as sedation and respiratory depression (Cousins et al., 1984). In 1976 Yaksh and Rudy provided clear evidence that spinal opioid receptors were associated with analgesia. Subsequent studies (see Yaksh and Noueihed, 1985) provided evidence that analgesia was produced by inhibition of 'neuron cells' in substantia gelatinosa by predominantly a presynaptic action and also possibly a postsynaptic action.

Leaving aside pain control at a peripheral level, for example by nonsteroidal anti-inflammatory drugs, there are now three major targets for control of severe pain: *brain, spinal cord neurons* and *blockade of axonal conduction*. Intravenous administration of opioids produces analgesia predominantly by effects on the brain; however, there is evidence that this is achieved by activation of descending inhibition and also to a lesser extent by opioid conveyed to spinal cord receptors. Spinally administered opioids may have a predominant analgetic effect on the spinal cord; however, administration of doses that infringe the 'therapeutic index' may progressively result in increasing effects on brain (Cousins, 1987). Local anesthetics injected spinally (epidurally or intrathecally) produce their effects predominantly by an action on axons of spinal cord nerve roots; however, there is also evidence that axons located in the spinal cord may be blocked

---

*Visiting Professor, Stanford University Medical Center, Stanford, CA, U.S.A.

(Cousins et al., 1984; Cousins and Bromage, 1987). In addition, large doses of local anesthetics given epidurally may be absorbed into the vasculature and may have an effect on primary afferent nociception in the spinal cord (Woolf and Wiesenfeld-Hallin, 1985).

Although local anesthetics have been in use for over 100 years, detailed studies of the pharmacology and physiology of their spinal administration were reported as recently as the period 1965–1985 (see Cousins and Bromage, 1987; Strichartz, 1987). In the case of spinal administration of opioids, substantial information is now available from animal studies (see Yaksh, 1981; Yaksh and Noueihed, 1985). However, as recently as 1984 it was concluded that data in humans were very meager (Cousins and Mather, 1984). Between 1984 and 1987 there has been very substantial progress in obtaining key pharmacokinetic and pharmacodynamic data to permit rational decisions concerning the safe and effective use of spinal opioids and to decide

upon the relative merits of this route of administration of opioids compared with other options for the control of acute and chronic pain. This chapter will concentrate on a presentation of such data and will mainly compare the spinal administration of opioids and local anesthetics. There will be a lesser emphasis on the spinal administration of non-opioid drugs, since these have only recently begun to be used in man.

Comparison of spinal administration of local anesthetics and opioids

Spinal administration refers to the injection of drugs outside the dural membrane into the fat-filled epidural space (epidural) and direct administration into the spinal fluid (intrathecal or subarachnoid). As discussed below, there is evidence that opioids administered at a lumbar level of the spine may produce a widespread area of pain relief (Gourlay

TABLE I

Comparison of actions and efficacy of spinally applied opioids and local anesthetics (reproduced with permission from Cousins, M.J. and Mather, L.E. (1984) Intrathecal and epidural administration of opioids. Anesthesiology, 61: 276–310)

	Opioids	Local anesthestics
Actions		
Site of action	Substantia gelatinosa of dorsal horn of spinal cord[a]	Nerve roots (and long tracts in spinal cord)
Type of blockade	Presynaptic and (postsynaptic) inhibition of neuron cell excitation	Blockade of nerve impulse conduction in axonal membrane
Modalities blocked	'Selective' block of pain conduction	Blockade of sympathetic and pain fibers, often also loss of sensation and motor function
Efficacy		
Type of pain and efficacy of blockade		
Surgical pain	Partial relief	Complete relief possible
Labor pain	Partial relief	Complete relief
Postoperative pain[b]		
Early first 24 h	Partial to complete relief (high dose)	Complete relief
24 h +	Complete relief (low dose)	Complete relief
Chronic pain	Complete relief	Impracticable (usually)

[a]And/or other sites where opioid receptors (binding sites) are present.

[b]Pain after major surgery requires higher doses (e.g., thoracotomy, 6 mg morphine) than pain after more minor surgery (e.g., lower abdominal, 4 mg morphine). Continuous infusion reduces dose in both situations.

et al., 1985, 1987) and thus lumbar epidural or intrathecal administration is the most common site; however, the clinical situation or the drug employed may sometimes dictate administration at a higher level. In the case of local anesthetics, the lumbar region is usually chosen for subarachnoid administration, but for epidural use it is preferable to place the local anesthetic as close as possible to the spinal nerve roots that it is desired to block (see Scott, 1987). Local anesthetics block the generation of an action potential in axons by interfering with the function of sodium channels in the axonal membrane (Table I). The presence of a local anesthetic makes it less likely for the sodium channel to open in response to a stimulating depolarization. It is now known that the proteins of the sodium channels are present in different states ('opened', 'closed' and 'inactive') (see Strichartz, 1987). Study of purified sodium channels is now yielding evidence of a local anesthetic receptor. If this is confirmed, molecular engineering may permit the design of agonists and antagonists which are highly specific for this receptor. Also there is evidence which raises the possibility that local anesthetic receptors may differ on sympathetic, sensory and motor fibers. Some support for this hypothesis is given by the clinical effects of the long-acting local anesthetic bupivacaine, which is capable of producing very profound sensory block without detectable motor block and often with minimal and very patchy sympathetic block (see Cousins and Bromage, 1987). This has previously been explained by drug physicochemical characteristics influencing the penetration of the drug to produce differential effects on fibers of different sizes. However, a review of such evidence indicates that this is an unsatisfactory explanation (see Strichartz, 1987). Development of a local anesthetic, or other drug, with a selective action on primary afferent nociceptive fibers would be a very desirable goal, since there is evidence that blockade of primary afferent transmission is a more potent method of producing pain relief than is activation of descending inhibitory systems or local inhibition in the spinal dorsal horn (Table I). For example, spinal opioids are not capable of producing com-

plete abolition of surgically induced pain, whereas local anesthetics can be used as the sole agent for surgical analgesia (see Table I). Also severe postoperative, obstetric and also cancer pain may sometimes be unresponsive to spinal opioids but may be relieved by spinal administration of local anesthetics (Arner and Arner, 1985; Cousins et al., 1987).

There are similarities in molecular weight and pK_a between local anesthetics and opioids. Also partition coefficients, which indicate lipid solubility, show considerable overlap among local anesthetics and opioids (Table II). Partition coefficients reflect-

TABLE II

Physicochemical properties of opioids and local anesthetics (reproduced with permission from Cousins, M.J. and Mather, L.E. (1984) Intrathecal and epidural administration of opioids. Anesthesiology, 61: 276–310)

	Molecular weight[a]	$\bar{p}K_a$ (25°C)	Partition coefficient[b]
Local anesthetics[c]			
Procaine hydrochloride	236	8.9	0.02[d]
Lidocaine hydrochloride	234	7.9	2.9[d]
Bupivacaine hydrochloride	288	8.1	27.5[d]
Etidocaine hydrochloride	276	7.7	141[d]
Opioids[c]			
Morphine sulfate	285	7.9[e]	1.42[f]
Meperidine hydrochloride	247	8.5	38.8[f]
Methadone hydrochloride	309	9.3	116[f]
Fentanyl citrate	336	8.4	813[f]
Sufentanil citrate	386	8.0	1.778[f]
(−)Lofentanil cis-oxalate	408	7.8	1.450[f]
β-Endorphin	3300	–	–

[a] Base.

[b] *n*-Heptane and octanol partition coefficients are strongly correlated for similar compounds in a log-log relationship.

[c] Commonly used forms.

[d] *n*-Heptane/pH 7.4 buffer, partition coefficient.

[e] Tertiary amino group.

[f] Octanol/pH 7.4 buffer partition coefficient.

TABLE III

Physicochemical properties of opioids (reproduced with permission from Cousins, M.J. and Mather, L.E. (1984) Intrathecal and epidural administration of opioids. Anesthesiology, 61: 276–310)

At pH 7.4 N³ group mostly ionized ∴ all H₂O-soluble

Morphine (M) OH groups → ↑ H₂O-soluble + ↓ lipid-soluble

Cord uptake of M and onset of analgesia is slow

Cord 'washout' of M is slow and analgesia prolonged

High residual levels of CSF M reach brain

Highly lipid-soluble opioids → rapid cord uptake, rapid onset (and offset) of analgesia,? low brain stem CSF levels

ing lipid solubility have been shown to be significant in the transfer of local anesthetics and opioids across the dural membrane into the CSF (Table III) (see Cousins and Mather, 1984).

Currently available local anesthetic drugs produce a relatively nonselective analgesia, since analgesia is usually associated with some degree of blockade of other sensory modalities, sympathetic function and motor function. In comparison, the pain relief that results from spinal administration of opioid drugs is a great deal more selective (see Table I). This led Cousins and associates to suggest the term 'selective spinal analgesia' to emphasize

TABLE IV

Effects and side-effects (reproduced with permission from Cousins, M.J., Cherry, D.A. and Gourlay, G.K. (1987) Acute and chronic pain. Use of spinal opioids. In M.J. Cousins and P.O. Bridenbaugh (Eds.), Neural Blockade in Clinical Anesthesia and Management of Pain, 2nd edition, J.B. Lippincott, Philadelphia, pp. 955–1029)

Effects and side-effects	Spinal opioids	Spinal local anesthetics
Cardiovascular	Minor heart rate changes	Low-block (below T10) sympathetic blockade: postural hypotension
	Usually not postural hypotension	High-block (above T4) sympathetic blockade: postural hypotension
	Vasoconstrictor response intact	Cardio-accelerator block: ↓ HR ↓ inotropic drive
Respiratory	Early depression[a,b] (0.1–1 h); systemically absorbed drug and? CSF-borne drug	Usually unimpaired unless cardiovascular collapse
	Late depression[a,b] (6–24 h); opioid in CSF migrating to brain	
CNS		
Sedation	May be marked*	Mild or absent, depending on agent
Convulsions	Usually not seen with clinical doses: theoretical possibility at high doses	Expected toxicity from two times overdose or with rapid vascular absorption
Other neurological abnormalities	Confusion, amnesia, catalepsy, hallucinations (reported with high doses intrathecally)	Not usually seen
Opioid withdrawal	If rapid discontinuation of systemic opioids	
Nausea	Yes[a]	Yes–low incidence
Vomiting	Yes[a]	Yes–low incidence
Pruritis	Yes[a]	No.
Miosis	Yes	No (unless Horner's syndrome)
Urinary retention	Yes[a,b]	Yes

[a]Antagonized by naloxone, but repeated doses may be required.
[b]Prevented by naloxone infusions, 5 μg/kg/h, without reversal of analgesic effects.

the differences between analgesia obtained with spinal administration of opioids and that which results from spinal administration of local anesthetics. This suggestion was made on the basis of simultaneous studies of pharmacokinetics and neurological function following spinal epidural administration of the opioid meperidine. Subsequent studies have confirmed that the sympathetic vasoconstrictor response remains intact (see Cousins and Mather, 1984) and motor function is unimpaired at clinical doses of spinal opioids (Willer et al., 1985). Evidence has subsequently emerged of a potential for effects of spinally administered opioids other than those on antinociception (see Yaksh and Noueihed, 1985) (Table IV). Most of these effects result from opioid migrating to the brain in the CSF or conveyed to the brain following vascular absorption. Such effects include sedation, respiratory depression, nausea and vomiting. Respiratory depression is antagonized by naloxone, usually without altering 'spinal' analgesia (Rawal et al., 1986). Other effects such as pruritis may be mediated partly at a spinal and brain level (see Cousins et al., 1987). Urinary retention results from decreased tone of the bladder detreusor muscle. This may be antagonized by naloxone, while retaining analgesia (Rawal et al., 1981, 1983). With the exception of urinary retention, all of the foregoing 'side-effects'

appear to be dose-related and can be minimized if minimal effective clinical doses are used (see Cousins et al., 1987). At very high doses it is possible for spinally administered opioids to cause either convulsions of a generalized nature or rather localized muscle contractions (Yaksh and Noueihed, 1985). Also at very high doses a bizarre syndrome of hyperalgesia has been reported (Yaksh et al., 1987). At minimally effective clinical doses, there may still be a variable incidence of some of the side-effects noted in Table IV; however, the analgesia is produced predominantly at a spinal level, and compared to that produced by local anesthetics is relatively selective. A summary of the evidence of a predominant spinal action of spinal opioids in man is given in Table V.

Spinal epidural and intrathecal routes: overview

In the case of acute pain, repeated intrathecal injection of opioid drugs is not a viable alternative to other methods. However, a single dose of approximately 0.25–0.5 mg of morphine can be injected at the same time as an intrathecal dose of local anesthetic, administered for surgical anesthesia. This combination of drugs results in a period of postoperative analgesia in the vicinity of 12–24 h (Nordberg, 1984). A similar dose of 0.25–0.5 mg morphine, given alone, has been used to provide satisfactory analgesia for labor pain and delivery in high-risk obstetrical patients (see Cousins et al., 1987; Cousins and Mather, 1984). In cancer pain, much more frequent use has been made of the intrathecal route, since it is possible to insert an indwelling silastic catheter and to connect the catheter to a totally implanted pump such as the Infusaid (Coombs, 1986). The intrathecal route theoretically has the advantage of a smaller dose of drug and thus lesser amounts of drug absorbed into the circulation. However, there is still the potential for the drug to migrate to the brain via the CSF. In the setting of acute pain, it has been reported that delayed respiratory depression occurs in approximately one in 300 patients following intrathecal administra-

TABLE V

Evidence of spinal action of opioids in humans (reproduced with permission from Cousins, M.J., Cherry, D.A. and Gourlay, G.K. (1987) Acute and chronic pain. Use of spinal opioids. In M.J. Cousins and P.O. Bridenbaugh (Eds.), Neural Blockade in Clinical Anesthesia and Management of Pain, 2nd edition, J.B. Lippincott, Philadelphia, pp. 955–1029)

Correlation of analgesic effects with CSF, but not blood, concentration of opioid

Antagonism of CNS side-effects, but not spinal analgesia, by naloxone intravenously

Analgesia without sedation with small doses spinally after sedation and poor analgesia owing to tolerance to high oral or intramuscular doses

Electrophysiological studies after intravenous and after epidural morphine

tion, compared to approximately one in 1200 following epidural administration (Rawal et al., 1987). This would seem to outweigh any advantage of the intrathecal route which results in a lesser degree of vascular uptake of drug.

Epidural administration offers a much more flexible approach to the treatment of acute pain than does the intrathecal route. An epidural catheter can be placed percutaneously and left in situ for many days to permit either repeated bolus doses or the infusion of drugs via an external infusion pump. In the case of cancer pain, epidural catheters have been tunneled under the skin and brought out through the subcutaneous tissue (Zenz, 1985), or connected to portals placed underneath the skin (Cherry et al., 1985) or to infusion pumps which are totally implanted (Coombs, 1986) (e.g., Infusaid). A problem with the long-term implantation of 'standard' epidural catheters is tissue reaction in the epidural space, which may form a fibrous tissue sheath around the epidural catheter (see Cousins et al., 1987; Durant and Yaksh, 1986a). This may cause pain on injection, may limit the effective spread of drug into the subarachnoid space, and may pose a rare risk of the formation of a fibrous tissue mass which could result in neurological sequela (Coombs et al., 1985a). Interpretation of pharmacokinetic studies in humans should be made in the light of the potential for fibrous tissue reaction and thus altered vascular and CSF absorption of drug. Such effects are likely to be minimal in single-dose studies immediately after the insertion of a catheter, but may become important as early as 24 h following the catheter insertion (see Durant and Yaksh, 1986a). The use of more inert catheter materials may help to solve this problem (see Dupen et al., 1987).

Transfer of opioid drugs across the dura
All opioid drugs appear to have physicochemical characteristics which permit transfer across the dural membrane into the CSF. It is possible that transfer may occur either directly across the dural membrane, across a greatly attenuated portion of the dural membrane in the region where the dura provides a small 'cuff' to the spinal nerve roots (the so-called dural cuff region) or at other as yet undetermined sites. In the region of the dural cuffs, there are a variable number of so-called 'arachnoid granulations' which are out-pushings of the dura with overlying epidural veins. In these areas there may be only a single layer of dural cells that separates the epidural space from the cerebral spinal fluid (see Figs. 1 and 2). Although such regions are plentiful in animals, there is currently debate about their prevalence and role in humans. This is of some importance, since the arachnoid granulations are capable of removing foreign debris and transferring large particles from CSF to epidural space or vice versa. This would have relevance for the potential of transport of high molecular weight agents, such as the peptides, from epidural space to CSF. Some anecdotal reports indicate that some peptides injected epidurally may produce a spinal analgesia; however, there is no evidence on the basis of measurements of peptides in CSF following epidural injection. Another theoretical route for transport of drugs from epidural space to spinal cord is via very small branches of the posterior radicular arteries. At most lumbar levels, these arteries are vestigial but have nevertheless been demonstrated to be patent. They have branches that pass directly into the substantia gelatinosa. The onset of analgesia following the epidural injection of highly lipid-soluble drugs has been reported in animal studies to be almost instantaneous. The most likely explanation for this rapid onset of action is direct vascular transport to the substantia gelatinosa (see Cousins and Mather, 1984). However, confirmation of this possible route has not yet been obtained (see Cousins et al., 1987). Because of the plentiful epidural plexus of veins, any drug injected into the epidural space will be subject to absorption into the epidural veins and then via the azygos vein will reach the general circulation. A further theoretical possibility is absorption into the so-called basivertebral venous plexus, which lies protected within the bony skeleton of the spine and is in direct communication with the cerebral venous sinuses. Absorption into this plexus would be a possibility during states where the epidural plexus and azygos vein are com-

pressed due to raised intraabdominal and intrathoracic pressure. In such a situation the flow in the basivertebral venous plexus may be reversed to favor flow towards the cerebral venous sinuses, raising the possibility of drug reaching brain by a very direct and rapid route. Evidence in support of this route of absorption has been provided by studies in which Yaksh made a rapid epidural injection of opioid and produced retching and vomiting in animals within seconds of injection. A similar-sized injection given directly into the femoral vein produced no such effects (see Yaksh, 1981). The epidural fat is another important factor influencing the disposition of epidurally injected drugs. Drugs

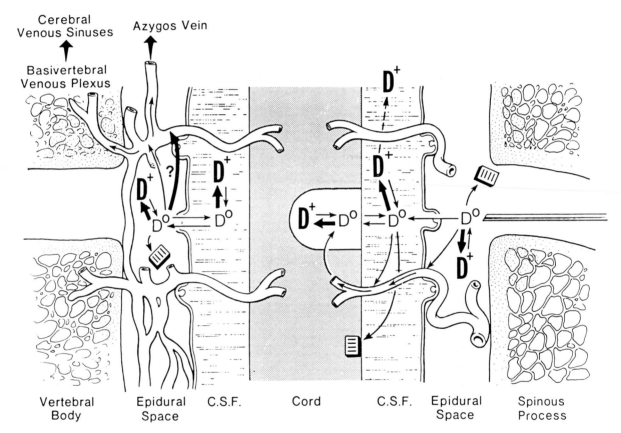

Fig. 1. Pharmacokinetic model: epidural injection of a hydrophilic opioid such as morphine. D^0 = un-ionized lipophilic drug; D^+ = ionized hydrophilic drug. An epidural needle is shown delivering drug to epidural space. The hatched squares in epidural space and spinal cord represent fat depots. Un-ionized drug is shown crossing dura via arachnoid granulations, in regions of dura where epidural veins are in close proximity to the dura. The semicircular areas in spinal cord represent spinal opioid receptors in dorsal horn. For convenience, epidural veins are shown draining into alternative channels, only in anterior epidural space. Arrows showing drug transport directly into spinal arteries and then spinal receptors are speculative. A hydrophilic drug such as morphine is present in epidural space predominantly as the ionized (D^+) species. Thus, transfer to cerebrospinal fluid (CSF) is slow, as is uptake into spinal cord. Egress from spinal cord is also slow, accounting for prolonged analgesia. Slow uptake into spinal cord and high water solubility result in high residual levels of ionized drug in CSF which migrates over the entire spinal cord to reach the brain in substantial amounts. Venous absorption occurs via veins in epidural space which drain to azygos vein. An alternative route is shown via basivertebral venous plexus to cerebral venous sinuses. This route is only possible with raised thoraco-abdominal pressure and reversal of direction of flow. (Reproduced with permission from Cousins, M.J., Cherry, D.A. and Gourlay, G.K. (1987) Acute and chronic pain. Use of spinal opioids. In M.J. Cousins and P.O. Bridenbaugh (Eds.), Neural Blockade in Clinical Anesthesia and Management of Pain, 2nd Edition, J.B. Lippincott, Philadelphia, pp. 955–1029.)

of high liposolubility may be deposited in epidural fat, depending upon the amount and composition of such fat. In the spinal cord, the target for antinociception is of course the spinal opioid receptors in the dorsal horn. This site lies several millimeters beneath the surface of the spinal cord and thus opioid drugs must penetrate lipid-rich tissue before reaching their site of action. It is also possible for opioid drugs to be deposited as a 'depot' in lipid tissue of spinal cord. Receptor kinetics for individual opioids at the spinal receptors will also determine the rapidity of association and dissociation of opioids with the spinal receptors and this will influence duration of action. This aspect is best described by the 'affinity of an opioid for its receptor in the spinal cord'. The ability of the opioid to activate the effector mechanism when bound to the spinal receptor is described by its 'efficacy' or intrinsic activity. In general it seems that physicochemical properties play a major part in the onset and offset of analgetic action of spinal opioids of the pure agonist type (e.g., morphine, meperidine). However, opioids of the partial agonist type such as buprenorphine have a very slow rate of dissociation from the spinal opioid receptors and this contributes to the long duration of action, in addition

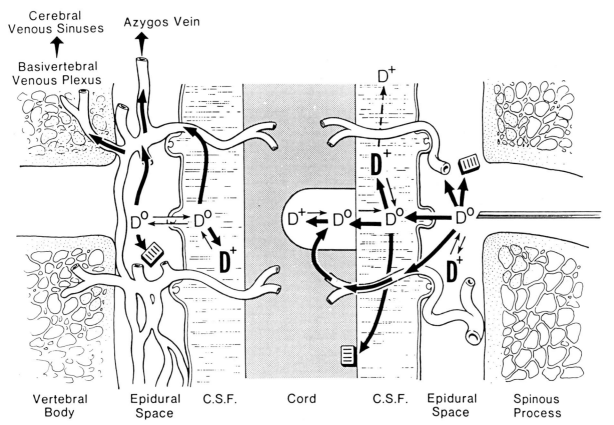

Fig. 2. Pharmacokinetic model: epidural injection of a lipophilic opioid such as meperidine or fentanyl. Symbols as in Fig. 1. Transfer into CSF is rapid, as is uptake into spinal cord. However, egress from spinal cord is also rapid. Residual amounts of ionized species in CSF are less than with morphine. Thus, concentrations of drug at higher levels of spinal cord and brain are less than for morphine. Vascular uptake may be very variable because of considerable competition between epidural fat and epidural veins. (Reproduced with permission from Cousins, M.J., Cherry, D.A. and Gourlay, G.K. (1987) Acute and chronic pain. Use of spinal opioids. In M.J. Cousins and P.O. Bridenbaugh (Eds.), Neural Blockade in Clinical Anesthesia and Management of Pain, 2nd Edition, J.B. Lippincott, Philadelphia, pp. 955–1029.)

to the high lipid solubility of this drug.

At physiological pH, all of the opioid drugs are mostly in an ionized state and exist as an equilibrium between an ionized water-soluble species and an un-ionized lipid-soluble species (see Figs. 1 and 2). It is the un-ionized lipid-soluble species that has the greatest facility for crossing lipid barriers such as the dural membrane and spinal cord lipid tissue. On the other hand, the ionized species, being highly water-soluble, is likely to remain in the cerebrospinal fluid, with a potential for migration over the spinal cord towards the brain (Bromage et al., 1982; Gourlay et al., 1985, 1987) with a potential for delayed respiratory depression (Glynn et al., 1979).

Pharmacokinetic model of epidural opioids
After epidural injection of a *highly ionized and hydrophilic drug* such as morphine, only low concentrations of lipid-soluble un-ionized drug will be present in solution in the epidural space. The high water solubility and low lipid solubility of morphine is due to the hydroxyl groups on the morphine molecule (see Tables II and III). The only other drug in clinical use with such high water solubility is the opioid hydromorphone. Because of the predominance of ionized species of morphine in the epidural space, the transfer of morphine across arachnoid granulations and dural membrane will be slow. This has been confirmed by measurements of morphine in CSF following lumbar epidural injection, which report that peak levels in lumbar CSF occur between 60 and 90 min following injection (Gustafsson et al., 1982; Nordberg, 1984; Nordberg et al., 1983). Interestingly, absorption into the venous system is rapid, with peak concentrations reached between 5 and 10 min after injection (Gourlay et al., 1985, 1987; Sjostrom et al., 1987a). Also the variability in peak plasma concentration of morphine is quite small, compared to other opioids (Sjostrom et al., 1987a,b). Both of these aspects may result from the minimal deposition of morphine in epidural fat due to its low lipid solubility. Thus, there is minimal competition for vascular absorption of the drug and the rich epidural venous plexus with a very large surface area

provides ample opportunity for such absorption, (see Sjostrom et al., 1987a; Gourlay et al., 1985, 1987). Delay in appearance of morphine in the CSF results in a rather low concentration gradient from CSF to spinal opioid receptors and this is reflected in a slow onset of analgesia. However, once morphine reaches spinal opioid receptors, the 'washout' of morphine from this lipid-rich area will be relatively slow (see Fig. 1). In the lumbar cerebrospinal fluid, morphine will be predominantly present as an ionized species and thus substantial amounts of drug will remain in the watery medium of the cerebrospinal fluid, with a potential for spread over a very wide area of the spinal cord and then to the brain. A substantial number of pharmacokinetic studies have now confirmed the proposals of this pharmacokinetic model (see Cousins et al., 1987; Durant and Yaksh, 1986; Gourlay et al., 1985, 1987; Max et al., 1985; Payne and Inturissi, 1985; Nordberg et al., 1983; Gustafsson et al., 1982a, 1984; Sjostrom et al., 1987a,b).

After epidural injection of a *mostly ionized lipophilic drug such as meperidine*, there will be substantial concentrations of lipid-soluble un-ionized drug in the epidural space, which will be rapidly transferred to the CSF, via the dural route and perhaps directly into spinal radicular arteries. Transfer from cerebrospinal fluid to spinal opioid receptors will also be rapid so that minimal concentrations of ionized species will remain in the CSF for spread to higher levels of the spinal cord and to the brain (Fig. 2). There will be a very significant potential for uptake of drug into epidural fat and also into lipid-rich areas of the spinal cord. These proposals are in keeping with pharmacokinetic data which indicate the rapid attainment of peak cerebrospinal fluid concentrations of drugs such as meperidine at 5–10 min after epidural injection (see Cousins et al., 1979; Glynn et al., 1982; Sjostrom et al., 1987a; Gustafsson et al., 1982a,b). The time course of CSF concentrations is closely paralleled by the onset and offset of analgesia. Vascular absorption is also rapid and this is reflected by the attainment of peak blood concentrations at 10–15 min following epidural injection of meperidine (Glynn et al., 1982; Sjostrom et al., 1987a). However, there is substantial competition for vascular absorption due to a variable uptake into epidural fat. This results in some delay in peak plasma concentrations and also a great variability in plasma concentrations (see Sjostrom et al., 1987a). The addition of a vasoconstrictor such as epinephrine would seem to potentially overcome this vascular absorption; however, this has proved to be clinically significant only for the highly lipid-soluble drugs such as fentanyl and sufentanil. The effect of epinephrine is also dependent upon the dose of opioid injected, the concentration of epinephrine used and the timing of administration of epinephrine (see Cousins et al., 1987). Recent evidence indicates that administration of epinephrine prior to the injection of opioid may result in the most pronounced effect. It should be acknowledged that epinephrine may also add to analgesia by a direct effect on spinal alpha-adrenergic receptors which are associated with antinociception. Additionally there is evidence that for the highly lipid-soluble opioids the volume of injectate may play an important part in determining the intensity and extent of analgesia achieved following epidural injection (see Cousins et al., 1987).

Comparative pharmacokinetic studies of lipid-soluble and water-soluble opioids
Sjostrom et al. (1987a,b) performed studies of CSF and blood pharmacokinetics following either epidural or subarachnoid injection of the lipid-soluble opioid meperidine or the water-soluble opioid morphine. Regardless of the drug used, they found that approximately 4% of an epidural dose was transferred across the dura into the spinal fluid. In the case of morphine, this corresponds nicely with estimates of the minimal effective epidural dose in the range 4–6 mg and the minimal effective subarachnoid dose in the range 0.25–0.5 mg. They confirmed the high degree of variability of transfer from epidural space to CSF of the order of 5–6-fold for both morphine and meperidine. The author's group have studied the time course and relative amounts of migration of opioid to the brain stem region; simultaneous epidural injections of morphine and meperi-

dine were made in the lumbar region and cerebrospinal fluid samples were obtained at the C7 T1 level (Gourlay et al., 1985, 1987) (Fig. 3). Peak concentrations of meperidine were measured in the cervical region within 60 min of epidural injection; however, these levels declined rapidly. In contrast, there was a delay of 120–180 min prior to the attainment of peak concentrations of morphine; these levels were then sustained at a relatively high level. A comparison of the amounts of morphine and meperidine in cervical CSF indicated that after approximately 60 min, the amounts of morphine were relatively much greater than those of meperidine. For example, the ratio of peak meperidine (60 min sample) to peak morphine (120 min sample) concentration in CSF samples was 1.6, which is considerably less than the equimolar amounts (ratio, 5) of the two opioids in the injection solution. This explains the greater potential for morphine to cause a delayed type of respiratory depression, which may be slow in onset and may persist for many hours after administration. In contrast, it would appear that lipid-soluble drugs such as meperidine may be capable of causing an early and transient respiratory depression at approximately 60 min after administration. However, the smaller amounts of drug in CSF in the region of the brain will result in this effect being transient. This is borne out by long-term studies of respiratory effects of lipid-soluble opioids such as fentanyl. Such studies indicate a peak respiratory depression at approximately 60 min after administration of the drug, with a rapid decline in this effect and no reappearance of respiratory depression over the ensuing 24 h (Lam et al., 1983). Contrary to previous thinking, it appears that this early respiratory depression is at least partly due to drug borne to the brain in the CSF rather than to drug absorbed into the vascular system, since peak vascular concentrations occur rather early at approximately 5–10 min after administration (Vella et al., 1985).

In a sheep ventriculocisternal perfusion model, Payne and Inturrisi (1985) administered morphine, methadone and [^{14}C]sucrose simultaneously by lumbar subarachnoid injection. They found that

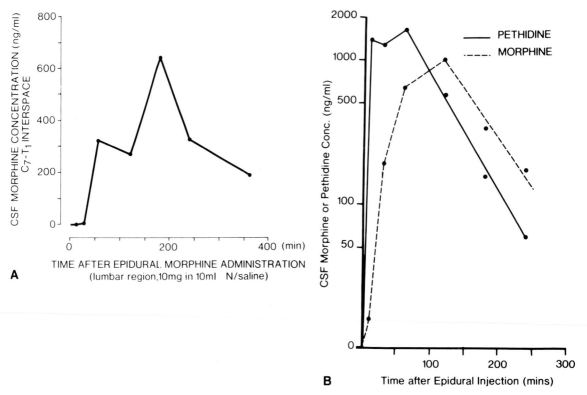

Fig. 3. A. Cervical cerebrospinal fluid (CSF) concentration of morphine. Cervical CSF samples were assayed for morphine at various times after lumbar epidural injection of morphine 10 mg in 10 ml saline. Note the early appearance of morphine in cervical CSF after 30 min and the peak concentration at about 3 h. (Data from Gourlay, G.K., Cherry, D.A. and Cousins, M.J. (1985) Cephalad migration of morphine in CSF following lumbar epidural administration in patients with cancer pain, Pain, 23: 317–326.) B. Cervical CSF concentrations of morphine and pethidine (meperidine) as a function of time following lumbar epidural administration. Morphine (10 mg) and pethidine (50 mg) in 10 ml of normal saline were administered simultaneously by means of a lumbar epidural catheter at L2–L3 interspace, and CSF samples were collected from the C7-T1 interspace at the times shown on the graph. Peak cervical CSF concentrations of pethidine were achieved earlier and declined sooner in comparison with those of morphine. Also the peak concentrations of pethidine were lower than those of morphine, considering the doses of the two drugs injected. The rapid appearance of pethidine in CSF is in keeping with rapid diffusion through the dura. (Reproduced with permission from Gourlay, G.K., Cherry, D.A., Armstrong, P.A., Plummer, J.L. and Cousins, M.J. (1987) The influence of drug polarity on the absorption of opioid drugs into CSF and subsequent cephalad migration following lumbar epidural administration: application to morphine and pethidine. Pain, 31: 297–305.)

morphine and [14C]sucrose were detected in peak concentrations in cisternal CSF at 180 min after injection. This is of interest, since both of these molecules have a high water solubility and the data are in very good agreement with those for morphine presented in Fig. 3. In contrast, the lipid-soluble opioid methadone was not detected in cisternal CSF. In unpublished studies the same group found that the opioids hydromorphone and DADL are distributed supraspinally. Methadone is much more lipid-soluble than morphine (see Table II) and this may explain the failure to detect it supraspinally. Unpublished studies from our own group indicate that epidural injection of the lipid-soluble opioid fentanyl is associated with extremely low concentrations or no detectable fentanyl in cervical CSF samples. Thus it seems that opioids with a high degree of water solubility will migrate readily to the brain and in large amounts. Opioids of intermediate lipid solubility such as meperidine migrate in moderate amounts to the brain but rapidly decline to concentrations that are devoid of clinical effects. Highly lipid-soluble opioids such as methadone and fentanyl have such a rapid uptake into lipid-rich structures of spinal cord that the residual amount of opioid remaining in CSF is undetectable in the cervical region. A fourth pharmacokinetic profile may be represented by lipophilic opioids with very high affinity for the spinal opioid receptors. One example may be the mu agonist lofentanil. As a result of the slow dissociation of lofentanil at mu receptors, its duration of action is longer than that of other lipid-soluble opioids. The partial agonist drugs and 'agonist-antagonist' drugs are mostly highly lipid-soluble and have a slow rate of dissociation from receptors; however, they suffer from a low intrinsic activity. Initial clinical studies indicate that the duration of action is much briefer than that of morphine; however, there may be a lesser incidence of side-effects mediated via the brain. At present pharmacokinetic data are not available to

provide insights into the migration of these drugs via the CSF in blood to the brain.

The spinal route in acute pain management

Clinical studies have now provided important data concerning dose-response relationships for analgesic effects of a number of opioids given by the spinal route (see Cousins and Mather, 1984; Cousins et al., 1987) and for side-effects (see Cousins et al., 1987). Pharmacokinetic studies have also provided strong evidence of a predominant spinal action of appropriate clinical doses of opioids administered at a spinal level. Recently, a substantial number of randomized prospective controlled studies have confirmed the analgesic efficacy of spinal opioids and have documented a superiority of analgesia for this route of administration compared with intramuscular opioid, oral opioid, intermittent intravenous bolus and 'patient-controlled intravenous ad-

TABLE VI

Epidural opioids: studies of efficacy (reproduced with permission from Cousins, M.J., Cherry, D.A. and Gourlay, G.K. (1987) Acute and chronic pain. Use of spinal opioids. In M.J. Cousins and P.O. Bridenbaugh (Eds.), Neural Blockade in Clinical Anesthesia and Management of Pain, 2nd edition, J.B. Lippincott, Philadelphia, pp. 955–1029)

Type of pain	Drug/regimen	Study design	Outcome	References[a]
Postoperative hip replacement	Meperidine 1 mg/kg i.m. versus 20, 60 mg EPI	RPDB	Kinetics of i.m. and EPI the same. Pain (VAS) less after EPI only for 0.25–1 h. Hyperalgesia to pinprick in some EPI patients for 2 h.	Gustafsson, 1982a, 1986
Knee arthrotomy	Morphine 0.05 $mg \cdot kg^{-1}$ EPI versus 0.1 $mg \cdot kg^{-1}$ i.m.	RPDB	Time to C_{max} less for EPI (12 min) and C_{max} dose greater for EPI. No correlation between plasma concentration and analgesia. Analgesia with EPI > i.m. 2 and 11 h. Maximum analgesia after 2 h.	Gustafsson, 1982a
Knee arthrotomy	EPI versus oral controlled-release morphine (CRM)	Controlled study	9/10 with EPI good relief. CRM not effective	Banning, 1986
Total knee replacement	EPI bupivacaine versus EPI + meperidine versus i.m. opioid	RPDB	Both epidural regimens superior to i.m. for analgesia and hospital stay. Less sensory/motor block with combination.	Raj, 1986

Abdominal surgery	EPI versus i.m. morphine	Controlled	Pain relief superior with EPI	Bonnet, 1984
Abdominal surgery	Morphine + bupivacaine EPI, versus morphine EPI, versus bupivacaine EPI, versus saline EPI by infusion	RPDB	Morphine + bupivacaine infusion superior for pain relief, mobilization and respiratory function.	Cullen, 1985
Thoracic surgery	EPI bupivacaine boli versus EPI morphine bolus versus EPI morphine infusion	Controlled study	EPI morphine infusion as effective as other two methods, but fewer side-effects	El-Baz, 1984
Abdominal surgery for obesity	EPI morphine versus i.m. morphine	RPDB	Analgesia same for both, but dose of morphine less for EPI. EPI superior for mobilization, pulmonary complications, bowel function, hospital stay	Rawal, 1984
Upper abdominal	EPI morphine versus intercostal local anesthetic versus i.v. fentanyl infusion + 'on-demand' boli	Controlled study	Pain at 2 and 24 h similar in all three groups. Efficacy rating similar. Time to supplemental analgesia longest in EPI morphine group. Pulmonary effects similar	Rosenberg, 1984
Thoractomy	EPI versus i.v. boli of morphine	RPDB	EPI, less pain at 2 and 8 h. No differences in pulmonary function.	Shulman, 1984
Abdominal surgery	EPI morphine versus EPI saline given intraoperatively	Double-blind multicenter	EPI morphine significantly longer analgesia, decreased requirements for i.m. morphine	Writer, 1985
Thoracotomy	EPI versus i.m. nicromorphine on patient demand	Controlled study	Both groups rapid and effective analgesia. Fewer pulmonary complications in epidural group	Hasenbos, 1985a,b
Laminectomy	EPI versus i.m. morphine	Controlled study	Pain relief superior with EPI, but dose of morphine same	Rechtine, 1984
Abdominal surgery	i.m. morphine versus EPI bupivacaine 1st 24 h then EPI morphine 72 h	Controlled study	Pain better controlled with epidural. No difference in pulmonary, cardiac, wound, metabolic, thrombotic indices. Convalescence not improved by epidural.	Hjorts, 1985
Postcesarean section	EPI morphine versus i.v. morphine	Controlled study	Excellent pain relief in 76% in epidural group, in 36% in i.v. group	Cohen, 1983
	EPI bupivacaine versus EPI meperidine versus i.m. meperidine	RPDB 'within patient'	Epidural regimens superior to i.m. Significant patient preference for EPI meperidine	Brownridge, 1985
During labor	EPI fentanyl versus i.v. fentanyl in patients receiving EPI bupivacaine	RPDB	EPI fentanyl produced more rapid, intense, and long-lasting analgesia than i.v. fentanyl despite higher plasma concentrations with i.v.	Vella, 1985

RPDB = randomized prospective double-blind; i.m. = intramuscular: EPI = epidural; VAS = visual analogue scale.
[a]Note only first author and year are given. See full reference in reference list.

ministration' (Banning et al., 1986; Bonnet et al., 1984; Brownridge and Frewin, 1985; Cohen and Woods, 1983; Cullen et al., 1985; El-Baz et al., 1984; Gustafsson et al., 1986; Hasenbos et al., 1985a,b; Hjorts et al., 1985; Raj et al., 1985; Rawal et al., 1984; Rechtine et al., 1984; Rosenberg et al., 1984; Shulman et al., 1984; Vella et al., 1985; Writer et al., 1985; Yeager et al., 1987) (Table VI, Fig. 4). In a number of studies the epidural administration of opioid was associated with analgesia which was similar to that provided by epidural local anesthetic. However, patients receiving epidural opioid could ambulate and did not have episodes of hypotension compared to those receiving epidural local anesthetic. Pharmacokinetic studies of epidural local anesthetics have provided guidance for the safe infusion of low doses of the long-acting drug bupi-

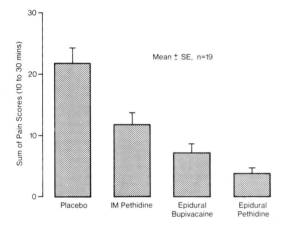

Fig. 4. Efficacy of epidural pethidine (meperidine) for relief of postoperative pain. A double-blind, within-patient comparison was made, with each patient receiving four treatments in random order. Each patient had an intramuscular 'butterfly' needle in situ and an epidural catheter. The following treatments were given in random order: intramuscular saline plus epidural bupivacaine; intramuscular saline plus epidural meperidine; intramuscular meperidine plus epidural saline; intramuscular saline plus epidural saline. The sums of the pain scores are shown for the time interval 10–30 min following injection. The epidural injections of bupivacaine or pethidine were superior to the intramuscular pethidine ($P > 0.01$). (Reproduced with permission from Brownridge, P. and Frewin, D.B. (1985) A comparative study of techniques of postoperative analgesia following cesarean section and lower abdominal surgery. Anaesth. Intens. Care, 13: 123–130.)

vacaine (Denson et al., 1983). Epidural infusion of opioid drugs has been reported to decrease the dose required to produce effective analgesia (El-Baz et al., 1984). It does seem logical to combine low doses of opioid and low doses of local anesthetic and indeed this has been reported to produce highly effective analgesia with a very low incidence of side-effects (Cullen et al., 1985). Adverse effects of pain on various organ systems are decreased by epidural opioids (Bonnet et al., 1984; Bromage et al., 1980). Such an approach has been reported to be useful for patients following very major and extensive surgery who are confined to bed during the initial 24–48 h and who require a very intense level of analgesia. The potential for effective pain control to influence the outcome of surgery has been underlined by a randomized prospective controlled study in high-risk surgical patients (Yeager et al., 1987). A control group received general anesthesia and standard intramuscular opioid postoperatively. The treatment group received supplementary epidural local anesthetic during general anesthesia and then postoperatively received epidural opioid. There was a striking decrease in the incidence of complications and in mortality in the group receiving epidural opioid (Table VII). In addition, the group receiving epidural opioid had substantially lower costs of medical treatment and hospitalization (Table VII). Because of the design of this study, it is unlikely that a type 1 error has been made. However, such important results need to be substantiated by further studies.

The spinal route for treatment of cancer pain

The first controlled study of the spinal administration of opioids concerned a single-dose study of intrathecal administration of morphine compared to placebo in cancer patients. This study clearly demonstrated the efficacy of intrathecal opioid (Wang et al., 1979). This study led to the insertion of chronically implanted intrathecal catheters which were connected to totally implanted pumps such as the 'Infusaid' (Coombs et al., 1984; Coombs, 1986).

TABLE VII

Acute pain relief with epidural local anesthetics and opioids: high-risk surgery (Yeager et al. 1987) Anesthesiology 66: 729

	Epidural (n = 25)	Control (n = 25)	P value
Mortality	0	4	0.04
Cardiovascular failure	4	13	0.007
Respiratory failure	1	8	0.009
Major infections	2	10	0.007
Complication rate	7/25	19/25	0.001
Cortisol 1st 24 h (μg/h)	37.2 ± 27.0	73.8 ± 61.9	0.025
Intubation time (h)	7.1 ± 10.1	81.8 ± 186.1	0.005
Mean costs	$15 019	$25 514	0.05

The authors included in their analysis three patients in the epidural group in whom an epidural catheter was not inserted despite randomization to receive one (their epidural group n = 28). In this analysis those three patients are excluded (n = 25). This affected the statistical analysis only for the total complication rate. In the author's original analysis the epidural group complication rate was 9/25, but this included 2 patients *without* an epidural catheter.

Opioids have also been administered in cancer patients by the epidural route (Cherry et al., 1985; Coombs, 1985; Zenz, 1985). Initially catheters were left in situ following a standard percutaneous placement, then by means of a catheter tunneled to the abdominal wall and exteriorized and then finally by an epidural catheter connected to a 'portal' which was totally implanted (Cherry et al., 1985). Epidural catheters have also been connected to an implanted Infusaid pump (Coombs, 1986). All of these approaches have been reported to be capable of producing effective relief of cancer pain for variable periods of time (Cherry et al., 1985; Coombs et al., 1984; Yentafridda et al., 1985). Unfortunately, there are no comparative data for the different methods of epidural insertion nor are there comparative studies for epidural versus intrathecal placement of catheters. The epidural route offers the advantage of retaining the protective functions of the dura; however, evidence has emerged of a fibrous reaction in the epidural space to conventional catheters

(Durant and Yaksh, 1986a). This may have been at least partly alleviated by the development of catheters made of silastic (Dupen, 1987) and other materials. Most appealing of these at the present time is a development of the Hickman and Broviac catheters, which have enjoyed over 100 patient years of use for intravenous feeding (Dupen, 1987). Ample clinical data now confirm that a catheter placed at the lumbar level is quite adequate for relief of cancer pain involving segmental distribution from cervical to sacral segments. This is because of the very wide dispersal of the water-soluble opioid morphine (see Cousins et al., 1987).

A critically important question relates to the relative efficacy of spinally administered opioids compared with alternative methods of relief of cancer pain such as the use of oral opioids and co-analgesic drugs, subcutaneous opioid infusion, transdermal opioid administration and other alternatives. It has been reported that in excess of 85% of cancer pain can be effectively managed by use of the 'WHO ladder' (Ventafridda et al., 1985). Subcutaneous infusion of opioid is now increasingly being used and has been reported to be effective. There is an urgent need for randomized prospective controlled studies of the comparative efficacy of spinal opioids and alternative methods of management.

Intuitively it would seem unlikely that administration of opioids by subcutaneous, transdermal or other routes would produce analgesia that was any different in efficacy or side-effects from a well-timed oral opioid regimen. This is because all of these methods rely upon the achievement and maintenance of effective blood concentrations of opioids. The only obvious advantage of subcutaneous and transdermal routes of administration would be in patients who were either unable or unwilling to take oral opioids. It seems quite likely that the superiority of the spinal route over other routes that has been demonstrated in the case of acute pain should also hold true in cancer pain. However, controlled data to answer this question are currently lacking. The problem of development of tolerance to spinal administration of opioids (Coombs et al., 1985) and the emergence of troublesome side-effects such as hyperalgesia at high doses of spinal opioids (Yaksh et al., 1987) require practical solutions. The availability of opioid drugs acting on different receptors (Onofrio and Yaksh, 1983; Yaksh, 1983) and non-opioid drugs (see Yaksh and Noueihed, 1985) appears to provide possible answers to these problems. There are currently no clear guidelines to indicate the advantages and disadvantages of sequential administration, co-administration or other regimens for use of these alternative agents by the spinal route in order to optimize the efficacy and to minimize side-effects.

Therapeutic index and individualization of therapy

A critical and neglected question in the spinal use of opioids relates to a clear identification of minimal effective dosage in each individual patient and documentation of the margin of safety between this dose and the emergence of side-effects (Cousins, 1987). Data available at the present time indicate that the ratio between a minimal effective epidural dose and a dose that will produce side-effects is approximately two (Cousins and Mather, 1984). In view of the substantial variability in transfer of opioid across the dura, in absorption of opioids into the blood stream (Glynn et al., 1982; Sjostrom et al., 1987a,b) and in individual requirements for analgesia, it is clear that careful titration of dose of spinal opioid in individual patients is critical. This is by no means surprising, since precisely the same situation exists for the administration of opioids by any other route. Indeed this is also the case for the administration of epidural local anesthetics, where the margin of safety is also in the vicinity of two (see Cousins and Bromage, 1987). Failure to pay

due attention to this therapeutic index will result in the administration of inappropriately large doses of spinal opioid in individual patients so that a predominant spinal action will be lost and any resultant analgesia will be as much determined by brain effects as by spinal effects (Cousins, 1987). This would negate any advantage of the spinal route of administration. Infusions of low doses of local anesthetics and opioids were developed in order to minimize the dose of both classes of drugs and presumably to decrease the potential for side-effects while retaining an efficacious spinal action. In the near future this will also lead to the co-administration of opioid and non-opioid drugs, such as alpha-agonists, to achieve analgesia but with the avoidance of the blockade of other neural modalities produced by local anesthetics. This approach is likely to achieve a further development of the concept of 'selective spinal analgesia' (Cousins et al., 1979).

Conclusion

In conclusion, the intrathecal and epidural routes for local anesthetics were introduced in 1898 and 1921, respectively. However, optimal clinical use closely paralleled detailed studies of the physiology and pharmacology of these techniques 50 years later in the decade 1970–1980. The spinal route for opioids was first used in 1979. It is likely that optimal use of spinal opioids and further refinements of 'selective spinal analgesia' will depend upon studies in man similar to those which permitted safe and effective use of local anesthetics by the spinal route. In this context the development of opioid and non-opioid drugs with more selectivity for spinal cord receptors associated with pain relief will likely permit major advances for this route of administration.

References

Arner, S. and Arner, B. (1985) Differential effects of epidural morphine in the treatment of cancer-related pain. Acta Anaesthesiol. Scand., 29: 32–36.

Banning, A.M., Schmidt, J.F., Chraemmer, J., et al. (1986) Comparison of oral controlled release morphine and epidural morphine in the management of postoperative pain. Anesth.

Analg., 65: 385–388.

Bonnet, F., Blery, C., Zatan, M., et al. (1984) Effects of epidural morphine on post-operative pulmonary dysfunction. Acta Anaesthesiol. Scand., 28: 147–151.

Bromage, P.R., Camporesi, E. and Chestnut, D. (1980) Epidural narcotics for postoperative analgesia. Anesth. Analg., 59: 473–480.

Bromage, P.R., Camporesi, E.M., Durant, P.A. and Nielsen,

C.H. (1982) Rostral spread of epidural morphine. Anesthesiology, 56: 431–436.

Brownridge, P. and Frewin, D.B. (1985) A comparative study of techniques of postoperative analgesia following cesarean section and lower abdominal surgery. Anaesth. Intens. Care, 13: 123–130.

Cherry, D.A., Gourlay, G.K., Cousins, M.J. and Gannon, B.J. (1985) A technique for the insertion of an implantable portal system for the long term epidural administration of opioids in the treatment of cancer pain. Anaesth. Intens. Care, 13: 145–153.

Cohen, S.E. and Woods, W.A. (1983) The role of epidural morphine in the post-cesarean patient: efficacy and effects of bonding. Anesthesiology, 58: 500–504.

Coombs, D.W. (1986) Management of chronic pain by epidural and intrathecal opioids. Newer drugs and delivery systems. In U.H. Sjostrand and N. Rawal (Eds.), Regional Opioids in Anesthesiology and Pain Management, Int. Anesthesiol. Clin., 24: 24–58.

Coombs, D., Maurer, L.H., Saunders, R.L. and Gaylor, M. (1984) Outcomes and complications of continuous intraspinal narcotic analgesia for cancer pain control. J. Clin. Oncol., 2: 1414–1420.

Coombs, D.W., Fratkin, J.D., Meier, F.A. et al. (1985a) Neuropathologic lesions and CSF morphine concentrations during chronic continuous intraspinal morphine infusion. A clinical and post-mortem study. Pain, 22: 337–351.

Coombs, D.W., Saunders, R.L., LaChance, D., Savage, S., Ragnarson, T.S. and Jensen, L. (1985b) Intrathecal morphine tolerance: use of intrathecal clonidine, DADLE, and intraventricular morphine. Anesthesiology, 62: 358–363.

Cousins, M.J. (Editorial) (1987) Comparative pharmacokinetics of spinal opioids in humans: a step toward the determination of relative safety. Anesthesiology, 67: 1–2.

Cousins, M.J. and Bromage, P.R. (1987) Epidural neural blockade. In M.J. Cousins Neural Blockade in Clinical Anesthesia and Management of Pain, 2nd edn., J.B. Lippincott, Philadelphia, pp. 253–360.

Cousins, M.J. and Mather, L.E. (1984) Intrathecal and epidural administration of opioids. Anesthesiology, 61: 276–310.

Cousins, M.J. and Phillips, G.D. (Eds.) (1986) Acute Pain Management, Churchill Livingstone, New York.

Cousins, M.J., Mather, L.E., Glynn, C.J., Wilson, P.R. and Graham, J.R. (1979) Selective spinal analgesia. Lancet, *i*: 1141–1142.

Cousins, M.J., Mather, L.E. and Gourlay, G.K. (1984) Axon, spinal cord and brain: Targets for acute pain control. In D.B. Scott, J. McClure and J.A. Wildsmith (Eds.), Regional Anaesthesia, J.H. Schultz, Copenhagen, pp. 120–132.

Cullen, M.L., Staren, E.D., el-Ganzouri, A., Logas, W.G., Ivankovich, A.D. and Economou, S.G. (1985) Continuous epidural infusion for analgesia after major abdominal operations: A randomized, prospective, double-blind study. Surgery, 98: 718–728.

Denson, D.D., Raj, P.P., Saldahna, F., Furnsson, R.A., Ritschel, W.A., et al. (1983) Continuous peridural infusion of bu-

pivacaine for prolonged analgesia. Pharmacokinetics considerations, Int. J. Clin. Pharmacol., 21: 591.

Dupen, S.L., Peterson, D.G., Bogosian, A.C., Ramsey, D.H., Larson, C. and Omoto, M. (1987) A new permanent exteriorized epidural catheter for narcotic self-administration to control cancer pain. Cancer, 59: 986–993.

Durant, P.A. and Yaksh, T.L. (1986a) Epidural injections of bupivacaine, morphine, fentanyl, lofentanil, and DADL in chronically implanted rats: a pharmacologic and pathologic study. Anesthesiology, 64: 43–53.

Durant, P.A. and Yaksh, T.L. (1986b) Distribution in cerebrospinal fluid, blood and lymph of epidurally injected morphine and inulin in dogs. Anesth. Analg., 65: 583–592.

El-Baz, N.M., Faber, L.P. and Jensik, R.J. (1984) Continuous epidural infusion of morphine for treatment of pain after thoracic surgery: a new technique. Anesth. Analg., 63: 757–764.

Glynn, C.J., Mather, L.E., Cousins, M.J., Graham, J.R. and Wilson, P.R. (1982) Peridural meperidine in humans: analgetic response, pharmacokinetics and transmission into CSF. Anesthesiology, 55: 520–526.

Glynn, C.J., Mather, L.E., Cousins, M.J., Wilson, P.R. and Graham, J.R. (1979) Spinal narcotics and respiratory depression. Lancet, ii: 356–357.

Gourlay, G.K., Cherry, D.A. and Cousins, M.J. (1985) Cephalad migration of morphine in CSF following lumbar epidural administration in patients with cancer pain. Pain, 23: 317–326.

Gourlay, G.K., Cherry, D.A., Plummer, J.L., Armstrong, P.J. and Cousins, M.J. (1987) The influence of drug polarity on the absorption of opioid drugs into CSF and subsequent cephalad migration following lumbar epidural administration: application to morphine and pethidine. Pain, 31: 297–305.

Gustafsson, L.L., Ackerman, S., Adamson, H., Garle, M., Rane, A. and Schildt, B. (1984) Kinetics of morphine in cerebrospinal fluid after epidural administration. Acta Anaesthesiol. Scand., 28: 535–538.

Gustaffsson, L.L., Friberg-Nielsen, S. and Garle, M. (1982) Extradural and parenteral morphine: kinetics and effects in postoperative pain. A controlled clinical study. Br. J. Anaesth., 54: 1167.

Gustafsson, L.L., Garle, M., Johannisson, J., Rane, A., Stenport, J. and Walson, P. (1982b) Regional epidural analgesia: kinetics of pethidine. Acta Anaesthesiol. Scand., 74 (Suppl.): 165.

Gustafsson, L.L., Johannisson, J. and Garle, M. (1986) Extradural and parenteral pethidine as analgesia after total hip replacement: effects and kinetics. A controlled clinical study. Eur. J. Clin. Pharmacol., 29: 529.

Hasenbos, M., Van Egmond, J., Gielen, M. and Crul, J.F. (1985b) Post-operative analgesia by epidural versus intramuscular nicomorphine after thoracotomy. Pt. I. Acta Anaesthesiol. Scand., 29: 572.

Hasenbos, M., Van Egmond, J., Gielen, M. and Crul, J.F. (1985) Post-operative analgesia by epidural versus intramuscular nicomorphine after thoracotomy. Pt. II. Acta Anaesthesiol. Scand., 29: 577.

Hjorts, N.C., Neumann, P., Frsig, F., Andersen, T., Lindhard,

A., Rogon, E. and Kehlet, H. (1985) A controlled study on the effect of epidural analgesia with local anaesthetics and morphine on morbidity after abdominal surgery. Acta Anaesthesiol. Scand., 29: 790.

Lam, A.M., Knill, R.I., Thompson, W.R., Clement, J.I., Varkey, G.P. and Spoerel, W.E. (1983) Epidural fentanyl does not cause delayed respiratory depression. Can. Anaesth. Soc. J., 30: 578.

Max, M.B., Inturrisi, C.E., Kaiko, R.F., Grabinski, P.Y., Li, C.H. and Foley, K.M. (1985) Epidural and intrathecal opiates: Cerebrospinal fluid and plasma profiles in patients with chronic cancer pain. Clin. Pharmacol. Ther., 38: 631–641.

Nordberg, G. (1984) Pharmacokinetic aspects of spinal morphine analgesia. Acta Anaesthesiol. Scand., 28 (Suppl. 79): 1–38.

Nordberg, G., Hedner, T., Mellstrand, T. and Dahlstrom, B. (1983) Pharmacokinetic aspects of epidural morphine analgesia. Anesthesiology, 58: 545–551.

Onofrio, B.M. and Yaksh, T.L. (1983) Intrathecal delta-receptor ligand produces analgesia in man. Lancet, i: 1386–1387.

Payne, R. and Inturrisi, C.E. (1985) CSF distribution of morphine, methadone and sucrose after intrathecal injection. Life Sci., 37: 1137–1144.

Raj, P.P., Knarr, D., Vigdorth, E., et al. (1985) Comparative study of continuous epidural infusions versus systemic analgesics in postoperative pain relief. Anesthesiology, 63: A238.

Rawal, N., Mollefors, K., Axelsson, K., Lingardh, G. and Widman, B. (1981) Naloxone reversal of urinary retention after epidural morphine. Lancet, ii: 1411–1412.

Rawal, N., Mollefors, K., Axelsson, K., Lingardh, G. and Widman, B. (1983) An experimental study of urodynamic effects of epidural morphine and of naloxone reversal. Anesth. Analg., 62: 641–647.

Rawal, N., Sjostrand, U., Christoffersson, E., Dahlstrom, B., Arvill, A. and Rydman, H. (1984) Comparison of intramuscular epidural morphine for postoperative analgesia in the grossly obese: influence on postoperative ambulation and pulmonary function. Anesth. Analg., 63: 583–592.

Rawal, N., Schott, U., Dahlstrom, B., Inturrisi, C.E., Tandon, B., Sjostrand, U. and Wennhager, M. (1986) Influence of naloxone on analgesia and respiratory depression following epidural morphine. Anesthesiology, 64: 194–201.

Rawal, N., Arner, S., Gustafsson, L.L. and Allvin, R. (1987) Present state of extradural and intrathecal opioid analgesia in Sweden. Br. J. Anaesth., 59: 791–799.

Rechtine, G.R., Reinert, C.M. and Bohlman, H.H. (1984) The use of epidural morphine to decrease postoperative pain in patients undergoing lumbar laminectomy. J. Bone Joint. Surg. (Am.), 66: 113–116.

Rosenberg, P.H., Heino, A. and Scheinin, B. (1984) Comparison of intrasmuscular analgesia, intercostal block, epidural morphine and on-demand-i.v. fentanyl in the control of pain after abdominal surgery. Acta Anaesthesiol. Scand., 28: 603–607.

Scott, D.B. (1987) Acute pain management. In M.J. Cousins and P.O. Bridenbaugh (Eds.), Neural Blockade in Clinical Anesthesia and Management of Pain, 2nd edn., J.B. Lippincott, Philadelphia, pp. 861–884.

Sjostrom, S., Hartvig, P., Persson, T. and Tamsen, A. (1987a) Pharmacokinetics of epidural morphine and meperidine in humans. Anesthesiology, 67: 877–888.

Sjostrom, S., Tamsen, A., Persson, P. and Hartvig, P. (1987b) Pharmacokinetics of intrathecal morphine and meperidine in humans. Anesthesiology, 67: 889–895.

Strichartz, G.R. (1987) Neural physiology and local anesthetic action. In M.J. Cousins and P.O. Bridenbaugh (Eds.), Neural Blockade in Clinical Anesthesia and Management of Pain, 2nd edn., J.B. Lippincott, Philadelphia, pp. 25–46.

Shulman, M., Sandler, A.N., Bradley, J.W., Young, P.S. and Brebner, J. (1984) Post-thoracotomy pain and pulmonary function following epidural and systemic morphine. Anesthesiology, 61: 569–575.

Vella, L.M., Willatts, D.G., Knott, C., Lintin, D.J., Justins, D.M. and Reynolds, F. (1985) Epidural fentanyl in labour. An evaluation of the systemic contribution of analgesia. Anaesthesia, 40: 741–747.

Ventafridda, V., Tamburini, M. and DeConno, F. (1985) Comprehensive treatment in cancer pain. In H. Fields et al. (Eds.), Advances in Pain Research and Therapy, Vol. 9, Raven Press, New York, p. 617.

Wang, J.K., Nauss, L.E. and Thomas, J.E. (1979) Pain relief by intrathecally applied morphine in man. Anesthesiology, 50: 149–151.

Willer, J.D., Bergeret, S. and Gaudy, J.H. (1985) Epidural morphine strongly depresses nociceptive flexion reflexes in patients with postoperative pain. Anesthesiology, 63: 675–680.

Woolf, C.J. and Wiesenfeld-Hallin, Z. (1985) The systemic administration of local anesthetics produces a selective depression of c-afferent fiber evoked activity in the spinal cord. Pain 23: 361–374.

Writer, W.D., Hurtig, J.B., Evans, D., Needs, R.E., Hope, C.E. and Forrest, J.B. (1985) Epidural morphine prophylaxis of postoperative pain: report of a double-blind multicentre study. Can. Anaesth. Soc. J., 32: 330–338.

Yaksh, T.L. (1981) Spinal opiate analgesia: characteristics and principles of action. Pain, 11: 293–346.

Yaksh, T.L. (1983) In vivo studies on spinal opiate receptor systems mediating antinociception. 1. Mu and delta receptor profiles in the primate. J. Pharmacol. Exp. Ther., 226: 303–316.

Yaksh, T.L. and Noueihed, R. (1985) The physiology and pharmacology of spinal opiates. Annu. Rev. Pharmacol. Toxicol., 25: 433–462.

Yaksh, T.L. and Rudy, T.A. (1976) Analgesia mediated by a direct spinal action of narcotics. Science, 192: 1357–1358.

Yaksh, T.L., Harty, G.J. and Onofrio, B.M. (1987) High doses of spinal morphine produce a non-opiate receptor mediated hyperesthesia. Practical and theoretical implications. Anesthesiology, in press.

Yeager, M.P., Glass, D.D., Neff, R.K. and Brinck-Johnsen, T. (1987) Epidural anesthesia and analgesia in high risk surgical patients. Anesthesiology, 66: 729–736.

Zenz, M. (1985) Epidural opiates: long-term experiences in cancer pain. Klin. Wochenschr., 63: 225–229.

R. Dubner, G.F. Gebhart & M.R. Bond (Eds.)
Proceedings of the Vth World Congress on Pain
© 1988 Elsevier Science Publishers BV (Biomedical Division)

CHAPTER 52

Analgesic effect of epidural clonidine

H. Germain, A. Néron and A. Lomssy

Department of Anesthesiology, St-Luc Hospital, 1058 St-Denis Street, Montreal, PQ H2X 3J4 Canada

Introduction

Although the analgesic effect of intrathecal clonidine has been demonstrated in animals, few authors have studied its usefulness and limitations in man at the spinal level (Lipman and Spencer, 1979; Reddy and Yaksh, 1980; Fielding et al., 1981; Yaksh and Reddy, 1981).

We have begun a study focusing on the quality of analgesia and the side-effects obtained by epidural clonidine. After the injection, we assessed the analgesic and hypotensive effects of clonidine given by this route and here report the preliminary results.

Methodology

Twenty-four patients, mean age 54 (range 21–80 years) and mean weight 62.8 kg (range 42.0–94.7 kg), suffering from acute or chronic pain were asked to participate in the study (see Table I). The protocol was approved and signed informed consent was obtained. Patients excluded from the study included those with neuropsychiatric problems (re: the psychotropic effect of clonidine), those with hypertensive or cardiac problems (re: the hemodynamic effect of clonidine), those with cerebrovascular accident or significant carotid stenosis and those who were breast-feeding (cases of post-caesarian pain).

All patients already had an epidural catheter in place and three subgroups were created: (i) obstetrical group, for postoperative pain relief; (ii) pain clinic group (outpatient), for steroid infiltration; (iii) surgical group, for postoperative pain relief.

Patients were closely observed for the first 100 min in the recovery room (monitoring of blood pressure and cardiac rhythm every 3 min) and then regularly on the care unit (by nursing staff) for the next 24–72 h. Patients on continuous infusion were monitored regularly until drug withdrawal. A subjective evaluation of the analgesic effect by a visual analogue scale (VAS) was performed. Side-effects were also noted. In postoperative cases other parameters were observed, namely early coughing, early movement, and facility in performing physiotherapy exercises.

The systolic blood pressure was recorded in standing and recumbent positions for some cases.

When possible, we measured the oxygen saturation because a decrease had been reported in one animal study (unpublished).

The pain was graded from 0 (no pain at all) to 100 (unbearable pain) by Huskisson's visual analogue scale (VAS). The baseline VAS was determined and an initial bolus dose of 4 μg/kg of clonidine HC1 (without preservative) in 10 ml of normal saline was injected (clonidine HC1 (Catapress®; 150 μg/ml)). After 30 min the VAS was noted and if greater than 30 the 4 μg/km dose was repeated. Thirty minutes after the second dose, the VAS was noted again and if greater than 30, a 2 μg/kg dose was given and repeated every 30 min until the VAS

TABLE I
Patients' characteristics

Sex	Age	Height (m)	Weight (kg)	Diagnosis
M	55	1.65	65.6	Arachnoiditis
M	34	1.72	76.0	Lumbar plexopathy
M	49	1.60	53.5	Lung carcinoma
M	61	1.65	42.0	Lung adenocarcinoma
M	61	1.72	60.0	Phantom limb
M	60	1.66	48.5	Leg ischemia
F	44	1.64	55.0	Breast adenocarcinoma
F	80	1.50	55.0	Post-op. cholecystectomy
M	63		75.0	Post-op. intestinal resection
M	67		55.0	Post-op. anterior resection
F	21		60.0	Cesarian section
M	56		75.0	Gastrectomy

was decreased to 0 or until the secondary effects compelled us to stop the drug (e.g., systolic blood pressure lower than 80 mmHg or a drop of 30% from the baseline).

During the study no other sedative or analgesic drug was infused concomitantly (only one patient with poor control was on morphine infusion).

In the outpatient group, no additional clonidine was injected after the first clinical effect had been achieved. In the obstetrical group, the efficient total bolus dose was repeated as soon as the VAS was greater than 30. In the postoperative group, as soon as the patient regained consciousness and had a VAS greater than 30, a volumetric infusion was begun (efficient dose/kg/hour as determined in the bolus dose).

Results

Since reports on the effects of clonidine administered epidurally in humans were scarce, we had little idea of the kind and amplitude of relief we could obtain with clonidine. In our experiment we observed an analgesic effect within minutes after to-

tal dose of 10 μg/kg of clonidine, lasting from 4 to approximately 72 h (mean 6–8 h). Analgesia was of sufficient magnitude in nearly all patients to bring the VAS near 0.

In four patients we maintained a constant infusion lasting from 5 to 23 days; two of four patients obtained an excellent analgesia (VAS = 0), while the two others were poorly controlled (VAS > 30) with clonidine or even other drugs (i.m. meperidine Demerol®).

The small sample and the qualitative nature of our study prevent us from making firm conclusions about the duration of the analgesic effect. Whatever the cause of pain, in no case did the pain recur within 4 h. We may infer that there is some evidence that clonidine given by the epidural route may produce a sustained analgesia.

Side-effects
No evidence of respiratory depression or decrease in blood oxygen saturation was observed. What we noted were sedation, dryness of the mouth, hypotension, headache (2 cases) and diaphoresis (1 case).

Sedation. All patients experienced moderate to deep sedation (many fell asleep) but were easily arousable (two patients were aroused with 2 doses of physostigmine 0.5 mg (Antilirium®)). Even when patients on continuous infusion received high doses of clonidine (up to 1.3 mg/day), they soon recovered from the initial sedation with an alert sensorium.

We had one patient who, at a dosage of 1.2 mg/day, experienced confusion and vivid dreams, which ceased with withdrawal of the clonidine and reappeared when we restarted the medication. No other patient manifested this reaction, which disappeared with the withdrawal of clonidine.

One patient on continuous infusion had somnolence that prevented him from following regular postoperative physiotherapy.

Dryness of the mouth. All patients reported and some complained about dryness of the mouth, which persisted during treatment and was alleviated

TABLE II

Systolic, diastolic and cardiac rhythm (11 patients, 33 measures)

(1) 729

112 120 114 118 108 105 96 87 92 88 84 82 82 79 80 77 74 85 82 78 73 77 76 76 80 74 78 77 82 83 77 86 91
 74 80 78 77 71 73 69 67 68 63 63 58 55 54 58 56 51 54 58 57 54 52 51 52 56 54 55 51 53 57 54 53 56
108 105 105 104 102 102 101 97 96 98 97 96 92 92 91 91 90 90 90 90 88 91 89 88 87 87 89 87 89 87 89 86 89

(2) 13788

118 114 107 113 110 106 103 99 101 104 104 99 102 100 97 97 110 86 99 102 99 103 106 108 101 106 102 99 104 95 107 103 99
 65 65 64 66 63 62 68 61 57 60 60 58 57 58 61 61 55 60 58 59 58 67 59 49 59 60 62 60 64 59 59 62 55
 85 82 83 84 80 78 79 70 80 73 73 75 72 75 72 72 69 70 70 73 72 70 76 70 70 70 75 72 71 70 74 71 75

(3) 45434

117 129 114 113 106 107 106 110 110 110 107 106 103 108 101 97 96 104 103 98 93 94 84 90 103 92 86 87 94 91 96 96 89
 74 78 74 73 71 71 68 72 66 66 69 66 65 65 67 60 60 57 51 57 54 60 65 56 53 58 56 56 59 53 72 72 54
 82 86 78 81 76 78 77 77 78 78 76 75 76 74 74 75 72 67 69 68 75 75 73 73 70 66 66 68 72 64 75 75 63

(4) 75563

151 144 161 127 137 139 118 137 121 121 116 119 123 107 119 114 117 108 105 103 108 106 107 108 98 110 118 113 108 107 105 108 103
 88 89 87 84 91 79 92 80 78 75 73 68 70 80 73 71 69 66 64 65 70 64 62 63 62 60 63 82 61 61 59 62 63
 78 76 75 72 80 77 81 77 77 78 77 75 76 82 72 72 72 74 74 73 74 73 74 72 73 75 74 73 72 71 72 72 70

(5) 105346

125 117 120 113 120 118 108 114 102 93 97 100 97 107 104 100 109 99 96 99 103 106 110 105 97 100 98 95 105 103 94 104 107
 80 71 84 73 70 60 63 70 58 63 62 64 61 57 58 58 60 53 57 54 60 58 60 71 62 61 61 62 57 64 61 57 60
 72 71 82 66 68 73 63 69 63 61 63 60 61 61 60 62 59 61 58 60 60 60 57 68 63 61 57 57 57 61 59 59 68

(6) 140752

127 137 128 118 115 119 105 113 109 106 99 93 93 103 90 100 103 95 100 91 96 94 98 100 99 97 91 103 94 94 98 102 93
 85 85 83 77 71 68 69 69 56 55 59 59 60 51 54 57 59 56 63 58 61 60 64 58 60 59 53 50 60 57 60 62 60
 78 74 66 74 68 70 69 68 66 66 64 65 65 63 64 64 64 63 61 60 59 60 59 60 60 60 59 64 57 57 58 60 55

(7) 168177

124 127 142 103 103 106 106 104 100 100 93 92 91 98 87 85 87 80 89 90 62 89 91 93 98 96 90 99 91 87 85 85 100
 58 49 38 55 60 52 53 50 48 47 42 46 44 38 46 43 31 37 49 42 42 44 49 51 46 44 48 43 49 46 37 45 50
117 121 121 115 119 117 119 103 111 115 108 103 106 105 106 97 103 103 97 102 99 103 106 108 105 105 103 96 108 108 103 95 103

(8) 215397

125 121 120 113 109 104 113 107 111 107 109 106 116 117 107 109 105 103 114 116 111 114 116 113 109 107 116 116 105 107 105 109 103
 80 78 72 73 71 71 69 70 69 67 70 72 70 66 70 71 68 71 70 70 65 70 68 67 68 71 71 70 64 63 65 68 69
 59 56 58 54 52 51 52 52 52 52 50 49 49 52 50 49 50 50 50 51 52 50 50 51 50 50 50 52 52 52 50 49 51

(9) 216581

135 129 135 122 118 116 114 112 110 113 110 103 103 108 106 111 109 104 98 104 104 100 107 112 102 101 101 109 110 96 105 102 108
 79 78 77 71 72 69 66 67 67 68 67 68 65 66 64 61 62 62 60 58 59 61 62 59 64 62 62 63 44 48 54 59 64
 78 76 77 75 77 75 75 74 75 75 73 75 72 72 70 69 70 71 73 72 71 67 65 64 66 64 65 64 64 60 63 63 62

(10) 227440

 87 81 79 73 84 75 72 73 81 78 75 76 71 61 68 92 92 92 90 93 94 96 89 92 88 85 94 89 92 90 92 91 88
 48 44 40 42 38 36 36 35 41 37 37 36 37 34 34 53 54 54 50 50 52 51 50 49 49 50 51 52 52 50 53 50 47
 72 70 62 66 65 64 63 63 65 62 55 61 61 59 61 58 57 57 55 53 53 52 53 55 55 55 54 53 55 55 57 55 55

(11) 239865

151 142 129 127 126 125 115 107 102 99 96 92 88 83 87 90 78 82 79 82 79 76 74 79 74 78 67 81 85 84 90 89 87
 85 88 84 81 78 73 74 70 64 63 58 53 52 54 47 51 49 49 47 45 42 46 45 45 46 43 45 48 51 50 55 49 51
131 115 113 110 110 110 113 108 105 108 105 105 104 111 101 100 97 100 98 97 98 97 96 96 96 94 93 89 88 87 87 88 88

after the drug had been stopped; one patient presented a parotiditis episode which subsequently necessitated antibiotic therapy.

Hypotensive effect. Before the injection, all patients received at least 500 ml of Ringer's lactate (R.L.) to ensure a good volemic status. Despite this fact, hypotensive episodes happened. In the eleven patients whose blood pressure and cardiac rhythm were suited for statistical analysis (Table II), the decreases in systolic and diastolic pressures and in cardiac rhythm were significant ($P < 0.0001$, analysis of variance). This effect was counteracted by R.L. bolus when necessary. Because of the initial screening, which excluded patients with atherosclerotic heart disease or cerebral deficit perfusion, no fall in blood pressure caused any clinical problem.

Headache. In two cases, headache was noted and disappeared spontaneously in a few hours.

Diaphoresis. This effect was transient and was seen in only one patient.

Blood oxygen saturation. In the majority of patients we noticed an initial change in skin coloration which tended to become grayish, but no coldness of extremities or decrease in blood oxygen saturation occurred in three patients who were observed with a saturometer.

Neurological exam. In all cases, the neurological examination was normal; there was no modification of tactile perception, motor strength or reflexes.

The side-effects observed with epidural clonidine are also encountered with the oral form of the drug. It is to be noted, however, that in no circumstance did we find a hypertensive rebound after completion of the treatment (infusion was tapered off slowly over two days).

Discussion

At first, we were impressed by reports stating that intrathecal clonidine could produce analgesia in a variety of animal models (Lipman and Spencer, 1979; Reddy and Yaksh, 1980; Fielding et al., 1981; Yaksh and Reddy, 1981). What we did not know was whether epidural clonidine was an acceptable alternative route and, if so, at what doses, and finally what side-effects would be encountered.

The epidural route seemed easier to adopt for practical reasons such as the lower risk of infection and the possibility of long-term use via an in situ catheter. A positive result would finally prove that this procedure could replace or complement the antinociceptive effect of epidural opioids for postoperative pain. Unfortunately, the early mobilization of patients was limited by the nature and number of side-effects encountered in our study. More studies are necessary to decide on the cost/benefit ratio of epidural clonidine for pain-relief purposes. Our study tended to demonstrate that clonidine, like other alpha-adrenergic receptor agonists, produces significant elevation of the nociceptive threshold if administered epidurally in humans. Because clonidine acts by a mechanism different from that of the opioids, it could be used in tolerant patients to allow their receptors to rest (Lopachin and Maixner, 1981).

Chronically hypertensive or atherosclerotic patients were excluded from our study, and so with the efficient 10 µg/kg bolus we observed no clinically dangerous hypotension. We do not know how much of the injected dose gained access to the systemic circulation and contributed to the hypotensive effect. We must certainly emphasize the fact that no respiratory depression was clinically observed and this allows clonidine to be considered for patients usually at risk for this complication.

Because each subject served as his own control and usually no other medication was given, there is no doubt that the analgesic effect was almost solely the result of clonidine's action on alpha-2 receptors. Some patients in the postoperative period had to receive intramuscular narcotics to ensure good analgesia. Clonidine appears to be a relatively weak analgesic agent for that particular purpose.

Due to the small number of continuous infusions, no conclusion can be drawn about the build-up of tolerance. In postoperative patients we had to increase the doses because the initial pain had not been brought under control. These should be interpreted as adjustments of the initial dose. There is still clearly a need for a non-opioid analgesic devoid of addictive or tolerance effects. Further studies could throw light on this point.

As it has been shown that intrathecal injection of clonidine and norepinephrine reduce lumbar sympathetic efferent activity, one could infer that at least some of the relief obtained is caused by chemical sympathectomy (Lopachin and Maixner, 1981).

Conclusion

The limited extent of our study precludes any conclusive statement, but we have observed that epidural clonidine can produce an analgesic effect of long duration. The main side-effect is hypotension and it requires close monitoring. It can be circumvented by conventional support in selected patients.

Many questions remain unanswered, namely the net effect (analgesia and side-effects) of mixing clonidine and opioids, the effect of introducing clonidine in a patient tolerant to epidural opioids, and the compatibility of mixing clonidine and opioids or clonidine and local anesthetics.

Acknowledgements

The authors wish to thank Carole Florence for technical assistance, Danielle Beaulieu, M.D., and Gérard Nault, M.D., for their valuable help in the preparation of the manuscript, and Mr. Delorme for statistical analysis.

References

Fielding, S., Spaulding, T.C. and Lal, H. (1981) Antinociceptive action of clonidine. In Psychopharmacology of Clonidine. Alan R. Liss, New York, pp. 225–242.

Lipman, J.J. and Spencer, P.S.J. (1979) Further evidence for a central site of action for the antinociceptive effect of clonidine-like drugs. Neuropharmacology, 18: 731–733.

Lo Pachin, A. and Maixner, W. (1981) The effects of intrathecal sympathomimetic agents on neural activity in the lumbar sympathetic chain of rats. Brain Res., 224: 195–198.

Reddy, S.V.R. and Yaksh, T.L. (1980) Spinal noradrenergic terminal system mediates antinociception. Brain Res., 189: 391–401.

Spaulding, T.C., Fielding, S., Venafro, J.J. and Lal, H. (1979) Antinociceptive activity of clonidine and its potentiation of morphine analgesia. Eur. J. Pharmacol., 58: 19–25.

Yaksh, T.L. and Reddy, S.V.R. (1981) Studies in the primate on the analgetic effects associated with intrathecal actions of opiates, α-adrenergic agonists and baclofen. Anesthesiology, 54: 451–467.

R. Dubner, G.F. Gebhart & M.R. Bond (Eds.)
Proceedings of the Vth World Congress on Pain
© 1988 Elsevier Science Publishers BV (Biomedical Division)

CHAPTER 53

Spinal cord ablation procedures for pain

Marc Sindou and Antonio Daher

Department of Neurosurgery, Hôpital Neurologique Pierre Wertheimer, Lyon 69003, France

Introduction

In the last two decades, neurostimulation and intrathecal morphine therapy have assumed an important place in the armamentarium of pain treatment. Clinical experience suggested that these methods were only effective in deafferentation syndromes with a sufficient integrity of the corresponding lemniscal pathways and in neoplasms with a short life expectancy. That is the reason why ablative procedures are still useful for some types of pain. Peripheral neurotomies or dorsal rhizotomies should only be applied to the treatment of pain in limited regions of the body, since extensive denervation could create or increase deafferentation phenomena. On the other hand, because of the wide dispersion of nociceptive projections to the cerebrum, ablative procedures at the brain level are associated with high rates of failure and recurrence. Therefore ablative procedures at the spinal cord level deserve consideration for the treatment of intractable pain.

In this report, the authors have analysed the results of their own series and those published in the literature.

Commissural myelotomy

First carried out by Armour in 1927, at the suggestion of Greenfield, and by Leriche in 1928, commissural myelotomy (CM) is aimed at dividing the nociceptive and thermoreceptive fibers which decussate from both sides of the body in the anterior white commissure, over the spinal cord segments corresponding to the painful territory. According to Guillaume et al. (1949), the myelotomy should be moved rostrally, on the assumption that the spino-reticulo-thalamic fibers cross the midline up to two or three segments above the level at which the corresponding dorsal roots enter the cord. Similarly, Lippert et al. (1974) have pointed out that the cord incision is better placed too high, i.e., above the estimated root level, than just at the estimated level.

CM has been mostly used at the thoraco-lumbar level for pain in the abdomen, pelvis and/or perineal region (95.7% of the reported cases); but the procedure has been also attempted at the cervical level for pain in the upper extemities and thorax (4.3%).

Opening of the dorsal fissure and interruption of the commissures may be performed either with a blunt instrument as classically described or with a CO_2-laser (Ascher, 1978; Fink, 1984) or an ultrasound probe (Richards et al., 1966). The use of microtechniques is of prime importance to avoid damaging the dorsal columns or injuring the anterior spinal artery.

In the 17 literature series that we have reviewed and which include 445 cases (see Ref. Note 1), CM was carried out for patients with advanced cancers in 86% and for pain from traumatic, inflammatory or degenerative origin in only 14%. Early pain relief was obtained in 67–100% of cases according to the authors, while late results, which were mentioned in only two of the 17 series, were favourable in 47–55%. The post-operative mortality rate ranged from zero to 14% (6% on average). Post-operative weakness was present in zero to 44% (12% on average), but in most cases was mild and transient. Permanent sphincter disturbances were reported in five of the 17 series, with an incidence of 11–33%. Persistent lemniscal sensory deficits were noticed in 5–13% of the patients. Post-operative dysesthesias or radicular-like pain were very frequent in the early post-operative period (more than 55% in all series), but remained important and long-lasting in only 6.4% of cases.

Because of the relatively low rate of long-lasting effects, CM has been used mainly for treatment of pain due to malignancies. The effectiveness of CM for limited midline rectal, perineal and sacral pain has been recognized by most of the authors, while it remains controversial for pain due to widespread invasion of the pelvic plexuses (Cook and Kawakami, 1977). Although rarely performed for bilateral upper limb and midline or bilateral thoracic pains, CM may be of some use for pain in such locations.

CM has the main advantage over bilateral antero-lateral cordotomy that a single incision may provide bilateral effects as long as the site of pain is limited. Pain relief can be achieved with CM with a lower morbidity in relation to permanent weakness and sphincterian disturbance than with bilateral cordotomy, but with a greater risk of at least transient hyperalgesia, dysesthesias and/or proprioceptive modifications.

All of the authors emphasize the difficulty in understanding: (1) the common finding of pain relief in areas not rendered analgesic to pin-prick in spite of a complete section of all the crossing fibers of the spino-thalamic tract and (2) the frequent analgesia extending downwards, far from the spinal cord segments operated on. To explain these facts, the effects of CM are hypothesized (Nathan et al., 1986) to be related to a combination of lesions, not only in the commissures, but also in deeper parts of the non-lemniscal system, especially the paleo-spino-re-ticular tracts and the slowly conducting multi-synaptic network lying in the central grey matter, as well as in some long second-order fibers situated at the base of the dorsal funiculi.

Extra-lemniscal myelotomy

Based on the postulated existence of a non-specific ascending pain pathway located around the central canal, Hitchcock (1970) and Schvarcz (1974) developed a new procedure, consisting of a radiofrequency (RF) lesion focused in the center of the spinal cord at the cervico-medullary junction, for treatment of pain throughout the body. An RF electrode with tip exposure of 1 mm is introduced percutaneously under local anesthesia, using a special stereotactic apparatus, through the atlanto-occipital ligament, into the cord, with impedance monitoring. The target is in the midline, 5 mm from the dorsal surface of the cord. The RF lesion, averaging 3 mm in diameter, is made fractionally at the site at which threshold stimulation evokes a tingling or electrical feeling in both distal lower limbs.

On the same basis, Gildenberg and Hirshberg (1984) carried out open central myelotomies with mechanical or RF lesions limited to a single segment at the thoraco-lumbar junction, for bilateral pelvic pain from cancerous origin.

In cancer pain, excellent or good results, for survival times ranging from 2 weeks to 24 months, were obtained in 87 and 78% of Hitchcock's (1970) and Schvarcz's (1978) 14 and 61 patients, respectively. Although Eiras et al. (1980) and Papo and Luongo (1976) had the same early good results, pain recurred after several months in five of the 12 cases of the former and in all of the nine patients for the latter. Gildenberg and Hirschberg (1984) obtained a 66.6% rate of good relief in their 18 patients, in whom four had a previous unilateral antero-lateral cordotomy. In his 14 patients with neurogenic pain (four causalgia, four post-herpetic neuralgia, three brachial plexus avulsions and three spinal cord lesions), Schvarcz (1978) reported a 64% rate of success with a 6 months to 4 year follow-up. All these results were achieved without mortality and with minimal side-effects, even in the sensory fields.

Extra-lemniscal myelotomy appears promising but larger series with better long-term follow-up are needed to provide a better estimate of its usefulness, especially for chronic pain of central origin. As with commissural myelotomy, the analgesic mechanisms of extra-lemniscal myelotomy remain speculative and puzzling (Nathan et al., 1986).

Antero-lateral cordotomy

Spiller's anatomo-clinical findings and Schuller's experimental work in monkey first demonstrated the role of the antero-lateral columns in conveying pain sensation. On the basis of this work, the first antero-lateral cordotomies (ALC) were carried out in 1911 by Martin at the cervico-thoracic level (Spiller and Martin, 1912) and in 1927 by Foerster at the high cervical level. Both authors used a similar open postero-lateral approach. Later on, Collis (1963) and Cloward (1964) described an anterior cervical approach.

In 1963, Mullan et al. pioneered the percutaneous method, using first a radioactive strontium needle inserted postero-laterally and then a unipolar electrode (Mullan et al., 1965). In 1965, Rosomoff et al. described an RF technique with an electrode induced through the C1–C2 interlaminar space. In 1966, Lin et al. proposed an anterior percutaneous approach at the lower cervical levels, in order to avoid damage to the descending respiratory pathways. Crue et al. (1968) and Hitchcock (1969) introduced a percutaneous posterior approach between the base of the skull and C1. Since these early studies several important technical and electrophysiological refinements have made ALC an increasingly popular procedure, especially for pain due to cancer.

Rationale
ALC aims to interrupt the spino-reticulo-thalamic ascending system, contralaterally to the painful

side, since at least 80% of fibers in this system cross the midline obliquely over 2 to 5 segments before entering the antero-lateral columns.

The antero-lateral tract consists of two anatomically different pathways (Bowsher, 1957): (1) the neo-spino-thalamic tract, which relays with the lemniscal pathways to the VPL thalamic nucleus and probably plays a major role in the topographical localization of painful stimuli, and (2) the paleo-spino-reticulo-thalamic tract, probably related to stimulus intensity and responsible for emotional reaction to pain, thanks to its diffuse central projections, particularly to the limbic system.

In the antero-lateral column, the fibers of the spino-thalamic tract have a relative somatotopic arrangement, with the sacral fibers being dorso-lateral, while the cervical ones are situated more deeply and ventrally (Walker, 1940).

Such a localization explains why ALC must be performed as posteriorly as possible for treatment of pain below the waist, whereas for pain in the upper part of the body ALC must be performed more anteriorly.

Of prime importance, when ALC is performed at high cervical levels (C1–C2), is the location of the descending respiratory pathways which lie just lateral to the ventral horn and are likely to be sectioned at the same time as the deeper nociceptive fibers. The descending autonomic pathways for vasomotor and genito-urinary control are situated in the intermedio-lateral columns at the equator of the cord, intermingled with the lumbo-sacral nociceptive fibers in the spino-thalamic tract. Bilateral interruption of these descending autonomic pathways may lead to transient or even permanent disturbances in blood pressure or sphincter control.

Methods
Open ALC may be carried out using different approaches. The traditional postero-lateral approach via laminectomy allows the procedure to be performed at any level of the cervical or thoracic spinal cord. Microtechniques allow the surgical approach to be as small as possible through a single hemilaminectomy with conservation of the spinous

and articular processes. For bilateral ALC, one or two spinal segments should intervene between the bilateral lesions in order to minimize the risk of spinal cord ischemia.

Although the anterior cervical approach via discectomy affords direct visualization of the anterior cord and spinal artery, this method is rarely used because of a number of other disadvantages. The procedure is restricted to the lower cervical levels; it does not provide sufficient landmarks to avoid the cortico-spinal tract and is performed through a narrow exposure which makes dural closure difficult.

The most common method for percutaneous ALC consists of introducing, under local anesthesia and X-ray control, an RF electrode through the C1–C2 interlaminar space (Rosomoff et al., 1965) into the antero-lateral column. Radioopaque contrast medium is used to identify the dentate ligaments and the anterior margin of the cord (Onofrio, 1971). The correct placement of the electrode is confirmed with impedance monitoring (Gildenberg et al., 1969) and electrical stimulation testing (Taren et al., 1969; Tasker, 1973).

For this report, we have analysed our 171 personal cases of open cordotomy and reviewed from the literature 22 series of open cordotomies (see Ref. note 2) and 15 series of percutaneous cordotomies (Onofrio, 1970; Gildenberg, 1973; Rosomoff, 1974; Lorenz et al., 1975; Bettag et al., 1975; Kuhner, 1975; Wepsic, 1975; Grote et al., 1978; Meglio and Cioni, 1981; Broggi et al., 1982; Mullan, 1983; Ischia et al., 1984; Mooij et al., 1984; Lipton, 1984; Tasker, 1985) regrouping 2306 and 3464 cases, respectively.

Results on pain

The effectiveness of pain relief after ALC was evaluated independently in the cancerous and the non-cancerous group.

In the cancer group (2022 cases), open ALC achieved early pain relief in 30–97% of patients (mean 70.9%), while with percutaneous ALC early pain relief was noted in 76–100% of patients (mean 88.3%). The length of follow-up was not precisely described in most publications. However, a majority of authors mentioned that – although analgesia was decreasing by the time – ALC was able to provide effective pain relief during the survival period in a significant number of patients, i.e. in 75% of patients at 6 months and in 40% after one year.

Long-term results in non-cancerous painful states could be evaluated in only 455 patients. Lasting good results were achieved in 21.4–75% of patients (mean 47%), whereas early pain relief was noted in 44–100% (mean 68.2%). The best results were obtained in pain related to lower spinal cord or cauda equina injuries and in painful amputation stumps or phantom limbs. About 60% of patients in these groups achieved pain relief.

Mortality

Complications related to the procedure were difficult to differentiate from those related to the evolution of the underlying disease, as most patients had advanced cancers and were in poor medical condition. This qualification holds particularly true for mortality, which averaged 5.1% for open and 3% for percutaneous ALC.

Concerning open cordotomy, there were marked differences in mortality rates according to the spinal level and whether the procedure was uni- or bilateral. In unilateral cervico-thoracic procedures, mortality was 4.3%, versus 14% when bilateral. In unilateral high cervical ALC, mortality was 9.1%, while bilateral open ALC above C4 has been abandoned by most authors, because of its high mortality rate (40%), mainly due to respiratory failures.

With regard to C1–C2 percutaneous ALC, mortality ranged from zero to 9% according to the series (2% on average) in unilateral procedures versus 11% (Ischia et al., 1984) to 50% (Broggi et al., 1982) when bilateral.

Morbidity

Motor complications were noticed in 14.4% of the patients who underwent an open ALC. Percentages were significantly different according to whether the procedure was unilateral (0–15%) or bilateral (12–39%). In unilateral percutaneous ALC, motor complications ranged from zero to 17% (3.5% on average). These complications attained the degree of a complete paraplegia in only a small percentage of cases, for instance 0.8% in Mansuy et al.'s series (1976).

Permanent urinary disturbances were frequent, but only after bilateral procedures, e.g., 46% after open cervico-thoracic ALC versus 22% after high cervical percutaneous procedures (Tasker, 1973). Urinary complications were more frequent in patients with pain due to cancer, which demonstrates the role played by pre-existing disorders in determining the frequency of complications after ALC. The latter holds true with respect to rectal and sexual dysfunctions after ALC.

Orthostatic hypotension was frequently seen after bilateral ALC. Ischia et al. (1984) reported an incidence of 36.1% in their percutaneous series, but only 5% of patients remained permanently disabled by orthostatic hypotension in most series.

Respiratory failure after unilateral high cervical ALC was observed in 3.5% of patients who underwent open ALC and 2.6% who underwent percutaneous ALC. Respiratory failure was especially frequent when phrenic paralysis or a pulmonary pathology was present on the painful side prior to ALC. The high frequency of sleep-apnea noticed after bilateral high cervical ALC led a large number of authors to stop performing ALC bilaterally above C4.

Dysesthesias after ALC usually appear after a several month post-operative delay. In White and Sweet's series (1969), they were present in 16.2% of their 80 non-cancerous patients but were severe in only 5%. The potential for distressing dysesthesias after ALC has led most surgeons to be very cautious in recommending ALC for pain due to non-cancerous diseases.

Horner's syndrome was frequently observed immediately after all types of cervical cordotomies, but in most cases it disappeared by the time of longer-term follow-up.

Discussion
Apart from cases with rapid extension of the carci-noma, initial failures and recurrences of pain cannot always be attributed to clear anatomical causes. In some instances, insufficient interruption of fibers could be demonstrated when complete pain relief was obtained with an additional section of the entire antero-lateral quadrant carried out at the same site. An inadequate height level can be demonstrated by achieving effective analgesia in redoing the procedure at a higher site. Unilateral ALC can be insufficient, especially in pelvic malignancies; as a matter of fact it is not infrequent for a pain ipsilateral to the procedure to appear post-operatively. Such a pain can be hypothesized as being pre-existent and hidden by predominant algias on one side and can be relieved by bilateral ALC. When no obvious anatomical factor can be found, explanations may lie in the possible development of new pain pathways or in the appearance of deafferentation phenomena.

Because ALC does not afford very long-lasting pain relief, most authors consider that it is best reserved for pain due to cancer. As for the choice of technical approaches, i.e., open (easier and more reproducible) or percutaneous (less invasive, in awake patients), an approximately equal number of surgeons are in favour of each of them. In 1973 Gildenberg revealed in a survey of 552 neurosurgeons that 275 performed percutaneous cordotomies and 300 open procedures, with a number performing both.

Lissauer's tractotomy and tractolysis

After entering the cord, most of the collaterals of the fine medullated and non-medullated fibers run longitudinally in Lissauer's tract before reaching the dorsal horn, some of them upward over three segments on average. On this basis, sections or destructions of this tract have been tried singly or in association with antero-lateral cordotomy in an attempt to achieve better analgesia.

In 1942, Hyndman proposed and performed a single transverse section of Lissauer's tract at the upper segment of the painful territory, in order to obtain analgesia in the subjacent metameres in two patients or in association with contralateral cordotomy, or in order to raise the level of analgesia in 13 others. The inconstant effects of such a tractotomy are not surprising, since some of the collaterals of the fine fibers reach the dorsal horn directly or through descending pathways.

In 1960, Rand investigated the effects of Lissauer's tractolysis with electrolytic lesions in 41 animal experiments, in an effort to produce analgesia in dermatomes of the upper and lower extremities and reported successful pain relief in a patient with arm pain, who underwent at the same time a C6–T1 tractolysis and a contralateral C2 cordotomy.

Cordectomy

Performed for the first time by McCarthy et al. in 1949 for pain associated with complete paraplegia of tumorous or traumatic origin, cordectomy consists of transection of the spinal cord or excision of one or a few segments above the level of the spinal injury. Cordectomy aims at removing the gliosis and the atrophic scar tissue considered to be the site of neurons which discharge abnormally and activate ascending sensory pathways. This rationale has received neurophysiological support from Loeser et al. (1968), who were able to record, in a patient with a complete traumatic paraplegia at the conus medullaris, neuronal hyperactivity, described as 're-miniscent of those seen in deafferented cat spinal cord or the primate cortical epileptic focus'.

The review of the literature series, of only 17 cases (see Ref. note 3), shows that in a majority of patients (58%) pain was not relieved or recurred. Cordectomy was particularly ineffective for the pain component located in the totally anesthetic territory, as experienced in three personal cases in whom the perineal, permanent, burning component was not relieved. In a critical analysis of the literature, Sweet and Poletti (1984) hypothesized that failures could be related to an insufficiently high transection of the cord, since in the few cases in which the surgical section reached a cord segment histologically demonstrated as normal, pain relief was long-lasting.

In a recent publication, Jefferson (1983) found cordectomy very effective in relieving pain due to traumatic lesions of the spine below T10, especially when the pain was episodic and located in the anterior thighs and over the knees. His clinical good results in 16 of 20 patients were similar to those obtained by others, with open (Sweet and Poletti, 1984) or percutaneous (Tasker, 1985) cordotomies.

With this background, cordectomy may be considered helpful for treating some of the 10–30% patients who develop severe intractable pain after paraplegia, particularly when pain is due to injury at the level of the conus medullaris and especially when the main painful component corresponds to the metameric level of the spinal cord lesion.

Surgery in the dorsal root entry zone

In the 1960s, a large amount of anatomical and physiological work on the dorsal horn, particularly as expressed in the 'Gate Control Theory' (Melzach and Wall, 1965), drew clinicians' attention to this site as the first level of modulation for pain sensation. These works convinced the authors of this article to consider the dorsal root entry zone (DREZ) as a possible target for pain surgery. Therefore, in 1972, we undertook anatomical studies and preliminary surgical trials in humans in order to determine whether a destructive procedure at this level was feasible (Sindou, 1972).

Rationale

We have proposed (Sindou, 1972; Sindou et al., 1974c; Mansuy and Sindou, 1978) that the DREZ – as an anatomical entity – includes the central portion of the dorsal roots, Lissauer's tract and laminae 1–5 of the dorsal horn where the afferent fibers articulate with the cells from which the ascending extra-lemniscal pathways originate.

The dorsal rootlets. Each dorsal root divides into 4–10 rootlets, of 0.25–1.50 mm diameter each. Corresponding to two embryologically different elements, each rootlet is formed from a peripheral and a central segment. The junction of the two portions called Tarlov's pial ring is on average 1 mm from the penetration of the rootlet into the dorso-lateral sulcus of the spinal cord (Fig. 1). As each rootlet has the same proportion of large- to small-diameter fibers as the root, each rootlet can be considered an anatomical-functional entity (see references in Sindou et al. (1975) and in Sindou and Goutelle (1983)), i.e. a root in miniature.

In the peripheral segment of the rootlet, the fibers have no particular organization according to size. However, on entering the spinal cord, most of the small-diameter fibers (considered nociceptive) are regrouped laterally before penetrating into

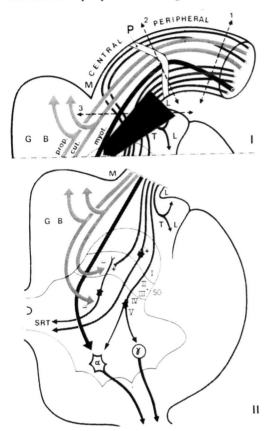

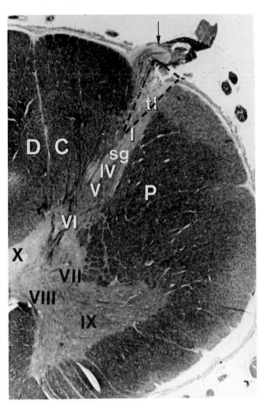

Fig. 1. *Left:* (I) Organization of fibers at the DREZ in humans. Each rootlet consists of a peripheral and a central segment, the junction of which constitutes the pial ring (P). Peripherally, the fibers have no organization. In the neighbourhood of the pial ring, the small fibers are situated under the rootlet surface, predominantly on its lateral side. In the central segment, they regroup laterally to enter the tract of Lissauer (TL). The large fibers are located centrally for the myotatic fibers and medially for the lemniscal ones. The black triangle indicates the proposed extent of the surgical lesion, i.e., the lateral and central bundles formed by the nociceptive and myotatic fibers, as well as the (excitatory) internal part of the TL and the apex of the dorsal horn. (II) Posterior rootlet projections to the spinal cord. The small fibers terminate on the spino-reticulo-thalamic (SRT) cells, which they activate, and through interneuronal pathways on the gamma and alpha neurons of the anterior horn. The short recurrent collaterals of the large fibers (of cutaneous or proprioceptive origin) terminate on the SRT cells, which they inhibit.

Right: Transverse hemisection of the spinal cord at the inferior cervical level, stained with luxol-fuschine, which darkens the myelin, showing the myelinated rootlet afferences reaching the dorsal column (DC) and Rexed's lamination. P, pyramidal tract. The arrow designates the pial ring of the posterior rootlet (diameter 1 mm). The dotted triangle shows the selective microsurgical lesion in the DREZ, which makes a 45° angle and extends 2 mm into the rootlet-spinal cord junction.

Lissauer's tract, while the large fibers run centrally (with respect to the myotatic fibers which penetrate the grey matter) and medially (with respect to the lemniscal fibers which reach the dorsal column), as shown in Fig. 1. This lateral regrouping of the small fibers should allow them to be preferentially interrupted without disturbing most of the large fibers.

Some authors have recently questioned whether all nociceptive fibers reach the spinal cord through the dorsal roots, for anatomical and electrophysiological studies in animals showed that about 30% of the fibers in the ventral roots were afferent C-axons, originating from the dorsal root ganglion cells and

projecting into the dorsal horn (Willis, 1985). These findings, challenging Bell and Magendie's law, were recently clarified. The majority (but not all) of the ventral root afferents would actually not enter the cord through the lamina cribrosa of the ventral root, but make a U-turn to reach the dorsal horn via the dorsal root (Willis, 1985).

Lissauer's tract. Lissauer's tract (LT), which is situated dorso-laterally to the dorsal horn, is composed of (1) a medial part which the small afferents enter and where they trifurcate to reach the dorsal horn, either directly or through a two metamere as-

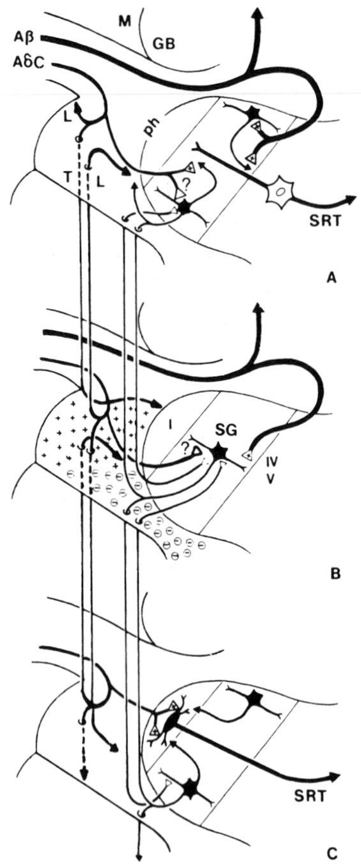

Fig. 2. Modulation of nociceptive radicular afferents in the DREZ. On entering the spinal cord, the nociceptive A delta and C fibres are lateral in the posterior rootlet to penetrate into the Lissauer's tract (TL) and reach the posterior horn (ph), either directly or through a 2 metamere ascending or descending trajec-

tory. There they relay onto the apical dendrites of the spino-reticulo-thalamic cells (SRT) of layer I marginal cells (part C) and layers IV and V nucleus proprius neurons (part A), whereas the lemniscal A beta fibres are medial in the posterior rootlet. They form long axons ascending in the dorsal column (DC) and short recurrent collaterals ending in the substantia gelatinosa (SG) where they relay onto the apical dendrites of the nucleus proprius neurons. These collaterals also activate the small cells constituting the SG, which is an inhibitory structure according to the gate control theory (part B). Thus, the lemniscal fibers prevent nociceptive A delta and C afferents from entering the SRT pathway. This constitutes a local segmental modulating system, which functions as a gate. On entering the cord, the afferents also undergo modulation from the neighboring roots through the TL associative fibers (part B). Its internal region (site of the ascending and descending collaterals of the nociceptive fibers) transmits the excitatory effects of the adjacent roots. In contrast, its external part (site of the SG longitudinal interconnecting axons called fasciculus proprius) presumably conveys the inhibitory influences of the neighboring metameres. We are dealing here with a regional plurisegmental modulating system which regulates metameric excitability from the adjacent levels. Thanks to its associative fibers which interconnect its constituent cells over a distance as long as 6 metameres, the SG can be considered a closed system with a mass effect. Thus, according to the gate theory, SG is able to work as a powerful inhibitory barrier against the entry of peripheral nociceptive afferents into the extralemniscal SRT pathway. This barrier can be reinforced by the A beta fibers at the same level and also those of adjacent metameres. Selective posterior rhizotomy in the DREZ interrupts the small nociceptive fibers and penetrates into the internal part of Lissauer's tract and the apex of the dorsal horn. It relatively preserves the following anatomical structures of the posterior root – spinal cord junction: (1) the lemniscal fibers and their recurrent collaterals to the posterior horn; (2) the SG interneurons; and (3) the SG interconnecting fibers which run through the external part of Lissauer's tract.

cending or descending pathway, (2) a lateral part through which a large number of longitudinal endogenous proprio-spinal fibers interconnect different levels of the substantia gelatinosa (SG) (Fig. 2).

According to Denny-Brown et al. (1973), the LT plays an important role in the intersegmental modulation of the nociceptive afferents, as its medial part would transmit the excitatory effects of each dorsal root to the adjacent segments and its lateral part would convey the inhibitory influences of the SG into the neighboring metameres. Thus, a selective destruction of the medial part of the LT could cause a reduction in the regional excitability of the nociceptive afferents.

The dorsal horn. Most of the fine nociceptive afferents which enter the cord through the LT medial part penetrate into the dorsal horn crossing the dorsal aspect of the SG, while the recurrent collaterals of the large lemniscal fibers (Ramon y Cajal, 1901) approach the dorsal horn through the ventral aspect of the SG (Szentagothai, 1964).

As the dendrites of some of the spino-reticulo-thalamic (SRT) cells make synaptic articulations with the primary afferents inside the SG layers, SG is most appropriate to exert a strong segmental modulating effect on the nociceptive input (Wall, 1964).

When the large lemniscal afferents within peripheral nerves or dorsal roots are altered, there is a reduction in the inhibitory control that they exert on dorsal horn mechanisms (Melzach and Wall, 1965). This situation presumably results in excessive firing of the dorsal horn neurons. This phenomenon, thought to be at the origin of deafferentation pain, has been identified in some human cases by electrophysiological recordings (Loeser et al., 1968) and reproduced in animal experiments (Loeser and Ward, 1967; Albe-Fessard and Lombard, 1983). Destruction of these hyperactive neurons might suppress the nociceptive impulses generated in the SRT pathways.

Surgical methods of DREZ lesions

Microsurgery. Based on this anatomical and physiological background, in 1972 we introduced the concept of surgery in the DREZ (Sindou, 1972; Sindou et al., 1974c) and began to make selective lesions in this target, using microsurgical techniques (Sindou et al., 1974a,b).

The procedure, which has been detailed elsewhere (Sindou and Goutelle, 1983), consists of microsurgical incision and bipolar coagulation performed ventro-laterally at the entrance of the rootlets into the dorso-lateral sulcus, along all the spinal cord segments selected to be operated on. The lesion, which penetrates the lateral part of the DREZ and the medial part of LT, extends down to the apex of the dorsal horn. The latter is recognized by its brown-grey color. The lesions are 2 mm deep and made at a 45° angle (Fig. 3).

The procedure is presumed: (1) to preferentially destroy the pain pathways, i.e., the small nociceptive fibers grouped in the lateral bundle of the dorsal rootlets when entering the DREZ, as well as the excitatory medial part of the LT; the upper layers of the dorsal horn are also destroyed if microbipolar coagulations are made inside the grey matter of the dorsal horn apex; and (2) to preserve, at least partially, the inhibitory structures of the DREZ, i.e., the lemniscal fibers reaching the dorsal column, as well as their recurrent collaterals to the dorsal horn and the SG proprio-spinal interconnecting fibers running through the lateral part of the LT.

The method, called selective posterior rhizotomy in the DREZ, has been conceived with a view to preventing complete abolition of tactile and proprioceptive sensations and avoiding deafferentation phenomena.

RF electrocoagulation. In 1974, Nashold and coworkers developed a new method using an RF electrode to destroy hyperactive neurons in the SG layers (1976) and later on the entire DREZ region (Nashold and Ostdahl, 1979). In their more recently modified technique (Nashold, 1981), the lesion is made with a 0.5 mm insulated stainless-steel elec-

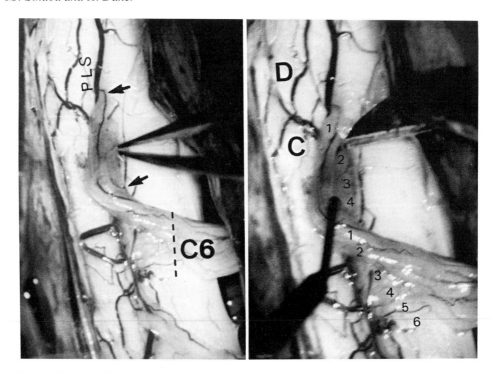

Fig. 3. Technique of microsurgical selective posterior rhizotomy in the DREZ (example at the cervical level). After identification of the segments to be operated on, the postero-lateral aspect of the spinal cord is approached under the microscope through a cervical hemilaminectomy (on the right side in this case). The exposed dorsal root (here the right C6 one, which has six rootlets) has been retracted backwards and toward the midline, to make the ventro-lateral region of the spinal cord–rootlet junction accessible (arrows). This region is the site of small pial vessels which are coagulated by means of a thin and sharp bipolar microforceps (left). The microsurgical lesion in the DREZ is made, continuously along the lateral edge of the dorso-lateral sulcus, using first a microscalpel made of a small piece of razor blade maintained in a blade-holder (right), and is then completed by micro-coagulations at a low intensity with the same bipolar microforceps, inside the incision, down to the dorsal horn apex recognized under the microscope by its brown-grey color. The lesion is 2 mm deep in the DREZ and makes a 45° angle internally oriented.

trode, with a tapered uninsulated 2 mm tip, introduced into the dorso-lateral sulcus for a distance of 1–3 mm and angled at 25° in the lateral medial direction. A series of RF coagulations are made under the microscope at a current of 35–40 mA (not over 75°C) for 10–15 s. The RF lesions are spaced at 2–3-mm intervals along the longitudinal extent of the dorso-lateral sulcus. The lesion observed under magnification is seen as a circular whitened area which extends 1–2 mm beyond the tip of the electrode.

Laser. Levy et al. in 1983 and Powers et al. in 1984 advocated a CO_2 and an argon laser, respectively, as the lesion maker. According to Levy et al.'s description, the pulse duration of the CO_2 laser

is 0.1 s and the power is adjusted to about 20 W, so that one or two single pulses create a 2 mm depression at a 45° angle in the DREZ. The lesions are probed with a micro-instrument marked at 1 mm increments to ensure that the depth of the lesions (1–2 mm) is adequate.

Experimental studies. The lack of information – with the exception of one autopsy study published in the proceedings of the First World Conference on DREZ (1984) – concerning the characteristics of the anatomical lesions produced by the various techniques directed at the DREZ target led several authors to undertake recent animal experiments. Powers et al. (1984) found that the argon laser produced precise and well-defined lesions in the

DREZ, while Walker et al. (1984) reported on the danger of creating extensive damage and syrinx cavities with the laser. Levy et al. (1985) compared experimental lesions made with the CO_2 laser and RF and concluded that the laser lesions were more circumscribed and less variable.

In a well-documented study evaluating the effects in dog spinal cord of DREZ lesions with RF and CO_2 or YAg laser, Young et al. (1988) found that the size and extent of the lesion related primarily to the magnitude of power used to make the lesion. They showed that, provided the procedures are performed with proper parameters, the lesions could be successfully localized to the DREZ, including the layers I–VI of the dorsal horn, and spare the dorsal columns and the cortico-spinal tract, using any of the three techniques. The main difference was that with laser the lesion was shaped like the letter 'V', with the maximum width at the surface, while with RF it tended to be more spherical. In both methods, in chronic animals, the same glial reactions were observed.

At present, no experimental study has been carried out using microsurgical incisions and bipolar coagulation as the lesion-maker. This technique is supposed to produce more selective destructive lesions in the DREZ, preserving its inhibitory structures. However, the unavoidable lesioning of perforating vessels located in the dorso-lateral sulcus (Sindou and Goutelle, 1983) probably increases the extent of the theoretical target.

Results

In malignant pain. Our first attempt at surgery in the DREZ was done in March 1972 for pain with Pancoast-Tobias syndrome. At the present time, our series consists of: (1) 26 patients operated on at the cervical or cervico-thoracic levels for malignant tumors limited to the superior pulmonary sulcus or even invading the brachial plexus, the axillary region and/or the lower cervical vertebrae, such as those encountered in carcinomas of lung (13 cases), breast (8 cases), oesophagus (3 cases) and cervical nodes (2 cases); (2) 28 patients operated on at the lumbar and/or sacral levels for cancers with very localized invasions of the pelvic floor or involvements of the lower limb nerves, as observed in neoplasms of rectum (13 cases), uterus (6 cases), bladder (4 cases) and also for radicular compressions by vertebro-epidural (2 cases) or sacral (3 cases) tumors.

Good results (i.e. complete relief of pain or a sufficient decrease to allow withdrawal of narcotics) was obtained in 87.5% of patients in the first group and 78.5% in the second, with survival times ranging from one month to 4 years (10 months on average). There were two post-operative deaths and two wound infections. When there was no marked pre-operative sensory deficit, the procedure allowed tactile and proprioceptive sensory capacities of a significant degree to be retained, avoiding complete functional sensory loss in the operated area. Because extensive operations at the lumbar and/or sacral segments would inevitably result in leg hypotonia and/or sphincterian disturbances, for pain below the waist the procedure must be restricted to the treatment of topographically limited carcinomas.

DREZ surgery has been occasionally carried out for cancer pain by others (Vlahovitch and Fuentes, 1975; Nashold and Ostdahl, 1979; Esposito et al., 1980) with successful results. Although there is still a lack of sufficient experience to precisely define its indications among the other destructive methods, it may be assumed that the procedure can be included in the armamentarium of pain surgery, provided it is reserved for patients with limited cancer extensions and reasonably long life expectancies.

In non-malignant pain. As the first results in cancer pain were encouraging, we decided the same year (i.e. in 1972) to attempt the procedure in patients with non-malignant pain syndromes, namely: painful paraplegia, amputation stump and brachial plexus injury (doing microcoagulations of the dorsal horn apex with a bipolar forceps at the avulsed root revels and selective ventro-lateral DREZ lesions in the remaining rootlets). Since then, only a small number of patients with neurogenic pain have been operated on, because of the need to observe the results for long periods of time before knowing whether this new procedure can be undertaken in a larger series. The results of this clinical trial (42 cases), as well as those obtained in pain associated with hyperspasticity in paraplegic or hemiplegic patients (57 cases), are given in Table I.

In the group of pure neurogenic pain (42 patients with a follow-up ranging from 6 months to 14 years), a good result (i.e. more than 50% relief) on the spontaneous electrical, burning, throbbing and/or aching painful components was obtained in 61%

TABLE I

Microsurgical DREZ lesions in non-malignant pain (Authors' series: 99 cases)

Etiologies	No. of cases	Results on spontaneous pain		Results on hyperalgesia		Follow-up range
		Good (>50%) n (%)	(<50%) n	Good (>50%) n	(<50%) n	
Group I (pure neurogenic pain): 42 cases						
Post-amputation (stump 3, stump + phantom 1)	4	3 (75%)	1	1	0	2 yr–14 yr
Periph. nerve inj. (trauma 2, post-surg. 2)	4	3 (75%)	1	2	0	16 m– 4 yr
Brach. plexus inj. (avulsion)	8	3 (37.5%)	5	2	1	15 m–13 yr
Brach. plexopathy (post-Rx)	3	1 (50%)	1	1	0	3 yr– 4 yr
Herpes zoster	4	0 (0%)	4	4	0	3 yr–13 yr
Cerv. (1) or Thor. (6) cord lesions	7	5	2	2	0	
Conus medullaris lesions	8	8	0	1	0	
Cauda equina lesions (origin: trauma 11, gun shot 1, tumor 2, Pott 1, post-surg. 1)	1	1	0	1	0	
Total:	16	14 (87.5%)	2	4	0	6 m– 7 yr
Misc.						
Idiopathic perineal pain	1	1	0	0	0	3 yr
Reflex symp. dystrophy	1	0	1	0	1	13 yr
Thalamic syndrome	1	0	1	1	0	4 yr
Total:	42	25 (61%)	16	15 (88%)	2	
Group II (pain associated with spasticity): 57 cases						
Lower limbs (bil. 39, unil. 3) (M.S., trauma. ,...)	42	40 (96%)	2	7	4	6 m–14 yr
Upper limb (unil.) (trauma, stroke, ...)	15	14 (93%)	1	1	0	13 m–13 yr
Total:	57	54 (94.7%)	3	8	4	
Overall results	99 cases	79 (80.6%)	19	23 (79%)	6	

of patients (31.7% with a relief of more than 75% of their pain), while the provoked hyperalgesic cutaneous component (present 17 times) was favourably influenced in 88.2% of patients (64.7% with a relief of more than 75% of their pain). The best results were achieved in spinal cord lesions in which the pain had a 'radiculo-metameric' distribution corresponding to or situated just below the level of the lesion (87.5% good results, with 56.2% achieving relief of more than 75% of their pain). In brachial plexus injuries and post-radiation plexopathies, a good result was obtained in only 37.5% and 50%, respectively. Pain after amputation, peripheral nerve injuries or herpes zoster was better alleviated when superficial hyperalgesia was predominant. Eighteen patients in the total group with neurogenic pain had a dorsal column stimulator implanted at the time of DREZ surgery. Of these, only 7 (39%) achieved 25% to maximum 50% pain relief directly related to the stimulation.

In the group with pain associated with spasticity, the results were excellent in 78.9% of patients and good in 15.8%, whether the presumed origin of pain was neurogenic, somatogenic or both (Sindou et al., 1982, 1985, 1986).

In these two groups of patients (i.e., with pain of neurogenic origin or associated with spasticity) two deaths occurred during the first month, both of them in patients with multiple sclerosis and severe respiratory insufficiency. There was no pyramidal or dorsal column deficit post-operatively except in one case with an incomplete Brown-Sequard syndrome.

The data from the literature concerning DREZ surgery with RF or laser, in neurogenic pain, are given in Table II. The results were considered good when at least 50% pain relief was obtained. In brachial (150 cases) and lumbosacral plexus (11 cases) injuries, good results averaged 75% and 82%, respectively. In spinal cord (92 cases) and cauda equina (6 cases) injuries, good pain relief was achieved in 47% and 83%, respectively. Better relief was obtained when pain was of a dermatomal type and situated at the junction between sensory loss and normal sensation (Young et al., 1988). Diffuse pain and

predominantly midline perineo-sacral pain responded not as well or not at all (Nashold and Bullit, 1981; Friedman and Nashold, 1986). In patients with amputations (40 cases), the phantom component was frequently relieved, but stump pain was often unaffected (Proc. 1st World Congr. DREZ, 1984; Saris et al., 1985; Young et al., 1988). In postherpetic neuralgias (25 cases), good results averaged 60% and surgery was more effective in alleviating the superficial burning pain and hyperesthesia than in relieving the deep ache (Friedman et al., 1984).

The most frequent complications encountered in the literature series included ipsi-lateral cortico-spinal tract and dorsal column deficits below the level of DREZ surgery, as summarized in Table II.

Discussion

The respective advantages and disadvantages of the different technical procedures applied to the DREZ target are difficult to analyse, because of the disparity in the pathological groups treated by the different authors and a lack of common criteria to assess the results. As shown in this study, DREZ surgery with the laser or with microsurgical incisions and bipolar coagulations was effective in a significant percentage of cases with a low rate of neurological deficits affecting the spinal tracts below the lesion: 11% and 1%, respectively. The proportion of pyramidal and dorsal column deficits provoked by the RF electrocoagulation technique has decreased from about 50% to 5%, without loss of efficacy, with the use of lower currents, applied for shorter periods of time and controlled by temperature monitoring, as recommended by Nashold in 1981 and demonstrated in Young et al.'s study (1988). As mentioned by all the authors using RF or laser, all sensation is lost in the cutaneous distribution of the nerve roots where the DREZ operation is performed. With the selective microsurgical procedure, which is carried out ventro-laterally in the DREZ, a complete abolition of tactile and proprioceptive sensations is often avoided in the operated area. This is explained by the fact that at least some of the lemniscal fibers are preserved, which is important in patients who retain motor and sensory functions in their painful limbs.

Whatever the technical modality used for DREZ procedures, there is still a need for further experimental work and larger clinical series to clarify the anatomical effects in the DREZ and to understand why certain painful states do not respond. Inappropriate levels or an insufficient extent of DREZ lesioning may explain failures, but more complex neurophysiological phenomena, such as those pointed out by Albe-Fessard and Lombard (1983) may also explain such failures. In recent animal experiments to evaluate the origin of deafferentation pain, they demonstrated that after dorsal root section abnormal spiking appeared not only in the dorsal horn, but also secondarily in more central structures such as thalamic nuclei and somesthetic cortex, through a kind of progressive kindling process. Thus chronic pain may be an evolving disease extending to affect neural structures more and more centrally.

Conclusions

In the developing field of functional neurosurgery for treatment of pain, a rigid protocol for management of individual patients cannot be given. For every surgeon, the choice of a particular procedure should be made after taking into account not only the etiology and site of the pain, but also its neurophysiological mechanisms (Gybels, 1984). The following guidelines are suggested.

In cancer patients, intrathecal morphine therapy

TABLE II

Literature results of DREZ surgery: number of good results/total number in the group (% good results) (good result = pain relief $\geq 50\%$)

Authors and follow-up	No. of cases	Tech.	Brach. plexus inj. (mostly avuls.)	Lumbo-sacral plex. inj. (avuls.)	Spinal cord injury	Cauda equina injury	Post-amputation	Post-herpetic	Miscellaneous	Complications below the lesions: motor weakness (M), propriocep. loss (P)
Nashold et al., 6 m–10 yr	153	RF	45/57 (80%) → 10 yr[a]	6/6 (100%)[a]	23/56 (50%) 6 m–6 yr. better results in conus med.[b]		8/22 (36%) 6 m–4 yr. phantom: 67% stump: 0% both: 28%[c]	8/12 (67%) 6 m–21 m. more effects on superficial pain.[d]		RF (amp) M: 50% P: 71% RF (t°) 5% (M, P)
Samii et al.[a] →4 yr	33	RF	20/22 (90%)		4/5 (80%)		1/2 (50%) phantom		m.s. = 1/1 periph.-nerv. 2/2 int.neuralg. 0.1	51% (M,P)

TABLE II (continued)

Literature results of DREZ surgery: number of good results/total number in the group (% good results) (good result = pain relief ≥ 50%)

Authors and follow-up	No. of cases	Tech.	Brach. plexus inj. (mostly avuls.)	Lumbo-sacral plex. inj. (avuls.)	Spinal cord injury	Cauda equina injury	Post-amputation	Post-herpetic	Miscellaneous	Complications below the lesions: motor weakness (M), propriocep. loss (P)
Richter et al.[a] 6 m–30 m	10	RF	6/8 (75%)		0/2 (0%)					44% (M,P)
Thomas et al. 4 m–44 m	34	RF	20/34 (58%)							50% (M,P)
Dieckmann et al. 2 m–16 m	18	RF	7/9 (78%)		0/2 (0%)		4/5 (80%) phantom	0/1 (0%)	arachn. 0/1	22% (M,P)
Young et al. →5 yr	21	RF (amp)	4/6 (67%)	1/2 (50%)	3/5 (60%)	2/2 (100%)	2/3 (67%)	2/3 (67%)		52% (M,P)
	26	RF (t°)	5/7 (71%)	2/2 (100%)	4/8 (50%)	2/2 (100%)	2/3 (67%)	3/4 (75%)		4% (M,P)
	20	CO$_2$ L	2/4 (50%)	0/1 (0%)	3/6 (50%)	1/2 (50%)	1/2 (50%)	2/5 (40%)		15% (M,P)
Powers et al. 2 m–19 m	21	Ar L	2/2 (100%)		6/7 (85%) bad results in back and coccyx pain		2/3 (67%)		arachn. 1/3; post-rhiz 2/2; periph.-nerv. 0/3; int.neuralg. 1/1	10% (P)
Levy et al.	3	CO$_2$ L	1/1 (100%)		0/1 (0%)				arachn. 1/1	0%
Total	339		112/150 (75%)	9/11 (82%)	43/92 (47%)	5/6 (83%)	20/40 (50%)	15/25 (60%)	8/15 (53%)	RF (amp) = 50% RF (t°) = 5% Laser = 0–10%

[a]Proc. 1st World Congr. DREZ, 1984.
[b]Friedman and Nashold, 1986.
[c]Saris et al., 1985.
[d]Friedman et al., 1984.

or ablative procedures may be considered. As the malignant lesions responsible have usually spread over large areas, invading many somatic and visceral sensory structures, DREZ surgery must be used only for pain due to topographically well-defined neoplasms. In more wide-spread lesions, myelotomies or antero-lateral cordotomies are preferable. The most common indications for commisural myelotomies are pelvic carcinomas with pain limited to the saddle region. For pain below the waist, cordotomies should not be done below the cervicothoracic junction and for chest or arm pain not below C2, so as to ensure a sufficiently high level of analgesia. For median bilateral pain, extralemniscal myelotomy may be an alternative to bilateral cordotomy.

When non-malignant pain does not respond to the neurostimulation methods, which should be attempted first, ablative procedures may be useful in some strictly selected cases. As clinical experience has shown that the effects of surgery at the level of the spino-thalamic tract usually do not last for more than one or two years and may generate secondary burning and painful dysesthetic manifestations, cordotomies and myelotomies are rarely indicated for treatment of non-malignant pain. The good preliminary results obtained with DREZ operations in certain types of non-malignant painful states indicate that they may be useful in some topographically limited neurogenic pain syndromes, which are resistant to non-narcotic medications and conservative treatments.

In pain treatment, the decision to undertake surgery and the choice of the procedure is difficult. As Tasker (1985) has ably expressed it: 'One must know the patient, dissect his pain syndrome, evaluate his disability, and only then embark on a program of surgical therapy beginning with the simplest measures and proceeding to the more complex, as far as the patient's disability warrants'.

Acknowledgement

This work was supported by 'La Ligue Nationale Française contre le cancer – Comité départemental du Rhône'.

Notes

For conciseness, all the articles reviewed for the analysis of the literature are not given in the reference section, but are cited in the following notes.

Note No. 1. The literature review concerning commissural myelotomy was compiled from the following 17 publications, referenced in the articles:

– by Tasker (1985): Wertheimer and Lecuire, 1953; Broager, 1974; Piscol, 1976; Sourek, 1977; McLaurin, 1977; Adams et al., 1982; Payne, 1984.

– by Sweet and Poletti (1984): Lembke, 1964; Grunert et al., 1970; Adams et al., 1977; King, 1977; Poletti and Sweet, 1982.

– and by Sindou and Daher (see this article): Mansuy, 1944; Lippert et al., 1974; Cook and Kawakami, 1977; Fascendini et al., 1979; Goedhart et al., 1984.

Note No. 2. The literature review concerning open antero-lateral cordotomy was compiled from the following 21 publications, referenced in the articles:

– by Sweet and Poletti (1984): Grant and Wood, 1958; Schwartz, 1960; Diemath et al., 1961; Frankel and Prokop, 1961; Porter et al., 1966; Falconer, 1966; Rasking, 1969; O'Connel, 1969; Nathan and Smith, 1972; French, 1974; Ehni, 1974; Piscol, 1975; Perneczky and Sunder-Plassman, 1975; Piotrowski and Passitz, 1975; Tasker, 1977; Guzman-Ramos et al., 1979; Cowie and Hitchcock, 1982.

– by Sindou and Daher (see this article): Hardy et al., 1974; Mansuy et al., 1976; Sindou and Lapras, 1982; Grunert and Sunder-Plassman, 1985.

Note No. 3. The literature review concerning cordectomy was made from the following 11 publications, referenced in the articles:

– by Sweet and Poletti (1984): Doris and Martin, 1947; Freeman and Heimburger, 1947; Botterel et al., 1954; Druckman and Lende, 1965; Druckman, 1966; Loeser et al., 1968; Melzack and Loeser, 1978; Durward et al., 1982.

– and by Sindou and Daher (see this article): White and Sweet, 1969; Jefferson, 1983.

References

Albe-Fessard, D. and Lombard, M.C. (1983) Use of an animal model to evaluate the origin of and protection against deafferentation pain. In J.J. Bonica et al. (Eds.), Advances in Pain Research and Therapy, Vol. 5, Raven Press, New York, pp. 691–700.

Armour, D. (1927) Surgery of the spinal cord and its membranes. Lancet, ii: 691–697.

Ascher, P.W. (1978) Longitudinal medial myelotomy with the laser. In R. Correa (Ed.), Proceedings of the Sixth International Congress of Neurological Surgery, Sao Paulo, Serie No. 433, Excerpta Medica Amsterdam, pp. 267–270.

Bettag, W., Wandt, H. and Roosen, K. (1975) Pain treatment of advanced malignant diseases by high cervical percutaneous cordotomy. Adv. Neurosurg., 3: 186–189.

Bowsher, D. (1957) Termination of the central pain pathway: the conscious appreciation of pain. Brain, 80: 505–522.

Broggi, G., Franzini, A., Lasio, G. and Servello, D. (1982) Cordotomie anterolaterale percutanée dans le traitement de la douleur d'origine cancéreuse. Med. Hyg., 40: 1962–1968.

Cloward, R.B. (1964) Cervical cordotomy by the anterior approach: technique and advantages. J. Neurosurg., 21: 19–25.

Collis, J.S., Jr (1963) Anterolateral cordotomy by an anterior approach: report of a case. J. Neurosurg., 20: 445–446.

Cook, A.W. and Kawakami, Y. (1977) Commissural myelotomy. J. Neurosurg., 47: 1–6.

Crue, B.L., Todd, E.M. and Canegal, E.J. (1968) Posterior approach for high percutaneous radiofrequency cordotomy. Confin. Neurol., 30: 41–52.

Denny-Brown, D., Kirk, E.J. and Yanagisawa, N. (1973) The tract of Lissauer in relation to sensory transmission in the dorsal horn of spinal cord in the macaque monkey. J. Comp. Neurol., 151: 175–200.

Dieckmann, G. and Veras, G. (1984) High-frequency coagulation of dorsal root entry zone in patients with deafferentation pain. Acta Neurochir., Suppl. 33: 445–450.

Eiras, J., Garcia, J., Gomez, J., Carcavalla, L.J. and Ucar, S. (1980) First results with extralemniscal myelotomy. Acta Neurochir., suppl. 30: 377–381.

Esposito, S., Canova, A. and Colangeli, M. (1980) Posterior radiculotomies in the treatment of the lumbo-sacral pain syndrome. Acta Neurochir., 53: 132–133.

Fascendini, A., Biroli, F. and Cassinari, V. (1979) Critical evaluation of commissural myelotomy in the treatment of intractable pain. J. Neurosurg. Sci., 23: 265–272.

Fink, R.A. (1984) Neurosurgical treatment of non-malignant intractable rectal pain: microsurgical commissural myelotomy with the carbon dioxide laser. Neurosurgery, 14: 64–65.

Foerster, O. (1927) Die Leitungsbahnen des Schmerzgefühls und die chirurgische Behandlung der Schmerzzustände, Urban & Schwarzenberg, Berlin, pp. 360.

Friedman, A.H., Nashold, B.S. and Ovelmen-Levitt, J. (1984) Dorsal root entry zone lesions for the treatment of post-herpetic neuralgia. J. Neurosurg., 60: 1258–1262.

Friedman, A.H. and Nashold, B.S. (1986) DREZ lesions for relief of pain related to spinal cord injury. J. Neurosurg., 65: 456–469.

Gildenberg, P.L. (1973) Percutaneous cervical cordotomy. Clin. Neurosurg., 21: 246–256.

Gildenberg, P.L., Zanes, C., Flitter, M.A., Lin, P.M. and

Lautsch, E.V. (1969) Impedance measuring device for detection of penetration of the spinal cord in anterior percutaneous cervical cordotomy. Technical note. J. Neurosurg., 30: 87–92.

Gildenberg, P.L. and Hirschberg, R.M. (1984) Limited myelotomy for the treatment of intractable cancer pain. J. Neurol. Neurosurg. Psychiatry, 47: 94–96.

Goedhart, L.D., Francariglia, N., Feirabend, H.K.P. and Voogd, J. (1984) Technical pitfalls in median commissural myelotomy for malignant sacral pain. Appl. Neurophysiol., 47: 216–222.

Grote, W., Roosen, K. and Bock, W.J. (1978) High cervical percutaneous cordotomy in intractable pain. Neurochirurgia, 21: 209–212.

Grunert, V.P. and Sunder-Plassmann, M. (1985) Ergebnisse der Zervikalen Chordotomie mit und ohne Rhizotomie bei Konservativ Therapieresistenten Schmerzen im Schulter-Arm-Bereich. Zbl. Neurochirurgie, 46: 267–271.

Guillaume, J., De Seze, S. and Mazars, G. (1949) Chirurgie cérebrospinale de la douleur, Presses Universitaires de France, Paris, pp. 192.

Gybels, J. (1984) The suggested mechanism of chronic pain and the rationale of neurosurgical treatment. Acta Neurochir., Suppl. 33: 397–406.

Hardy, J., Leclercq, T.A. and Mercky, F. (1974) Microsurgical cordotomy by the anterior approach. Technical note. J. Neurosurg., 41: 640–643.

Hitchcock, E.R. (1969) Stereotaxic spinal surgery. A preliminary report. J. Neurosurg., 31: 386–392.

Hitchcock, E.R. (1970) Stereotactic cervical myelotomy. J. Neurol. Neurosurg. Psychiatry, 33: 224–230.

Hyndman, O. (1942) Lissauer's tract section. A contribution to chordotomy for the relief of pain (preliminary report). J. Int. Coll. Surgeons, 5: 394–400.

Ischia, S., Luzzani, A., Ischia A. and Maffezzoli, G. (1984) Bilateral percutaneous cervical cordotomy: immediate and long-term results in 36 patients with neoplastic disease. J. Neurol. Neurosurg. Psychiatry, 47: 141–147.

Jefferson, A. (1983) Cordectomy for intractable pain. In S. Lipton and J. Miles (Eds.), Persistent Pain, Vol. 4, Grune & Stratton, New York, pp. 115–132.

Kuhner, A. (1976) La cordotomie cervicale percutanée. Neurochirurgie, 22: 261–280.

Leriche, R. (1936) Du traitement de la douleur dans les cancers abdominaux et pelviens inopérables ou récidives. Gaz. Hop. Civ. Mil., 109: 917–922.

Levy, W.J., Nutkiewicz, A., Ditmore, M. and Watts, C. (1983) Laser induced dorsal root entry zone lesions for pain control. Report of three cases. J. Neurosurg., 59: 884–886.

Levy, W.J., Gallo, C. and Watts, C. (1985) Comparison of laser and radiofrequency dorsal root entry zone lesions in cats. Neurosurgery, 16: 327–330.

Lin, P.M., Gildenberg, P.L. and Polakoff, P.O. (1966) An anterior approach to percutaneous lower cervical cordotomy. J. Neurosurgery, 25: 553–560.

Lippert, R.G., Hosobuchi, T. and Nielsen, S.L. (1974) Spinal commissurotomy. Surg. Neurol., 2: 373–377.

Lipton, S. (1984) Percutaneous cordotomy. In P.D. Wall and R. Melzach (Eds.), Texbook of Pain, Churchill Livingstone, Edinburgh, pp. 632–638.

Loeser, J.D. and Ward, A.A., Jr. (1967) Some effects of deafferentation of neurons of the cat spinal cord. Arch. Neurol., 17: 629–636.

Loeser, J.D., Ward, A.A., Jr. and White, L.E., Jr. (1968) Chronic deafferentation of human spinal cord neurons. J. Neurosurg., 29: 48–50.

Lorenz, R., Gumme, T.H., Hermann, D., Palleske, H., Kuhner, A., Steude, U. and Zierski, J. (1975) Percutaneous cordotomy. Adv. Neurosurg., 3: 178–185.

Mansuy, L. and Sindou, M. (1978) Physiology of pain at the spinal cord level: neurosurgical aspects. In R. Carrea (Eds.), Neurological Surgery, International Congress Series, no. 433, Excerpta Medica, Amsterdam, pp. 257–263.

Mansuy, L., Lecuire, L. and Acassat, L. (1944) Technique de la myelotomie commissurale postérieure. J. Chir., 60: 206–213.

Mansuy, L., Sindou, M., Fischer, G. and Brunon, J. (1976) La cordotomie spino-thalamique dans les douleurs cancéreuses. Neurochirurgie, 22, 5: 437–444.

McCarthy, C.S. and Kiefer, E.J. (1949) Thoracic, lumbar and sacral spinal cordectomy: preliminary report. Mayo Clin. Proc., 24: 108–115.

Meglio, M. and Cioni, B. (1981) The role of percutaneous cordotomy in the treatment of chronic cancer pain. Acta Neurochir., 59: 111–121.

Melzach, R. and Wall, P.D. (1965) Pain mechanism. A new theory. Science, 150: 971–979.

Mooij, J.J.A., Bosch, D.A. and Beks, J.W.F. (1984) The cause of failure in high cervical percutaneous cordotomy: an analysis. Acta Neurochir., 72: 1–14.

Mullan, S. (1983) Cordotomy and rhizotomy for pain. Clin. Neurosurg., 31: 344–350.

Mullan, S., Harper, P.V., Hekmatpanach, J., Torres, H. and Dobbin, G. (1963) Percutaneous interruption of spinal pain tracts by means of a strontium 90 needle. J. Neurosurg., 20: 931–939.

Mullan, S., Hekmatpanach, J., Dobbin, G. and Beckman, F. (1965) Percutaneous intramedullary cordotomy utilising the unipolar anodal electrolytic lesion. J. Neurosurg., 22: 548–553.

Nashold, B.S. (1981) Modification of DREZ lesion technique, (letter). J. Neurosurg., 55: 1012.

Nashold, B.S. and Ostdahl, P.H. (1979) Dorsal root entry zone lesions for pain relief. J. Neurosurg., 51: 59–69.

Nashold, B.S. and Bullit, E. (1981) Dorsal root entry zone lesions to control central pain in paraplegia. J. Neurosurg., 55: 414–419.

Nashold, B.S., Urban, B. and Zorub, D.S. (1976) Phantom relief by focal destruction of substantia gelatinosa of Rolando. In J.J. Bonica and D. Albe-Fessard (Eds.), Advances in Pain Research and Therapy, Vol. 1, Raven Press, New York, pp. 959–963.

Nathan, P.W., Smith, M.C. and Cook, A.W. (1986) Sensory effects in man of lesions of the posterior columns and of some other afferent pathways. Brain, 109: 1003–1041.

Onofrio, B.M. (1970) Recent results with percutaneous cordotomy. Mayo Clin. Proc., 45: 689–694.

Onofrio, B.M. (1971) Cervical spinal cord and dentate delineation in percutaneous radiofrequency cordotomy at the level of the first to second cervical vertebrae. Surg. Gynecol. Obstet., 133: 30–34.

Papo, J. and Luongo, A. (1976) High cervical commissural myelotomy in the treatment of pain. J. Neurol. Neurosurg. Psychiatry, 39: 705–710.

Powers, S.K., Adams, J.E., Edwards, S.B., Boggan, J.E. and Hosobuchi, Y. (1984) Pain relief from dorsal root entry zone lesions made with argon and carbon dioxide microsurgical lasers. J. Neurosurg., 61: 841–847.

Proceedings of the First World Conference on Dorsal Root Entry Zone (DREZ), Mainz, FRG, March 10–11 (1984) Neurosurgery, 15: 887–970.

Ramon y Cajal, S. (1901) Histologie du système nerveux. Vol. 1, Maloine, Paris, pp. 986.

Rand, R. (1960) Further observations on Lissauer's tractolysis. Neurochirurgia, 3: 151–168.

Richards, D.E., Tyner, C.F. and Shealy, C.N. (1966) Focused ultrasonic spinal commissurotomy. Experimental evaluation. J. Neurosurg., 24: 701–707.

Rosomoff, H.L. (1974) Percutaneous radiofrequency cervical cordotomy for intractable pain. Adv. Neurol., 4: 683–688.

Rosomoff, H.L., Carroll, F., Brown, J. and Sheptak, P. (1965) Percutaneous radiofrequency cervical cordotomy: technique. J. Neurosurg., 23: 639–644.

Saris, S.C., Iacono, R.P. and Nashold, B.S. (1985) Dorsal root entry zone lesions for post-amputation pain. J. Neurosurg., 62: 72–76.

Schvarcz, J.R. (1974) Spinal cord stereotactic surgery. In K. Sano and S. Ishii (Eds.), Recent progress in Neurological Surgery, Excerpta Medica, Amsterdam, pp. 234–241.

Schvarcz, J.R. (1978) Spinal cord stereotactic techniques re trigeminal nucleotomy and extralemniscal myelotomy. Appl. Neurophysiol., 41: 99–112.

Sindou, M. (1972) Etude de la jonction radiculo-médullaire postérieure: la radicellotomie posterieure sélective dans la chirurgie de la douleur. Thèse Med., Lyon, p. 182.

Sindou, M. and Lapras, C. (1982) Neurosurgical treatment of pain in the Pancoast-Tobias syndrome: selective posterior rhizotomy and open antero-lateral C2-cordotomy. In J.J. Bonica, V. Ventafrida and C.A. Pagni (Eds.), Advances in Pain Research and Therapy, Vol. 4, Raven Press, New York, pp. 199–209.

Sindou, M. and Goutelle, A. (1983) Surgical posterior rhizotomies for the treatment of pain. In H. Krayenbühl (Ed.), Advances and Technical Standards in Neurosurgery, Vol. 10, Springer-Verlag, Wien, pp. 147–185.

Sindou, M., Fischer, G., Goutelle, A. and Mansuy, L. (1974) La radicellotomie postérieure sélective. Premiers résultats dans la chirurgie de la douleur. Neurochirurgie, 20: 391–408.

Sindou, M., Fischer, G., Goutelle, A., Schott, B. and Mansuy, L. (1974) La radicellotomie postérieure sélective dans le traitement des spasticités. Rev. Neurol., 130: 201–215.

Sindou, M., Quoex, C. and Baleydier, C. (1974) Fiber organization at the posterior spinal cord-rootlet junction in man. J. Comp. Neurol., 153: 15–26.

Sindou, M., Fischer, G. and Mansuy, L. (1976) Posterior spinal rhizotomy and selective posterior rhizidiotomy. In H. Krayenbühl, P.E. Maspes and W.H. Sweet (Eds.), Progress in Neurological Surgery, Vol. 7, Karger, Basel, pp. 201–250.

Sindou, M., Millet, M.F., Mortamais, J. and Eyssette, M. (1982) Results of selective posterior rhizotomy in the treatment of painful and spastic paraplegia secondary to multiple sclerosis. Appl. Neurophysiol., 45: 335–340.

Sindou, M., Abdennebi, B. and Sharkey, P. (1985) Microsurgical selective procedures in the peripheral nerves and the posterior root–spinal cord junction for spasticity. Appl. Neurophysiol., 48: 97–104.

Sindou, M., Mifsud, J.J., Boisson, D. and Goutelle, A. (1986) Selective posterior rhizotomy in the dorsal root entry zone for treatment of hyperspasticity and pain in the hemiplegic upper limb. Neurosurgery, 18: 587–595.

Spiller, W.G. and Martin, E. (1912) The treatment of persistent pain of organic origin in the lower part of the body by division of the antero-lateral column of the spinal cord. JAMA, 58: 1489–1490.

Sweet, W.H. and Poletti, C.E. (1984) Operations in the brain stem and spinal canal, with an appendix on open cordotomy. In P.D. Wall and R. Melzach (Eds.), Textbook of Pain, Churchill Livingstone, Edinburgh, pp. 615–631.

Szentagothai, J. (1964) Neuronal and synaptic arrangement in the substantia gelatinosa. J. Comp. Neurol., 122: 219–239.

Taren, J.A., Davis, R., and Crosby, E.C. (1969) Target physiologic corroboration in stereotaxic cervical cordotomy. J. Neurosurg., 30: 569–584.

Tasker, R.R. (1973) Percutaneous cordotomy. Physiological identification of target site. Confin. Neurol., 36: 110–117.

Tasker, R.R. (1985) Surgical approach to the primary afferents and the spinal cord. In H.L. Fields et al. (Eds.), Advances in Pain Research and Therapy, Vol. 9, Raven Press, New York, pp. 799–824.

Vlahovitch, B. and Fuentes, J.M. (1975) Resultats de la radicellotomie sélective postérieure à l'étage lombaire et cervical. Neurochirurgie, 21: 29–42.

Walker, A.E. (1940) The spino-thalamic tract in man. Arch. Neurol. Psychiatry, 43: 284–298.

Walker, J.S., Ovelmen-Levitt, J., Bullard, D.E. and Nashold, B.S., Jr. (1984) Dorsal root entry zone lesions using a CO_2 laser in cats with neurophysiologic and histologic assessment. Neurosurgery, 15: 265.

Wall, P.D. (1964) Presynaptic control of impulses at the first central synapse in the cutaneous pathway. In J.C. Eccles and J.P. Schadé (Eds.), Physiology of Spinal Neurons, Elsevier, Amsterdam, pp. 92–118.

Wepsic, J.G. (1976) Complications of percutaneous surgery for pain. Clin. Neurosurg., 23: 454–464.

Willis, W.D. (1985) The pain system, Karger, Basel, pp. 346.

White, J.C. and Sweet, W.H. (1969) Pain and the Neurosurgeon. A. Forty Year Experience. Charles C. Thomas, Springfield, IL, pp. 1000.

Young, R.F., Foley, K., Israel Chambi, V. and Rand, R.W. (1988) Dorsal root entry zone lesions: Part I: a comparison of radiofrequency and laser techniques; Part II: clinical experience in 67 patients over five years. J. Neurosurg: (in press).

Epidemiology of Pain

R. Dubner, G.F. Gebhart & M.R. Bond (Eds.)
Proceedings of the Vth World Congress on Pain
© 1988 Elsevier Science Publishers BV (Biomedical Division)

Epidemiology of temporomandibular disorders. I. Initial clinical and self-report findings

Samuel F. Dworkin[1,2,3], Michael Von Korff[4], Linda LeResche[1] and Edmond Truelove[1]

[1]*Department of Oral Medicine, SC-63,* [2]*Department of Psychiatry and Behavioral Sciences, School of Medicine,* [3]*Multidisciplinary Pain Center, University of Washington, Seattle WA 98195, and* [4]*Group Health Cooperative of Puget Sound, Seattle, WA, USA*

Results are presented from a large U.S.A. population-based epidemiological study of temporomandibular disorders (TMD). The study population is a representative sample of the enrolled population ($n = 320000$) of a large health maintenance organization.

Our research plan includes a screening phase, training of reliable field examiner/interviewers, conducting a first-wave field examination and interview and a one-year follow-up examination and interview. Clinical findings were available to allow comparisons among the following groups: (1) clinic cases receiving treatment (CLCA, $n = 232$); (2) currently symptomatic community cases, defined as having experienced TMD pain within the past six months which was not of a trivial or fleeting nature, most of whom were not under treatment within the last six months (COCA, $n = 110$); (3) TMD pain free community controls (COCO, $n = 130$). Selected analyses divided community cases into those who had received TMD treatment some time in the past (COCATX, $n = 53$) and symptomatic community cases who had never received TMD treatment (COCANTX, $n = 57$).

The data presented result from initial descriptive analyses of clinical findings for TMD clinic cases, community cases and controls. The early results indicate that TMD clinic cases are distinguishable from controls in amount of pain reported spontaneously and in response to palpation of the masticatory muscles and the TMJ as well as in the range of vertical jaw opening possible, with and without assistance. Other excursions of the jaw, such as lateral and protrusive excursions, do not seem to distinguish cases from controls. Clinic cases and controls do not appear distinguishable based on prevalence of non-clicking type joint sounds or findings related to occlusion.

Further detailed analyses of our extensive data should identify clinical variables that may or may not reliably distinguish clinic cases from symptomatic persons in the community not under treatment and from pain-free controls.

Introduction

Epidemiological studies (Helkimo, 1976; Solberg et al., 1979) confirm the presence in countries around the world of temporomandibular disorders (TMD). Reviews of these studies, by Greene and Marbach (1982) and Rugh and Solberg (1985), have been critical on several grounds. Many studies have not been population-based but have tended to focus on description and analysis of TMD signs and symptoms exclusively within symptomatic patient populations seeking treatment.

There are no published epidemiological studies

of TMD in the United States, for example, which have used identical study methods to compare the following groups of subjects; (1) those who are both symptomatic and seeking treatment; (2) those from the same community who are asymptomatic; and (3) those who are symptomatic but either are not currently seeking treatment or have never sought treatment.

The present report presents the first clinical data from a large, population-based epidemiological study of TMD designed to address some of these shortcomings. Our study has four research objectives: (1) to develop descriptive epidemiological data on clinical signs and symptoms associated with TMD as well as a descriptive assessment of psychological, psychosocial and demographic factors; (2) to develop diagnostic criteria; (3) to identify prog-

nostic factors which may influence the natural history and clinical course of TMD for treated and untreated cases; and (4) to identify risk factors which influence the probability of developing TMD pain as well as factors that influence treatment seeking.

Methods

The study population is a representative sample of the enrolled population of the Group Health Cooperative of Puget Sound, one of the largest health maintenance organizations in the United States, with 320000 enrollees served by more than 500 physicians.

Our research plan includes a screening phase, training of reliable field examiner/interviewers, and

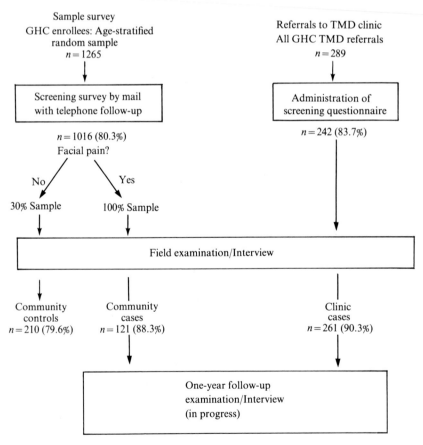

Fig. 1. Epidemiological studies of temporomandibular disorder study design.

conducting a first-wave and one-year follow-up field examination and interview. The overall research scheme is depicted in Fig. 1.

Responses to the screening survey were used to identify representative samples of community cases (COCA) and community controls (COCO). Since GHC provides treatment for TMD to its enrollees, we were also able to identify from the same population clinic cases (CLCA) referred for treatment. All three groups (COCO, COCA and CLCAs) were clinically examined and interviewed in the field by carefully trained and calibrated registered dental hygienist field examiners. The clinical examination included assessment of range of motion, joint sounds measured both by palpation and stethoscope, pain assessment in response to muscle and joint palpation, classification of occlusion, dental and oral health status and other clinical variables suggested as of possible theoretical or clinical significance.

Results

Data presented in this report relate to our first research objective. We present initial descriptive analyses of representative clinical findings drawn from the field examination and incorporate findings for selected self-reported associated symptoms. Examination procedures were conducted in accord with written specifications. Results of our extensive efforts to ensure reliability of clinical examiners have been previously reported (Dworkin et al., 1986; Truelove et al., 1987).

For the present report, data were available from completed clinical examinations as follows: (1) clinic cases receiving treatment (CLCA, $n = 232$); (2) currently symptomatic community cases, defined as having experienced TMD pain within the past six months which was not of a trivial or fleeting nature (COCA, $n = 110$); (3) community controls free of TMD pain (COCO, $n = 130$). Selected analyses divide the community cases into those who have received TMD treatment at some time in the past (COCATX, $n = 53$) and currently symptomatic

community cases who have never received TMD treatment (COCANTX, $n = 57$).

Overall TMD pain levels

Overall prevalence of TMD pain experienced in the prior 6 months was 12.1%. Pain intensity recorded by subjects on visual analogue scales indicated much variability. Average (SD) TMD pain intensity reported was 39.7 (25.8) for CLCA, 32.5 (24.3) for COCATX and 25.1 (21.5) for COCANTX. Pain intensity at its worst was comparable for COCATX and COCANTX, e.g., 63.2 (26.5), vs. 56.3 (27.6), and somewhat higher, e.g. 70.5 (26.0), for CLCA.

Range of motion

Vertical jaw opening Measures of vertical jaw opening (mm) included unassisted pain-free opening, maximum unassisted opening (with or without pain) and maximum assisted opening. Results are summarized in Table I.

A consistent pattern was observed for all measures of vertical jaw opening. For example, COCO showed the largest amount of mean jaw opening and CLCA the smallest, as was expected, with COCA taking intermediate values. For example, mean unassisted openings (SD) for CLCA, COCA and COCO were 37.5 (10.7) mm, 41.9 (9.2) mm, and 47.9 (7.6) mm, respectively. COCATX and COCANTX were comparable on these measures. Only 46% of COCO reported pain associated with maximum assisted jaw opening compared to 67.1% for COCA and 79.1% of CLCA.

Jaw opening patterns Inconsistent relationships among the subject groups were observed for measures of jaw opening patterns. A straight (no deviation) pattern of jaw opening was observed in 42.5% CLCA, with COCATX showing a lower rate (35.8) and COCANTX a higher rate (52.6%), while 65.5% COCO demonstrated a straight jaw opening pattern. CLCA and COCO demonstrated comparable rates for opening patterns associated with self-corrected deviations (27.1% vs 21.6% respectively) but differed on percent of subjects who showed un-

TABLE I

Range of motion: vertical jaw opening (mm)

Vertical Jaw Opening	CLCA (n = 232)	COCATX (n = 53)	COCANTX (n = 57)	COCO (n = 232)
Unassisted				
Mean	37.5	41.0	43.0	47.9
SD	10.7	9.6	8.7	7.6
Maximum unassisted (with pain)				
Mean	45.1	48.0	49.8	52.1
SD	9.0	7.2	6.1	7.5
Maximum assisted (with pain)				
Mean	47.4	50.6	51.3	53.4
SD	8.6	8.3	6.4	7.4
% S's with pain	79.1	64.2	73.7	46.0

CLCA, Clinic cases; COCA TX, community cases previously treated; COCA NTX, community cases not previously treated; COCO, community controls.

corrected deviations (CLCA = 27.5% vs COCO = 11.6%). The highest and lowest rates of self-corrected deviations were observed in COCATX (41.5%) and COCONTX (17.5%), respectively.

Jaw excursions CLCA, COCA and COCO were fairly consistent in extent (mm) of lateral excursions (range across all groups = 9.4–10.3 mm), protruded movement (range across all groups = 4.9–6.1 mm) and protrusive opening (range across all groups = 38.1–42.6 mm). By contrast, the prevalence of pain report was much higher for CLCA than for COCO during lateral jaw excursions (41.9% vs 8.8%), protruded movement (46.9% vs. 12.1%) and protrusive opening (50.2% vs. 7.2%). For COCAs, pain prevalence ranged from 22.7% to 28.6% for these jaw excursions.

Occlusion variables
Classification of occlusion was assigned for each subject. Table II presents the prevalence for posterior and anterior occlusion types as well as for crossbite and open-bite.

TABLE II

Classification of occlusion (% of subjects)

Occlusion	CLCA (n = 232)	COCATX (n = 53)	COCANTX (n = 57)	COCO (n = 138)
Class I	23.1	26.4	24.6	20.7
II	5.2	2.9	9.7	4.4
III	4.2	2.9	3.5	4.7
Posterior X-bite	11.7	12.3	19.3	20.0
Anterior X-bite	5.0	5.7	12.3	11.1
Posterior open-bite	8.1	8.5	3.6	5.8
Anterior open-bite	6.7	3.8	0.0	7.7

Abbreviations as in Table I.

As can be seen from Table II, CLCA, COCA and COCO are not distinguishable based on rates observed for the classification of posterior occlusion or for other occlusal variables. Class III occlusion and cross-bites appear more prevalent in COCO than in CLCA. Clinical examiners were least able to classify anterior occlusion reliably.

Joint sounds

Joint sounds in the temporomandibular joint (TMJ) were assessed using both palpation and stethoscope methods according to rigid measurement specification developed by our study team of clinical investigators. Results for CLCA, COCA and COCO are depicted in Fig. 2.

It is interesting to observe that the estimated prevalence of clicking and popping TMJ noises is about the same whichever method is used. However, large discrepancies appear between the methods when soft crepitus and hard grating sounds are assessed. Clicking or popping TMJ noises are detected in about 28–32% of CLCA, whether palpation or stethoscope methods are used; by contrast, crepitus sounds are detected in 7.1% of CLCA using palpation and 32.0% using the stethoscope. The prevalence of non-clicking joint sounds detected by stethoscope appeared comparable for CLCA, COCO and COCA groups (see Fig. 2).

When self-report data for joint sounds were examined, it was observed that CLCA and COCA consistently overestimated the presence of sounds in the TMJ, while COCO tended to under-report joint sounds, compared to findings on clinical examination. For example, 54% of CLCA reported clicking noises, while palpation examination revealed only 28% with detectable clicks or pops, for a 2:1 over-reporting discrepancy; on the other hand, 6% of COCO reported TMJ clicks, while 17% were detected by clinical examination, for an almost 3:1 under-reporting discrepancy.

In our extensive reliability studies of TMD measurement, we consistently observed that joint sounds were associated with the poorest reliability of measurement of all clinically relevant variables even though our calibrated examiners were con-

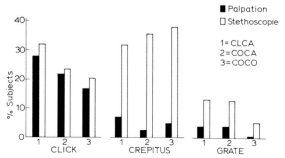

Fig. 2. Assessment of temporomandibular joint sounds: palpation and stethoscope (% of subjects).

sistently more reliable than uncalibrated but experienced clinical TMD specialists (Dworkin et al., 1988).

Palpation pain

Palpation of extra- and intra-oral muscles as well as palpation of the TMJ is consistently associated with a higher prevalence of pain for CLCA than for any other group. Table III summarizes the prevalence of pain elicited by palpation of the masticatory muscles and the TMJ.

In most instances, the differences in prevalence of palpation elicited pain between CLCA and COCO are appreciable (e.g., 39.3% CLCA compared to 9.5% COCO reported pain on palpation of the superficial masseter; palpation of the lateral pole of the TMJ elicited pain in 41.0% CLCA but 5.8% COCO). While COCATX and COCANTX fell between these extremes, it is also interesting to note that the differences between treated (COCATX) and non-treated (COCANTX) community cases is often negligible (e.g., 30.2% vs, 34.2%, respectively, for the superficial masseter; 22.7% vs. 28.1%, respectively, for the lateral pole of the TMJ). Pain was elicited in 13.6% of the CLCA and 10.4% COCATX but only 1.1% of COCO in response to palpation of a theoretically non-TMD-involved (i.e. 'placebo') anatomic site, the mastoid process.

Overall, pain report on palpation ranged between mild and moderate. Severe ratings for palpation pain were elicited only from CLCA and only in response to palpation of certain intra-oral muscles or palpation of the TMJ, and, even then, in only a small proportion of subjects (Table III).

Discussion

The data presented result from initial descriptive analyses of clinical findings for TMD clinic cases, community cases and controls. The early results indicate that TMD clinic cases are distinguishable from controls in the range of vertical jaw opening possible, with and without assistance. Other excursions of the jaw, such as lateral and protrusive excursions, do not seem to distinguish cases from controls.

Clinic cases and controls do not appear distinguishable based on prevalence of joint sounds except for the possibility that both palpation and stethoscope examination reveal more clicking and popping TMJ noises among cases than controls. However, findings regarding joint sounds must be interpreted with caution, both because differences among groups seem small and because recording of joint sounds may not be reliable.

Classification of occlusion and assessment of other variables related to tooth or occlusal arch relationship do not appear to distinguish clinic cases from controls.

Community cases, for the most part, fall between clinic cases and controls on many variables assessed. For many clinical variables, these initial analyses did not appear to reveal important differences between community cases who received treatment compared to community cases who never received treatment.

In summary, these clinical findings parallel an earlier preliminary report (Dworkin et al., 1987) regarding the frequency of TMD-associated symptoms as gleaned from self-report questionnaires. Clinic cases seem to report more symptoms and react with greater intensity to most examination and self-report items than do community cases or controls. While it seems undeniable that clinic cases report more pain, both spontaneously and in response to palpation examination, and they experience greater limitations in vertical jaw excursions, they may not be as readily distinguishable from controls or untreated community cases on many clinical variables. Further detailed analyses of our extensive data sets promise to shed further light on clinical variables that may or may not reliably distinguish clinic cases from treated and untreated symptomatic persons in the community not under treatment and from TMD pain free community controls.

TABLE III

Palpation pain: extra- and intra-oral muscles and temporomandibular joint (TMJ) patient self-report (mild + moderate + severe) (% of subjects)

Palpation site	CLCA (n = 232)	COCATX (n = 53)	COCANTX (n = 57)	COCO (n = 138)
Posterior temporalis	12.1	8.5	8.8	1.5
Ant. temporalis	22.9	9.4	14.9	3.3
Superf. masseter	39.3	30.2	34.2	9.5
Frontalis	10.8	3.8	6.2	0.7
Trapezius	32.2	23.6	28.9	6.7
Mastoid process	13.6	10.4	7.9	1.1
TMJ*: lateral pole	41.0	22.7	28.1	5.8
Intrameatal	24.2	8.5	10.5	4.7
Lat. pterygoid**	63.4	47.2	50.1	40.0
Tendon of tempor.**	59.5	40.6	56.2	29.7
Tongue	15.9	9.4	10.5	4.0

Severe pain reported by: *4–6%; **9–12%.

References

Dworkin, S.F., Von Korff, M., Truelove, E., Sommers, E. and LeResche, L. (1986) Reliability of examiners assessing TMD signs and symptoms. 64th General Session International Association for Dental Research, The Hague, Netherlands.

Dworkin, S.F., Von Korff, M., LeResche, L. and Kruger, A. (1987) TMD and other pain complaints: initial screening results from a population-based epidemiologic study. 65th General Session, International Association for Dental Research, Chicago, Illinois.

Dworkin, S.F., Le Resche, L. and DeRouen, T. (1988) Reliability of clinical measurements in temporomandibular disorders. Clin. J. Pain, in press.

Greene, C.S. and Marbach, J.J. (1982) Epidemiologic studies of mandibular dysfunction. J. Prosth. Dent., 48: 184–190.

Helkimo, M. (1976) Epidemiologal surveys of dysfunction of the masticatory system. Oral Sci. Rev., 1: 54–69.

Rugh, J.D and Solberg, W.K. (1985) Oral health status in the United States: Temporomandibular disorders. J. Dent. Educ. 49: 398–405.

Solberg, W.K., Woo, M.W. and Houston, J.B. (1979) Prevalence of mandibular dysfunction in young adults. J. Am. Dent. Assoc., 98: 25–34.

Truelove, E., LeResche, L., Sommers, E., Dworkin, S., Huggins, K., Reay, B. (1987) Reliability of TMJ sounds in patients and controls. 65th General Session International Association for Dental Research, Chicago, Illinois.

R. Dubner, G.F. Gebhart & M.R. Bond (Eds.)
Proceedings of the Vth World Congress on Pain
© 1988 Elsevier Science Publishers BV (Biomedical Division)

Epidemiology of temporomandibular disorders. II. TMD pain compared to other common pain sites

Michael Von Korff[1], Samuel Dworkin[2], Linda LeResche[2] and Andrea Kruger[1]

[1]*Center for Health Studies, Group Health Cooperative of Puget Sound, 200 15th Avenue East, Seattle, WA 98112, and*
[2]*Department of Oral Medicine, University of Washington School of Dentistry, Seattle, WA, USA*

Summary

An epidemiological survey concerning temporomandibular disorder (TMD) pain and four other chronic pain conditions (back pain, headache, abdominal pain and chest pain) was carried out among a probability sample of 1265 adult enrollees of a large Seattle area health maintenance organization. Completed questionnaires were obtained for 1016 persons (80.3% response rate). Each of the pain conditions was common. TMD pain, headache and abdominal pain were associated with younger age and female gender. Prevalent cases of each pain condition typically had a long-standing pain problem which was intermittent and of mild to moderate intensity. TMD pain was less likely to be associated with activity limitation than the other pain conditions. Back pain and headache were the leading sources of pain-related disability, accounting for 1.6 and 1.0 activity limitation days per capita in the six month prevalence period. A history of use of health care for each pain condition was reported by 52–66% of current cases, but only 20–35% reported use of health care for the pain problem in the previous six months.

Each pain condition was associated with elevated Hopkins Symptoms Checklist (SCL) scores for somatization, anxiety and depression relative to persons with no current pain. Current pain was also associated with an increased prevalence of an algorithm diagnosis of DSM-III major depression. Examination of SCL scores and major depression by number of pain problems revealed that the excess of psychological impairment was limited to persons with multiple pain conditions. For example, the prevalence of major depression was 2.0% for persons with no pains, 1.5% for persons with a single pain, and 9.9% for persons with two or more current pain conditions.

Introduction

Most epidemiological studies of chronic pain have investigated pain occurring at a single anatomical site, for example back pain (Nagi et al., 1973; Reisborg and Greenland, 1985; Frymoyer et al., 1983), headache (Linet and Stewart, 1984; Newland et al., 1978; Ekbom et al., 1978), irritable bowel (Whitehead et al., 1982; Drossman et al., 1982), or temporomandibular disorder (TMD) pain (Greene and Marbach, 1982; Solberg et al., 1979; Agerberg and Carlsson, 1972). Recently, Sternbach (1986a, b) reported results of a survey of chronic pain in the U.S. population which examined the occurrence and correlates of a number of different types of chronic pain. This methodological innovation provides a basis for comparative study of chronic pain conditions. In this report, we use the comparative method to shed light on the aspects of chronic pain that are unique to particular pain conditions, and aspects that are common to chronic pain irrespective of site. Our main focus is on TMD pain, which was not examined in Sternbach's study. We compare TMD pain to four other pain conditions: back pain, headache, abdominal pain and chest pain.

The specific aims of this research are to estimate the prevalence in the general population of each of these five pain conditions in a representative sample of adults, and to compare prevalent cases of each pain condition in terms of their age and sex distribution, lifetime incidence, duration and recurrence, pain intensity, activity limitation, use of health care for pain, and psychological status. This report presents a brief overview of initial results.

Methods

The population surveyed consisted of adult residents of the greater Seattle area enrolled in a large health maintenance organization. A probability sample of 1265 persons was identified and standardized questionnaires were administered through a mail survey with telephone follow-up of non-respondents. The questionnaires included uniform sets of items for each of the five pain conditions, a 60-item version of the Hopkins Symptoms Checklist (SCL) (Derogatis et al., 1974) and other items.

Completed questionnaires were obtained from 1016 persons, for a response rate of 80%.

Persons were asked to report pain conditions which had lasted a whole day or more or which had recurred several times in a year. They were instructed to exclude fleeting or minor aches and pains. This report focuses on pain conditions reported as occurring within the six months prior to the survey date.

Results

Our results are consistent with previous epidemiological surveys in that each of the five pain conditions was found to be common among adults. The six month prevalence of TMD pain was 12% (Fig. 1). The most common pain condition was back pain, followed by headache, abdominal pain, TMD pain and chest pain. TMD pain was almost twice as common among females as males. This two to one ratio is substantially less than the five to one predominance of females observed among persons seeking specialty treatment for TMD in this population. Headache and abdominal pain were found to be more common among females than males as well. TMD pain, headache and abdominal pain were also similar in that prevalence decreased with age, which was not the case for back pain or chest pain.

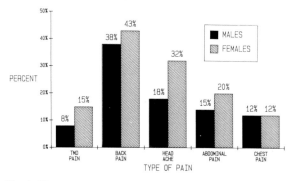

Fig. 1. Six month prevalence (percent) of selected pain conditions.

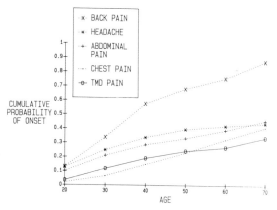

Fig. 2. Life-table estimate of the cumulative probability of developing selected pain conditions by age.

Based on the respondents' self-reported lifetime history of each pain condition and initial age of onset, we estimated the probability of the occurrence of each pain condition by a given age using life-table methods (Fig. 2). Among persons surviving to age 70, 85% are projected to have experienced a problem with back pain. The lifetime occurrence of headache, abdominal pain and chest pain are each projected to exceed 40%, while about one-third of all persons surviving to age 70 would have experienced an episode of TMD pain.

Table I reports data on the usual pain intensity of each pain condition during the six month prevalence period. Intensity was rated on a ten-point anchored scale. The mean intensity rating for TMD pain was 4.3, corresponding to moderate intensity. The usual intensity of TMD pain was similar to the ratings for the other conditions, with the exception of headache. The percentage of headache cases reporting usual pain as severe was 39%, compared to 15–21% for the other pains.

Comparison of the temporal dimensions of each pain condition also revealed similarities and differences (Table I). Prevalent cases of TMD pain, on average, had an interval of eight years since initial onset. This was within the range of the other pain conditions. While the pain conditions were typically long-standing problems, most cases experienced several brief episodes over the six month prevalence period rather than persistent pain. Only about one-quarter of the TMD cases reported pain on more than half the days, which was similar to back pain. Headache, abdominal pain and chest pain were less likely to be persistent. In terms of usual daily duration, back pain, headache and TMD pain were the most persistent. About 30% of persons with these conditions reported pain lasting more than eight hours a day, whereas this was the case for less than 15% of persons with abdominal pain and chest pain.

In summary, while there were differences in temporal pattern between the different pain conditions,

TABLE I

Pain conditions present in previous six months: usual intensity, duration and frequency of prevalent cases

	TMD pain	Back pain	Head-ache	Abdominal pain	Chest pain
Intensity rated on a ten-point anchored scale					
Mean	4.3	4.7	5.9	5.1	4.3
S.D.	2.3	1.9	2.1	2.1	2.5
Percent severe	16.4%	15.3%	39.3%	20.9%	21.1%
Duration					
Mean years since initial episode	8.3	10.5	13.9	10.2	6.2
Pain for 9+ hours per day	27.3%	32.2%	29.4%	14.5%	13.0%
Frequency in previous six months					
Single brief episode	9.8%	9.1%	9.7%	11.8%	17.4%
Two or more episodes	66.4%	62.0%	74.0%	72.9%	68.7%
Pain on more than half the days	23.7%	28.8%	16.4%	15.3%	13.9%

TABLE II

Pain conditions present in previous six months: activity limitation and use of health care services of prevalent cases

	TMD pain	Back pain	Head-ache	Abdominal pain	Chest pain
Activity limitation days					
Mean days per case	0.5	3.8	3.9	1.2	1.3
Percent with 1 + days	9.1%	23.6%	39.6%	28.6%	15.3%
Mean days per capita	0.1	1.6	1.0	0.2	0.2
Use of health care for pain condition					
Percent of cases using services in previous 6 months	23.1%	26.8%	20.9%	29.1%	34.7%
Percent of cases ever using services	61.9%	66.2%	51.7%	62.8%	63.5%
Percent of total population using services for pain condition in previous 6 months	2.8%	10.9%	5.4%	4.9%	4.1%

each of the five pain conditions was typically long-standing and intermittent, with substantial individual variation in pain pattern among cases.

Each case was asked the number of days pain kept them from usual activities, including work, school or housework, during the six month prevalence period (Table II). For TMD, the mean number of activity-limitation days per case was half a day. Only 9% of TMD cases reported one or more activity-limitation days. In contrast, prevalent cases of back pain and headache reported almost four activity-limitation days per case. About 40% of head-ache cases and 24% of back pain cases had at least one activity-limitation day. On a per capita basis, back pain and headache were by far the leading causes of disability, accounting for 1.6 and 1.0 activity-limitation days per person, respectively.

Large differences between pain conditions were not observed for use of health care services (Table II). About one-quarter of all prevalent TMD cases had sought health care services for TMD pain in the previous six months. The percentage of persons seeking health care in the previous six months was similar for the other pain conditions. Over 60% of

TABLE III

Adjusted odds ratios for major depression estimated by logistic regression: persons with one, two and three or more pain conditions in the previous six months

Variable	Beta	Odds ratio	Chi square	P value
Age (years)	−0.029			
Sex (Female)	0.440			
One pain*	−0.339	0.71	0.33	0.570
Two pains*	1.478	4.38	10.39	0.000
Three pains* or more	1.805	6.08	12.72	0.000

*Odds ratios, adjusted for age and sex, are relative to persons with no pain condition.

current TMD cases had sought health care for TMD pain at some time. Again, persons with the other pain conditions reported similar percentages. On a per capita basis, about 3% of the adult population had sought care for TMD pain in the previous six months, compared to 11% for back pain and 4 to 5% for the other pain conditions.

We now turn from pain experience and behavior to the association of psychological distress with each pain condition. We examined age–sex adjusted and standardized SCL scale scores for somatization, anxiety and depression. Each of the five pain conditions was associated with significantly elevated somatization, anxiety and depression relative to persons with none of the five pain conditions.

Applying an algorithm (Uhlenhuth et al., 1983) based on DSM-III (American Psychiatric Association, 1980) criteria to the symptom data, we estimated the percentage of subjects meeting criteria for major depression. Two percent of the persons with no pain condition met DSM-III criteria for major depression, compared to 11% of persons with TMD pain. The prevalence of major depression varied from 6 to 10% for the other four pain conditions.

Since each of the pain conditions was associated with psychological impairment, we examined the association of SCL scale scores with number of pain conditions. We found that persons with a single pain condition had an SCL profile below the population mean and only slightly higher than persons with no pain condition. Persons with two pain conditions had substantially elevated SCL scores and the presence of three or more pain conditions was associated with an additional statistically significant increment in SCL scores.

The increased prevalence of major depression was also limited to persons with multiple pain conditions. Among persons with a single pain condition the prevalence of major depression was 1.5%, less than the prevalence of major depression among persons with no pain condition (2.0%), whereas the prevalence of major depression among persons with two or more pain conditions was almost 10%.

This association of major depression with multiple pain conditions, but not a single pain problem, held after adjusting for age and sex using a logistic regression model (Table III). Relative to persons with no pain condition, the age–sex-adjusted odds ratio was less than 1 for persons with a single pain condition. Relative to pain-free persons, those with two pain conditions were over four times as likely to meet criteria for major depression, and persons with three or more pain conditions were about six times as likely.

Conclusions

Our initial results indicate that TMD pain, back pain, headache, abdominal pain and chest pain are all common complaints in the general population. TMD is similar to headache and abdominal pain in that it is more common among females and younger persons. Persons with TMD pain, like other kinds of pain, typically had a long-standing, intermittent pain problem of mild to moderate intensity. While back pain and headache are important sources of activity limitation, this is less characteristic of TMD pain. Most TMD cases had sought treatment for TMD pain at some time, but most cases of TMD in this population were not currently under treatment. This was also the case for each of the other pain conditions.

In terms of psychological impairment, each pain condition was associated with increased likelihood of emotional disorder. The excess of psychological impairment, though, was limited to persons reporting multiple pains.

Our initial results show many similarities among different pain conditions, and some differences. They also indicate that persons with mutiple pain complaints may differ from persons with a single pain condition. Our comparative studies of chronic pain will be pursued further with more refined analyses of cross-sectional data and analyses of longitudinal data now being collected.

References

Agerberg, G. and Carlsson, G.E. (1972) Functional disorders of the masticatory system: I. Distribution of symptoms according to age and sex as judged from investigation by questionnaire. Acta Odont. Scand., 30: 596–613.

American Psychiatric Association (1980) Diagnostic and Statistical Manual, Third Edition, APA, Washington DC.

Derogatis, L.R., Lipman, R.S., Covi, L. et al. (1974) The Hopkins Symptom Checklist (HSCL); A self report inventory. Behav. Sci., 19: 1–15.

Drossman, D.A., Sandler, R.S., McKee, D.C. and Lovitz, A.J. (1982) Bowel patterns among subjects not seeking health care. Gastroenterology, 82: 529–534.

Ekbom, K., Ahlborg, B. and Schele, R. (1978) Prevalence of migraine and cluster headache in Swedish men of 18. Headache, 18: 9–19.

Frymoyer, J.W., Pope, M.H., Clements, J.H. et al. (1983) Risk factors in low-back pain: An epidemiological survey. J. Bone Joint Surg., 65:213–218.

Greene, C.S. and Marback, J.J. (1982) Epidemiologic studies of mandibular dysfunction. J. Prosth. Dent., 48: 184–190.

Linet, M.S. and Stewart, W.F. (1984) Migraine headache: Epidemiologic perspectives. Epidemiol. Rev., 6: 107–139.

Nagi, S.Z., Riley, L.E. and Newby, L.G. (1973) A social epidemiology of back pain in a general population. J. Chron. Dis., 26: 769–779.

Newland, C.A., Illis, L.S., Robins, P.K. et al. (1978) A survey of headache in an English city. Headache, 5: 1–20.

Reisbord, L.S. and Greenland, S. (1985) Factors associated with self reported back-pain prevalence: A population-based study. J. Chron. Dis., 38: 691–702.

Solberg, W.K., Woo, M.W. and Houston, J.B. (1979) Prevalence of mandibular dysfunction in young adults. J. Am. Dent. Assoc., 98: 25–34.

Sternbach, R.A. (1986a) Pain and hassles in the United States: findings of the Nuprin Pain Report. Pain, 27: 69–80.

Sternbach, R.A. (1986b) Survey of pain in the United States: the Nuprin Pain Report. Clin. J. Pain,, 2: 49–53.

Uhlenhuth, E.H., Balter, M.B., Mellinger, G.D, et al. (1983) Symptom Checklist syndromes in the general population: Correlations with psychotherapeutic drug use. Arch. Gen. Psychiatry, 40: 1167–1173.

Whitehead, W.E., Winget, C., Fedoravicius, A.S. et al. (1982) Learned illness behavior in patients with irritable bowel syndrome and peptic ulcer. Digest. Dis. Sci., 27: 202–208.

R. Dubner, G.F. Gebhart & M.R. Bond (Eds.)
Proceedings of the Vth World Congress on Pain
© 1988 Elsevier Science Publishers BV (Biomedical Division)

CHAPTER 56

Etiology of cranio-facial pain and headache in stomatognathic dysfunction

Franco Mongini, Franco Ventricelli and Enrico Conserva

Center for Gnathology and Cranio-Facial Pathophysiology, University of Turin, Italy

Summary

In order to examine the relationship between cranio-facial pain and headache and the different etiologic factors of stomatognathic dysfunction 162 females and 34 males referred for dysfunction of the stomatognathic system were examined. For each patient the 'Dysfunction Index System' (Mongini, 1986) was constructed, which quantifies (score 0 to 10) etiologic and consequential factors. Etiologic factors considered are: occlusal alterations, mandibular displacement, abnormal tooth contact in movements, muscle parafunction and psychogenic stress. Consequential factors are: TMJ impairment, restriction of movements, muscle tenderness, tenderness of cranial sites, headache and facial pain. Three statistical approaches were used: each factor was correlated to the other by means of the Pearson correlation coefficient; the canonical correlation analysis was performed and subgroups of patients with severe headache and/or facial pain were collated and their mean scores for etiologic factors were examined. The data showed that in stomatognathic dysfunction facial pain and headache are more related to neuromuscular and psychogenic factors

than to structural ones. In some females, however, headache is probably mixed in nature, with tension headache superimposed on vascular migraine.

Craniofacial pain and headache are frequent findings in patients with stomatognathic dysfunction and their etiology is still debated. One reason for lack of consensus is that a precise assessment of such dysfunction is still missing, so that it is often referred to in different ways, such as temporomandibular disorders (TMD) or myofacial pain dysfunction syndrome (MPDS). There is a fairly general agreement that the etiology of stomatognathic dysfunction may be multifactorial (Solberg et al., 1972; Mikhail and Rosen, 1980; Kopp, 1982; Wedel and Carlsson, 1985) but disagreement persists as to how different factors (structural, neuromuscular psychosocial) are relevant in causing such disorders (Laskin, 1969; Farrar, 1982; De Boever and Adriaens, 1983). On the other hand, not only may inputs different in nature be present, to various extents in the same patient but, in different individuals, the same input may lead to different consequential factors through a large variety of pathogenic mechanisms (Mongini, 1984). Therefore, correlation studies on craniofacial pain and headache in such patients need a system for assessing and quantifying inputs and outputs. Several indexes to evaluate the degree of dysfunction have been proposed (Helkimo, 1974; Smith, 1981; Rieder and Martinoff, 1983) which usually provide a good means for epidemiological studies, but are less ef-

Correspondence: Franco Mongini, M.D., D.D.S., Ph. D., Director, Center for Gnathology and Cranio-Facial Pathophysiology, University of Turin, Corso Polonia 14, I–10126 Torino, Italy.

fective in quantifying separately the different etiologic and consequential factors. For this purpose a 'Dysfunction Index System' (DIS) has been developed and tested for a period of three years (Mongini, 1986).

Our present purpose was to employ this index in a consistent number of patients with stomatognathic dysfunction in order to examine the relationship between craniofacial pain and headache and the different etiologic factors and to identify some pathogenic mechanisms leading to such symptoms.

Material and methods

Patient assessment

One hundred and ninety-six patients referred for dysfunction of the stomatognathic system were considered. After history and clinical examination, transcranial radiographs and/or polytomography of the temporo-mandibular joint (TMJ) were performed.

For each patient the DIS was constructed from the data obtained. In this system different etiologic factors are considered: structural (occlusal disorders, mandibular displacement, abnormal tooth contact in movement), neuromuscular (muscle hyperfunction and parafunction) and psychogenic. Consequential factors considered are: TMJ impairment, restriction of motility, tenderness of cranial sites at palpation, headache and facial pain. The index for each factor is constructed on the basis of a score given to several parameters obtained from the patient's history and clinical and instrumental examination (Table I). The score is fixed in some cases and variable in others: for instance, a cross-bite is scored 2 to 5 depending on the number of teeth involved; since a cross-bite of canines is more severe than that of other teeth, one or two points are added if one or two canine pairs are involved. Some parameters are considered under different factors: tooth attrition is a parameter for 'occlusion' and for 'muscle hyperfunction and parafunction' (as a sign of tooth clenching and grinding). Similarly, condylar displacement (as evaluated from TMJ radio-

graphs) is a parameter for the TMJ factor and for mandibular displacement in intercuspal position (ICP). The total of the scores for the single parameters gives the actual score for any given index; the maximum score considered is 10. The guidelines for the computation of all indexes have been extensively reported elsewhere (Mongini, 1986). Depending on the final score obtained, the following distinctions are made: 0–1.5 = no problem; 2–4.5 = mild problem; 5–7.5 = moderate problem; 8–10 = severe problem. Thus any single factor is quantified on the basis of a scale (from 0 to 10) and of categories of increasing severity. For instance, a severe (score 3) facial pain, lasting between one and two hours (score 2) but occurring less than once a month (score −1) is a 'mild' problem (total score 4). If the frequency or duration increases the corresponding scores will be higher and the total score will fall into the 'moderate' or 'severe' categories.

Statistical evaluation

The data obtained from the DIS of all patients were evaluated by means of three different statistical approaches. First, the Pearson correlation coefficient was used to correlate each factor with the other. Second, the canonical correlation analysis was performed. Through this procedure a collection of variables is distributed between two sets, an x-set and a y-set, and the possible relationship between the two sets is sought. For this purpose linear combinations of the variables of each set are calculated (i.e. $\eta = a'x$ and $\varphi = b'y$) and then all pairs of linear combinations of the two sets which show some correlation to each other are determined: thus, pairs of 'canonic variables' ($\eta_1 \varphi_1$, $\eta_2 \varphi_2$, $\eta_3 \varphi_3$ and so forth) are found (Fig. 1). Finally, those canonic variables which belong to pairs having a sufficient degree of correlation are related to the original variables (that is, the η canonic variables with the original variables of the x-set and the φ canonic variables with the original variables of the y-set) to find the weight of the latter inside the set. In our case the variables of the x-set were the etiologic factors and the variables of the y-set were the consequential factors, and through this method we could

TABLE I

DIS scores of a patient with mixed headache, burning pain at the right cheek and restriction of mandibular movements

Occlusion		Mandibular displacement		Abnormal tooth contact in movements		Muscle parafunction and hyperfunction		Psychogenic stress	
Overjet > 4 mm (2)	2	Inferior midline displacement in ICP (2–5)	3	Anterior or lateral hyper-balance (6 × 1–2)		Tooth attrition (1–4)	3	Nervous breakdown (2)	2
Open bite (2–5)		Vertical displacement (2–5)	3	Balancing contact on attrition facet (2 × 1–2)		Bruxing or clenching incidental (1) regular (2) regular and severe (3)	3	Frequent tension (2)	2
Deep bite (2–5)	2	Condylar displacement (1–4)	3	Tooth guidance or group contact without cuspids (3 × 1–2)		Muscle tension or pain after waking up (3)		Sleeping difficulty (2)	2
Cross-bite (2–5)+(1–2)		Face asymmetry 1–5	3	With one cuspid (2 × 1–2)		Muscle hypertrophy (4)	2	Intake of tranquilizers (2)	2
Class 2,3 (3)				Unilateral contact in protrusion (2)	2	Increased tooth sensitivity (1)		Onset of symptoms in a period of tension probably (2) surely (3)	2
Missing or not occluding teeth (0.5–1×)	10					Other parafunctional habits (2)	2	Stress worsens symptoms sometimes (2) always (3)	2
Tooth attrition (1–4)	3							Clinician's evaluation (2–4)	2
Total	10	Total	10	Total	2	Total	10	Total	10

TMJ	R	L
Condylar displacement (1–2)	2	1
Change in shape (2–4)		
Arthrotic degeneration (8)		
Disc-condyle incoordination (3–7)		
Locking (8)		8
Articular noise independent of arthrotic degeneration or disc-condyle incoordination (2)	2	
Intra-auricular pain at palpation (2)		
Total	4	9

Restriction of motility	
Mouth opening (1–8)	3
Protrusive and lateral border movements (1–2×)	1
Deviation at opening independent of opening click (1–3)	3
Total	7

Muscle tenderness		Tenderness of cranial sites (1×)
Lateral pterygoid (2×)	3	2
Other masticatory muscles (1×)	1	6
Paramasticatory muscles (1×)	3	5
Total	7	10

Headache, Facial pain		
Pattern (1–3)	2	2
Duration (1–3)	3	3
Frequency (−1–4)	4	4
Total	9	9

Most etiologic factors (upper line) reach the maximum level of severity, indicating a multifactorial etiology in this case. As a consequence a left articular locking is present, together with severe muscle tenderness, headache and facial pain. × means that the score must be multiplied for the number of times the factor is present. The maximum total score considered is 10 even in the event that a higher figure is obtained.

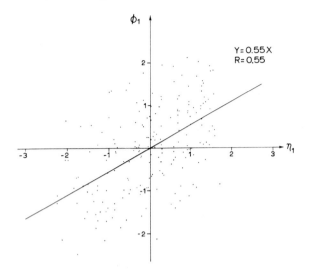

Fig. 1. Correlation between canonic variables η_1 and φ_1.

Y = 0.55 X
R = 0.55

assess combinations of etiologic factors which to-gether led to combinations of consequential factors: moreover, the relevance of the single factors within the group could be evaluated. Computations were performed as described in classical textbooks (see, for instance, Mardia et al., 1979) by means of specific software (BMDP GM, BMPD Statistical Software, Los Angeles, CA). By the third statistical ap-

proach subgroups of patients were constructed in which preselected consequential factors (headache and/or facial pain, headache only, facial pain only) always fell into the 'severe' category (score 8 to 10) and the distribution of the etiologic factors in these subgroups was examined.

Results

In the group examined there were 162 females (82.65%) and 34 males (17.35%). Mean age was 29.22 yr ($\pm$ 11.52), with no significant differences between sexes.

In Table II the DIS data are given for the whole group and for females and males separately. Several etiologic and consequential factors reached the moderate problem range. It is noteworthy that all etiologic factors except psychogenic stress were higher in males than in females: however, none of these differences was statistically significant. Headache had a significantly higher score in the female group as compared to the male group. Fifty-three patients (27.04%) had only severe (score 8 to 10) structural factors, 33 of them (16.84%) had only severe neu-

TABLE II Mean scores ($\pm$ S.D.) of etiologic (upper section) and consequential (lower section) factors for all patients, males and females

	All patients (*n* = 196)	Males (*n* = 34)	Females (*n* = 162)
Occlusion	7.27($\pm$2.70)	7.66($\pm$2.25)	7.23($\pm$2.80)
Mandibular displacement	5.22($\pm$2.60)	5.44($\pm$2.51)	5.04($\pm$2.61)
Abnormal tooth contact	4.38($\pm$3.81)	5.32($\pm$3.71)	4.20($\pm$3.83)
Muscle parafunction	6.51($\pm$3.10)	7.35($\pm$2.83)	6.22($\pm$3.19)
Psychogenic stress	5.59($\pm$3.12)	5.35($\pm$3.72)	5.67($\pm$3.06)
TMJ	6.60($\pm$2.61)	6.69($\pm$2.75)	6.53($\pm$2.64)
Restriction of motility	3.42($\pm$2.99)	2.88($\pm$2.81)	3.54($\pm$3.03)
Tenderness of cranial sites	2.68($\pm$2.39)	3.00($\pm$2.61)	2.62($\pm$2.36)
Muscle tenderness	5.52($\pm$3.25)	5.5 ($\pm$3.36)	5.54($\pm$3.24)
Headache	3.76($\pm$3.62)	2.52($\pm$3.62)	4.36($\pm$3.61)
Facial pain	4.83($\pm$3.36)	4.22($\pm$3.52)	5.08($\pm$3.37)

Headache is significantly higher in females than in males (P < 0.05). Note also that all etiologic factors, except psychogenic stress, are higher in males.

TABLE III Significant correlations between the single factors

Factors	r
A	
Psychogenic stress and facial pain	0.40
Muscle parafunction and facial pain	0.36
Psychogenic stress and muscle tenderness	0.35
Psychogenic stress and headache	0.28
Mandibular displacement and TMJ	0.25
Muscle parafunction and muscle tenderness	0.25
B	
Psychogenic stress and muscle parafunction	0.34
Occlusion and mandibular displacement	0.31
C	
Restriction of motility and TMJ	0.39
Facial pain and muscle tenderness	0.36
Headache and muscle tenderness	0.33
Facial pain and restriction of motility	0.31
Facial pain and tenderness of cranial sites	0.26
Headache and tenderness of cranial sites	0.25

A, correlations between etiologic factors and consequential factors; B, correlation between etiologic factors; C, correlation between consequential factors. Only r values with $P < 0.0009$ are shown because α critical = 0.05. The critical values take into account that 55 correlations have been tested (0.05/55 = 0.0009).

romuscular and/or psychogenic factors and 79 (40.31%) had factors of both sorts. Conversely, 37 patients (18.9%) had severe TMJ problems as consequential factors, 79 patients (40.3%) had severe cephalalgia (headache and/or facial pain) and 33 patients (16.84%) had both TMJ impairment and cephalalgia at severe level.

Table III shows the significant correlations between single factors: psychogenic stress was significantly correlated with facial pain, muscle tenderness and headache; parafunction with facial pain and muscle tenderness; mandibular displacement with TMJ impairment. Etiologic factors which significantly correlated with each other were: psychogenic stress with parafunction, occlusal alterations with mandibular displacement. Between the consequential factors muscle tenderness and tenderness of cranial sites were both significantly correlated with headache and facial pain; restriction of motil-

ity with TMJ impairment and facial pain.

Five possible pairs of canonic variables were found with the following correlation degrees: η_1, φ_1: 0.55; η_2, φ_2: 0.38; η_3, φ_3: 0.26; η_4, φ_4: 0.18; η_5, φ_5: 0.06. The pairs η_1, φ_1 and η_2, φ_2 had the highest correlation: the correlation of these canonic variables with the variables originally considered were then plotted (Table IV). In the first pair of canonic variables (η_1, φ_1) η_1 showed a high correlation with psychogenic stress ($r = 0.92$) and a weaker correlation with parafunction ($r = 0.66$). No other significant correlation was present. φ_1 correlated with facial pain ($r = 0.83$), with muscle tenderness ($r = 0.69$) and, more weakly, with headache ($r = 0.48$) and tenderness of cranial sites at palpation ($r = 0.45$). In the second pair of canonic variables (η_2, φ_2), η_2 correlated with mandibular displacement ($r = 0.94$) and, to a lesser extent, with occlusion ($r = 0.57$), φ_2 correlated with TMJ impairment ($r = 0.72$) and, weakly, with tenderness of cranial sites ($r = 0.40$).

When groups with preselected severe consequential factors were collated, parafunctions and psychogenic stress (as etiologic factors) were significantly higher in the group with only headache and/or facial pain at the severe level. Significantly enough, the latter trend was confirmed for the

TABLE IV Correlation of canonic variables η_1, η_2, φ_1, φ_2 with the original variables

1st set variables	η_1	η_2
Occlusion	−0.053	0.576
Mandibular displacement	−0.099	0.94
Abnormal tooth contact	0.098	0.29
Muscle parafunction	0.659	0.083
Psychogenic stress	0.921	−0.024

2nd set variables	φ_1	φ_2
TMJ	−0.19	0.721
Restriction of motility	0.167	−0.029
Tenderness of cranial sites	0.453	0.403
Muscle tenderness	0.694	0.037
Headache	0.488	0.166
Facial pain	0.834	0.051

TABLE V Mean scores (±S.D.) of etiologic factors in subgroups of patients with severe headache and/or facial pain, severe facial pain only and severe headache only

	Headache and/ or facial pain (n = 79)	Rest of the patients (n = 117)	Facial pain (n = 36)	Rest of the patients (n = 160)	Headache (n = 17)	Rest of the patients (n = 179)
Occlusion	7.32(±2.74)	7.37(±2.62)	7.40(±2.36)	7.34(±2.73)	6.47(±3.38)	7.43(±2.59)
Mandibular displacement	5.37(±2.76)	5.19(±2.4)	4.97(±2.65)	5.32(±2.56)	5.47(±2.58)	5.17(±2.58)
Abnormal tooth contact	4.43(±3.71)	4.38(±3.82)	4.19(±3.78)	4.46(±3.83)	5.59(±3.47)	4.24(±3.83)
Muscle parafunction	7.95(±2.62)[b]	5.57(±3.08)	7.92(±2.79)[a]	6.10(±3.14)	7.59(±3.26)	6.35(±3.13)
Psychogenic stress	6.99(±2.73)[b]	4.72(±3.07)	6.94(±2.84)[a]	5.25(±3.1)	5.65(2.87)	5.56(±3.16)

As compared to the rest of the patients, scores for muscle parafunction and psychogenic stress are significantly higher in the headache and/or facial pain subgroups and in the facial pain subgroups. This trend is not confirmed in the headache group. [a] $P < 0.01$; [b] $P < 0.001$.

group with only severe facial pain but not for the group with only severe headache (Table V).

Discussion

The data at hand confirm that the etiology of stomatognathic dysfunctions is multifactorial. Mean data from the whole group showed that several etiologic factors reached the moderate problem range (Table II). Moreover, 40.31% of the patients had severe etiologic factors of different natures (structural and neuromuscular and/or psychogenic).

Regarding the problem of etiology of cranio-facial pain in such patients, all data indicate that this symptom is strictly related to psychogenic stress. In the pair of canonic variables (η_1, φ_1) with the highest reciprocal correlation, psychogenic stress had the highest correlation degree with η_1, followed by muscle parafunction, and facial pain the highest correlation degree with φ_1, followed by muscle tenderness (Table IV). This confirms the study of single factors (Table III) and the subgroup study (Table V).

Therefore, one possible mechanism leading to facial pain seems to be the following; psychogenic pain elicits or increases the tendency to muscle hyperfunction and parafunction which in turn causes muscle tenderness and facial pain as a final consequence. However, since psychogenic stress and fa-

cial pain showed the highest correlations, other more direct mechanisms are probably present, such as a lower pain threshold in stressed patients.

The question could be raised as to whether chronic facial pain is a cause rather than an effect of psychogenic stress. However, the factors considered to quantify psychogenic stress in our system tend to provide evidence for its presence prior to or independently of facial pain (history of nervous breakdown, frequent tension, sleeping difficulties) or its causative relation to pain (pain started during or after a period of stress, pain is worsened by stress).

The study of single factors and, particularly, the canonical correlation analysis show that headache could also be a consequence of muscle hyperfunction and parafunction in stressed patients (Tables III and IV). This is actually a generally accepted mechanism for 'tension headache'. However, the correlation scores for headache were lower than those for facial pain, and in the subgroup study the subgroup with severe headache only did not show higher scores for muscle parafunction and psychogenic stress than did the two other subgroups (Table V). Moreover, headache was the only consequential parameter significantly different between males and females (the latter having a higher headache score) (Table II). These data seem to indicate that in a certain amount of female patients headache was mixed in nature, with muscle tension headache superimposed on vascular migraine, which, in fact, prevails in females (Dalsgaard Nielsen et al., 1970; Lance, 1973). This hypothesis was indeed confirmed by history data from several patients.

Structural factors do not seem to be a major determinant of facial pain and headache, but rather for TMJ impairment: in the study of single factors, TMJ impairment correlated with mandibular displacement as an etiologic factor. Occlusal disorders did not correlate with any consequential factor but did correlate with mandibular displacement (Table III). These data are in agreement with those from the canonical correlation analysis: here in the pair of canonic variables (η_2, φ_2), η_2 was highly correlated with mandibular displacement and, more weakly, with occlusion, and φ_2 was correlated with TMJ impairment (Table IV). It seems therefore that occlusal disorders are detrimental for TMJ function only in that they trigger other structural anomalies, notably mandibular displacement.

Conclusions

From the data obtained the following conclusions may be drawn:

(1) In stomatognathic dysfunction, different etiologic factors (structural, neuromuscular, psychogenic) may be superimposed in a group of patients and in the single patient: this explains the large variety of symptoms.

(2) Facial pain and headache seem to be related to neuromuscular and psychogenic factors rather than to structural factors. Psychogenic stress may trigger muscle hyperfunction and parafunction and hence muscle tenderness, facial pain and/or tension headache. However, psychogenic stress probably elicits facial pain also through more direct mechanisms.

(3) In a certain number of female patients, tension headache is superimposed on vascular migraine.

(4) TMJ impairment seems to relate more to structural factors, and to mandibular displacement in particular.

Acknowledgement

We wish to express our gratitude to Dr. A. Piazza, Professor of Human Genetics, University of Turin, for his decisive assistance in the statistical evaluation of the data.

References

Dalsgaard-Nielsen, T., Engberg-Pedersen, H. and Holm, H.D. (1970) Clinical investigations of the epidemiology of migraine. Dan. Med. Bull., 17: 138–148.

De Bouver, J.A. and Adriaens, P.A. (1983) Occlusal relationship in patients with pain-dysfunction in the temporomandibular joint. J. Oral Rehabil., 10: 1–7.

Farrar, W.B. (1982) Craniomandibular practice: the state of the art; definition and diagnosis. J. Craniomandib. Pract., 1: 5–12.

Helkimo, M. (1974) Studies in function and dysfunction of the masticatory system. II. Index for anamnestic and clinical dysfunction and occlusal state. Swed. Dent. J., 67: 101–121.

Kopp, S. (1982) Pain and functional disturbances of the masticatory system — A review of etiology and principles of treatment. Swed. Dent. J., 6: 49–60.

Lance, J.W. (1973) Mechanism and management of headache. Sandoz Butterworths, London, p. 97.

Laskin, D.M. (1969) Etiology of the pain-dysfunction syndrome. J. Am. Dent. Assoc., 79: 147–153.

Mardia, K.V., Kent, J.T. and Bibby, J.M. (1979) Multivariate analysis. Academic press, London, New York, pp. 281–299.

Mikhail, M. and Rosen, H. (1980) History and etiology of myofacial pain dysfunction syndrome. J. Prosthet. Dent., 44: 438–444.

Mongini, F. (1984) The Stomatognathic System. Function, Dysfunction and Rehabilitation. Quintessence, Inc., Chicago, pp. 133-141.

Mongini, F. (1986) An index system to quantify etiopathogenetic factors in oral dysfunction. J. Craniomandib. Pract., 4: 179–189.

Rieder, C.E. and Martinoff, J.T. (1983) The prevalence of mandibular dysfunction. Part II: a multiphasic dysfunction profile. J. Prosthet. Dent., 50: 237–244.

Smith, J.P. (1981) Symptoms and signs of the mandibular pain dysfunction syndrome — a symptom index. Community Dent. Oral. Epidemiol., 9: 236–238.

Solberg, W.K., Flint, R.T. and Brantner, J.P. (1972) Temporomandibular joint pain and dysfunction: a clinical study of emotional and occlusal components. J. Prosthet. Dent., 28: 412–422.

Wedel, A. and Carlsson, G.E. (1985) Factors influencing the outcome of treatment in patients referred to a temporomandibular joint clinic. J. Prosthet. Dent., 54: 420–426.

R. Dubner, G.F. Gebhart & M.R. Bond (Eds.)
Proceedings of the Vth World Congress on Pain
© 1988 Elsevier Science Publishers BV (Biomedical Division)

CHAPTER 57

Microcomputer documentation for pain clinics

A. Weyland[1], J.U. Wieding[2], M. Bautz[1], and J. Hildebrandt[1]

Departments of [1] Anaesthesiology and [2] Medical Informatics, Göttingen University Hospital, Göttingen, FRG

Summary

In pain clinics a thorough documentation of patient-related data is essential for analyses of patient histories, long-term evaluation of diagnostic and therapeutic procedures, and research on the etiology and epidemiology of chronic pain syndromes. We developed a set of questions for pain patients, a medical record for formatted and encoded data entry, and a microcomputer documentation system which is based on a commercial database software concept. High compatibility for computers under MS-DOS® operating system, flexible data management, a comfortable dialogue system for users due to the application of a programmable data base system, and rapid data access by an index sequential access mode are important features of our computerized documentation system. The present experience with data from 2627 patients, including 14 959 follow-up sets, showed effective support in administration, evaluation of treatment outcome and research on chronic pain as well as good user acceptance and satisfactory adaptability of the system.

Correspondence: Dr. Andreas Weyland, Schmerzambulanz, Zentrum Anaesthesiologie, Universitätsklinik Göttingen, Robert-Koch-Str. 40, 3400 Göttingen, F.R.G.

Introduction

Pain clinics and pain centers require a thorough documentation of patient-related data to ensure a detailed analysis of patient histories, to allow an evaluation of diagnostic and therapeutic procedures in follow-ups, and to supply necessary data for research on the epidemiology and etiology of chronic pain syndromes. Immediate access to patient-related data for these objectives can be obtained by a computer-assisted documentation system.

The realization of an electronic data-processing system (EDP) for storage and analysis of these data required:

(1) development of suitable patient questionnaires,

(2) development of medical records for EDP-supported documentation,

(3) development and modification of software concepts for the specific requirements of the pain center.

We therefore developed a standardized set of items and a problem-oriented medical record for both formatted and unformatted data entry, as had already been described previously (Klar et al., 1984). In the beginning of this project the program was realized on a DEC® PDP 11 minicomputer and the software was based on the operating system RT 11 with the Shareplus multiuser system and the application language BASIC as interpreter and compiler (Hildebrandt et al., 1987). Due to the high

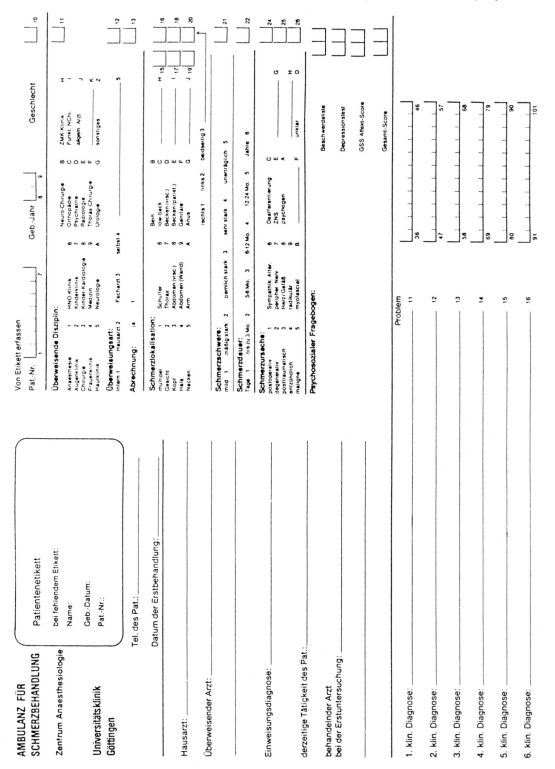

Fig. 1. Medical record. Documentation of identification and basic data, including patient history, diagnostic findings and diagnoses.

costs for additional hardware, marked dependence on expert programming advice for maintenance and inadequate compatibility of this system, the EDP-assisted documentation is now realized on an AT microcomputer with MS-DOS operating system (640 kilobyte internal memory, 20 megabyte hard disk).

System design

The list of items for the medical record is based on an extract of our patient questionnaire, which all patients are requested to fill out prior to their first appointment. This questionnaire elicits information on the socio-biographical and pathological background, and the history, localization, intensity and quality of pain. It also contains information on illness behaviour and preliminary psychometric tests. These include a depression scale and a list of unspecific somatic complaints according to von Zerssen as well as an extended form of Cziske's RMSS (a multidimensional pain scale) (Cziske, 1983; von Zerssen, 1976).

This information and the additional follow-up data are encoded for formatted data entry (see Figs. 1 and 2). The keys of diagnoses are based on the KDS system, which is the standard code of the general information system in the University of Göttingen (Ehlers and Klar, 1982); a transcription to the ICD code is currently carried out.

The medical record contains three sections of documentation: data for identification, basic data concerning patient history and diagnostic results, and treatment-related follow-up data (see Table I).

Program design

The present software concept is based on a dBASE III plus® database system which offers a rapid access to even larger data pools due to the index sequential access mode (ISAM). We developed program files for a completely menu-controlled management of user admittance, data entry, data access, search conditions, back-up of data and additional utilities. Format files generate screen displays for all parts of the program (see example in Fig. 4).

According to the structure of the medical record the patient-related data with different update frequencies are stored in three different data files (ID.dbf, BASDAT.dbf, FOLUP.dbf). These different sections of documentation are linked to each other by the patient's ID No. Treatments and follow-up data are related to one of the diagnoses via a problem key, which also guarantees the correct evaluation of diagnostic and therapeutic procedures for patients with multiple medical problems.

TABLE I

Structure of data for the medical record

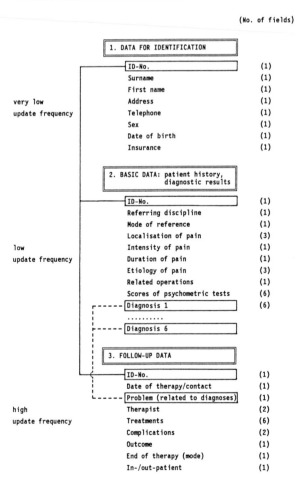

Patientenetikett:

bei fehlendem Etikett

Name:

Geb.-Datum:

Pat.-Nr.:

Ergebnisse:

sehr gut	1
gut	2
mäßig	3
keine Besserung	4
Verschlechterung	5
_____	6
_____	7

Behandlungsende:

unkontrolliert (Patient)	1
vereinbart (Arzt/Pat.)	2
erfolgreich	3
_____	4
_____	5

Follow-up:

nötig	1

Therapeuten-Nr.:

1 2 3 4 5

Behandlungen:

Nervenblockaden:

Plexus cerv.	01
Plexus brach.	02
Plexus lumb.	03
Trigeminus periph.	04
Ggl sphenopalatinum	19
Ggl. Gasseri	20
andere Hirnnerven	21
Intercostalis	05
and. periph. Nerven	06
Facett cerv.	07
Facett thorak.	22
Facett lumb.	08
Infiltration:	
Muskel	09
Bänder/Sehnen	10
Gelenke	23
Bursa	25
perivaskulär	11
intracutan	26
Ggl. coeliacum	12
Ggl. stellatum	13
Sympathik. lumb.	14

Sympathik. thorak.	24
Spinal	15
Epidural	16
Caudal	17
Wurzelblockade	18
Subdural	27
ISG	28
_____	29

Chirurgische:

Neurektomie (offen)	30
Neurektomie (percutan)	44
Rhizotomie (offen)	31
Rhizotomie (percutan)	32
perc. Facett-Rhiz. cerv.	33
perc. Facett-Rhiz. thorak.	45
perc. Facett-Rhiz. lumb.	34
Thermoläs. Ggl. Gasseri	35
Chordotomie (percutan)	36

Chordotomie (offen)	37
Myelotomie	38
Hypophysektomie	39
Thalamotomie	40
zentrale Stimulation	41
epidurale Stimulation	42
operat. Dekompression	43
Nashold (DREZ)	46
Spondylodese	47
perc. Den. ISG	48
_____	49

sonstige:

Chirurgie	50
Radiotherapie	51
Kryo	52
TNS	53
Akupunktur	54
Biofeedback	55
Psychotherapie	56
Physiotherapie	57
Hypnose	58
Entspannung	59
Gespräch	60
Test	61
psycholog. Anamnese	62
autogen. Training	63
Chirotherapie	64
Disographie	65
Schmerztherapie	66
R-F-Läsion	67

medikamentös:

Tranquilizer	70
Hypnotika	71
Analg. (Asp., Nov., Ben.)	72
Cod., Prop., Tram., Temg.	73
Morphin u. Deriv.	74
Antidepressiva	75
Neuroleptika	76

Lokalanästhetika	77
Neurolytika	78
Steriode	79
i.v.-Lösungen	80
Hormone	81
Chemotherapie	83
Muskelrelaxantien	84
Guanethidin/Reserpin	85
Secale-Alkaloide	86
Tryptophan	87
Beta-Blocker	88
Clonidin	89
Alpha-Bl (Praz./Reg.)	90
Serotonin-Antag.	91
Ca-Antag.	93
Antiarrhyth.	93
_____	94

Komplikationen:

Paresen	01
RR-Abfall	02
Blutung	03
Parästhesien	04
Neuritis	05
Harninkontinenz	06
Darminkontinenz	07
Durapunktion	08
Pneumothorax	09
Kopfschmerz	10
Deafferentierung	11
totale Spinal A.	12
_____	13
_____	14
_____	15
_____	16

Follow up:

1 = 1 Mon.	
2 = 1 Quartal	
3 = 1/2 Jahr	
4 = 1 Jahr	

Fig. 2. Medical record. Documentation of follow-up.

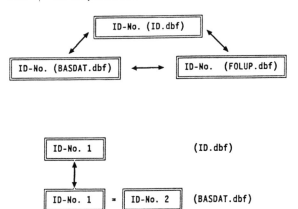

Fig. 3. Relation of multiple data files for complex evaluations and data listings. Upper: Switch of relations: Lower: Combination of two (or more) fixed relations by duplication of ID No. in different fields.

```
                                        ═══ B A S I C   Data ═══

  Identification-No:   461034X


  referring department ..... 3       complaints - score ........ 35
  mode of reference ........ 1       depression - score ........ 12

                                     'number of words chosen'... 28
  localization of pain 1 ... 62      affective items ........... 20
  localization of pain 2 ...         sensory-discrim. items .... 090
  localization of pain 3 ...
                                     No. of related operations . 1
  intensity of pain......... 4
  duration of pain.......... 4
                                     diagnosis 1 ....... 89641001001
  etiology of pain 1 ....... 2       diagnosis 2 ....... 86811000001
  etiology of pain 2 ....... 1       diagnosis 3 ....... 14611003001
  etiology of pain 3 .......         diagnosis 4 .......
                                     diagnosis 5 .......
  questionnaire completed ? 1        diagnosis 6 .......
```

Fig. 4. Screen display for entry of basic data.

Program files control the sequence of screen displays and menus during data entry and data access for every patient according to these data file relations.

Different levels of user admittance control limitations of data access and evaluation with regard to the user's qualification and task.

A modification of the data structure or the installation of new data fields can easily be accomplished, e.g., when new psychometric tests are employed in the initial patient evaluation or new results on the validation of items suggest a modification of the medical record.

The simultaneous relation of more than two data files as required for complex evaluations is not sufficiently supported by dBASE III plus in all situations. However, analyses and listings concerning all three sections of the medical record simultaneously can be realized in two different ways (see Fig. 3).

Applications

Up to now data from 2627 patients have been entered on the microcomputer documentation system, including 14 959 follow-up set which are continually updated. The data pool from our initial DEC PDP 11 computer which had been entered under the operating system RT 11 and a BASIC program could be transferred when the present database system was installed.

The microcomputer documentation system offers listings for administration as well as effective patient scheduling by a recall system according to the date of the last contact, selected therapeutic procedures and any other optional item of the medical record. A mailmerge service can be applied, particularly for follow-up studies.

Immediate access to all important patient-related data facilitates the long-term evaluation of diagnostic and therapeutic procedures. Filter conditions can be employed on the data pool for any combination of items of the medical record and have been used for epidemiological investigations. Further applications include studies on the relationships of psychological and somatic data not only from our standardized list of items but also from additional data from our patient questionnaire and additional test results which may be entered for special inquiries.

Conclusions

– The computerized documentation for our pain center showed effective support in administration, evaluation of treatment outcome and research on chronic pain.

– Low hardware costs and high compatibility could be realized by use of a microcomputer with MS-DOS operating system.

– Flexible data management and a comfortable dialogue system for users could be obtained by application of a programmable data base system.

– The present experience showed good user accept-

ance. Changes in the staff of our pain center so far suggest a satisfactory adaptability of the system.

– Compared to our former program on a DEC PDP 11 with the RT 11 operating system and the application language BASIC, the present documentation system is based on a commercial software concept and showed several advantages concerning the maintenance, flexibility and compatibility of the system. However, a multi-user system with a PC network has not yet been realized.

References

Cziske, R. (1983) Faktoren des Schmerzerlebens und ihre Messung: Revidierte Mehrdimensionale Schmerzskala. Diagnostica, 29: 61–74.

Ehlers, C.T. and Klar, R. (1982) The information system of the Göttingen Hospital. In R.R. O'Moore, B. Barber, P.L. Reichertz and F.H. Roger, (Eds.), Medical Informatics Europe 82: Springer, Berlin.

Hildebrandt, J., Klar, R., Weyland, A. and Wieding, J.U. (1987) A computerized information system for a pain clinic. Methods Inf. Med., 2: 97–101.

Klar, R., Waschke, K. and Hildebrandt, J. (1984) Problem- and source-oriented medical records for a pain clinic. In F.H. Roger, J.L. Willems, R.R. O'Moore and B. Barber (Eds.), Medical Informatics Europe 84: Springer, Berlin.

von Zerssen, D. (1976) Klinische Selbstbeurteilungsskalen (Ksb-S) aus dem Münchener Psychiatrischen Informations-System, Beltz, Weinheim.

Nociception and Pain

R. Dubner, G.F. Gebhart & M.R. Bond (Eds.)
Proceedings of the Vth World Congress on Pain
© 1988 Elsevier Science Publishers BV (Biomedical Division)

CHAPTER 58

Hypothesis for novel classes of chemoreceptors mediating chemogenic pain and itch

Robert H. LaMotte, Donald A. Simone, Thomas K. Baumann, Carole N. Shain and Meenakshi Alreja

Department of Anesthesiology, Yale University School of Medicine, 333 Cedar St., New Haven, CT 06510, USA

Summary

Capsaicin and histamine dihydrochloride, injected intradermally into the human forearm, each produced a different quality of sensation. Capsaicin elicited pain without itch, whereas histamine produced itch but not pain. Each substance also elicited a different quality of hyperesthesia within a large area of skin surrounding the injection site. Lightly stroking the skin within this area elicited tenderness (allodynia) after capsaicin but itch ('alloknesis') after histamine. Experimental evidence suggested that the hyperesthesias were neurogenic and of peripheral origin. Most C- and A-fiber mechanoheat nociceptive afferent fibers recorded from peripheral nerve in anesthetized monkey did not respond to either capsaicin or histamine injected inside or outside their cutaneous receptive fields; those that did respond usually did so weakly and transiently. Two novel classes of C-fiber thermal nociceptors responded weakly or not at all to mechanical stimuli. One type responded readily to noxious heat and to capsaicin, the other only to noxious cold. None of the nociceptors studied became mechanically sensitized. It was hypothesized that two additional classes of 'chemonociceptive' afferents exist, one contributing to capsaicin pain and allodynia, the other to histamine itch and alloknesis.

The purpose of this study was twofold: first, to obtain psychophysical measurements of chemically induced cutaneous pain and itch in humans, and then, using the monkey as a physiological model for the human, to search for the cutaneous receptors whose responses to these chemicals might help to explain our psychophysical observations. Although this search has proven to be quite difficult, the available evidence does allow some interesting working hypotheses to be made.

All human subjects gave informed consent to protocols approved by the Human Investigation Committee at Yale University School of Medicine. In our studies of chemical pain, capsaicin was injected intradermally into the volar forearm in a dose of 100 μg in 10 μl of Tween-saline. Subjects judged the magnitude of pain every 15 s using proportional numbers of their own choosing according to the method of magnitude estimation (Stevens, 1975). The magnitude estimates were normalized and averaged for 10 subjects (see Simone et al., 1987a). The mean magnitude estimates for pain are plotted in Fig. 1A as a function of time after injection. Upon injection, the pain was immediate and severe and its quality was characterized as burning.

Correspondence: Robert LaMotte, Department of Anesthesiology, Yale University School of Medicine, 333 Cedar St. New Haven, CT 06510, U.S.A.

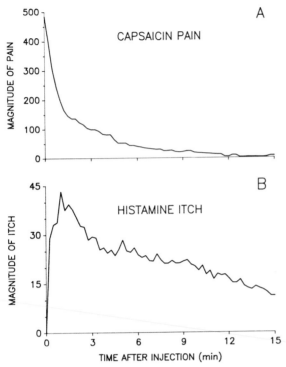

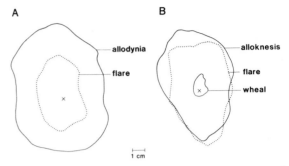

Fig. 1. The time course of the magnitude of pain or itch in humans after an intradermal injection of 100 µg of capsaicin or histamine. Each subject's magnitude estimate, obtained every 15 s, was normalized and the estimates of all subjects were averaged. A: The mean magnitude estimate of pain after injection of capsaicin. B: The mean magnitude of itch after injection of histamine.

Fig. 2. Skin reactions and the areas of hyperesthesia after an intradermal injection of capsaicin or histamine into the volar forearm of a human subject. The solid line in each panel encloses an area of hyperesthesia to lightly stroking the skin with a cotton swab. The dotted line encloses an area of redness (flare) and the 'x' marks the injection site. A: The area of mechanical tenderness (allodynia) and flare after an injection of capsaicin. B: the area of mechanically evoked itch (alloknesis), wheal and flare after an injection of histamine.

The pain then declined exponentially to a low level which persisted for 5–10 min. Based on comparative data from other experiments the maximal pain from capsaicin was judged to be 3–5 times more intense than that produced by a 5 s heat stimulus of 51°C.

In contrast, an intradermal injection of 0.1, 1 or 100 µg of histamine in 10 µl of physiological saline produced a sensation of itch without pain. The magnitude of itch was judged in the manner described for capsaicin pain. The mean normalized magnitude estimates of itch, based on data for 8 subjects, using a dose of 100 µg, are plotted in Fig. 1B as a function of time after injection. The itch began after a latency of 10–20 s, reached maximum at 1–2 min and then gradually declined over the next 15–20 min (Simone et al., 1987c).

Immediately after capsaicin or histamine, a hyperesthesia to light mechanical stimulation developed in a large area of skin surrounding the injection site, as shown in Fig. 2. The area of hyperesthesia was mapped with a cotton swab. After capsaicin, light stroking within the area elicited pain or tenderness, which was termed allodynia. In contrast, after histamine, a similar stroking elicited itch. We coined the word 'alloknesis' to describe the itch from light mechanical stimulation ('knesis' is the ancient Greek word for 'itching'). The itch from light stroking around the site of exposure to a pruritic chemical is also referred to as 'itchy skin' and was studied earlier by Bickford (1938) and Graham et al. (1951). The alloknesis from histamine and the allodynia from capsaicin persisted long after the primary sensation (itch or pain) from the injection had ceased.

Both capsaicin and histamine produced a flare (histamine but not capsaicin also produced a wheal) but the hyperesthesias were independent of the flare and differed from the flare in spatial distribution.

Studies were made of the mechanisms underlying these hyperesthesias. Cooling the injection site for 1–3 min with a 1 cm thermode (5°C) greatly reduced or in some cases eliminated the area of allodynia produced following a capsaicin injection,

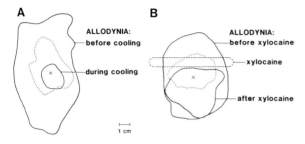

Fig. 3. Demonstration that allodynia from capsaicin is mediated by a peripheral neurogenic mechanism. The solid line in each panel encloses an area of allodynia resulting from a capsaicin injection into the volar forearm of a human subject. The dotted line encloses the area of the flare and the 'x' marks the injection site. A: Area of allodynia before and after cooling the skin to 5°C for several minutes with a 1 cm thermode centered over the injection site. B: A mediolateral strip of xylocaine (area enclosed with the dashed line) eliminated the allodynia which had developed on the side of the strip away from the injection site.

while rewarming brought it back (Fig. 3A). This sequence could be repeated. In addition, an injection of local anesthetic directly into the injection site abolished the allodynia. Thus, allodynia was maintained by neural activity at the injection site. Further, this neural activity probably spread by way of a cutaneous axon reflex because a mediolateral strip of local anesthetic eliminated the allodynia on the side of the strip away from the injection site, but not on the other side (Fig. 3B). Similar results were obtained for alloknesis after histamine.

When we repeated these experiments during a selective conduction block in A or C fibers, the results demonstrated that capsaicin pain, allodynia, histamine itch and alloknesis were mediated by C fibers and slowly-conducting A-delta fibers (Simone et al., 1986, 1987b, and unpublished observations). Based on these psychophysical observations we conclude the following: (1) capsaicin pain and histamine itch are served by different cutaneous receptors, and (2) allodynia from capsaicin and alloknesis from histamine are each maintained by neural activity at the injection site and neurogenically mediated by different cutaneous axon reflexes (or chains of axon reflexes electrically or chemically coupled together (cf. Lewis, 1937).

Although our psychophysical observations sug-

gest that the hyperesthesias are *maintained* by neural activity originating at the injection site and spread via a cutaneous neural mechanism (such as an axon reflex), they do not tell us whether the neurons that become mechanically sensitized are located in the peripheral or the central nervous system. One hypothesis is that sensitization occurs in the central nervous system (cf. Hardy et al., 1950; Graham et al., 1951). For example, there may be two sets of dorsal horn neurons, one mediating allodynia and the other alloknesis, each receiving convergent input from two types of peripheral nerve fiber: (1) those responsible for the spread and maintenance of the hyperesthesia in the periphery (e.g., nociceptive afferents which are chemically or electrically coupled in the periphery via axon reflexes) and (2) nociceptive afferents which normally respond to light mechanical stroking (see below) but do not become mechanically sensitized after chemical injection. Then, mechanical sensitization would result from ongoing activity in the first type of nerve fiber which facilitates the discharge of the dorsal horn neuron to the mechanically evoked activity in the second type of nerve fiber. The first type of afferent input would be facilitory but not capable of directly evoking discharges in the dorsal horn neuron receiving mechanically evoked input, since the hyperesthesias persist long after spontaneous pain or itch have disappeared and occur only in response to mechanical stimulation. Thus, a peripheral mechanism would mediate the spread and maintenance of the hyperesthesia but the neurons that are mechanically sensitized would reside in the dorsal horn.

An alternative hypothesis is that the mechanically sensitized neurons are peripheral receptors. For example, the nerve fibers maintaining allodynia might release a chemical substance that mechanically sensitizes other fibers which, once sensitized, evoke tenderness when mechanically stimulated. Nerve fibers mediating alloknesis might release a different chemical that sensitizes fibers which evoke itch when mechanically stimulated.

Indirect evidence for peripheral sensitization was obtained in a recent experiment in which intraneural electrical stimuli were delivered through a microelectrode inserted into the common or superficial peroneal nerve in the awake human subject (LaMotte et al., 1987, and unpublished observations). Brief electrical test stimuli produced moderate pain referred to a localized area of skin on the dorsum of the foot (the 'projection field'). Then a sustained and intensely painful conditioning stimulus was delivered through the same electrode. This typically produced erythema and allodynia (tenderness to lightly stroking the skin) within the projection field. Yet when the same intraneural test stimuli were again delivered they were typically perceived as no more painful than they were prior to the conditioning stimulus. The same result was obtained if, instead of the electrical conditioning stimulus, a capsaicin injection was given adjacent to or within the projection field. These results suggest that the neuronal sensitization responsible for allodynia was in the peripheral and not the central nervous system.

A search was begun for peripheral nerve fibers contributing to chemogenic pain, itch and the accompanying hyperesthesias. In electrophysiological experiments, recordings were made from single peripheral nerve fibers innervating the hairy skin in anesthetized monkeys. C-fiber and A-fiber mechanoheat nociceptive afferents, which we term CMHs and AMHs, respectively, were given an injection of either capsaicin or histamine into or outside their receptive fields in the skin. Injections outside the receptive field were 1–7 mm away. In addition we studied C-fiber heat nociceptors which responded readily to noxious heat but poorly or not at all to noxious mechanical stimuli. The proportion of units tested that responded to 100 μg of capsaicin or 0.1 or 1 μg of histamine is shown in Table I (not included in the table is one C-fiber cold nociceptive afferent which responded readily to noxious cold ($<10°C$) but not at all to heat, mechanical or chemical noxious stimuli). Only 1 AMH responded to capsaicin. Only about a third of the CMHs responded to an injection outside their receptive fields and slightly less than one-half to an injection inside. Fibers that did respond usually did so tran-

TABLE I
Proportion of fibers responding

	Outside	Inside
Capsaicin		
CMH	6/21	10/24
AMH	1/16	0/19
CH	3/ 3	3/ 3
Histamine		
CMH	0/11	0/14
AMH	0/ 4	0/ 6

siently (e.g. less than 2 min) and weakly, i.e., with a maximum discharge rate typically less than that evoked by a 5 s heat stimulus of $51°C$. In contrast, all of the C-heat nociceptors responded to capsaicin with a much greater discharge rate than that of the CMHs. Further, the response durations of some of the C-heat nociceptors were nearly as long as the duration of pain from capsaicin injection in humans. Thus, although a larger population of these fibers must be studied before more definitive conclusions can be made, the C-heat nociceptors seem more likely than the CMHs to contribute to the pain from intradermal capsaicin.

None of the mechanoheat nociceptors responded to histamine (Table I). (We are currently testing the responses of the C-heat nociceptors to histamine.) We conclude that either there is a species difference between monkey and human in fiber sensitivity to the histamine injection or the CMHs and AMHs do not make a significant contribution to histamine-evoked itch.

Anecdotal observations were also made of what might be an additional class of nociceptor which we call a 'chemical nociceptor' or 'chemonociceptor'. None of these fibers responded to thermal or mechanical noxious stimuli prior to chemical injection and each was discovered by its spontaneous discharges after an intradermal injection of capsaicin or histamine during an experiment carried out with a mechanoheat or C-heat nociceptor. Six of them began firing after injection of capsaicin and 1 after histamine. We obtained conduction velocities on a few such fibers and they were in the C-fiber range.

Thus we propose that there exist separate chemo-nociceptive afferents: one contributing to chemogenic pain and the other to chemogenic itch.

The question that follows is: what are the afferent fibers that might mediate the spread and maintenance of allodynia or alloknesis over a large area of skin surrounding the injection site? The available information is as yet insufficient to answer this question. A few of the CMHs, C-heat and 'chemical' nociceptive afferents responded with prolonged low rates of discharge but we have not yet ascertained whether these discharges last as long as the mechanical hyperesthesias in humans. Emphasis is now on mapping out the chemically responsive receptive fields of the 'chemonociceptors' and in determining whether the C-heat nociceptors (which had relatively small receptive fields) could be remotely activated by an injection beyond 1 mm outside their receptive fields. Present findings show that only a few CMHs and 1 AMH responded to an outside injection of capsaicin. Such responses are interesting because they suggest regional differences in transducer sensitivity to chemical and mechanical noxious stimuli (the mechanical being used to map the receptive field). Yet the responses of these fibers did not appear to be sufficiently prolonged to be able to maintain the long duration of allodynia. One possibility is that chemically responsive afferent fibers such as certain CMHs stop sending action potentials centrally but continue to propagate some form of neural activity for a prolonged period of time along remote branches of the parent axon that arborizes within the skin outside the sensory receptive field.

It seems unlikely that mechanoheat nociceptive afferents contribute to an axon reflex mediating hyperesthesia; these fibers respond less to capsaicin or histamine than they do to mechanical or heat stimuli which when applied to human skin, produce neither a flare nor hyperesthesia. We therefore hypothesize that the spread and maintenance of the mechanical hyperesthesias are served by the terminal branches of two sets of chemonociceptive afferents, one responding best to algesic chemicals and mediating allodynia, the other responding to pruritic substances and mediating alloknesis. (The flare may be mediated by still another set of chemonociceptive afferents that responds to both algesic and pruritic chemicals or perhaps it is mediated by a separate effector mechanism in the first two fiber types.) Each axon reflex might involve the branches of only one parent axon, arborizing widely within the skin, or a series of axons whose endings are electrically or chemically coupled in such a way that activity in one triggers activity in its neighbor. There is recent evidence that C-fiber afferents in monkey can be physiologically coupled in the periphery, that most of these do not have mechanical receptive fields, and that some of them respond to pruritic or algesic chemicals injected into a local area on the skin (Meyer et al., 1985; Meyer and Campbell, 1987).

Which neurons become mechanically sensitized to light mechanical stimulation of the skin sur-

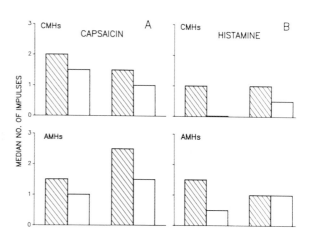

Fig. 4. The responses of CMH and AMH nociceptive afferent fibers to light mechanical stroking before and after intradermal chemical injection. The median number of impulses evoked by a stroke of a cotton swab across the cutaneous receptive field was obtained before (hatched bars) and after (open bars) an intradermal injection outside vs. inside (left vs. right two bars in each panel) the receptive field. Responses are shown only for those fibers responding with 1 or more impulses to stroking before injection. A: Median responses of CMHs and AMHs to capsaicin (number of fibers contributing to each median was, from left to right, 6 and 12 for CMHs and 12 and 14 for AMHs). B: Median responses of CMHs and AMHs to histamine (number of fibers: 5 and 4 for CMHs and 2 and 2 for AMHs).

rounding an injection of capsaicin or histamine? To search for mechanical sensitization in CMHs and AMHs we recorded the number of impulses evoked in each fiber by a cotton swab stroked across its cutaneous receptive field. Of those mechanoheat nociceptive afferents injected with histamine or capsaicin (Table I) 55% of the CMHs and 89% of the AMHs responded with 1 or more impulses prior to injection. The median number of impulses per stroke, averaged for several strokes and for only those fibers which responded initially to stroking, are plotted before vs. after an injection of capsaicin (Fig. 4A). Typically responses averaged only 1 or 2 impulses per stroke prior to injection and the same or less after. Certainly neither the CMHs nor the AMHs increased their responses after an injection inside or outside the receptive field. Thus allodynia cannot be accounted for by the mechanical sensitization of these nociceptors. A similar negative result was obtained with histamine (Fig. 4B). Finally, only two of the candidate chemonociceptive afferents, those responding to capsaicin, developed a response, which was transient, to mechanical stimuli. This finding needs replication before any definitive statement can be made.

There is always the possibility of species differences between monkeys and humans as to the functional properties of nociceptive afferents. One apparent difference is the absence of a visible flare in monkey skin after an injection of capsaicin or histamine. However, recent recordings from single peripheral nerve fibers in awake humans suggest no important species differences, at least in the responses of CMHs to capsaicin (LaMotte et al., 1987). About half of the CMH afferents tested in humans responded weakly and transiently when capsaicin was injected inside or close to ($\leq$ 8 mm) their cutaneous receptive fields. Still fewer re-

sponded (weakly and transiently) to injections further outside the receptive field. Also, there was no significant sensitization to mechanical stimuli even though the usual area of allodynia enveloped the fiber's receptive field.

Recently, recordings were made from multireceptive (wide dynamic range) and nociceptive-specific neurons in the dorsal horn of the cat before and after an injection of capsaicin (100 μg) into their cutaneous receptive fields (D.A. Simone in collaboration with J.G. Collins, unpublished observations). Both types of neuron exhibited vigorous and sometimes prolonged discharges and both became mechanically sensitized. For example, nociceptive-specific neurons which were initially insensitive to light mechanical stroking responded with multiple discharges to stroking subsequent to the capsaicin injection.

While these preliminary results provide central neuronal correlates with some of our psychophysical observations, they do not provide a clue as to the types of primary afferent fibers mediating the chemically evoked sensations and accompanying hyperesthesias; these fibers are almost certainly diverse in their chemical sensitivities and probably also differ as to the chemicals that they release from their peripheral and central terminal endings. We do not think it plausible that chemogenic pain and allodynia and chemogenic itch and alloknesis can all be served by a single class of afferent fibers each having the same peripheral transducer(s) and effector mechanism. Instead we propose that chemogenic pain and itch with their accompanying mechanical hyperesthesias are each served in large part by at least two types of chemonociceptor, each possessing in its terminal endings a different sensitizing chemical substance responsible for maintaining and spreading the hyperesthesia within the skin.

References

Bickford, R.G. (1938) Experiments relating to the itch sensation, its peripheral mechanism and central pathways. Clin. Sci., 3: 377–386.

Graham, D.T., Goodell, H. and Wolff, H.G. (1951) Neural

mechanisms involved in itch, 'itchy skin,' and tickle sensations. J. Clin. Invest., 30: 37–49.

Hardy, J.D., Wolff, H.G. and Goodell, H. (1950) Experimental evidence on the nature of cutaneous hyperalgesia. J. Clin. Invest., 29: 115–140.

LaMotte, R.H., Torebjörk, E. and Lundberg, L. (1987) Neural

mechanisms of cutaneous hyperalgesia in humans: peripheral or central? Neurosci. Abstr., 13: 189.

Lewis, T. (1937) The nocifensor system of nerves and its reactions. I and II. Br. Med. J., 1: 431–437 and 491–494.

Meyer, R.A. and Campbell, J.N. (1987) A novel electrophysiological technique for locating cutaneous nociceptors and chemospecific receptors. Brain Res., in press.

Meyer, R.A., Raja, S.N. and Campbell, J.N. (1985) Coupling of action potentials between unmyelinated fibers in the peripheral nerve of the monkey. Science, 227: 184–187.

Simone, D.A., Baumann, T.K., Shain, C.N. and LaMotte, R.H. (1986) The common polymodal nociceptor does not contribute to hyperalgesia produced by intracutaneous injection of capsaicin. Soc. Neurosci. Abstr., 12: 331.

Simone, D.A., Baumann, T.K., Shain, C.N. and LaMotte, R.H. (1987a) Magnitude scaling of chemogenic pain and hyperalgesia in humans. Soc. Neurosci. Abstr., 13: 109.

Simone, D.A., Ngeow, J.Y.F., Putterman, G.J. and LaMotte, R.H. (1987b) Hyperalgesia to heat after intradermal injection of capsaicin. Brain Res., 418: 201–203.

Simone, D.A., Ngeow, J.Y.F., Whitehouse, J., Becerra-Cabal, L., Putterman, G.J. and LaMotte, R.H. (1987c) The magnitude and duration of itch produced by intracutaneous injections of histamine. Somatosens. Res., 5: 81–92.

Stevens, S.S. (1975) Psychophysics, John Wiley & Sons, New York.

R. Dubner, G.F. Gebhart & M.R. Bond (Eds.)
Proceedings of the Vth World Congress on Pain
© 1988 Elsevier Science Publishers BV (Biomedical Division)

CHAPTER 59

A reliable model of experimental itching by iontophoresis of histamine

W. Magerl and H.O. Handwerker

Institut für Physiologie und Biokybernetik, Universitätsstraße 17, D-8520 Erlangen, FRG

Summary

Histamine$^+$ ions were iontophoresed from a gel store in a small perspex probe (5 mm in diameter) to the ventral forearm skin of 22 volunteers of both sexes using 10-s constant-current pulses. The method of constant stimuli was used for psychophysical evaluations. Perceived itching was expressed at 10-s intervals by means of a visual analogue scale (VAS). The objective signs of the triple response, wheal and flare, were measured by planimetry and laser Doppler flowmetry (flux) respectively. VAS ratings of perceived itch sensations were correlated to the logarithm of stimulus strength ($r = 0.45$). Prediction of itch intensity by wheal and flux responses was superior ($r = 0.55$ and 0.58, respectively). Analysis of variance revealed a significant impact of the factors 'stimulus intensity', 'gender' and 'subjects' ($P < 0.0001$, $R^2 = 0.80$) on the itch responses. Standardizing the ratings on the basis of an anchor stimulus and introduction of wheal and flux as covariates abolished gender differences and improved the correlations between the itch ratings and the diameters of the wheals. Discrimination of the stimulus levels could be achieved in all but two levels ($p = 0.05$, Duncan's Multiple Range Test). The sense of itch may therefore hold at least 3 bits of information.

Introduction

Research on the mechanisms of nociception in the past gained much profit from the introduction of precisely controlled stimulation procedures. This, however, does not apply to the sensation of itch, where sensory physiology is still on the level of qualitative demonstrations and threshold studies (Cormia, 1952; Shelley and Arthur, 1957). This retardation is at least partly due to a marked lack of rigidly controlled models of itching in animals as well as in humans (Woodward et al., 1985).

In this study we attempted to introduce a controlled and reliable model of itching in humans and to analyse its psychophysical characteristics. Several parameters of the responses to histamine iontophoresis were quantified. This agent stored in mast cells of the skin is commonly believed to be the main natural mediator of itching.

Methods

Histamine$^+$ ions were delivered to the skin of young healthy volunteers by iontophoresis. A drop of a 1% aqueous solution of histamine dihydrochloride stabilized as a gel by methylcellulose (2.5%) was stored in the cavity of a small hand-held perspex rod, 5 mm in diameter, containing a volume of 50 μl, under a silver plate electrode and directed to the skin of the ventral forearms. A sponge-covered larger electrode (3 × 3 cm) near the wrist moistened with tyrode served as a reference. The histamine$^+$ ions were driven from the gel store into the skin using 10-s constant-current pulses from an isolated stimulation unit (WPI 305B). Stimulus intensity could be varied by changes in the current. The effective stimulus was calculated as the transport of charged molecules, i.e. the product of time and current. The following charges were delivered in this study: 0.156, 0.625, 2.5 and 10 mC.

Histamine iontophoresis usually resulted in a local wheal surrounded by a flare, both reactions developing slowly after termination of the stimulus. Both wheal and flare were marked with water-resistant pens 10 min after each stimulus and redrawn on translucent paper for planimetric evaluation. For assessing time courses and the relative increases in blood flow in the course of the flare reaction, a laser Doppler flowmeter (Periflux/PF 1d) was used,

the probe of which was positioned 8 mm from the iontophoresed spot.

In a pilot study on the ventral forearm skin of 48 subjects (27 male, 21 female) various levels of stimulation were used. In a subsequent study, five levels of stimulation, including a zero control stimulus and four charge levels (see above), were applied in random order to the forearm skin of 22 young volunteers of either sex (10 male, 12 female). In addition, every subject was made familiar with the procedure by means of a medium-sized training stimulus of 1.25 mC. All our subjects gave their informed consent to participate in these experiments.

Iontophoretic stimuli usually elicited sensations of itching within about 20 s, which lasted for several minutes. Their actual strength was expressed by the subject via an electronically controlled horizontal visual analogue scale (VAS) at 10-s intervals for 10 min. The left and right ends of the scale were defined as 'threshold' and as 'maximal itch imaginable', respectively. Ratings were given by the subjects on an acoustic signal.

Data were sampled by a microcomputer (Sorcus) and analysed off-line on a main-frame computer using Statistical Analysis Systems (SAS).

Results

In a pilot study on 48 subjects (27 male, 21 female) interrelations of stimulus size (charges) and the parameters of the triple responses (wheal and flare) were evaluated. The diameters of the respective areas of both wheal and flare were found to be the relevant parameters of the responses. These were linearly related to the logarithms of stimulating charges. The respective correlation coefficients were 0.88 in both cases. Threshold doses were 0.04 mC for the flare and 0.05 mC for the wheal responses (Fig. 1).

Almost all of the stimuli were followed by itching of various extents and durations. These sensory impressions were more precisely analysed in the second psychophysical study. Itching usually started after long latencies of about 10 s and then rose

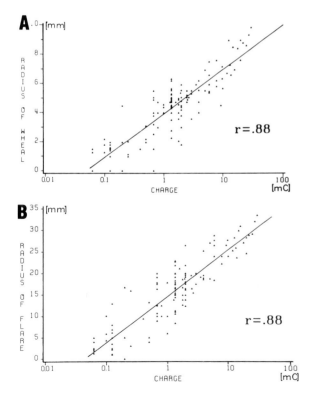

Fig. 1. Correlation of wheal (A) and flare responses (B) to logarithm of stimulus intensities (charges).

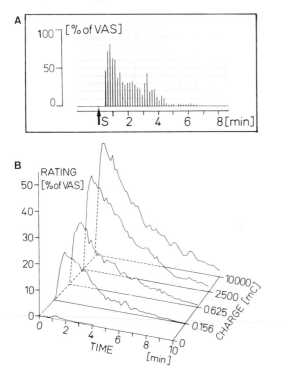

Fig. 2. Typical itch response to the iontophoretic stimulation as measured on the visual analogue scale. B: Mean ratings of 22 subjects to respective doses of histamine iontophoresis and to placebo stimulation.

sharply to a maximum reached at about 1 min. Thereafter the itch sensation declined exponentially, with time constants of about 3 min (range: 155–205 s) (Fig. 2). Apart from this uniform mean time course, itch sensations were typically waxing and waning.

Fig. 2B shows the mean itch responses depending on charge. For correlation statistics mean itch ratings obtained in 2 min after the onset of itching were computed. The correlation coefficient to the logarithm of charges was 0.45 (Fig. 3A). However, prediction of itch responses was better accomplished by using flare and wheal responses as predictors, providing correlations of 0.55 and 0.58, respectively (Fig. 3B and C).

Analysis of variance revealed a significant impact of the factors 'stimulus intensity', 'gender' and 'subject' on itch ratings ($P < 0.0001$, $R^2 = 0.80$). There

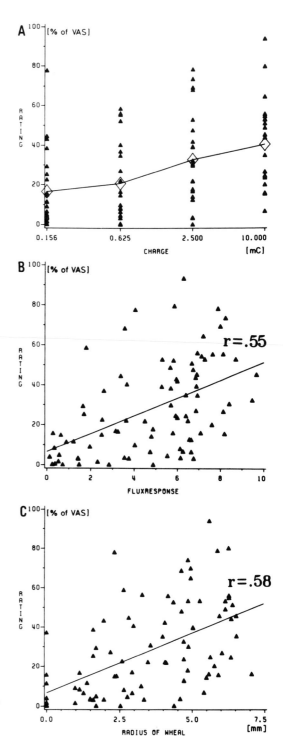

Fig. 3. Relation to subjective estimates (itch ratings) to stimulus intensities (charges (A) (triangles represent single responses, mean values are given as diamonds connected by solid lines) and correlations of itch ratings to flare (B) and wheal responses (C).

was a consistent tendency in females towards higher itch ratings over the whole stimulus range.

Influence of the 'subjects' factor was eliminated when 'wheal' and 'flux' were used as covariates, indicating that different susceptibility to histamine could be largely attributed to differences in local skin responses rather than to those of central nervous disposition. However, influence of 'gender' was then still present, indicating that different responsiveness in male and female can only partly be explained by differences in the thickness of the skin. Probably these persistent gender differences can be attributed to a response bias in the female subjects. This hypothesis is emphasized by the fact that females significantly more often perceived itching after application of the zero control stimulus than did male subjects ($P < 0.05$, chi-square test). When the rating data were normalized on the basis of the training stimulus (see 'Methods') the gender differences were diminished. Introducing 'wheal' and 'flux' as covariates in a variance analysis on the normalized data abolished the gender differences. The normalized rating data could be better predicted by the radius of the wheals, indicated by correlation coefficients of 0.66 in the whole population and of 0.71 in the male subgroup.

Discrimination of the five stimulus levels could be achieved in all but two stages on a 5% level of significance (Duncan's Multiple Range test). The sense of itch may therefore hold at least 3 bits of information.

A special point of interest arises from the question of the quality of sensation elicited, as it is commonly thought that itching will turn to burning pain with increases in the intensity of stimuli, suggesting that itching is a form of subthreshold pain (Rothman, 1941; von Frey, 1922). In our experiment, we asked the subjects for descriptions of the sensation as percentages of different distinguished sensations. A variety of pain descriptors (Mumford and Bowsher, 1976) were offered besides itching. Though the subjects used descriptors such as 'brennen' (burning) and 'stechen' (stinging), 'jucken' (itching) appeared to be the predominant descriptor. In the stimulus range used there was no indica-

tion of a shift towards a more frequent use of 'burning' or 'stinging' as descriptors ($P > 0.20$, F test).

Discussion

It was the objective of this study to approach a quantitative analysis of the sensation of itch. This could be realized by the iontophoretic histamine stimulation of the skin. Subjects were well able to distinguish different levels of itching related to different stimulus strengths. Itching appears to hold more information than was believed in the past.

The method described provides several features that make it feasible for the study of sensory mechanisms of the skin. It is quantitatively controlled, noninvasive and minimizes unspecific stimulus effects. There is no damage to the epidermal barrier, since permeability is not altered (Siddiqui et al., 1985). There are also no difficulties with buffering and stabilization of the agent, as occur with the injection technique (Broadbent, 1955). Moreover, iontophoresis is particularly suitable for reaching the itch sensors located in the outermost skin layers, mainly in the stratum papillare and stratum basale (Keele and Armstrong, 1964; Shelley and Arthur, 1957). On the other hand, transport to deeper layers, though minor, cannot be totally prevented (Glass et al., 1980). This is illustrated by the fact that even small stimuli are able to pass to the vascular region, thus inducing wheal responses. Deposition of histamine in the deeper layers of the skin, e.g. by jet injection, invariably leads to pain (Lindahl, 1961). The portion of histamine ions migrating to deeper tissues may thus be responsible for adding components such as 'burning' and 'stinging' to the itch sensations of some subjects. The latter also occur in various other models such as intradermal injection and the blister base (Broadbent, 1955; Keele and Armstrong, 1964; Shelley and Arthur, 1957). Iontophoresis of histamine avoids inherent troubles associated with these models such as unreliability of the depth of injection and hyperalgesia. Results are always uniform, provided that analogous skin regions are compared. However, care has to be taken to control the influence of objective and subjective experimental factors. Registration of the wheal responses may provide some information about the amount of histamine deposited, while monitoring flare vasodilation gives an indirect measure of neuronal excitation via the 'axon reflex' mechanism (Lewis, 1927). We have shown previously that the flare induced by histamine iontophoresis is indeed due to afferent neurogenic vasodilatation (Handwerker et al., 1987). Using wheal and flare as indices of the effectiveness of stimulation improved the prediction of subjective itch responses.

The use of reference and zero stimuli was effective in this study in controlling a gender-related rating bias that is also likely to occur in other pain-associated sensations, as recently demonstrated (Rollman et al., 1987).

Regarding the qualitative side of the sensation, no changes of the pattern were observed with increasing stimulus strength. Contrary to the assumption of itch as subthreshold pain (Rothman, 1941; von Frey, 1922), itching did not turn into burning. This finding is in agreement with a previous report on electrically induced itching (Tuckett, 1982).

The data presented suggest that iontophoresis of histamine is a reliable model of experimental itching in humans, giving qualitatively stable and quantitatively discernible perceptions.

Acknowledgements

This work was supported by the DFG grant Ha 831/8. We wish to thank Mr. K. Burian for the preparation of the figures and Ms. D. Bechtle for editing the manuscript.

References

Broadbent, J.L. (1955) Observations on histamine-induced pruritus and pain. Br. J. Pharmacol., 10: 183–185.

Cormia, F.E. (1952) Experimental histamine pruritus I. Influence of physical and psychological factors on threshold reactivity. J. Invest. Dermatol., 19: 21–34.

Glass, J.M., Stephen, R.L. and Jacobson, S.C. (1980) The quantity and distribution of radiolabelled dexamethasone delivered to tissue by iontophoresis. Int. J. Dermatol., 19: 519–525.

Handwerker, H.O., Magerl, W., Klemm, F., Lang, E. and Westerman, R.A. (1987) Quantitative evaluation of itch sensation. In R.F. Schmidt, H.–G. Schaible, C. Vahle-Hinz (Eds.), Fine afferent nerve fibers and pain, VCH Verlagsgesellschaft, Weinheim, pp. 461–473.

Keele, C.A. and Armstrong, D. (1964) Substances Producing Pain and Itch, E. Arnold, London, pp. 10–29 and 124–151.

Lewis, T. (1927) The Blood Vessels of the Human Skin and their Responses, Shaw & Sons, London, 1927.

Lindahl, O. (1961) Experimental skin pain. Acta Physiol. Scand., 51: Suppl. 179.

Mumford, J.M. and Bowsher, D. (1976) Pain and protopathic sensibility. A review with particular reference to the teeth. Pain, 2: 223–243.

Rollman, G.B., Clohosey, L.K., Harris, G. and Scudds, R.A. (1987) Sex of subject and responsiveness to experimental pain. Pain, Suppl. 4: S11.

Rothman, S. (1941) The physiology of itching. Physiol. Rev., 21: 357–381.

Shelley, W.B. and Arthur, R.P. (1957) The neurohistology and neurophysiology of the itch sensation in man. Arch. Derm., 76: 296–323.

Siddiqui, O., Roberts, M.S. and Polack, A.E. (1985) The effect of iontophoresis and vehicle pH on the in-vitro permeation of lignocaine through human stratum corneum. J. Pharm. Pharmacol., 37: 732–735.

Tuckett, R.P. (1982) Itch evoked by electrical stimulation of the skin. J. Invest. Dermatol., 79: 368–373.

von Frey, M. (1922) Zur Physiologie der Juckempfindung. Arch. Neerland. Physiol., 7: 142–145.

Woodward, D.F., Conway, J.L. and Wheeler, L.A. (1985) Cutaneous itching models. In H.I. Maibach and N.J. Lowe (Eds.), Models in Dermatology, Vol. 1, S. Karger, Basel, pp. 187–195.

R. Dubner, G.F. Gebhart & M.R. Bond (Eds.)
Proceedings of the Vth World Congress on Pain
© 1988 Elsevier Science Publishers BV (Biomedical Division)

CHAPTER 60

Characterization and projection of nociceptive input from the nasal cavity of the cat

Gregory E. Lucier* and Rita Egizii

University of Calgary, Faculty of Medicine, Department of Physiology, 3330 Hospital Drive N.W., Calgary, Alberta T2N 4N1, Canada

Summary

The purpose of the study reported here was to characterize the second-order neurones in the trigeminal nucleus which receive nasal afferent information of a nociceptive nature. Results show, for the first time, that nociceptive information from the nasal cavity is relayed in the ethmoidal nerve to the trigeminal sub-nuclei, and that the second-order neurones which receive this input are those which receive nociceptive information from other trigeminal subdivisions. Previous electrophysiological studies have demonstrated that these neurones have direct projections to thalamus, cerebellum, spinal cord and subnucleus oralis. We have been unable to demonstrate that there is a direct projection from the nasal mucosa to areas in the brain stem, such as the solitary tract, which play a major role in respiration and upper airway protective reflexes. How nociceptive information from the nasal cavity is conveyed eventually to the respiratory system to elicit these protective reflexes remains the subject of further investigation.

Introduction

In addition to being the site of olfactory reception, the nose is the portal of the respiratory system. Inspired air must be conditioned (i.e., warmed, humidified and, to a lesser degree, filtered) before reaching the lungs. The nose may also be regarded as the sentinel of the airway, since one of its chief jobs is to protect the respiratory system from foreign invasion. It is not surprising, therefore, that the nose is the site of a number of protective reflexes (i.e., sneezing, apnea, coughing) designed to stop potentially harmful material from entering the lungs and to expel foreign substances. This system operates quite independently of the olfactory sense and is mediated by branches of the trigeminal nerve (V), which contain predominantly small diameter, myelinated and unmyelinated axons (Biedenbach et al., 1975). The primary prerequisite of such a reflex mechanism is a receptor which is capable of responding to a potentially harmful or noxious input. Although the sensory receptors involved with nasal reflexes have not been anatomically identified, free nerve endings have been observed throughout the nasal mucosa and are thought to constitute the sensory receptors involved (Cauna 1982). Previous anatomical and electrophysiological studies have shown that afferents from the laryngeal mucosa of the cat, capable of initiating respiratory protective reflexes, project directly to respiratory neurones in

*To whom correspondence should be addressed.

the vicinity of the solitary tract (Sessle et al., 1978; Lucier et al., 1978; Lucier et al., 1986). Recent anatomical studies in our laboratory using horseradish peroxidase (HRP) tracing techniques (Lucier and Egizii, 1986) have shown that the ethmoidal nerve which innervates the nasal mucosa of the cat does not project directly to the solitary tract but to the trigeminal nucleus (spV). The purpose of the study reported here was to characterize these second-order neurones in spV which receive nasal afferent information of a nociceptive nature.

Methods

A total of 15 adult cats were used in this study. Each cat was anaesthetized with chloralose (60 mg/kg, i.v.). Blood pressure was monitored, end-tidal CO_2 was maintained at 3.5–4.0%, and rectal temperature was maintained at 37–38°C. In addition to a conventional tracheal cannula, a second cannula was inserted into the trachea and directed upward into the larynx, so that air delivered to the nasal cavity could be expelled. In addition, the oral cavity was blocked with a gauze pad saturated with physiological saline. The animal's head was placed in a stereotaxic apparatus which was then rotated so that the animal lay on its back. The following nerves were dissected on the right side for subsequent stimulation: glossopharyngeal (IX), exposed distal to its carotid body branch; internal branch of the superior laryngeal (iSLN); hypoglossal (XII); and vagus (X), 5 mm caudal to the cricoid cartilage. Each nerve was placed on a bipolar hook electrode, enclosed within a polyethylene sleeve and covered with low-melting-point wax to minimize stimulus spread. Bipolar stimulating electrodes were also placed in the ipsilateral maxillary and mandibular canine tooth pulps. The animal was then returned to a prone position. The ipsilateral ethmoidal nerve was exposed by complete enucleation of the eyeball, using standard veterinary surgical procedures (Hickman and Walker, 1973). The nerve was separated from its accompanying blood vessels as it emerged from the nasal cavity through the ethmoi-

dal foramen. Bipolar stimulating electrodes were applied as described above. An occipital craniotomy was carried out to expose the caudal brain stem. The extracellular activity of single, ipsilateral brain stem neurones was recorded with tungsten microelectrodes placed stereotaxically with co-ordinates referenced to the obex. Obex is defined as that point at which the central canal first opens into the fourth ventricle. Medical air was delivered through the nasal cavity at a constant pressure and flow rate. A series of gas-washing bottles containing test substances were connected to the input side of the system and controlled by valves so that various odorants could be introduced into the air flow and directed to the nasal cavity. In addition, trigeminal receptive fields were determined by using: light mechanical stimulation with hand-held von Frey probes and an electronically driven servo-controlled probe; harsh mechanical stimulation with serrated forceps; and radiant heat stimuli judged as noxious when applied to the experimenter's skin. During brain stem microelectrode recordings, the animal was paralysed with gallamine triethiodide and artificially ventilated. Recording sites were later verified histologically.

Results

The results reported here follow from a primary afferent study (Lucier and Egizii, 1983; Lucier and Egizii, in preparation) designed to characterize the types of nasal receptors (i.e., chemosensitive, pressure, flow- and temperature-sensitive) and will therefore concentrate on cells receiving nociceptive input from the nasal cavity. The spV may be divided functionally and histologically into three subnuclei: subnucleus oralis (5.0 mm to 8.2 mm rostral to obex), subnucleus interpolaris (obex to 5.0 mm rostral to obex) and subnucleus caudalis (obex to 5.0 mm caudal to obex) (Gobel and Purvis, 1972). Results from previous anatomical studies (Lucier and Egizii, 1986) showed that the ethmoidal nerve projected primarily to interpolaris and caudalis, and therefore we limited our study to these areas. One of the major problems encountered was that of gaining access to the nasal mucosal receptive field. If the field could be localized close to the external nares, it could be easily probed with von Frey hairs. Tactile receptors further back in the nasal cavity could sometimes be stimulated with brief puffs of air. We discovered very early in the experiments that probing about deep in the nasal cavity only caused damage and shortened the life of the preparation. In addition, the bulk of the receptors lie in regions of the nasal cavity not only inaccessible to mechanical probes, but also not reached during laminar airflow through the nose.

Interpolaris

Using ethmoidal nerve stimulation as our search stimulus, we began exploring the region of the brain stem rostral to obex. One hundred and thirteen cells located in the ventrolateral portion of the sub-nucleus were found to receive input from the ethmoidal nerve. Of these, 98 responded to innocuous mechanoreceptive input from within the nasal cavity (i.e., air flow, pressure or light tactile stimulation). The latency of these cells to ethmoidal input ranged between 3 and 18 ms, with most having an input latency less than 10 ms (Fig. 1A). Twenty-two received input from iSLN, 28 from IX, 8 from XII and 1 from tooth pulp. In addition, most of these neurones had discrete ipsilateral non-noxious tactile facial receptive fields around the nose and eye. A second, much smaller group of cells representing only 15 of the interpolaris cells receiving input from the ethmoidal nerve responded to noxious input from within the nasal cavity (i.e., ammonia vapour, heavy pressure). All of these cells had latencies to ethmoidal nerve input greater than 10 ms (Fig. 1C). Four received input from iSLN, 5 from IX and 2 from XII. In addition, over one-half of these cells also received ipsilateral tooth pulp input. All of these cells were encountered between obex and 2 mm anterior. Many of these neurones had discrete ipsilateral facial receptive fields around the nose and eye which responded to either noxious or non-noxious stimuli. Fig. 2A shows the characteristics of one of these cells. It had a long latency (16 ms) to

ethmoidal and to the ipsilateral maxillary tooth pulp (17 ms) stimulation as well as responding to ammonia vapour applied to the nasal cavity. In ad-

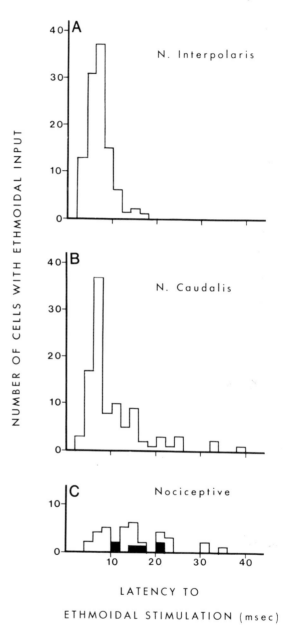

Fig. 1. Distribution of response latencies to ipsilateral ethmoidal nerve stimulation of non-nociceptive neurones in interpolaris (A) and in caudalis (B). C. Response latencies to ipsilateral ethmoidal nerve stimulation of neurones in caudalis (open area) and interpolaris (shaded area) which also received a nociceptive input.

dition, this cell had a non-noxious tactile receptive field located just inside the nose.

Caudalis

Moving caudally into sub-nucleus caudalis, 138 neurones receiving input from the ethmoidal nerve were studied. Latency to ethmoidal input ranged from 3 to 40 ms, with most having an input latency less than 10 ms (Fig. 1B). Of these cells, 102 received non-noxious mechanoreceptive input from within the nasal cavity. Twenty-three received input from iSLN, 21 from IX, 9 from XII and 6 from tooth pulp. These cells could often be activated by light tactile stimulation of the nasal receptive field or by air flow through the nasal cavity. Often these cells had a facial receptive field limited to the ipsilateral ophthalmic division of V. All of these mechanoreceptive neurones were recorded from deeper layers of the nucleus. Thirty six cells received nociceptive ethmoidal input (i.e., responded to noxious substances applied to the nasal cavity). The majori-

ty of these nociceptive cells had latencies to ethmoidal stimulation greater than 10 ms (Fig. 1C). Four received input from iSLN, 5 from IX, and 2 from XII. All of these were found to have tooth pulp input. Fig. 2B illustrates the characteristics of one of these cells. In addition to receiving long latency input from ethmoidal stimulation (18 ms) and from the ipsilateral maxillary tooth pulp (18 ms), this cell also responded to heavy pressure applied to the nasal mucosa and noxious radiant heat applied to the facial receptive field. Most of these cells were located within layers I and II of caudalis (Fig. 3A). These layers were defined as set out by the cytoarchitectonic criteria of Gobel and Purvis (1972).

Discussion

Although it had been known for a long time that irritation of the nasal cavity was capable of producing protective reflexes (e.g., sneezing, apnea, cough-

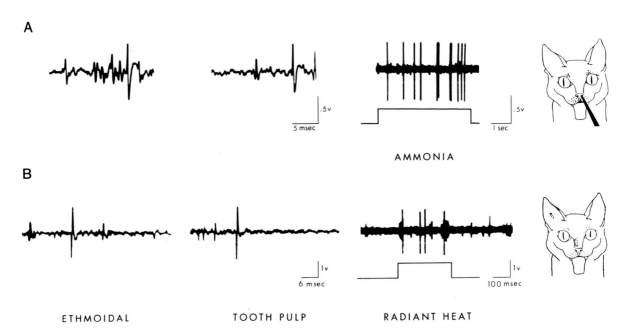

Fig. 2. Characteristics of interpolaris and caudalis neurones receiving ethmoidal input. A. Neurone recorded extracellularly in interpolaris having a long-latency input from ethmoidal (16 ms) and from the ipsilateral maxillary tooth pulp (17 ms). This unit was also stimulated by ammonia applied to the nasal cavity and had a tactile receptive field just inside the nose. B. Neurone recorded extracellularly in caudalis with a long-latency input from ethmoidal (18 ms) and from the ipsilateral maxillary tooth pulp (18 ms). This unit also responded to noxious radiant heat applied to the receptive field indicated by the cross-hatched area on the nose.

ing) in a wide variety of species, it was not known to where in the brain stem this information was relayed. As mentioned in the introduction, previous studies of the projection of laryngeal receptor afferents in the cat, capable of producing similar reflexes (e.g., coughing, apnea, swallowing) had been found to project directly onto respiratory neurones in the vicinity of the nucleus tractus solitarius (nTS) (Lucier et al., 1986). On the basis of these findings, one would have predicted that nasal mucosal afferents would also project to this same region of the brain stem. However, anatomical tracing of the ethmoidal nerve in the cat revealed that nasal afferents projected to the trigeminal nucleus and primarily to the sub-nuclei interpolaris and caudalis, with minimal projection to sub-nucleus oralis (Lucier and Egizii, 1986). These findings were in agreement with previous electrophysiological studies in the cat (Beuerman, 1975) and the rat (Van Buskirk and

Erickson, 1977). Van Buskirk and Erickson, using electrical stimulation of the ethmoidal nerve, had observed electrophysiological projection of ethmoidal afferents to subnucleus oralis. However, the latencies encountered in this study suggested that many of the neurones in oralis receive multi-synaptic input from the ethmoidal nerve relayed via other brain stem areas. If this were the case, it would account for the sparse labelling in nucleus oralis following the application of HRP to the ethmoidal nerve, since HRP is not carried trans-synaptically. Beuerman's earlier study in the cat demonstrated that the ethmoidal nerve projected to all divisions of the spinal trigeminal complex. In his more detailed study of the region of sub-nucleus caudalis, he failed to find cells which have a chemosensory input. However, neither the chemical nor the mechanical inputs employed by Beuerman could be considered noxious in nature (e.g., gentle touching,

A

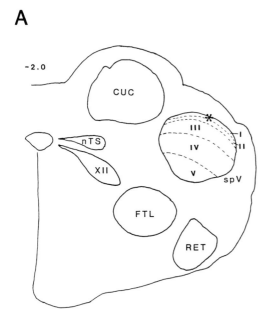

B

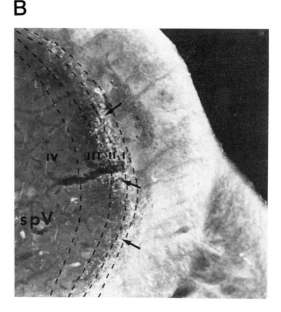

Fig. 3. Location of ethmoidal projection in nucleus caudalis. A. Schematic representation of the cat brain stem at the level of caudalis, 2.0 mm caudal to obex. Dashed lines delineate layers I to V of caudalis. Asterisk represents the site at which the neurone described in Fig. 1B was recorded from. B. Dark-field photomicrograph of horseradish peroxidase (HRP) reaction product in the spinal trigeminal nucleus (spV) at the same level as A but not in the same animal, resulting from the application of HRP to the ipsilateral ethmoidal nerve. Dashed lines delineate the layers of caudalis. Arrows indicate the presence of HRP reaction product in layers I and II. CUC, cuneate nucleus; FTL, lateral tegmental field; nTS, nucleus of the solitary tract; RET, lateral reticular nucleus; XII, hypoglossal nucleus. Magnification 80 × .

amyl acetate).

The results reported here show, for the first time, that nociceptive information from the nasal cavity is relayed in the ethmoidal nerve to the trigeminal sub-nuclei, and that the second-order neurones which receive this input are those which receive nociceptive information from other trigeminal subdivisions. A number of very thorough studies have characterized the cells receiving both nociceptive and innocuous cutaneous inputs in interpolaris (Hayashi et al., 1984) and caudalis (Price et al., 1976; Hayes et al., 1979; Hu et al., 1981; Sessle et al., 1981; Amano et al., 1986). Briefly, these cells may be divided into three classifications: low-threshold mechanoreceptive neurones (LTM), which receive light tactile input and are not nociceptive; wide-dynamic-range neurones (WDR), which receive both noxious and non-noxious stimuli; and nociceptive-specific neurones (NS), which do not respond to non-noxious stimuli but require noxious stimuli for their activation.

Interpolaris

The observation that the majority of cells in interpolaris which received ethmoidal input were found in the ventrolateral portion of the nucleus is in agreement with our previous anatomical study. In addition, Hayashi et al. (1984) observed that neurones in this area of interpolaris had receptive fields restricted to the ophthalmic division of spV, of which the ethmoidal is a subdivision. In addition, Hayashi et al. (1984) found that LTM neurones accounted for over 75% of a 220 neurone sample of cells in interpolaris receiving cutaneous stimuli. Clearly, 87% of the neurones in interpolaris which received innocuous input from within the nasal cavity can be classified as LTM neurones, and, as such, represent the general population of interpolaris cells receiving mechanoreceptive input from the oral facial region. Only 13% of the neurones sampled in our study received nociceptive input from the nasal mucosa, as opposed to 20% in the cutaneous afferent study of Hayashi et al. In addition, all of the cells in interpolaris receiving noxious input via the ethmoidal nerve can be classified as

belonging to the WDR type. Our inability to detect NS neurones receiving nasal input may be due in part to our inability to use nociceptive nasal stimulation as a search stimulus. Indeed, often during the application of ammonia to test the response of a neurone responding to ethmoidal nerve stimulation, we would observe smaller background units start to discharge with a long latency to the ammonia stimulus. However, we found this too damaging to the nasal mucosa to be used continuously as a search stimulus.

Caudalis

Seventy-four percent of the cells in caudalis receiving ethmoidal input could be classified as LTM neurones. These results are in agreement with an earlier study of cutaneous afferent projections to caudalis which reported approximately 71% of the cells sampled as being LTM neurones (Hu et al., 1981). These authors also observed, as we did, that the neurones were located in the deeper layers of the nucleus. As for the neurones receiving nasal mechanoreceptive input, those receiving cutaneous mechanoreceptive input exhibited light von Frey force thresholds and receptive fields usually limited to one ipsilateral V division. As observed for the interpolaris neurones, those cells in caudalis receiving noxious nasal input (26%) can be classified as WDR neurones. Again, our inability to detect NS neurones receiving ethmoidal input may be the result of our sampling procedure. Our observation that most of the cells receiving nociceptive ethmoidal input are located in layers I and II of caudalis are in agreement with previous electrophysiological cutaneous afferent studies (Hu et al., 1981) and our own study of the projection of the ethmoidal nerve (Fig. 3B).

Our findings indicate that, contrary to expectations, nociceptive information from the nose is conveyed to neurones in nucleus interpolaris and caudalis which are known to receive noxious cutaneous input from other oral facial regions. Previous electrophysiological studies (Hayashi et al., 1984; Hu et al., 1981) have demonstrated that these neurones have direct projections to thalamus, cerebellum, spinal cord and subnucleus oralis. We have been unable to demonstrate that there is a direct projection from the nasal mucosa to areas in the brain stem, such as the solitary tract, which play a major role in respiration and upper airway protective reflexes. This raises a critical question: how does the nervous system distinguish between nociceptive input coming from oral facial cutaneous receptors which initiate escape responses such as withdrawal, and that coming from receptors in the nasal mucosa which elicit responses such as sneezing and apnea?

How nociceptive information from the nasal cavity is conveyed eventually to the respiratory system to elicit these protective reflexes remains the subject of further investigation.

Acknowledgements

The authors wish to acknowledge Mr. F.S. Chivers for technical assistance, Mr. J.D. Naylor for critical review of the manuscript and the Medical Research Council of Canada for support of this work.

References

Amano, N., Hu, J.W. and Sessle, B.J. (1986) Responses of neurons in feline trigeminal subnucleus caudalis (medullary dorsal horn) to cutaneous, intraoral, and muscle afferent stimuli. J. Neurophysiol., 55: 227–243.

Beuerman, R.W. (1975) Neurons in trigeminal nucleus and reticular formation excited by ethmoidal nerve stimulation. Brain Res., 92: 479–484.

Biedenbach, M.A., Beuerman, R.W. and Brown, A.C. (1975) Graphic-digitizer analysis of axon spectra in ethmoidal and lingual branches of the trigeminal nerve. Cell Tissue, Res., 157: 341–353.

Cauna, N. (1982) Blood and nerve supply of the nasal lining. In D.F. Proctor and I.B. Andersen (Eds.), The Nose: Upper Airway Physiology and the Atmospheric Environment, Elsevier, Amsterdam, pp. 45–69.

Gobel, S. and Purvis, M.B. (1972) Anatomical studies of the organization of the spinal V nucleus: the deep bundles and the spinal V tract. Brain Res., 48: 27–44.

Hayashi, H., Sumino, R. and Sessle, B.J. (1984) Functional organization of trigeminal subnucleus interpolaris: nociceptive and innocuous afferent inputs, projections to thalamus, cerebellum, and spinal cord, and descending modulation from periaqueductal gray. J. Neurophysiol., 51: 890–905.

Hayes, R.L., Price, D.D. and Dubner, R. (1979) Behavioural and physiological studies of sensory coding and modulation of trigeminal nociceptive input. In J.J. Bonica, J.C. Liebeskind and D.G. Albe-Fessard (Eds.), Advances in Pain Research and Therapy, Vol. 3, Raven, New York, pp. 219–243.

Hickman, J. and Walker, R. (1973) Atlas of Veterinary Surgery, T.A. Constable Ltd., Edinburgh, pp. 123–124.

Hu, J.W., Dostrovsky, J.O. and Sessle, B.J. (1981) Functional properties of neurons in cat trigeminal subnucleus caudalis (medullary dorsal horn). I. Responses to oral facial noxious and nonnoxious stimuli and projections to thalamus and subnucleus oralis. J. Neurophysiol., 45: 173–192.

Lucier, G.E. and Egizii, R. (1983) Characterization of cat nasal respiratory protective reflexes. Can. Fed. Biol. Soc. Proc., 26: PA242.

Lucier, G.E. and Egizii, R. (1986) Central projections of the ethmoidal nerve of the cat as determined by the horseradish peroxidase tracer technique. J. Comp. Neurol., 247: 123–132.

Lucier, G.E., Daynes J. and Sessle, B.J. (1978) Laryngeal reflex regulation: peripheral and central neural analysis. Exp. Neurol., 62: 200–213.

Lucier, G.E., Egizii, R. and Dostrovsky, J.O. (1986) Projections of the internal branch of the superior laryngeal nerve in the cat. Brain Res. Bull., 16: 713–721.

Price, D.D., Dubner, R. and Hu, J.W. (1976) Trigeminothalamic neurons in nucleus caudalis responsive to tactile, thermal, and nociceptive stimulation of monkey's face. J. Neurophysiol., 39: 936–953.

Sessle, B.J., Greenwood, L.F., Lund, J.P. and Lucier, G.E. (1978) Effect of upper respiratory tract stimuli on respiration and single respiratory neurones in the adult cat. Exp. Neurol., 61: 245–259.

Sessle, B.J., Hu, J.W., Dubner, R. and Lucier, G.E. (1981) Functional properties of neurons in cat trigeminal subnucleus caudalis (medullary dorsal horn). II. Modulation of responses to noxious and nonnoxious stimuli by periaqueductal gray, nucleus raphe magnus, cerebral cortex, and afferent influences, and effect of naloxone. J. Neurophysiol., 45: 193–207.

Van Buskirk, R.L. and Erickson, R.P. (1977) Responses in the rostral medulla to electrical stimulation of an intranasal trigeminal nerve: convergence of oral and nasal inputs. Neurosci. Lett., 5: 321–326.

R. Dubner, G.F. Gebhart & M.R. Bond (Eds.)
Proceedings of the Vth World Congress on Pain
© 1988 Elsevier Science Publishers BV (Biomedical Division)

CHAPTER 61

The spinohypothalamic and spinotelencephalic tracts: direct nociceptive projections from the spinal cord to the hypothalamus and telencephalon

Rami Burstein, Kenneth D. Cliffer and Glenn J. Giesler, Jr.

Department of Cell Biology and Neuroanatomy, University of Minnesota, Minneapolis, MN 55455, USA

Summary

Somatosensory input to the hypothalamus has been thought to ascend via an indirect pathway. However, we have antidromically identified nociceptive spinal cord neurons which project directly to the lateral hypothalamus in rats. Retrograde tracers injected into lateral hypothalamus labelled many spinal neurons bilaterally within marginal zone, lateral reticulated area, lateral spinal nucleus, and the area surrounding the central canal. An anterograde tracer injected into these spinal cord areas labelled fibers and terminals in the lateral and medial hypothalamus and, surprisingly, in the basal forebrain, the medial septal nucleus, and the nucleus accumbens. A retrograde tracer injected into each of these areas labelled cells in the same areas of the spinal cord as the cells labelled after injections into the lateral hypothalamus. These findings demonstrate a direct nociceptive projection from the spinal cord to the hypothalamus and a direct projection from nociceptive areas of the spinal cord to several telencephalic regions.

Correspondence: Glenn J. Giesler, Jr., Department of Cell Biology and Neuroanatomy, University of Minnesota, Minneapolis, MN 55455, U.S.A.

It is known that a variety of somatosensory stimuli can cause marked changes in the firing of hypothalamic neurons. Of particular interest in the present context, painful stimuli can activate hypothalamic neurons (Kanosue et al., 1984). In many studies a direct input from the spinal cord to the hypothalamus was not seen (e.g. Mehler, 1969). It has been generally believed, therefore, that the afferent pathway of somatosensory information from the spinal cord to the hypothalamus is indirect. However, during an electrophysiological study of the termination of the spinothalamic tract, we found that nociceptive neurons in the spinal cord dorsal horn could be antidromically activated from the lateral hypothalamus.

Initially, we antidromically activated six neurons in the lumbar spinal cord from the contralateral ventrobasal complex (VBC) in rats. We then used antidromic activation techniques to explore the diencephalon for projections of these axons outside the VBC (Burstein et al., 1987). Five of the six neurons antidromically activated from the VBC were found to have axons that could be followed toward or into the hypothalamus. Two additional neurons were antidromically activated from electrodes in the lateral hypothalamus exclusively. Antidromic thresholds were less than 50 μA. The cell bodies of the antidromically activated neurons were located within the marginal zone, nucleus proprius, or lat-

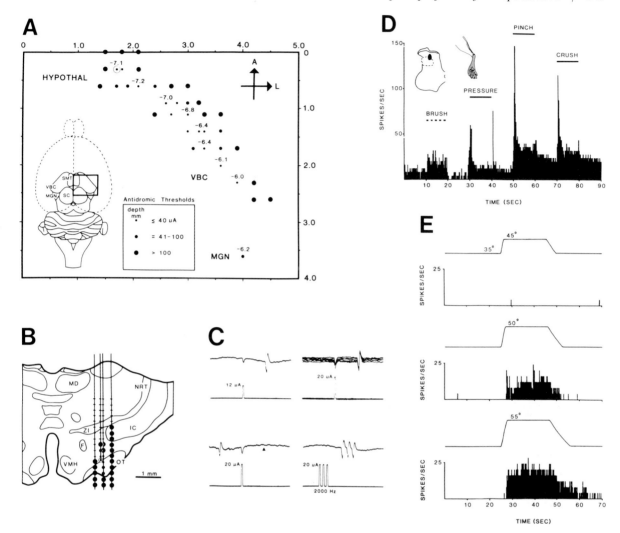

Fig. 1. Characterization of a spinohypothalamic tract neuron. (A) The large square represents a dorsal view of the brain. The position of the square is indicated in the drawing of the brain at left. Within the square, the positions are illustrated of 37 penetrations through the diencephalon with an antidromic stimulating electrode. The distance caudal to bregma is indicated at right and the distance from the midline is indicated at top. The size of each dot is related to the minimum level of current required to activate the neuron within the track (inset). The depth below the cortical surface of the point with the lowest threshold in each anterior-posterior plane is indicated. The axon was followed to progressively more anterior, medial and ventral positions within the diencephalon. The location of the most anterior track in which a small antidromic threshold was encountered is circled. A = anterior, L = lateral, MGN = medial geniculate nucleus, SC = superior colliculus, SMT = stria medullaris thalami, VBC = ventrobasal complex. (B) The location in transverse section of the track circled in A. Each penetration of the stimulating electrode is indicated by a vertical line. The sizes of the dots on the vertical lines reflect the same antidromic threshold values as in A. Dashes on the vertical lines indicate positions at which antidromic activation could not be produced using 500-μA pulses. The position of the point at which the threshold was lowest in this plane is circled. F = fornix, IC = internal capsule, MD = medial dorsal nucleus, NRT = nucleus reticularis thalami, OT = optic tract, VMH = ventral medial hypothalamic nucleus, ZI = zona inserta. (C) Antidromic responses of the neuron to stimulation at the low-threshold point illustrated in A and B. In each panel, the intensity of the antidromic stimulus is indicated in the lower record. The latency of the response was 4.2 ms. Upper left: response of the neuron to a single 12-μA shock in the lateral hypothalamus. Upper right: overlapping traces of responses to several shocks in the hypothalamus; note the stable latency of the response. Lower left: Collision of an orthodromic spike with the antidromic spike. The point at which the antidromic response would have occurred is indicated by an

arrowhead. Lower right: Responses of the neuron to a train of three pulses delivered at 2000 pulses per second. (D) Peristimulus-time histogram (bin width = 250 ms) of the response of the unit to mechanical stimulation within its peripheral receptive field (insert). The period of each stimulus is indicated by lines above the histogram. Note that the largest responses were produced by noxious stimuli. A drawing of the lesion made to mark the recording site within the lumbar dorsal horn is at upper left. (E) Responses of the unit to thermal stimulation of its receptive field. The period and intensity of each stimulus are indicated in the record above the histogram. Note the increasing responses to more intense noxious thermal stimuli. Reproduced with permission from Burstein et al., 1987.

Fig. 2. (A) Locations of cells of origin of the spinohypothalamic tract. Injection of Fluoro-Gold into the hypothalamus labelled a large number of neurons bilaterally throughout the length of the cord. The rostral (top) and caudal (bottom) limits and the center of the injection site are depicted. The total numbers of labelled neurons in each side of the cord within the illustrated segments are indicated. Scale bar = 1 mm. LV = lateral ventricle, SN = septal nucleus, CPu = caudate putamen, AC = anterior commissure, LPO = lateral preoptic area, MTT = mamillothalamic tract, VBC = ventrobasal complex, IC = internal capsule, ZI = zona inserta, IIIV = third ventricle, OT = optic tract, A = amygdala, F = fornix. (B–E) Fibers and terminals in the hypothalamus and telencephalon labelled with PHA-L following unilateral injections into the cervical enlargement of the spinal cord. (B) Contralateral lateral hypothalamus. (C) Contralateral nucleus of the diagonal band of Broca. (D) Ipsilateral medial septal nucleus adjacent to midline. (E) Ipsilateral nucleus accumbens. Note that many axons have labelled varicosities that apparently are apposed to counterstained cell bodies. Scale bar = 10 μm. Reproduced with permission from Burstein et al., 1987.

→

eral reticulated area of the dorsal horn.

Results obtained from a neuron which was antidromically activated from the hypothalamus are illustrated in Fig. 1. Antidromic thresholds were determined at more than 600 points. It is clear from this figure that the axon was followed to progressively more anterior, medial and ventral positions within the diencephalon. The most anterior point (circled in Fig. 1A) at which a small current activated the neuron is illustrated in a transverse section through the diencephalon in Fig. 1B (circled dot). This low-threshold point was located within the lateral hypothalamus.

The antidromic response of this neuron to stimulation in the lateral hypothalamus is illustrated in Fig. 1C. Antidromic responses of all recorded neurons had constant latencies, followed high-frequency stimulus trains, and collided with orthodromic spikes.

The antidromic threshold for the illustrated neuron at the lesion site was less than 12 μA, indicating that this stimulation point was close to the axon. The effective spread of a 12 μA current pulse is less than 120 μm (Abzug et al., 1974; Ranck, 1975). The point was surrounded medially, laterally, dorsally, ventrally and anteriorly by locations at which considerably more current was required to activate the neuron. These findings suggest that this low-threshold point was near the terminal region of the axon.

The illustrated neuron responded to innocuous mechanical stimuli but was more strongly activated by noxious mechanical stimuli (Fig. 1D) within its receptive field (inset). It was, therefore, classified as a wide dynamic range (WDR) neuron. It also responded incrementally to noxious thermal stimuli (Fig. 1E).

Six of the seven recorded cells were classified as WDR neurons. The remaining neuron responded only to noxious stimuli. All examined neurons responded incrementally to increasingly intense noxious thermal stimuli. The incrementing responses of these neurons to graded noxious thermal stimuli strongly suggest that these neurons receive inputs which originate in primary afferent nociceptors; nociceptors are the only type of primary afferent fiber capable of responding incrementally to increasingly intense noxious thermal stimuli (Fitzgerald and Lynn, 1977; LaMotte and Campbell, 1978; Hallin et al., 1981).

Retrograde tracing techniques were used to determine more completely the locations of spinal cord neurons that project to the hypothalamus. Tracers were injected stereotaxically into the lateral hypothalamus through a glass micropipette attached to the needle of a microsyringe (Burstein et al., 1987). Three retrograde tracers were used:

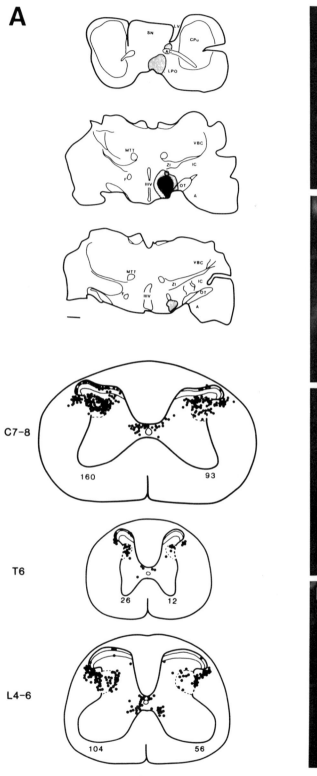

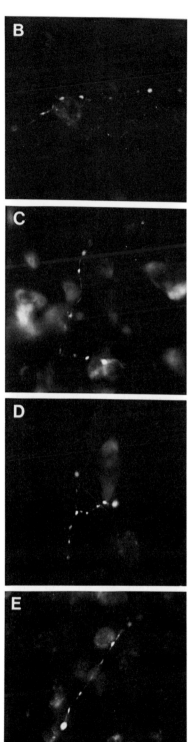

Fluoro-Gold (2%; Schmued and Fallon, 1986), horseradish peroxidase conjugated to wheat germ agglutinin (0.2%; Graham and Karnovsky, 1966; Mesulam, 1978), and a suspension of rhodamine-labelled microspheres (Katz et al., 1984).

An example of an injection of Fluoro-Gold restricted to the hypothalamus is illustrated in Fig. 2A. This and nine other comparable injections each labelled many neurons bilaterally throughout the length of the spinal cord (Fig. 2A). About 25% of the labelled neurons were found in the lateral spinal nucleus. Approximately half of the labelled neurons were located in the lateral reticulated area. Roughly 10% of the labelled neurons were found in the gray matter surrounding the central canal. An additional 10% were found in the marginal zone. The last three areas are all thought to be significantly involved in nociceptive processing in the spinal cord. They receive direct inputs from primary afferent nociceptors, contain large percentages of nociceptive second-order neurons, and contribute axons to other ascending nociceptive pathways (Willis, 1985).

The distribution within the spinal cord of the cells of origin of what we will call the spinohypothalamic tract (SHT) is in some ways similar to the distribution of spinothalamic tract (STT) neurons. For example, many of the cells of origin of both tracts are located within the lateral reticulated area (Giesler et al., 1979; Kevetter and Willis, 1983). However, the distributions of the cells of origin of these two tracts also differ in several ways. For example, approximately 40% of SHT neurons project ipsilaterally whereas fewer than 10% of STT neurons project ipsilaterally (Giesler et al., 1979; Kevetter and Willis, 1983). Also, the lateral spinal nucleus and the neurons adjacent to the central canal frequently project to the hypothalamus but do not contribute prominently to the spinothalamic tract (Giesler et al., 1979; Kevetter and Willis, 1983).

The projections of spinal cord neurons within the hypothalamus were examined using the anterograde transport of *Phaseolus vulgaris* leuco-agglutinin (PHA-L), a technique which reveals the detailed morphology of labelled axons and terminals (Ger-

fen and Sawchenko, 1984). In 11 rats multiple iontophoretic injections of PHA-L were made into the cervical enlargement. In all 11 animals, terminal varicosities were seen within the lateral hypothalamus (Fig. 2B). Additional labelled fibers and varicosities were encountered within the medial hypothalamus and, unexpectedly, in a number of nuclei in the basal forebrain and other telencephalic areas. For example, labelled fibers and terminals were seen contralaterally in the nucleus of the diagonal band of Broca (nDBB; Fig. 2C), bilaterally in the medial septal nuclei (MS; Fig. 2D) and ipsilaterally in the medial nucleus accumbens (Fig. 2E). Frequently, labelled varicosities in all of these areas could be seen in apparent contact with counterstained neurons (Fig. 2B–E). Labelled decussating axons were also observed in the supraoptic decussation including the caudal-most portion of the optic chiasm.

We were able to confirm direct spinal projections to the medial hypothalamus, basal forebrain, septal nuclei and nucleus accumbens using retrograde tracing techniques. Injections of Fluoro-Gold that were restricted to each of these areas labelled spinal neurons bilaterally throughout the length of the spinal cord within the lateral spinal nucleus, the marginal zone, the lateral reticulated area, and the area around the central canal. These findings indicate that at all segmental levels of the spinal cord, neurons in nociceptive areas of the gray matter project not only to medial and lateral hypothalamus, but also to a number of telencephalic regions. To our knowledge, such projections have not been previously reported. Interestingly, the locations of axons and varicosities anterogradely labelled with PHA-L in the MS and nDBB after injections in the spinal cord correspond precisely to those in which nociceptive neurons projecting to the hippocampus have been found (Dutar et al., 1985).

The three independent techniques used in this study demonstrate that a direct projection carries somatosensory information from the spinal cord to the hypothalamus in the rat. It appears that a spinohypothalamic tract may also be present in other species. Ring and Ganchrow (1983) reported that spinal lesions produced degeneration in the lateral hypothalamus of hedgehogs. Ju (1984) found that injections of HRP into the spinal cord of rabbits produced what he interpreted to be anterograde labelling in the hypothalamus. Anderson and Berry (1959) noted that spinal lesions in cats caused degeneration of fibers in the lateral hypothalamus. Several of the reconstructions in a paper by Chang and Ruch (1947) appear to show degenerating axons in the supraoptic decussation following spinal lesions in monkeys. Kerr (1975) reported that lesions of the ventral funiculus produced terminal degeneration in the medial hypothalamus of monkeys.

The hypothalamus, septal nuclei and nucleus accumbens are all believed to participate in the expression of a large number of emotional behaviors, including rage and aggressive responses (Panksepp, 1971; Blanchard et al., 1977; Albert et al., 1982). It will be important to determine whether direct spinal nociceptive projections to these areas play a role in the production of such responses to nociceptive stimulation.

Acknowledgements

This is a shortened version of a paper published in the Journal of Neuroscience (Burstein et al., 1987). Supported by grants BNS84187878 and DA02148.

References

Abzug, C., Maeda, M., Peterson, B.W. and Wilson V.J. (1974) Cervical branching of lumbar vestibulospinal axons. J. Physiol. (Lond.), 243: 499–522.

Albert, D.J., Walsh, M.L., Ryan, J. and Siemens Y. (1982) Mouse killing in rats: A comparison of spontaneous killers and rats with lesions of the medial hypothalamus or the medial accumbens nucleus. Physiol. Behav., 29: 989–994.

Anderson, F.D. and Berry, C.M. (1959) Degeneration studies of long ascending fiber systems in the cat brain stem. J. Comp. Neurol., 111: 195–230.

Blanchard, D.C., Blanchard, R.J., Takahashi, L.K. and Takahashi, T. (1977) Septal lesion and aggressive behavior. Behav. Biol. 21: 157–161.

Burstein, R., Cliffer, K.D. and Giesler, G.J., Jr. (1987) Direct somatosensory projection from the spinal cord to the hypothalamus and telencephalon. J. Neurosci., 7: 4159–4164.

Chang, H.T. and Ruch, T.C. (1947) Topographical distribution of spinothalamic fibers in the thalamus of the spider monkey. J. Anat. (Lond.) 81: 150–164.

Dutar, P., Lamour, Y. and Jobert, A. (1985) Activation of identified septo-hippocampal neurons by noxious peripheral stimulation. Brain Res., 328: 15–21.

Fitzgerald, M. and Lynn, B. (1977) The sensitization of high threshold mechanoreceptors with myelinated axons by repeated heating. J. Physiol. (Lond)., 365: 549–563.

Gerfen, C.R. and Sawchenko, P. (1984) An anterograde neuroanatomical tracing method that shows the detailed morphology of neurons, their axons and terminals: immunohistochemical localization of an axonally transported plant lectin, *Phaseolus vulgaris* leucoagglutinin (PHA-L). Brain Res., 290: 219–238.

Giesler, G.J., Jr., Menetrey, D. and Basbaum, A.I. (1979) Different origins of spinothalamic tract projections to medial and lateral thalamus in the rat. J. Comp. Neurol., 184: 107–126.

Graham, R.C. and Karnovsky, M.J. (1966) The early stages of absorption of injected horseradish peroxidase in the proximal tubules of mouse kidney: ultrastructural cytochemistry by a new technique. J. Histochem. Cytochem., 11: 291–302.

Hallin, R.G., Torebjork, H.E. and Wiesenfeld, Z. (1981) Nociceptors and warm receptor innervated by C fibers in human skin. J. Neurol. Neurosurg. Psychiatry, 44: 313–319.

Ju, G. (1984) Direct connections between hypothalamus and lumbar spinal cord in rabbits. Scientia Sinica, 27: 789–799.

Kanosue, K., Nakayama, T., Ishikawa, Y. and Imai-Matsumura, K. (1984) Responses of hypothalamic and thalamic neurons to noxious and scrotal thermal stimulations in rats. J. Therm. Biol., 9:11–13.

Katz, L.C., Burkhalter, A. and Dreyer, W.J. (1984) Fluorescent latex microspheres as a retrograde neuronal marker for in vivo and in vitro studies of visual cortex. Nature, 310: 498–500.

Kerr, F.W.L. (1975) The ventral spinothalamic tract and other ascending systems of the ventral funiculus of the spinal cord. J. Comp. Neurol., 159: 335–356.

Kevetter, G.A. and Willis W.D. (1983) Collaterals of spinothalamic cells in the rat. J. Comp. Neurol., 215: 453–464.

LaMotte, R.H. and Campbell, J.N. (1978) Comparison of responses of warm and nociceptive C-fibers in monkey with human judgment of thermal pain. J. Neurophysiol., 41: 509–529.

Mehler, W.R. (1969) Some neurological species differences – a posteriori. Ann. NY. Acad. Sci., 167: 424–468.

Mesulam, M.M. (1978) Tetramethyl benzidine peroxidase neurohistochemistry: A non-carcinogenic blue reaction product with superior sensitivity for visualizing neural afferents and efferents. J. Histochem. Cytochem., 26: 106–117.

Panksepp, J. (1971) Aggression elicited by electrical stimulation of the hypothalamus in albino rats. Physiol. Behav., 6: 321–329.

Ranck, J.B. (1975) Which elements are excited in electrical stimulation of mammalian central nervous system: A review. Brain Res., 98: 417–440.

Ring, G. and Ganchrow, D. (1983) Projections of nucleus caudalis and spinal cord to brainstem and diencephalon in the hedgehog (*Erinaceus europaeus* and *Paraechinus aethiopcus*): A degeneration study. J. Comp. Neurol., 216: 132–151.

Schmued, L.C. and Fallon, J.H. (1986) Fluoro-Gold: a new fluorescent retrograde axonal tracer with numerous unique properties. Brain Res., 377: 147–154.

Willis, W.D., Jr. (1985) The Pain System: The Neural Basis of Nociceptive Transmission in the Mammalian Nervous System (Pain and Headache, Vol. 8), Karger, Basel.

R. Dubner, G.F. Gebhart & M.R. Bond (Eds.)
Proceedings of the Vth World Congress on Pain
© 1988 Elsevier Science Publishers BV (Biomedical Division)

CHAPTER 62

Distribution of trigeminal nociceptive neurons in nucleus ventralis posteromedialis of primates

Toshikatsu Yokota, Yasuo Nishikawa and Natsu Koyama

Department of Physiology, Medical College of Shiga, Seta, Otsu 520–21, Japan

Summary

Distribution of trigeminal nociceptive-specific (NS) and wide-dynamic-range (WDR) neurons in the somatosensory part of the nucleus ventralis posteromedialis (VPM proper) was studied in Japanese macaques anesthetized with urethane-chloralose. Trigeminal NS and WDR neurons were found in the VPM part of the shell region around the ventrobasal complex of the thalamus except for the concave medial edge of the VPM proper just adjacent to the convex lateral margin of the interposing nucleus centrum medianum or pars oralis of the pulvinar. Trigeminal NS neurons were found in the caudal part of the VPM proper, while trigeminal WDR neurons were found in a narrow zone just rostral to the NS zone wherein trigeminal NS neurons were found.

Introduction

The nucleus ventralis posterior of the monkey's thalamus consists of four parts: nucleus ventralis posteromedialis (VPM proper), nucleus ventralis posteromedialis parvocellularis (VPMpc), nucleus ventralis posterolateralis (VPL) and nucleus ventra-

lis posterior inferior (VPI). The VPL is further subdivided into pars oralis (VPLo) and pars caudalis (VPLc) (Olszewski, 1952). The ventrobasal (VB) complex of the thalamus comprises somatosensory parts of the nucleus ventralis posterior. In the monkey, it is coextensive with the VPM proper and VPLc, exclusive of the VPMpc and VPLo (Jones, 1985).

Perl and Whitlock (1961) first observed that when projections from dorsal columns and one dorsolateral quadrant are eliminated, a somatotopically organized excitation of the VPLc is demonstrable, with some neurons responding to innocuous stimuli and others only to noxious stimuli. Almost 2 decades later, Kenshalo et al. (1980) discovered nociceptive neurons in the VPLc of the monkey with intact ascending pathways. Their observations led to the general proposition that the spinothalamic system projects to the VPLc and the postcentral gyrus, and may play a role in pain sensibility. The present study was undertaken to explore another part of the VB complex, the VPM proper, for trigeminal nociceptive neurons in the monkey.

Methods

A total of 30 anesthetized Japanese macaques (*Macaca fuscata*, 4.3–9.4 kg) were used. The animals were pretreated with ketamine (20 mg/kg) and were then anesthetized with 3.5 ml/kg of urethane-chlor-

---

Correspondence: Toshikatsu Yokota, Department of Physiology, Medical College of Shiga, Seta, Otsu 520–21, Japan.

alose solution (urethane 125 mg/ml and chloralose 10 mg/kg). Supplementary doses of urethane-chloralose solution were administered to maintain a proper anesthetic level. After a tracheotomy, the animals were paralysed with pancuronium bromide (2–4 mg/kg/h), and ventilation was maintained with a respirator.

A craniotomy was performed on the right side to allow introduction of a recording microelectrode into the thalamus. Glass capillary microelectrodes filled with 2% pontamine sky blue in 1 M sodium acetate were used for recording single unit activities. Single unit potentials were amplified and fed into a window discriminator. The output pulses of the window discriminator were used by a spike counter to compile peristimulus time histograms.

Once well-isolated unitary activity had been recorded from the thalamus, the receptive field of the neuron was examined and mapped using mechanical stimuli. The mechanical stimuli included displacement of hairs, stroking and probing the skin, firm but innocuous pressure exerted by picking up a fold of skin with flattened forceps or an arterial clip, and noxious pinch with small serrated forceps or an alligator clip. In some units, graded radiant heat stimulation was applied to the center of the receptive field defined by mechanical stimulation. Precisely controlled skin temperatures were obtained by a servo-controlled thermostimulator. Recording sites of nociceptive neurons were marked by passing 5 μA cathodal current through the micro-electrode tip for 10 min. At the termination of each experiment, the brain was cleared of blood and fixed in situ by perfusing 1000 ml of normal saline through the beating heart, followed by 3000 ml of 10% formalin-saline. After at least one week, the brain was frozen and cut into 50-μm sections and stained with cresyl-violet. Dye marks were identified in stained sections, and sections containing dye marks were photographed.

Results

A total of 1242 units were recorded from the VPM proper. They were activated by mechanical stimulation of the trigeminal integument, and were divided into 3 classes using the same criteria as employed in previous studies in the cat (Yokota et al., 1985). The first class was called low-threshold mechanoreceptive (LTM) units. They maximally responded to gentle mechanical stimulation, either hair movements or light pressure on the trigeminal integument. A total of 1124 units belonged to this class. They had a clearly defined receptive field on the contralateral side, except for 4 units which had a receptive field on the ipsilateral tongue surface. The remaining 118 units were nociceptive-specific (NS) or wide-dynamic-range (WDR) units. In the following, results obtained with these two classes of nociceptive units will be described.

Nociceptive-specific units
A total of 108 units were identified as NS units. They were unresponsive to weak forms of mechanical stimulation, but discharged when intense mechanical stimuli were applied to a circumscribed area of the contralateral trigeminal integument (Fig. 1). A great majority of them responded with

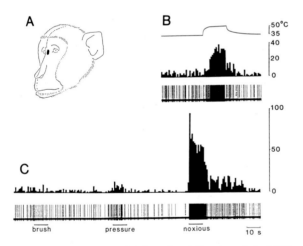

Fig. 1. An NS unit recorded from the shell region of the VPM proper. A: Receptive field indicated by a black area. B: Responses to heat stimulation of the receptive field. The upper trace indicates skin temperature. The middle record is the peristimulus time histogram. The bin width is 1 s. The lower trace shows spike discharges. C: Responses to 3 different types of mechanical stimuli applied to the receptive field.

a maintained discharge to noxious mechanical stimuli. Some of them responded to application of firm but innocuous pressure, but discharged more vigorously when noxious stimuli were applied. Of these, 9 units had a peripheral receptive field in the ophthalmic division of the face, 24 units in the maxillary skin, 42 units in the mandibular skin, 18 units in the gum, and 15 units in the tongue.

Trigeminal NS units were found in the marginal rim of the caudal VPM proper, but they were absent along the border between the VPM proper and VPLc. In other words, they were found in the VPM part of the shell region around the VB complex.

Fig. 2 illustrates locations of NS and LTM units in a transverse plane near the caudal end of the VPM proper. At this level, the ventral aspect of the VPM proper is surrounded by the VPLc. Trigeminal NS units were found in the dorsal shell region of the VPM proper just ventral to the pars oralis of the pulvinar (PuO). They had a receptive field in the ophthalmic or maxillary division of the face.

Fig. 3 illustrates results obtained at a more rostral transverse plane. In the lateral microelectrode track, NS units were found at dorsal and ventral ends of a row of VPM units. At this level, the ventral part of the VPM proper extends medially underneath the nucleus centrum medianum (CM). The medial microelectrode track passed through this ventromedial part of the VPM proper. In this track, NS units were found at dorsal and ventral ends of a row of VPM proper units. The middle microelectrode track passed through the medial part of the VPM proper, adjacent to the lateral margin of the CM. In this part, the VPM proper is separated into dorsal and ventral parts by the interposing CM. An NS unit was found at the dorsal margin of the dorsal VPM proper and another NS unit at the ventral margin of the ventral VPM proper. In five other experiments, 10 microelectrode tracks

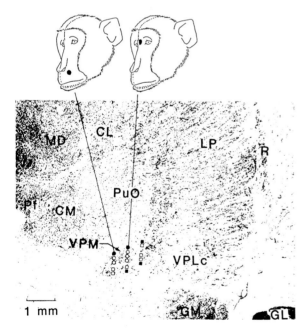

Fig. 2. Locations of LTM and NS units in a transverse plane near the caudal end of the VPM proper and receptive fields of trigeminal NS units. Open circles, solid circles, open squares and solid squares indicate locations of trigeminal LTM, trigeminal NS, spinal LTM and spinal NS units, respectively.

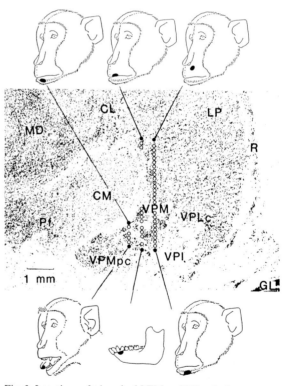

Fig. 3. Locations of trigeminal LTM and NS units in a transverse plane corresponding to the rostral NS zone of the VPM proper, and receptive fields of trigeminal NS units. Open circles indicate locations of trigeminal LTM units, while solid circles indicate locations of trigeminal LTM units.

passed through dorsal and ventral parts of the VB complex separated by the interposing CM or PuO. In these microelectrode tracks, NS units were found either at the dorsal margin of the dorsal VB complex or at the ventral margin of the ventral VB complex. No NS units were encountered at the concave medial edge of the VPM proper just adjacent to the convex lateral margin of the interposing CM or PuO.

In general, NS units having a receptive field in the gum were encountered in the rostral part of the NS zone. In the ventral shell region of the rostral NS zone, the tongue, gum and mandibular skin were mediolaterally represented in this order.

Wide-dynamic-range units
Ten units were identified as WDR units. They had

a graded response to brush, pressure and noxious pinch applied to the center of the receptive field (black area in Fig. 4), and responded best to noxious pinch. Outside this zone (cross-hatched area in Fig. 4), they were unresponsive to low-intensity mechanical stimuli, but responded differentially to firm pressure and noxious pinch. Finally, the latter area was surrounded by an area in which only noxious pinch resulted in unit discharges (shaded area in Fig. 4). The receptive field was confined to the ipsilateral half of the trigeminal integument.

Of 10 WDR units recorded, 5 units had the center of the receptive field in the maxillary skin. The remaining 5 units had the center of the receptive field in the mandibular skin.

Fig. 5 illustrates locations of trigeminal NS, WDR and LTM units recorded from a sagittal plane 7.3 mm lateral to the midline. It can be seen that WDR units were located at the dorsal or ventral end of a row of trigeminal units, and that WDR units were located in a narrow zone of the shell region of the VPM proper just rostral to the NS zone.

Discussion

It has been well established that the VB complex receives specific mechanoreceptive and thermoreceptive input, but whether it also receives nociceptive

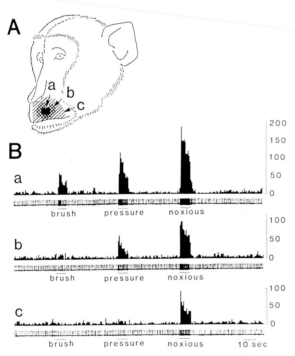

Fig. 4. A WDR unit recorded from the shell region of the VPM proper. A: Receptive field. In the black area, the unit had a graded response to brush, pressure and noxious pinch. In the cross-hatched area, the unit did not respond to brush, but differentially responded to pressure and noxious pinch. In the shaded area, the unit exclusively responded to noxious pinch. B: Responses of the unit to mechanical stimulation of three different areas of the receptive field. Records a, b and c represent responses to stimulation of corresponding areas in A.

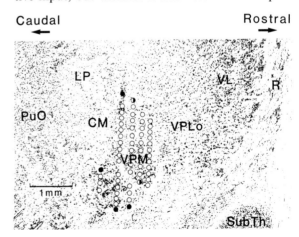

Fig. 5. Locations of trigeminal NS, WDR and LTM units recorded from the VPM proper in a sagittal plane 7.3 mm lateral to the midline. Solid circles, half solid circles and open circles indicate locations of trigeminal NS, WDR and LTM units, respectively.

input was uncertain. Poggio and Mountcastle (1960, 1963) did not find nociceptive neurons in the VB complex of the cat and monkey. Instead, they found that the majority of neurons recorded in the posterior nuclear group (PO) of the thalamus were sensitive to noxious stimuli in the cat, and suggested that the PO plays a significant role in central pain mechanisms. Subsequent analysis cast doubt on the nociceptive role of PO neurons (Curry, 1972; Nyquist and Greenhoot, 1974), and nociceptive neurons were found in the VB complex in cat and monkey in which the dorsal part of the spinal cord had been transected (Perl and Whitlock, 1961; Pollin and Albe-Fessard, 1979).

During the past decade, nociceptive neurons have been found in the VPL in rat (Mitchell and Hellon, 1977; Peschanski et al., 1980), cat (Honda et al., 1983; Kniffki and Mizumura, 1983) and monkey (Kenshalo et al., 1980; Chung et al., 1986) with an intact neuraxis. Nociceptive neurons in the cat VPL were located in the shell region (i.e., dorsal, ventral and lateral boundaries). In the monkey, however, locations of cutaneous neurons in the VPLc showed little correlation with the response characteristics of the neurons (Chung et al., 1986).

Previously, Yokota et al. (1985) had discovered trigeminal NS and WDR neurons in the VPM part of the shell region around the VB complex in the cat. Trigeminal NS neurons were found in the caudal third of the VPM proper, whereas trigeminal WDR neurons were found in a narrow band of the shell region about 300 μm wide, just rostral to the NS zone. Both NS and WDR neurons showed a somatotopic organization. In the present study, trigeminal NS and WDR neurons were found in the VPM part of the shell region around the VB complex in the Japanese macaque. It was also confirmed that trigeminal NS and WDR neurons were spatially segregated in the Japanese macaque, WDR neurons being located more anteriorly. However, there was a minor difference between cats and Japanese macaques. In the cat, nociceptive neurons are distributed over the whole surface of the caudal VB complex, so that there is no interruption in the location of nociceptive neurons in the shell region around the VB complex in a transverse plane. In the Japanese macaque, nociceptive neurons were missing along the concave medial edge of the VPM proper just adjacent to the convex lateral margin of the interposing CM or PuO.

References

Chung, J.M., Lee, K.H., Surmeier, D.J., Sorkin, L.S., Kim, J. and Willis, W.D. (1986) Response characteristics of neurons in the ventral posterior lateral nucleus of the monkey thalamus. J. Neurophysiol., 56: 370–390.

Curry, M.J. (1972) The exteroceptive properties of neurons in the somatic part of the posterior group (PO). Brain Res., 44: 439–462.

Honda, C.N., Mense, S. and Perl, E.R. (1983) Neurons in ventrobasal region of cat thalamus selectively responsive to noxious mechanical stimulation. J. Neurophysiol., 49: 662–673.

Jones, E.G. (1985) The Thalamus, Plenum Press, New York.

Kenshalo, D.R., Jr., Giesler, G.J., Jr., Leonard, R.B. and Willis, W.D. (1980) Responses of neurons in primate ventral posterior lateral nucleus to noxious stimuli. J. Neurophysiol., 43: 1594–1614.

Kniffki, K.-D. and Mizumura, K. (1983) Responses of neurons in VPL and VPL-VL region of the cat to algesic stimulation of muscle and tendon. J. Neurophysiol., 49: 649–661.

Mitchel, D., and Hellon, R.F. (1977) Neuronal and behavioral responses in rats during noxious stimulation of the tail. Proc. R. Soc. Lond. Ser. B., 197: 169–194.

Nyquist, J.K. and Greenhoot, J.H. (1974) Unit analysis of non-specific thalamic responses to high-intensity cutaneous input in the cat. Exp. Neurol., 42: 609–622.

Olszewski, J. (1952) The Thalamus of the *Macaca mulatta*, Karger, Basel.

Perl, E.R. and Whitlock, D.G. (1961) Somatic stimuli exciting spinothalamic projections to thalamic neurons in cat and monkey. Exp. Neurol., 3: 256–296.

Peschanski, M., Guilbaud, G., Gautron, M. and Besson, J.M. (1980) Encoding of noxious heat messages in neurons of the ventrobasal complex of the rat. Brain Res., 197: 401–413.

Poggio, G.F. and Mountcastle, V.B. (1960) A study of the functional contributions of the lemniscal and spinothalamic systems to somatic sensibility. Bull. Johns Hopkins Hosp., 106: 266–316.

Poggio, G.F. and Mountcastle, V.B. (1963) The functional properties of ventrobasal thalamic neurons studied in unanesthetized monkeys. J. Neurophysiol., 26: 775–806.

Pollin, B. and Albe-Fessard, D. (1979) Organization of somatic thalamus in monkeys with and without section of dorsal spinal tracts. Brain Res., 173: 431–441.

Yokota, T., Koyama, N. and Matsumoto, N. (1985) Somatotopic distribution of trigeminal nociceptive neurons in ventrobasal complex of cat thalamus. J. Neurophysiol., 53: 1387–1400.

R. Dubner, G.F. Gebhart & M.R. Bond (Eds.)
Proceedings of the Vth World Congress on Pain
© 1988 Elsevier Science Publishers BV (Biomedical Division)

CHAPTER 63

Responses of thermosensitive tooth pulp driven neurons in the cat cerebral cortex

Koichi Iwata*, Hiroyuki Muramatsu, Yoshiyuki Tsuboi and Rhyuji Sumino

Department of Physiology, School of Dentistry, Nihon University, 1-8-13 Kandasurugadai, Chiyoda-Ku, Tokyo 101, Japan

Summary

Distribution and response properties of SI neurons driven by thermal stimulation of the tooth pulp were studied by recording single neuronal activities from the cat cerebral cortex. A total of 103 neurons responding to electrical stimulation of the tooth pulp (TPNs) were tested by thermal stimulation (20–55°C) of the tooth pulp. Eighteen of them were thermosensitive (Ts-TPNs). All Ts-TPNs were distributed in the cytoarchitectonic area 3b, while thermo-insensitive TPNs (Tins-TPNs) were in area 3a as well as 3b. About 50% of Ts-TPNs received noxious cutaneous inputs from the orofacial regions, while only 15% of Tins-TPNs received them. Ts-TPNs were further divided into two groups according to their input pattern. Results suggest that Ts-TPNs may be involved in the perception of tooth pain as well as cutaneous pain in the trigeminal region.

Introduction

Cortical projection areas of tooth pulpal afferents have been studied by recording field potentials (Melzack and Haugen, 1957; Keller et al., 1974; Vyklicky and Keller, 1974; Dong and Chudler, 1984) or single unit activity (Lund and Sessle, 1974; Andersson et al., 1977; Roos et al., 1982; Matsumoto, 1984; Iwata et al., 1986). The focal projection area was located in the lateral part of the coronal gyrus, suggesting that the coronal gyrus is closely related to the perception of pain in the trigeminal system. In these experiments, however, the results were based mainly on the data obtained by electrical stimulation of the tooth pulp, which might produce unnatural impulses in the pulpal nerve. It is also known that in man low intensity electrical stimulation of the tooth pulp produces prepain sensation which is a different sensation from pain (Shimizu, 1964).

In order to clarify the role of the coronal gyrus in pain sensation of tooth pulp, we used a thermal stimulation which produced pain but no other sensation (Matthews, 1977; Narhi, 1985). Various properties of the thermosensitive TPNs were compared with those of thermo-insensitive TPNs.

Methods

This study was performed on 26 young adult cats that were initially anesthetized with ketamine-HCl (50 mg/kg) and given supplemental doses (20 mg/kg) every hour. End-tidal CO_2 concentration was continuously monitored and maintained at a level

---

*To whom correspondence should be addressed.

of 3.5–4.5%. Femoral arterial blood pressure was continuously monitored, experiments being terminated if the systolic pressure fell below 80 mmHg. Rectal temperature was maintained at 37–39°C with a thermostatically controlled heating pad. The maxillary and mandibular canine teeth on both sides were prepared for electrical and thermal stimulation of the pulp. Small holes were drilled into the dentine along the long axis and silver ball electrodes were embedded with EMG electrode paste and fixed with dental wax and acrylic resin. Using a slow running burr under constant isotonic saline, the enamel and outermost layer of dentine were removed from the labial side of the tooth crown. Each pulp was stimulated electrically with single pulses (0.2 ms duration, 0.01–1 mA) delivered via constant-current pulse generator. Thermal stimulation (20–55°C, 10–30 s duration) was applied by a controlled thermal probe attached to the exposed tooth surface. The skull was opened over the coronal gyrus and adjacent regions, and an acrylic chamber was placed on the opening and filled with mineral oil. The animal's head was mounted on a non-traumatic head-holder and lidocaine-HCl was periodically applied to wound margins. Natural stimuli (tactile with brush, pinching with forceps and heating with the controlled heating probe) were also applied to intra- and peri-oral regions and facial skin. The threshold value for the pulp-evoked jaw opening reflex was measured as the first visible movement evoked in the digastric muscle by the lowest intensity of pulp stimulation (before the cat was immobilized). Glass coated tungsten microelectrodes were inserted deep into the coronal gyrus to record single unit activity. During the recording sessions, the animals were immobilized with pancronium bromide (about 1 mg/kg, i.v., every hour) and artificially ventilated. In each experiment, one to five recording points were marked by passing a direct current (10 μA, 10 s) and verified histologically subsequent to the experiment.

Results and Discussion

Landgren and Olsson (1980) showed that the ante-

rior part of the coronal gyrus was exclusively the oral projection area, and the neurons in this area received inputs from the intra- and/or peri-oral regions. We recorded 103 TPNs from the anterior part of the coronal gyrus. Only 18 of them responded to heating of the tooth pulp, and were all located in the same oral projection area as in the previous report (Landgren and Olsson, 1980).

Most of these neurons also received inputs from

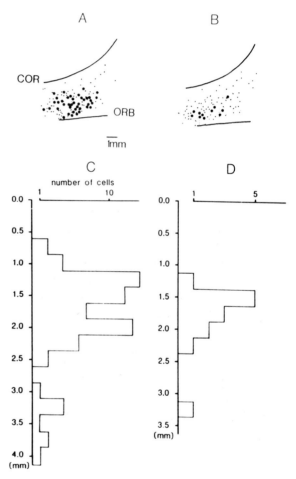

Fig. 1. Penetration tracks for recording response of TPNs and intracortical distribution of TPNs. A. Thermo-insensitive TPNs were encountered in the anterior part of the coronal gyrus and are illustrated as solid circles. B. Thermosensitive TPNs were encountered in the ventral part of the anterior coronal gyrus. The small dots indicate the tracks where no TPNs could be encountered. COR, coronal sulcus; ORB, orbital sulcus. C and D show the depth profiles of thermo-insensitive and thermosensitive TPNs, respectively.

mucosa and skin in the oral region. In the present experiment, we focused on the Ts-TPNs which responded to heating the tooth pulp and did not analyse cold-sensitive TPNs. Figure 1 illustrates the penetration tracks and depth profiles of Ts-TPNs and Tins-TPNs. In the upper part of this figure, the large solid circles indicate the penetration points in which Tins-TPNs (Fig. 1A) and Ts-TPNs (Fig. 1B)

were encountered. Tins-TPNs were more widely distributed within the anterior part of the coronal gyrus than Ts-TPNs. The depth profiles of Ts-TPNs and Tins-TPNs were not different from each other (Fig. 1C,D). Figure 2 shows the representative records of a Ts-TPN and a Tins-TPN. The Ts-TPN driven by the ipsilateral upper canine tooth pulp was located at a depth of 1.7 mm from the

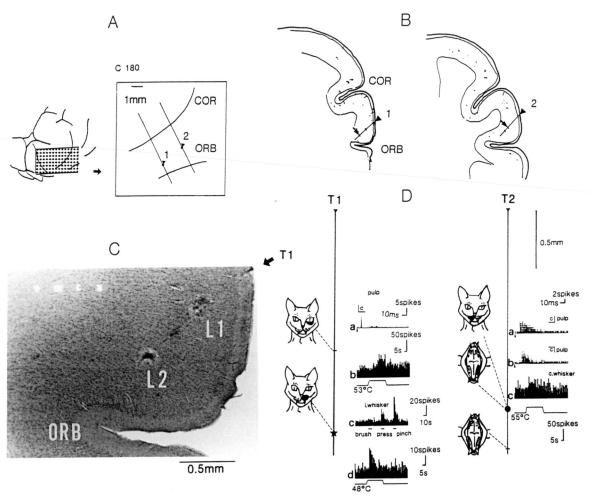

Fig. 2. Reconstruction of the tracks where neuronal activity of Ts-TPNs were encountered. A. Penetration tracks (T1 and T2) and sectional orientation are shown. Penetration tracks were plotted on the coronal gyrus. Inset shows the frontolateral view of the cat cortex. B. Drawing of the sectional plane of tracks 1 and 2. C. Photograph indicates two lesions (L1 and L2) marking track 1. D. In Track 1, the Ts-TPN was encountered at the point indicated by the solid star. This neuron responded to electrical (a) and heat (b) stimulation of the ipsilateral lower canine tooth pulp and also to pressure, pinching (c) and noxious heating (d) of the ipsilateral whisker pad. Peristimulus time histograms of the response of the Ts-TPN to each stimulation are illustrated on the right side along each track. In track 2, the Tins-TPN was encountered at the point of the solid circle. This neuron responded to electrical stimulation of the contralateral upper (a) and lower (b) canine tooth pulps, and also responded to heating of the contralateral whisker pad.

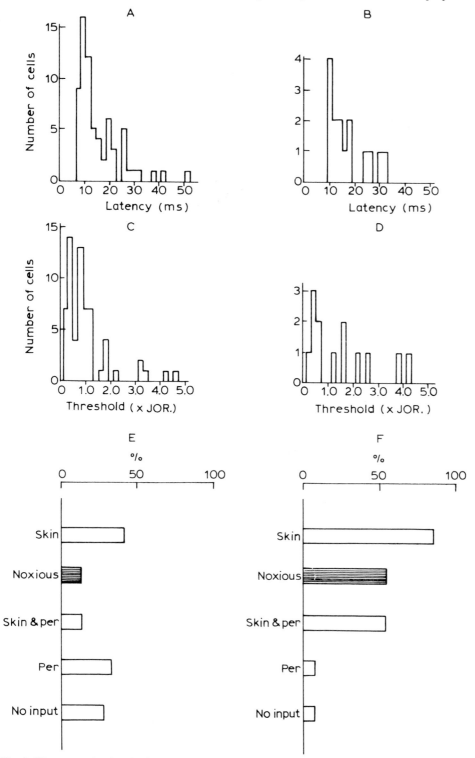

Fig. 3. Histograms showing the frequency distribution of the peak latency (A,B), threshold intensity (C,D) and convergence pattern (E,F). Those of Tins-TPNs are illustrated in A,C and E, and those of Ts-TPNs are illustrated in B,D and F.

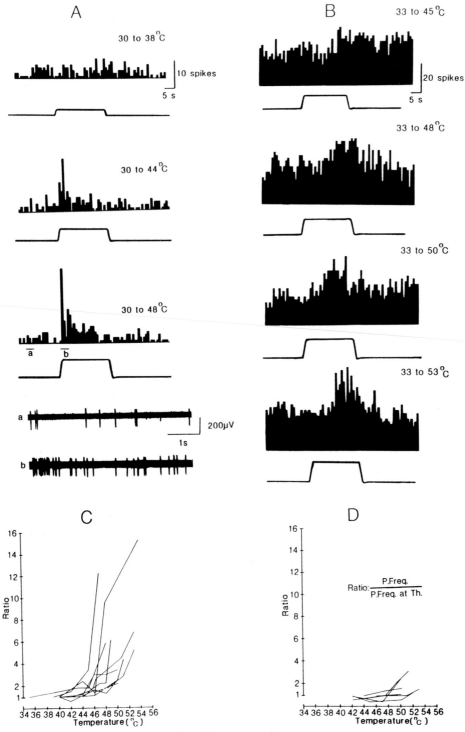

Fig. 4. Sample peristimulus time histograms (A and B) and stimulus–response functions (C and D) of two different types of Ts-TPNs. The ratio of peak frequency to peak frequency at threshold intensity is plotted as a function of stimulus intensity in C and D. Histograms and graphs of innocuous skin/mucosa inputs converging Ts-TPNs are illustrated in A and C, and those of noxious skin/mucosa inputs converging Ts-TPNs are illustrated in B and D. In A, a and b are expanded scales of activity shown in response to 30–48°C temperature change.

cortical surface in track T1. This Ts-TPN also responded to pressing, pinching (c) and noxious heating (d) of the ipsilateral whisker pad (Fig. 2, T1). In track T2 (Fig. 2), the Tins-TPN driven by the contralateral upper (a) and lower (b) canine tooth pulps was encountered at a depth of 1.5 mm from the cortical surface. This Tins-TPN also responded to noxious heating of the contralateral whisker pad (c) and tactile stimulation of the tooth (activation of the periodontal receptor), and of the perioral mucosa and whisker pad. Cytoarchitectonically, Ts-TPNs recorded in the present experiment were in laminae III–IV of area 3b, while Tins-TPNs were in laminae III–IV of areas 3a and 3b, according to Hassler and Muhs-Clement (1964). Therefore, we propose that area 3b of the anterior part of the coronal gyrus is involved in the perception of trigeminal pain. Kenshalo et al. (1983) also suggested that cortical areas 1, 2 and 3b play a role in the cortical processing of noxious information to the body surface. Response properties and convergence patterns of Tins-TPNs and Ts-TPNs are illustrated in Fig. 3. The peak latency of Tins-TPNs was 14.2 ± 8.8 ms (Mean $\pm$ SD, $N = 81$) and that of TS-TPNs was 14.0 ± 6.7 ms ($N = 18$). About 70% of Tins-TPNs responded to electrical stimulation of an intensity less than the threshold for the tooth pulp-evoked jaw opening reflex, but only 40% of Ts-TPNs responded to the same weak stimulation. The later results suggest that Ts-TPNs are driven by smaller intrapulpal fibers than those driving Tins-TPNs. Furthermore, the convergence pattern was different between these two types of TPNs. Forty-five per cent of Tins-TPNs received low threshold cutaneous inputs from the oro-facial region and 10% of them also responded to noxious pressure, pinching and heating of the facial skin. On the other hand, 89% of Ts-TPNs received low threshold cutaneous inputs and 50% of them responded to noxious stimulation of the skin. These convergent patterns of cutaneous afferents were similar to those described in the caudal region of the spinal trigeminal nucleus (Hu and Sessle, 1984; Amano et al., 1986) and the thalamus (Yokota et al., 1985). These results further suggest that Ts-TPNs have important roles in the perception of tooth pain produced by heating as well as in the perception of cutaneous pain in the orofacial regions.

Figure 4 illustrates the sample peristimulus time histograms (A,B) and stimulus–response relationships (C,D) of two Ts-TPNs. The Ts-TPN shown in A responded to light touch and noxious stimulation of the facial skin, as well as to heating of the tooth pulp. On the other hand, the Ts-TPN in B responded only to noxious skin stimulation in addition to heating the tooth pulp. The pattern of response to thermal stimulation of tooth pulp was also different between these two types of Ts-TPNs. Ts-TPNs receiving innocuous skin/mucosa inputs showed a rapid rise to a peak frequency of discharge and graded responses to increasing stimulus temperature. On the contrary, Ts-TPNs receiving only noxious skin/mucosa inputs showed a gradual increase in firing frequency following heating of the tooth pulp, and did not alter their response frequency until very high temperatures. It seems that those Ts-TPNs with innocuous inputs are involved in the intensity coding of pain sensation produced by heat stimulation of the tooth pulp as well as cutaneous pain sensation, while noxious skin/mucosa inputs converging on those Ts-TPNs with only noxious inputs may signal the quality of the stimulus applied to the tooth pulp.

References

Amano, N., Hu, J.W. and Sessle, B.J. (1986) Responses of neurons in feline trigeminal subnucleus caudalis (medullary dorsal horn) to cutaneous, intraoral, and muscle afferent stimuli. J. Neurophysiol., 55:227–243.

Andersson, O., Keller, A., Roose, A. and Rydenhag, B. (1977) Cortical projection of tooth pulp afferents in the cat. In D.J. Anderson and B. Matthews (Eds.), Pain in Trigeminal Region, Elsevier, Amsterdam, pp. 335–364.

Dong, W.K. and Chudler, E.H. (1984) Origins of tooth pulp-evoked far-field and early near-field potentials in the cat. J. Neurophysiol., 51:859–889.

Hassler, R. and Muhs-Clement, K. (1964) Architectonisher Aufbau des sensomotorischen und parietalen cortex der Katze. J. Hirnforsch., 6:377–420.

Hu, J.W. and Sessle, B.J. (1984) Comparison of responses of cutaneous nociceptive and nonnociceptive brain stem neurons in trigeminal subnucleus caudalis (medullary dorsal horn) and subnucleus oralis to natural and electrical stimulation of tooth pulp. J. Neurophysiol., 52:39–53.

Iwata, K., Itoga, H., Ikukawa, A., Tamura, K. and Sumino, R. (1986) Cortical cells driven by the low threshold tooth-pulpal afferent in cats. Brain Res., 368:399–403.

Keller, O., Butkhuzi, S.M. Vyklicky, L. and Brozek, G. (1974) Cortical responses evoked by stimulation of tooth pulp afferents in the cat. Physiol. Bohemoslov. 23:45–53.

Kenshalo, D.R. Jr., and Isensee, O. (1983) Responses of primate SI cortical neurons to noxious stimuli. J. Neurophysiol., 50:1479–1496.

Landgren, S. and Olsson K.A. (1980) Low threshold projections from the oral cavity and the face to the cerebral cortex of the cat. Exp. Brain Res., 39:133–147.

Lund, J.P. and Sessle, B.J. (1974) Oral-facial and jaw muscle afferent projections to neurons in cat frontal cortex. Exp. Neurol., 45:324–331.

Matsumoto, N. (1984) Functional difference of tooth pulp-driven neurons in oral and facial areas of somatosensory cortex (SI) of the cat. Exp. Neurol., 85:437–451.

Matthews, B. (1977) Responses of intradental nerves to electrical and thermal stimulation of teeth in dogs. J. Physiol., 264:641–664.

Melzack, R. and Haugen, F.P. (1957) Responses evoked at the cortex by tooth stimulation. Am. J. Physiol., 190:570–574.

Narhi, M. (1985) The characteristics of intradental sensory units and their responses to stimulation. J. Dent. Res., 64:564–571.

Roos, A., Rydenhag, B. and Andersson, S.A. (1982) Cortical responses evoked by tooth pulp stimulation in the cat. Surface and intracortical responses. Pain, 14:247–265.

Shimizu, T. (1964) Tooth pre-pain sensation elicited by electrical stimulation. J. Dent. Res., 43:467–475.

Vyklicky, L. and Keller, O. (1974) Cortical representation of tooth pulp primary afferents in the cat. Adv. Neurol., 4:233–240.

Yokota, T., Koyama, N. and Matsumoto, N. (1985) Somatotopic distribution of trigeminal nociceptive neurons in ventrobasal complex of cat thalamus. J. Neurophysiol., 53:1387–1400.

R. Dubner, G.F. Gebhart & M.R. Bond (Eds.)
Proceedings of the Vth World Congress on Pain
© 1988 Elsevier Science Publishers BV (Biomedical Division)

CHAPTER 64

Reliability and validity of ultra-late cerebral potentials in response to C-fibre activation in man

Rolf-Detlef Treede and Burkhart Bromm

Institute of Physiology, University Hospital Eppendorf, University of Hamburg, 2000 Hamburg 20, FRG

Summary

To study evoked cerebral potentials (EP) mediated by slowly conducting cutaneous afferents, a CO_2 laser delivering non-contact radiant heat pulses causing rapid increases in temperature (1 °C/ms) on the skin was used. Due to its superficial absorption, the stimulus is confined to epidermis and superficial dermis (100 μm) even with strong energy. With microneurographic techniques in awake humans it was shown that the CO_2 laser predominantly activates Aδ and C nociceptors.

The CO_2 laser EP is maximal at the vertex. It is biphasic, with a negativity at 240 ms and a positivity at 370 ms. This potential can be related to Aδ-fibre input. The C-fibre EP in humans is most clearly shown when earlier activity is suppressed by a preferential A-fibre block. It is biphasic or mainly positive, with a latency of about 1250 ms, and has a shape and scalp topography similar to those of the Aδ-fibre EP. Both potentials may therefore stem from the same generator. The coactivation of cutaneous Aδ and C fibres leads to a double afferent volley with an approx. 900 ms interval. With CO_2 laser double pulses of 900ms interval, the second response is markedly reduced. Correspondingly, without block the amplitude of the C-fibre EP is very low due to the preceding Aδ-fibre EP.

Reprint requests to Prof. Dr. Dr. B. Bromm.

Introduction

CO_2 laser radiant heat pulses are able to induce marked changes in skin temperature within very short times of a few ms (Bromm and Treede, 1983). The peripheral fibre spectrum and the dorsal horn neuronal population activated by these stimuli were shown to be similar to those activated by conventional long-lasting heat pulses (Devor et al., 1982; Bromm et al., 1984). The late vertex potential after CO_2 laser stimulation of the hairy skin of the hand appears about 100 ms later than with mechanical or electrical stimuli (Bromm et al., 1983). This delay can be related to the slow conduction velocity of about 10–14 m/s in the Aδ afferents involved (Kenton et al., 1980). The afferent volley may thus be expected to arrive at the cerebral cortex about 80 ms after the stimulus. Hence these potentials represent secondary information-processing of Aδ-fibre input.

Selective C-fibre activation in the skin, after application of a pressure nerve block, led to the detection of ultra-late cerebral potentials with long latencies of more than one second (Bromm et al., 1983). Up to then such potentials had not been described unequivocally in the literature, despite intense efforts to identify them, especially in animal experiments (for review see Chudler and Dong, 1983). The present paper reports a comparison of late and ultra-late evoked potential waveforms and addresses the question of why the ultra-late potentials are usually masked in the electroencephalogram.

Methods

The subjects (healthy male volunteers, 21–29 years old) were familiarized with CO_2 laser stimuli and EEG recordings in a preceding session. They gave written informed consent according to the Declaration of Helsinki and were free to withdraw at any time.

A 300 mm^2 area of the hairy skin supplied by the superficial branch of the left radial nerve was stimulated with radiant heat pulses of 20 ms duration, generated by a CO_2 laser stimulator (10.6 μm wavelength, 5–60 W output power, 5 mm beam diameter). The stimuli were delivered by a microprocessor with randomized interstimulus intervals of between 20 and 40 s, and both the experimenter and the subjects were blind with respect to stimulus onset and strength.

Pre- and post-stimulus electroencephalogram (EEG) segments were recorded from vertex versus linked earlobes (bandpass 0.1–30 Hz), digitized by an LSI 11/23 (sampling rate 100/s) and stored on disc for off-line evaluation. For artefact control the vertical component of the electro-oculogram (EOG) was recorded from supra- and infra-orbital electrodes. The interelectrode impedance was reduced to less than 1 kohm (10 Hz) by scratching the skin with an abrasive paste. Evoked potentials (EP) were averaged over blocks of 40 stimulus repetitions. Latency-corrected averaging was accomplished by a modified Woody filter (for details see Bromm and Treede, 1987). In order to prevent incidental phase locking of the filter with the EEG activity, the data segments were digitally bandpass-filtered (0.5–7 Hz, 40 dB per octave) and template length and maximum shift were kept as narrow as possible around the expected EP latency.

Ultra-late EPs were studied in two samples of 12 (experiment 1) and 16 subjects (experiment 2) with a preferential A-fibre block. For this purpose the superficial branch of the radial nerve was subjected to pressure by means of two 700-g weights hanging on both sides of 2-cm-wide ribbon. The build-up of the block was monitored by electroneurography (ENG) with surface electrodes (500 weak electrical pulses, repetition rate 2/s), examination of cutaneous sensitivity (v.Frey bristles, cold and warm probes, pin-pricks) and evaluation of the subjects' reaction time to laser stimuli. The latter was measured either simultaneously with the EP ($n = 6$) or separately ($n = 22$). In experiment 1, subsequent injection of 2–3 ml lidocaine (1%) also interrupted the remaining C-fibre conduction for about 30 min. In experiment 2, the EEG was recorded from 14 electrodes over both hemispheres. The subjects were instructed to focus on second pain, which resulted in small ultra-late EPs in 7 cases.

In four subjects the late EP was not blocked by either pressure or lidocaine. These subjects showed only minimal sensory loss in spite of ENG disappearance. Apparently they did not have an autonomous innervation area of the radial nerve on the back of their hands.

Results

C-fibre-related ultra-late evoked potential components

Fig. 1 illustrates grand mean evoked potentials from both nerve-block experiments. In the first trace, with unaffected nerve, there is a marked response of about 15 μV peak-to-peak amplitude. The mean latencies were 240 ms for the vertex negativity (N240) and 370 ms for the adjacent positivity (P370). This is the 'late' EP reported in the literature (Kenton et al., 1980). Although the subjects perceived two pain sensations after each single laser stimulus, only minimal activity can be seen in the C-fibre latency range (right).

The second trace shows measurements during A-fibre block. The disappearance of the surface ENG was usually accompanied by a loss in cold sensitivity, increase in tactile threshold and loss of two-point discrimination. Warm and painful stimuli could still be perceived; pin-pricks were sometimes more painful than without block, especially with repeated pricks. In this state the late EP disappeared; instead there was a delayed ultra-late vertex positivity with a maximum of about 8 μV at 1300 ms (second trace). Simultaneously, the CO_2 laser-induced sensation lost its pricking component; its intensity was reduced but the time course was prolonged and it was described as burning and dull. The reaction time of the subjects was prolonged by about 900 ms from 420 ms to 1300 ms ($n = 24$). There were only C fibres left to conduct the information that there was a stimulus, and thus the ultra-late EP is assumed to be triggered by peripheral C-fibre activity.

After injection of lidocaine around the peripheral nerve, the ultra-late potential disappeared (third trace, left). Under this condition no stimulus-locked EEG activity could be detected at all, since all cutaneous afferents were blocked. Correspondingly, the CO_2 laser stimuli were no longer perceived by the subjects. This indicates that the ultra-late potential was triggered by cutaneous afferents. All changes were fully reversible after release of the pressure block (last trace).

Single-trial late and ultra-late evoked potential components

The averages in Fig. 1 indicate that there is stimulus-locked ultra-late activity during A-fibre block, but what is the shape of this EP? In order to answer this question, we looked at the single-trial post-stimulus EEG segments. Fig. 2 shows sample single-trial evoked responses to CO_2 laser stimuli from one subject. The evoked cerebral responses are contaminated to a variable degree by EEG activity (mainly in the alpha frequency range). Generally, the signal-to-noise ratio (SNR) is too bad to identify the evoked part in the single post-stimulus EEG. Therefore, the single trials had to be selected for good SNR. Even in these selected epochs, obviously the commonly regarded 'late' potentials (200–400 ms) exhibited a higher SNR than the 'ultra-late' potentials (beyond 1000 ms) illustrated here. The latency jitter in the late responses was smaller than their width. Therefore, averaging led to a comparable waveform in the mean (bottom trace, left). In contrast, the single-trial ultra-late responses (right) did not look at all like their average (bottom trace, right). Instead, the selected ultra-late potentials

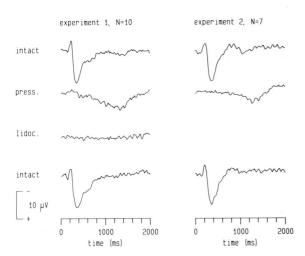

Fig. 1. Ultra-late components in the CO_2 laser evoked potential. Each trace shows the average over 40 stimuli and 10 subjects (left) or 7 subjects (right), respectively. Vertex negativity upward. With intact nerve the usual late EP appears. After total block of the A fibres (pressure) the late EP is gone. It is replaced by an ultra-late vertex positivity. After lidocaine injection (experiment 1 only) the ultra-late EP is also wiped out. The bottom trace shows the recovery immediately after release of block. (left-hand part from Bromm and Treede, 1987).

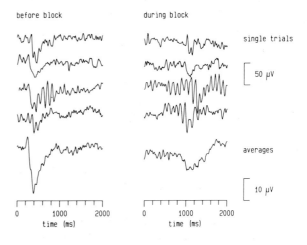

Fig. 2. Single-trial evoked responses from one subject. Late (before block) and ultra-late EPs (during pressure block) were selected for best signal-to-noise ratios. Vertex records, negativity up. The corresponding averages are given below. Note the enormous latency jitter of the ultra-late potentials in contrast to the relatively constant latency of the late potentials.

were surprisingly similar to their (earlier) 'late' counterparts. Their latencies were spread over a broad range, larger than the width of the individual potentials. Such latency jitter explains the smeared appearance in the conventional average.

Late and ultra-late evoked potentials after latency correction

To achieve a better average, the single trials should be adjusted according to their latency shifts. We chose an adaptive procedure, based on an iterative latency correction filter, where the template is continually modified according to the waveforms present in the single trials. Template length and maximum shift were chosen as 300 ± 150 ms for late and 600 ± 300 ms for ultra-late EPs. The latencies of the last iteration step were used to calculate a shifted time-varying filtered average per stimulus block.

Fig. 3 shows examples of latency-corrected averages from three subjects. As in the single trials, the late (left) and ultra-late waveforms (right) are rather similar. Subject W.M. who exhibited the largest negativity before block, had a large negativity during block as well. Subject S.S., whose EP before block was rather broad, also generated a broad ultra-late EP. Hence the similarity stated for single trials was also found for latency-corrected averages. The mean latency of the ultra-late vertex positivity after latency correction was 1252 ± 121 ms (Table I) and the mean intra-individual latency jitter 154 ± 23 ms. In addition, a small vertex negativity at 1049 ± 104 ms could be observed. The corresponding values for the latency-corrected late EPs are 243 ± 20 ms for the negativity and 371 ± 40 ms for the positivity with 55 ± 17 ms intra-individual jitter. In summary, the latencies of ultra-late EPs exhibit about 3-times-larger variability within and across subjects than the late EPs.

Scalp topography of late and ultra-late evoked potentials

The similarity of late and ultra-late potentials is also true with respect to the spatial distribution on the scalp. This is shown by multilead recordings (experiment 2). For each time point a potential map

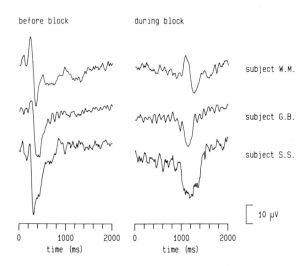

Fig. 3. Latency-corrected EPs in three subjects. Before block, late EP; during block, ultra-late EP. Negativity upwards. Note the striking similarity of late and ultra-late EP waveforms.

can be generated by interpolation between the measured electrode positions (Coppola et al., 1982). Fig. 4 shows the topography 400 ms after the stimulus (late EP) and 1200 ms after the stimulus (ultra-late EP during nerve block) from one subject. These time points correspond to the maxima of the positive components. The amplitude of the ultra-late potential is lower than for the late potential. The spatial distributions, however, are similar. Both potentials are maximal around the vertex and spread into the centro-parietal region.

Discussion

The single CO_2 laser pulse elicited two pain sensations with mean latencies of about 420 ms and 1300 ms. Correspondingly, two EP waveforms were observed: the late components N240/P370 and the ultra-late components N1050/P1250. The ultra-late EP was found after peripheral A-fibre block. Its shape was reproducible in two independent samples of healthy subjects. We interpret it to be a cerebral response to C-fibre activation, accomplished by the exclusion of conduction in all other fibres (Bromm et al., 1983; cf. Harkins et al., 1983).

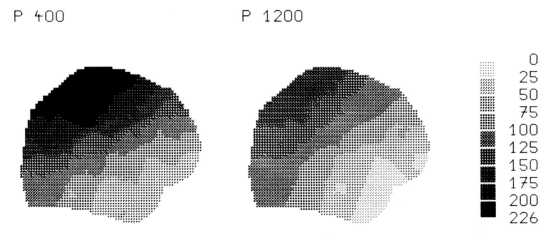

Fig. 4. Scalp topography of late (P400) and ultra-late evoked cerebral potentials (P1200). The spatial distributions were interpolated between data from 12 leads, measured from standard 10-20-system positions over the right hemisphere versus linked earlobes. Frontal regions are to the right. The grey scale indicates amplitudes in 1/10 μV for both maps. The maps indicate the distributions for the time points of maximal scalp positivity. Latency-corrected averages over 40 stimuli in one subject. (from Treede, 1987).

TABLE I
Evoked potentials after latency correction (from Bromm and Treede, 1987)

Subject	Late EP				Ultra-late EP			
	L_N (ms)	L_P (ms)	sL (ms)	δA (μV)	L_N (ms)	L_P (ms)	sL (ms)	δA (μV)
1	240	360	48	23.38	1050	1420	133	16.91
2	220	320	40	31.44	900	1090	166	9.85
3	230	350	40	34.61	1100	1280	121	18.61
4	260	380	46	23.66	1180	1330	125	6.55
5	220	350	43	24.13	1050	1250	175	11.41
6	280	410	64	27.60	1030	1180	178	21.25
7	260	360	76	17.87	1240	1410	147	13.34
8	240	450	91	12.05	960	1100	185	8.35
9	230	330	55	33.83	950	1320	144	8.95
10	250	400	47	22.75	1030	1140	163	11.98
Mean	243.0	371.0	55.0	25.13	1049.0	1252.0	154.0	12.72
SD	19.5	39.6	17.0	7.05	103.8	121.0	22.9	4.80
SD/mean	0.08	0.11	0.31	0.28	0.10	0.10	0.15	0.38

L_N, vertex negativity latency; L_p, vertex positivity latency;
sL, standard deviation of template shift;
δA, peak-to-peak amplitude difference.

Because of the enormous intra- and interindividual latency jitter of the ultra-late EP, conventional stimulus-locked averaging was found to distort its waveform. The observed latency jitter may in part arise peripherally; even a single C fibre does not conduct at a constant velocity upon repeated stimulation (Vallbo et al., 1979) and the afferent populations activated by consecutive stimuli may vary in mean conduction velocity. A considerable contribution of the central nervous system to the variability has to be assumed in addition. Even auditory evoked potentials, where the conduction distance is extremely short, exhibit a marked latency jitter (Michalewski et al., 1986). Lastly, the superposition of evoked potentials and EEG induces phase distortions, mimicking additional latency jitter. This factor alone, however, does not explain the amount of latency jitter of the late EP (McGillem et al., 1985), let alone that of the ultra-late EP.

The average ultra-late EP was rather similar to the average late EP, if the single trials were aligned in order to compensate for the latency jitter. Since convergence of myelinated and unmyelinated fibre input is known at all levels of the pain pathways, Aδ- and C-fibre input may trigger a common generator. This suggestion is confirmed by preliminary experiments examining the distribution of potentials on the scalp, which revealed a similar topography of late and ultra-late EP components. The large amplitude of the ultra-late EP makes it highly unlikely that it reflects the primary projection of C-fibre input, in the sense of early nearfield potentials. Instead, it should be considered, in analogy to the well-investigated late EPs, as an expression of cognitive processing of sensory input, now conducted by unmyelinated cutaneous afferents.

If similar cerebral mechanisms are involved in the generation of late and ultra-late EPs, the latter should also be subject to attention and distraction.

This explains why we usually do not see an ultra-late potential without A-fibre block, although the laser heat pulses activate C-fibres. When stimulating the upper limb the latency difference between first and second pain is relatively small and both sensations may apparently merge. An unexperienced observer directs his attention entirely to the first painful sensation and thus misses the second. Furthermore, since the stimuli are applied at randomized intervals, first pain always comes as a surprise, whereas second pain is announced by the first. EPs are smaller, if the subjects know the stimulus timing (Schafer et al., 1981). In this context the often described dependence of late vertex potentials on the interstimulus interval (ISI) becomes important, which leads to a considerable reduction in amplitude if the ISI is reduced to 1000 ms or less (Angel et al., 1985). With CO_2 laser double pulses of 900 ms ISI, we found a mean amplitude decrement of 42% for the second response (Bromm and Treede, 1987). All these factors render the C-fibre response without block smaller than with block, when C fibres conduct the only information about the stimulus.

In conclusion, EPs elicited by CO_2 laser radiant heat pulses promise to provide a non-invasive means of studying cutaneous Aδ – and C-fibre function. Whether this technique can successfully be applied to the examination of patients with dissociated sensory loss such as in syringomyelia or other affections of the central and peripheral nervous system is currently being evaluated (Zangemeister et al., 1987).

Acknowledgements

Supported by the Deutsche Forschungsgemeinschaft (SFB 115 and Schwerpunktprogramm 'Nociception und Schmerz').

References

Angel, R.W., Quick, W.M., Boylls, C.C., Weinrich, M. and Rodnitzky, R.L. (1985) Decrement of somatosensory evoked potentials during repetitive stimulation. Electroenceph. Clin. Neurophysiol., 60: 335–342.

Bromm, B. and Treede, R.D. (1983) CO_2 laser radiant heat pulses activate C nociceptors in man. Pflügers Archiv., 399: 155–156.

Bromm, B. and Treede, R.D. (1987) Human cerebral potentials evoked by CO_2 laser stimuli causing pain. Exp. Brain Res., 67: 153–162.

Bromm, B., Neitzel, H., Tecklenburg, A. and Treede, R.D. (1983) Evoked cerebral potential correlates of C fibre activity in man. Neurosci. Lett., 43: 109–114.

Bromm, B., Jahnke, M.T. and Treede, R.D. (1984) Responses of human cutaneous afferents to CO_2 laser stimuli causing pain. Exp. Brain Res., 55: 158–166.

Chudler, E.H. and Dong, W.K. (1983) The assessment of pain by cerebral evoked potentials. Pain, 16: 221–244.

Coppola, R., Buchsbaum, M.S. and Rigal, F. (1982) Computer generation of surface distribution maps of measures of brain activity. Comput. Biol. Med., 12: 191–199.

Devor, M., Carmon, A. and Frostig, R. (1982) Primary afferent and spinal sensory neurons that respond to brief pulses of intense infrared radiation: a preliminary survey in rats. Exp. Neurol., 76: 483–494.

Harkins, S.W., Price, D.D. and Katz, M.A. (1983) Are cerebral evoked potentials reliable indices of first or second pain? In J.J. Bonica (Ed.), Advances in Pain Research and Therapy, Vol. 5, Raven Press, New York, pp. 185–191.

Kenton, B., Coger, R., Crue, B., Pinsky, J., Friedman, Y. and Carmon, A. (1980) Peripheral fibre correlates to noxious thermal stimulation in humans. Neurosci. Lett., 17: 301–306.

McGillem, C.D., Aunon, J.I. and Yu K.B. (1985) Signals and noise in evoked brain potentials. IEEE Trans. Biomed. Engn., 32: 1012–1016.

Michalewski, H.J., Prasher, D.K. and Starr, A. (1986) Latency variability and temporal interrelationships of the auditory event-related potentials (N1, P2, N2, P3) in normal subjects. Electroenceph. Clin. Neurophysiol., 65: 59–71.

Schafer, E.W.P., Amochaev, A. and Russell, M.J. (1981) Knowledge of stimulus timing attenuates human evoked cortical potentials. Electroenceph. Clin. Neurophysiol., 52: 9–17.

Treede, R.D. (1987) C-Faser Aktivität und evozierte cerebrale Potentiale beim Menschen. In B. Bromm and H.P. Koepchen (Eds.), Physiologie aktuell, Vol. 3, Fischer, Stuttgart, pp. 167–175.

Vallbo, A.B., Hagbarth, K.E., Torebjörk, H.E. and Wallin, B.G. (1979) Somatosensory, proprioceptive, and sympathetic activity in human peripheral nerves. Physiol. Rev., 59: 919–957.

Zangemeister, W.H., Treede, R.D., Kunze, K. and Bromm, B. (1987) Painful dysaesthesias due to dissociated sensory loss: clinical and neurophysiological findings. Pain, Suppl. 4: S308.

Modulation of Nociception and Pain

R. Dubner, G.F. Gebhart & M.R. Bond (Eds.)
Proceedings of the Vth World Congress on Pain
© 1988 Elsevier Science Publishers BV (Biomedical Division)

CHAPTER 65

Peripheral conditioning stimulation produces differentially greater antinociceptive effect on noxious thermal response in the cat

J.M. Chung, K.S. Paik and S.C. Nam

Marine Biomedical Institute and Departments of Anatomy and Neurosciences and of Physiology and Biophysics, University of Texas Medical Branch, Galveston, TX 77550, USA

Summary

To see whether peripheral nerve conditioning stimulation produces an antinociceptive effect and to find the most sensitive method of detecting the effect, we applied conditioning stimulation to a peripheral nerve while observing the activity of dorsal horn cells and motor axons in the lumbar spinal cord in 16 decerebrate-spinal cats. The activity of spinal neurons was evoked by noxious and innocuous mechanical stimuli and by noxious thermal stimuli applied to the receptive fields. The peripheral conditioning stimulation was applied to the tibial nerve with repetitive electrical pulses (2 Hz) at an intensity suprathreshold for either $A\delta$ or C fibers for 5 min. Applying conditioning stimulation to a peripheral nerve produced a powerful inhibition of the responses elicited by noxious stimuli, suggesting that this inhibition is an antinociceptive effect. The inhibition produced by peripheral conditioning stimulation was differentially greater on the responses to noxious than to innocuous stimuli. It was further concluded that the most sensitive method to detect the antinociceptive effect is by way of recording the reflex activity in motor axons that is elicited by noxious thermal stimuli.

Introduction

Peripheral nerve conditioning stimulation has been widely used in clinical practice to relieve pain. Procedures involving peripheral nerve stimulation include transcutaneous electrical nerve stimulation and acupuncture. Although both procedures are effective in producing analgesia (Andersson et al., 1973; Chang, 1979; Long and Hagfors, 1975; Wall and Sweet, 1967), the reported effectiveness and methodology of application vary greatly between studies. The lack of a standard method of application and the inconsistency of the effects between studies are primarily due to a poor understanding of the mechanisms of analgesia produced by peripheral nerve conditioning stimulation.

In an attempt to study mechanisms of analgesia produced by peripheral nerve conditioning stimulation, we developed two experimental animal models (Chung et al., 1983, 1984) which are based primarily on the inhibitory effect of peripheral nerve conditioning stimulation on electrically evoked responses to peripheral nerve stimulation. Therefore, it is not

Correspondence: Jin Mo Chung, Ph.D., Marine Biomedical Institute, University of Texas Medical Branch, 200 University Boulevard, Galveston, TX 77550, U.S.A.

absolutely certain that the elicited responses are 'nociceptive responses' and that the effects produced by peripheral conditioning stimulation are 'antinociceptive'.

By observing the activity of spinal neurons evoked by natural forms of stimuli applied to the receptive fields, we attempted to: (1) see if conditioning stimulation of the peripheral nerve produced an antinociceptive effect; (2) test whether the inhibition produced is differentially greater for the responses to noxious than to innocuous stimuli; and (3) find the most sensitive method of detecting the antinociceptive effect produced by peripheral conditioning stimulation.

Methods

A total of 16 adult cats weighing 2.2–4.0 kg were decerebrated by sectioning the midbrain at the mid-collicular level under a gaseous anesthesia. Animals were ventilated artificially and immobilized with an intravenous injection of gallamine triethiodide. The end-tidal CO_2 concentration was monitored and maintained between 3.5 and 4.5% throughout the experiment. Rectal temperature was maintained near 37°C with a heating blanket. The spinal cord was transected at the T11 level after laminectomy. The common peroneal and tibial nerves were dissected free from surrounding connective tissue and placed on pairs of platinum bipolar electrodes for stimulation. Mineral oil pools were made around the exposed spinal cord and peripheral nerves to prevent drying, and the temperature of the pools was maintained by heating coils.

The activity of dorsal horn cells was recorded with carbon-filament-filled glass microelectrodes at the lumbosacral spinal cord level where the largest cord dorsum potential could be recorded by stimulation of the common peroneal nerve. Single-unit activity of motoneurons was recorded with a pair of platinum bipolar recording electrodes from a filament of rootlet dissected from the L7 or S1 ventral root. The recorded activity was amplified and fed into a window discriminator, the output of which

was used by a computer to compile peristimulus time histograms.

Activity of spinal neurons was evoked by applying mechanical and thermal stimuli to the skin within the receptive fields. As a form of innocuous stimulus, the skin was brushed repeatedly with a camel's hair brush. Noxious mechanical stimulation was delivered by applying a small arterial clip to a fold of skin (583 g/mm^2); this stimulus is felt as painful to humans. In addition, various intensities of noxious thermal pulses were applied to the skin for 15 s by a thermostimulator equipped with a contact thermode.

Conditioning stimuli delivered to the tibial nerve were square-wave electrical pulses at 2 Hz for 5 min. Cord dorsum potentials were recorded with a monopolar platinum ball electrode to determine the threshold (T) for activation of the largest A fibers. Threshold ranged from 20 to 40 and 10 to 20 μA with 0.1 and 0.5 ms pulses, respectively. To activate just A fibers (including Aδ fibers), the intensity was adjusted to 20 T with 0.1 ms pulses since the threshold for Aδ fibers ranged from about 3 to 5 T. For activation of both A and C fibers, 0.5 ms pulses at an intensity of 500–1000 T (usually 10 mA) were delivered since the threshold for C fibers was found to be about 200 T in previous studies (Kim et al., 1987; Shin et al., 1986).

Unit activity was evoked repeatedly with a test stimulus at 5 min intervals until the evoked responses were stable within 10% for three consecutive trials. The average of these three responses was used as the control response. Unit activity was evoked again with an identical stimulus just after application of 5 min of conditioning stimulation to the tibial nerve. The evoked activity was compared before and after conditioning stimulation. Statistical analyses were performed using Student's t test. Two-tailed P values less than 0.05 were considered significant.

Results

Recordings were made from a total of 20 dorsal

dynamic-range and 5 high-threshold cells. The responses of dorsal horn cells evoked by mechanical stimuli applied to the receptive field were inhibited by conditioning stimulation of a peripheral nerve. As shown in Fig. 1, a wide-dynamic-range cell responded to both brushing the skin and application of a small arterial clip (pinch) to the skin within the receptive field. The responses to brush and pinch were both reduced moderately after application of conditioning stimulation to the tibial nerve for 5 min (2 Hz) at an intensity suprathreshold for Aδ fibers. However, with higher-intensity conditioning stimulation (to include activation of C fibers), the response to pinch was almost abolished, whereas the response to brushing was only slightly inhibited. These data suggest that although conditioning stimulation of the peripheral nerve with a low intensity produced the same degree of mild inhibition of responses to both innocuous and noxious stimuli, stimulation with a higher strength to include C-fiber activation produced differentially greater inhibition of responses to noxious than to innocuous stimulation.

Peripheral nerve conditioning stimulation inhibited the responses of dorsal horn cells evoked not only by mechanical but also by thermal stimuli. Fig. 2 shows the effect of peripheral nerve conditioning stimulation on the responses of two dorsal horn cells evoked by thermal stimulation. The activity of these cells was evoked by application of noxious thermal pulses (15 s) applied to the skin within the receptive field with a contact thermode. After conditioning stimulation of the tibial nerve for 5 min (2 Hz) at an intensity suprathreshold for Aδ fibers, the evoked response decreased to less than half the control response. The activity decreased further after conditioning stimulation with a higher intensity (suprathreshold for C fibers).

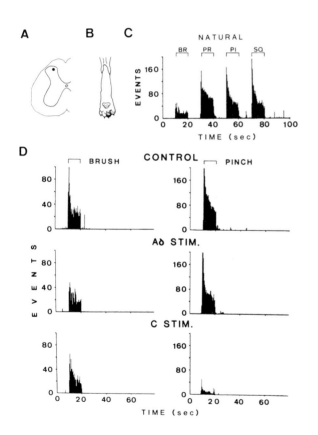

←

Fig. 1. Effect of peripheral conditioning stimulation on the activity of a dorsal horn cell evoked by mechanical stimuli. A: The location of the recording site in the dorsal horn. B: The location of the receptive field of the cell is indicated by the shaded area (the darkened area is the most sensitive spot). C: Single-pass peristimulus time histogram of the responses of the cell to graded mechanical stimuli. This cell responded to both innocuous and noxious mechanical stimuli applied to the receptive field. Innocuous tactile stimuli applied by repetitive brushing of the skin within the receptive field (BR) elicited sustained activity. The cell responded more vigorously to various degrees of noxious mechanical stimuli such as application of a large (PR) or a small (PI) arterial clip to a fold of skin, or squeezing the skin (SQ) with a pair of serrated forceps. In D, brush and pinch (application of a small arterial clip) stimuli were selected to represent innocuous and noxious mechanical stimuli, respectively. The responses of the cell to these stimuli were tested for the effect of conditioning stimulation of a peripheral nerve. Stimulation of the tibial nerve at an intensity suprathreshold for Aδ fibers for 5 min (2 Hz) reduced the responses to brush and pinch stimuli to 74.6 and 83.6% of prestimulus control, respectively. The stimulation was repeated at a higher intensity (suprathreshold for C fibers) and the response to brush was inhibited to a level similar to that with a lower intensity (75.6%). However, conditioning stimulation with a high intensity produced a much more powerful inhibition of the response to a pinch stimulus (10.9%). All records in C and D are single-pass peristimulus time histograms with bin widths set at 400 ms. (Reproduced from Paik et al., 1987.)

Unlike dorsal horn cells, sustained reflex activity in a ventral root filament usually required intense mechanical or thermal stimuli, making it difficult to test for effects on responses evoked by innocuous stimuli. Fig. 3 shows an example of the reflex activity of a motor axon elicited by natural forms of stimulus and its modification by peripheral conditioning stimulation. The reflex activity of this motor axon was elicited by applying strong mechanical stimuli (Fig. 3B) to a small area of the skin on the central pad of the foot (Fig. 3A). The responses eli-

cited by both intense mechanical and thermal stimuli were markedly reduced by conditioning stimuli suprathreshold for Aδ fibers applied to the tibial

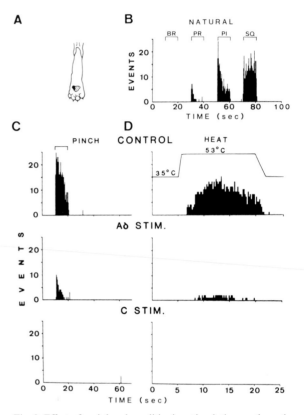

Fig. 3. Effect of peripheral conditioning stimulation on the activity of a motor axon evoked by noxious stimuli. The activity of a motor axon was recorded from a filament of the L7 ventral root and evoked by various stimuli applied to the receptive field (shown in A as a shaded area; the darkened area is the most sensitive spot). B: Unit activity could only be elicited with noxious stimuli, such as applying a small arterial clip to a fold of the skin (PI) or squeezing the skin with a pair of serrated forceps (SQ). Weaker stimuli such as brushing the skin (BR) or application of a large arterial clip to a fold of the skin (PR) did not elicit a sustained response. C: The response elicited by noxious mechanical stimuli was decreased to 19.1% of the control after conditioning stimulation of the tibial nerve for 5 min (2 Hz) at Aδ strength. Stimulation at C-fiber strength completely abolished the response. D: the activity evoked by noxious heat stimuli (53°C) was reduced to 9.0% after conditioning stimulation of the tibial nerve at Aδ-fiber strength and abolished after stimulation at C strength. All records in B, C and D are single-pass peristimulus time histograms. Bin widths in B and C are set at 400 ms, and in D at 200 ms. (Reproduced from Paik et al., 1987.)

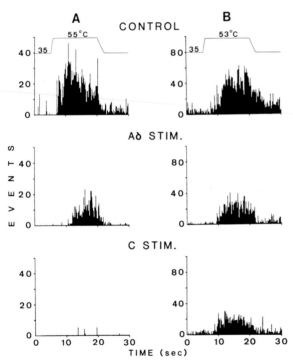

Fig. 2. Effect of peripheral conditioning stimulation on the activity of dorsal horn cells evoked by noxious thermal stimuli. A and B are the results obtained from two different cells. The temperature of the skin within the receptive field was adapted at 35°C with a contact thermode and the response was elicited by applying a 15-s-long heat pulse of 55 or 53°C (for A or B) as shown by the temperature tracings at the top. After application of conditioning stimulation to the tibial nerve for 5 min (2 Hz) at Aδ strength, the evoked responses decreased to 33.2 and 44.8% of the control values in A and B, respectively. The evoked responses after conditioning stimulation at C-fiber strength were 1.0 and 38.0% of the controls in A and B, respectively. All records were single-pass peristimulus time histograms with bin widths set at 200 ms. (Reproduced from Paik et al., 1987.)

nerve for 5 min. Increasing the intensity of conditioning stimulation to an intensity suprathreshold for C fibers completely abolished the responses.

Fig. 4 summarizes the effect of conditioning stimulation on the responses of all recorded dorsal horn cells and motor axons in this study. Four conclusions can be drawn from these results. First, conditioning stimulation at an intensity suprathreshold for C fibers is more effective in reducing the activity of spinal neurons than is a weaker stimulus which activates just A fibers. Second, nociceptive responses are inhibited more than innocuous responses, at least with strong conditioning stimulation. Third, the response elicited by noxious heat is very sensitive to peripheral conditioning stimulation, so that stimulation with an intensity suprathreshold for C fibers almost abolishes the response to noxious heat. Fourth, the reflex activity recorded in motor axons is more sensitive than the evoked activity of dorsal horn cells for demonstrating antinociceptive effects.

Discussion

There was greater inhibition of the activity of dorsal horn cells evoked by noxious stimuli than that evoked by innocuous stimuli. Following electroacupuncture in the cat, Pomeranz and Cheng (1979) observed a selective reduction of nociceptive responses of dorsal horn cells. Responses to innocuous stimuli were unaffected. Although the results of the present study are similar to those of Pomeranz and Cheng (1979) in terms of a differentially greater inhibition of nociceptive responses by peripheral stimulation, there are some differences. The two most important differences are: (1) the magnitude of inhibition was much greater in the present experiment in that we have commonly observed reduction in activity of 50% or more, as opposed to their observation of reductions of 15% at most; and (2) the inhibition they observed was reversed by naloxone, developed slowly and lasted a long time, whereas the inhibition we studied is mainly a non-naloxone-reversible inhibition which developed

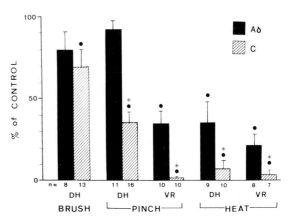

Fig. 4. Summary graph showing effect of peripheral conditioning stimulation on the activity of dorsal horn cells and motor axons evoked by mechanical and thermal stimuli in the spinal cat. Data are expressed as mean percent of the control value (bars indicate standard errors of means). Dots indicate values significantly different from the controls. Asterisks indicate values significantly different from those obtained after conditioning stimulation at Aδ strength. DH, dorsal horn cells; VR, ventral root motor axons. (Modified from Paik et al., 1987.)

quickly and lasted a short time (Chung et al., 1983, 1984; Lee et al., 1985). The differences between our results and those of Pomeranz and Cheng (1979) are likely due to the use of a different animal preparation and methods of peripheral stimulation. Because of the different procedures, it is possible that the results of the two studies are different in that Pomeranz and Cheng might have produced an effect comparable to acupuncture, while the present study produced an effect similar to transcutaneous electrical nerve stimulation.

Although the slowly developing, naloxone-reversible inhibition is interesting because it suggests an involvement of endogenous opioid mechanisms, it is very small in magnitude, making it difficult to differentiate from the baseline noise. On the other hand, the short-lasting, naloxone-resistant inhibition which is the focus of this study is attractive because it is powerful enough to abolish the response completely in many instances. The results of previous studies suggested that the most suitable preparation for the study of the powerful, non-naloxone-reversible antinociceptive effect is an unanesthetized, spinal preparation (Chung et al.,

horn cells. These included 5 low-threshold, 10 wide-
1983, 1984; Martin et al., 1964).

In summary, the present study demonstrated that a powerful antinociceptive effect mediated by spinal mechanisms was produced by conditioning stimulation of a peripheral nerve. Both A and C fibers in the peripheral nerve seem to contribute to the production of the antinociceptive effect. For testing of an antinociceptive effect, the activity evoked by noxious thermal stimuli is more sensitive than that evoked by noxious mechanical stimuli. Although a direct comparison may be difficult to make because the magnitudes of responses in dorsal horn cells and motoneurons produced by pinch and heat are different and the corresponding mechanisms may also differ, proportionally greater inhibition was observed in the reflex activity evoked by noxious stimuli in motor axons than in the activity recorded from dorsal horn cells. Therefore, the most sensitive method of detecting antinociceptive effects produced by conditioning stimulation of a peripheral nerve seems to be the recording of reflex activity of motoneurons elicited by noxious thermal stimuli. Perhaps because of this sensitivity, many successful antinociceptive effects have been demonstrated using the tail flick test (D'Amour and Smith, 1941; Irwin et al., 1951; Sandkühler and Gebhart, 1984; Yeung et al., 1977), a form of reflex motor activity elicited by noxious thermal stimuli.

Acknowledgements

This work was supported by National Institutes of Health grants NS21266, NS11255, and a Research Career Development Award NS00995. We thank Heidi Freeborn for the artwork and photography.

References

Andersson, S.A., Ericson, T., Holmgren, E. and Lindqvist, G. (1973) Electroacupuncture. Effect on pain threshold measured with electrical stimulation of teeth. Brain Res., 63: 393–396.

Chang, H. (1979) Acupuncture analgesia today. Chin. Med. J., 92: 7–16.

Chung, J.M., Fang, Z.R., Cargill, C.L. and Willis, W.D. (1983) Prolonged, naloxone-reversible inhibition of the flexion reflex in the cat. Pain, 15: 35–53.

Chung, J.M., Fang, Z.R., Hori, Y., Lee, K.H. and Willis, W.D. (1984) Prolonged inhibition of primate spinothalamic tract cells by peripheral nerve stimulation. Pain, 19: 259–275.

D'Amour, F.E. and Smith, D.L. (1941) A method for determining loss of pain sensation. J. Pharmacol. Exp. Ther., 72: 74–79.

Irwin, S., Houde, R.W., Bennett, D.R., Hendershot, L.C. and Seevers, M.H. (1951) The effects of morphine, methadone and meperidine on some reflex responses of spinal animals to nociceptive stimulation. J. Pharmacol. Exp. Ther., 101: 132–143.

Kim, J., Shin, H.K., Nam, S.C. and Chung, J.M. (1987) Proportion and location of spinal neurons receiving ventral root afferent inputs in the cat. Exp. Neurol., in press.

Lee, K.H., Chung, J.M. and Willis, W.D. (1985) Inhibition of primate spinothalamic tract cells by TENS. J. Neurosurg., 62: 276–287.

Long, D.M. and Hagfors, N. (1975) Electrical stimulation in the nervous system: the current status of electrical stimulation of the nervous system for relief of pain. Pain, 1: 109–123.

Martin, W.R., Eades, C.G., Fraser, H.F. and Wikler, A. (1964) Use of hindlimb reflexes of the chronic spinal dog for comparing analgesics. J. Pharmacol. Exp. Ther., 144: 8–11.

Paik, K.S., Nam, S.C. and Chung, J.M. (1987) Differential inhibition produced by peripheral conditioning stimulation on noxious mechanical and thermal responses of different classes of spinal neurons in the cat. Exp. Neurol., in press.

Pomeranz, B. and Cheng, R. (1979) Suppression of noxious responses in single neurons of cat spinal cord by electroacupuncture and its reversal by the opiate antagonist naloxone. Exp. Neurol., 64: 327–341.

Sandkühler, J. and Gebhart, G.F. (1984) Characterization of inhibition of a spinal nociceptive reflex by stimulation medially and laterally in the midbrain and medulla in the pentobarbital-anesthetized rat. Brain Res., 305: 67–76.

Shin, H.K., Kim, J. and Chung, J.M. (1986) Inhibition and excitation of the nociceptive flexion reflex by conditioning stimulation of a peripheral nerve in the cat. Exp. Neurol., 92: 335–348.

Wall, P.D. and Sweet, W.H. (1967) Temporary abolition of pain in man. Science, 155: 108–109.

Yeung, J.C., Yaksh, T.L. and Rudy, T.A. (1977) Concurrent mapping of brain sites for sensitivity to the direct application of morphine and focal electrical stimulation in the production of antinociception in the rat. Pain, 4: 23–40.

R. Dubner, G.F. Gebhart & M.R. Bond (Eds.)
Proceedings of the Vth World Congress on Pain
© 1988 Elsevier Science Publishers BV (Biomedical Division)

CHAPTER 66

Is modulation of the stimulus a way to increase the efficacy of conventional TENS? An experimental study

Ulla Ekström and Bengt H. Sjölund*.

Medical Board of the Armed Forces, Karolinen, S-651 80 Karlstad, Sweden

Summary

Transcutaneous electrical nerve stimulation (TENS) is a well-established technique for the alleviation of chronic pain. The stimulation parameters used are based on subjective reports from patients. Recently, it has been claimed that frequency or intensity modulation of the stimulus may give better analgesia than stimulation at constant parameters. In the present study, a systematic investigation has been performed with modulated conditioning stimulation of different parameters of a dissected skin nerve in the lightly anesthetized rat, utilizing the size of a C-fibre-evoked flexion reflex as a measure of transmission from nociceptive afferent fibers in the spinal cord. Frequency modulation did not produce better suppression of the nocifensive reflex than stimulation at a fixed frequency. Intensity modulation did not produce any suppression at all. The implications for clinical treatment are discussed.

Introduction

Transcutaneous electrical nerve stimulation (TENS) is now widely used for the alleviation of

chronic pain. (Wall and Sweet, 1967; Loeser et al., 1975; Long, 1976; Sjölund and Eriksson, 1980; Eriksson et al., 1984). With the original technique (conventional TENS), mainly superficial nerve fibers are stimulated at 10–120 Hz at an intensity evoking a tingling sensation in the painful region. It has been hypothesized that this stimulation closes a 'gate' to the nociceptive information entering the human spinal cord (Melzack and Wall, 1965). It is known that various afferent nerves can mutually inhibit each other at the presynaptic level (Schmidt, 1971). It may therefore be that such mechanisms are at least partly responsible for the effects observed; however, the optimal parameters for producing presynaptic and other forms of long-standing inhibition of afferent impulse in man are not well defined. Only subjective reports of what feels 'pleasant' or is preferred by small numbers of patients undergoing TENS have been published (Picaza et al., 1975; Linzer and Long, 1976).

In a previous study (Sjölund, 1985), a systematic experimental investigation was undertaken of the most suitable parameters for conditioning stimulation of a skin nerve to elicit maximal suppression of a C-fibre-evoked flexion reflex in a nearby spinal segment. The present study was performed with the same technique to examine the claim that frequency or intensity modulation of the TENS stimuli would be more effective than stimulation with constant parameters in suppressing nociception.

---

*Present and correspondence address: The Pain Clinic, Department of Anesthesiology, Malmö General Hospital, S-21401 Malmö, Sweden.

Methods

151 Wistar rats, weighing 250–300 g each, were used for the present study. The method of preparation has been described elsewhere (Schouenborg and Sjölund, 1983). Briefly, the rats were anesthetized with 1–1.5% halothane in a moistened nitrous oxide/oxygen mixture (2:1). A tracheostomy was

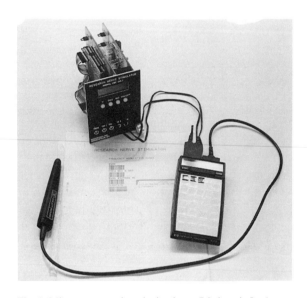

Fig. 1. Microprocessor-based stimulator (Medtronic Inc.), programmable with bar codes via wand, and Hewlett Packard 41 C calculator, customized to fit Neurolog^R constant-current output stage and power supply.

made, and one external jugular vein and one carotid artery were cannulated. In one hindlimb, the plantar and sural nerves were dissected for stimulation and the common peroneal and sciatic nerves were exposed for flexion reflex and nerve volley recordings, respectively.

During nerve measurements the animals were paralysed with gallamine and artificially ventilated. The halothane concentration was lowered to 0.4%, still allowing stable anesthesia with constricted pupils and no blood pressure variations or spontaneous motor nerve discharges. Blood pressure, end-expiratory CO_2 concentration and rectal temperature were monitored continuously and kept at 120–140 mmHg, 3.5–4%, and 37–38.5°C, respectively.

The test reflex discharges were elicited by stimulation with 5 shocks at a stimulus amplitude of 100-times nerve threshold (see below) at 10–ms intervals and were recorded bipolarly as neurograms. They were rectified, integrated (time constant 20 ms) and displayed on a storage oscilloscope for photographic recording. Usually five sweeps were superimposed at 1 Hz stimulation frequency. The maximal amplitude in the interval 100–500 ms was used as an index of size of C-fibre-evoked activity in the flexor motoneurones. The strength used for stimulation was expressed as multiples of that just giving a barely visible nerve volley in the sciatic nerve (Eccles and Lundberg, 1959). The stimulation pulses were monophasic square waves of 150 μs duration.

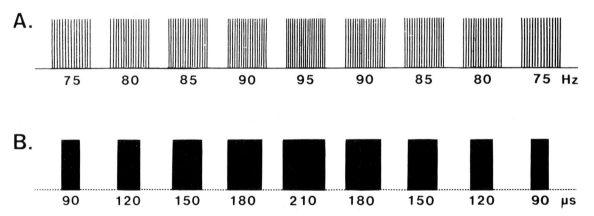

Fig. 2. Modulation modes employed. A, frequency modulation 75–95 Hz. B, intensity (pulse duration) modulation 90–210 μs. Periods of modulation 2, 6 or 15 s (continuous).

Preparations where the dissected nerves had a threshold of more than 20 μA were discarded.

Modulation of the stimuli was achieved by using a specially designed stimulus generator (Fig. 1; Medtronic Inc.), based on a microprocessor. The unit could be programmed in code form, utilizing a Hewlett Packard 41C calculator with a wand and bar codes. Further, it was customized to drive a Neurolog[R] pulse buffer and constant-current output stage for stimulation of the nerves.

Two modulation modes were used in the study. With frequency modulation, variations around a centre frequency of 85 Hz (cf. Sjölund, 1985) of ± 10 Hz and ± 20 Hz were employed, each in 2, 6 or 15 s periods (Fig. 2A). The stimulus duration was then constant at 150 μs. With intensity modulation, a centre impulse duration of 150 μs was used with variations of ± 60 μs and ± 90 μs, similarly in 2, 6 or 15 s periods (Fig. 2B). The simulus frequency was here kept constant at 85 Hz.

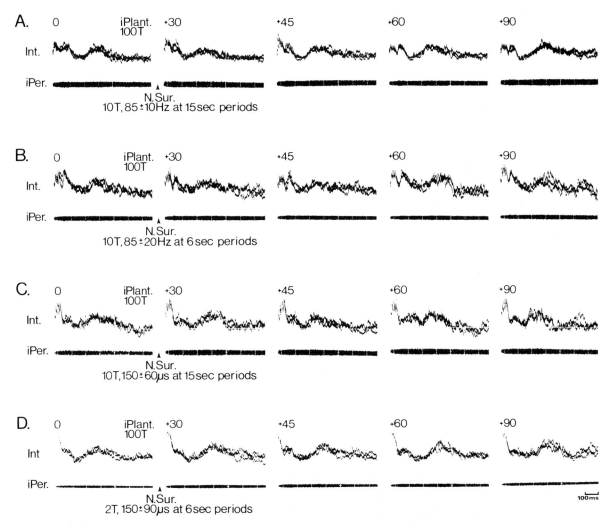

Fig. 3. Sample records from four different experiments. A and B, frequency modulation as indicated. C and D, intensity modulation as indicated. iPlant 100T, test stimulation of ipsilateral plantar nerve at 100-times nerve threshold evoking flexion reflex in ipsilateral peroneal (iPer) nerve, integrated in upper traces (Int). nSur, conditioning modulated stimulation for 30 min of ipsilateral sural nerve. Digits in upper left corners give time in minutes. Sweep calibration in lower right corner for all records.

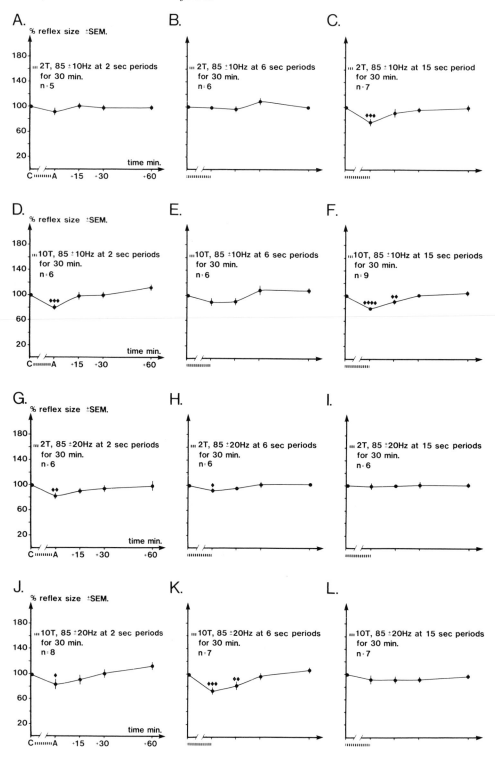

Student's t-test. ♦♦♦♦ p<0,0005 ♦♦♦ p<0,005 ♦♦ p<0,025 ♦ p<0,05

Fig. 4. Summary of results of frequency modulation at ±10 Hz (A–F) and ±20 Hz (G–L). *n*, number of experiments (and animals). C, control, normalized to 100%; all integrated reflex sizes are expressed in percent thereof. A, reflex size after 30 min of modulated conditioning stimulation.

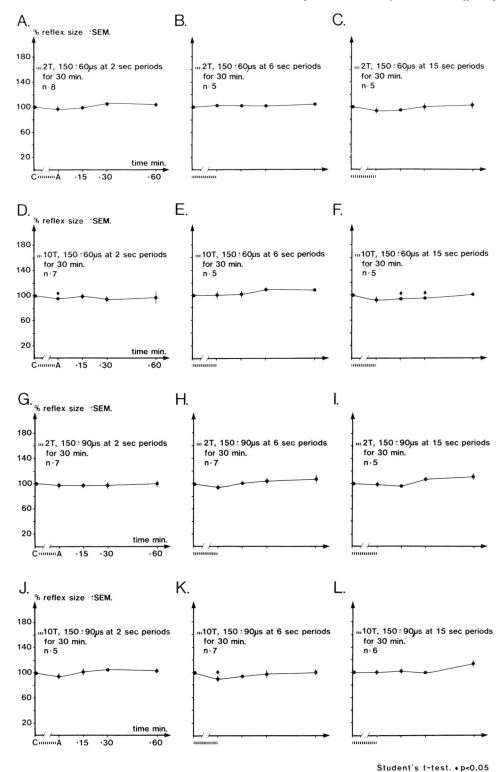

Student's t-test. ◆p<0,05

Fig. 5. As Fig. 4 but after intensity modulation at $\pm 60\ \mu s$ (A–F) and $\pm 90\ \mu s$ (G–L).

Results

As can be seen in Fig. 3 A–D (left traces), a long-latency discharge is evoked at a stimulation strength recruiting C fibres (upper integrated sweeps, Int). This discharge has properties similar to those of a subgroup of class two neurones in the dorsal horn (Menétrey et al., 1977; Schouenborg and Sjölund, 1983) and is very sensitive to morphine in the cat (Koll et al., 1963).

Samples from four typical experiments are illustrated in Fig. 3. In all experiments, the ipsilateral plantar nerve was stimulated at 100-times T (threshold) at the intervals given (min) in upper left corners. Between 0 and +30 min, the ipsilateral sural nerve was stimulated at the frequencies, impulse durations and amplitudes (expressed in multiples of the nerve thresholds) given. It can be seen that after conditioning stimulation with frequency modulation there is a transient decrease of the C-fibre-evoked discharge, returning to control levels 30 min after the end of the conditioning stimulation (A–B). With modulation of intensity (pulse duration) of the conditioning stimulation almost no changes were seen (C–D).

In Figs. 4 and 5 summaries are given of the results from all the rats at the two modulation modes, each at three period lengths and at stimulation amplitudes recruiting A beta fibres only (2 T) or A beta fibres and some A delta fibres (10 T; Lloyd, 1943). Each combination was tested in at least five rats and after normalization to 100% of reflex control values (stable and measured at least twice with an interval of 15 min) the mean size of the integrated reflex size is given at times indicated. It can be seen that a significant depression of the reflex discharge is seen only in the frequency modulation experiments (Fig. 4) and there mainly with the higher stimulus intensity (10 T; D, F, J, K). Modulation

of stimulus duration, on the other hand, gives practically no depression at all (Fig. 5).

Discussion

Firstly, the present results confirm that a C-fibre-evoked flexion reflex in the rat may be susceptible to a long-lasting (30 min) conditioning stimulation of afferents in an ipsilateral cutaneous nerve, adjacent to that used for eliciting the reflex (Sjölund and Eriksson, 1979; Cervero et al., 1981; Chung et al., 1983; Sjölund, 1985, 1987).

However, our study shows that a modulation of the stimulus, whether of its frequency or of its intensity (duration), does not give a more efficient suppression of the transmission of nociceptive stimuli than stimulation at constant parameters (Sjölund, 1985). In fact, stimulation at constant stimulus duration and frequency produced more effective depression (down to 55% of control; Sjölund, 1985) than in the present study.

The depression of the C-fibre-evoked flexion reflex in this mammal by long-lasting conditioning stimulation of skin afferents in a nerve adjacent to that used to elicit the reflex may well be related to the pain relief in man after TENS. If so, the present results do not favour modulation modes for TENS, especially not of stimulus intensity (duration). On the other hand, a modulation of the stimulus frequency might possibly be more readily accepted by some patients, allowing a more consistent use of the TENS treatment.

Acknowledgements

This study was supported by grants from Medtronic Inc., Minneapolis, MN, and from the Swedish Medical Research Council (No. 05658).

References

Cervero, F., Schouenborg, J. and Sjölund, B. (1981) Effects of conditioning stimulation of somatic and visceral afferent

fibres on viscero-somatic and somato-somatic reflexes. J. Physiol., 317: 84 P.

Chung, J.M., Fang, Z.R., Cargill, C.L. and Willis, W.D. (1983) Prolonged naloxone-reversible inhibition of the flexion reflex in the cat. Pain, 15: 35–53.

Eccles, R.M. and Lundberg, A. (1959) Synaptic actions in moto-neurones by afferents which may evoke the flexion reflex. Arch. Ital. Biol. 97: 199–220.

Eriksson, M., Sjölund, B. and Sundbärg, G. (1984) Pain relief from peripheral conditioning stimulation in patients with intractable facial pain. J. Neurosurg., 61: 149–155.

Koll, W., Haase, J., Block, G. and Muhlberg, B. (1963) The predilective action of small doses of morphine on nociceptive spinal reflexes on low spinal cats. Int. J. Pharmacol., 2: 57–65.

Linzer, M. and Long, D.M. (1976) Transcutaneous neural stimulation for relief of pain. IEEE Trans. Biomed. Eng., 23: 341–345.

Lloyd, D.P.C. (1943) Reflex action in relation to the pattern and peripheral source of afferent stimulation. J. Neurophysiol., 6: 111–119.

Loeser, J.D., Black, R.G. and Christman, A. (1975) Relief of pain by transcutaneous stimulation. J. Neurosurg., 42: 308–314.

Long, D.M. (1976) Cutaneous afferent stimulation for relief of pain. Progr. Neurol. Surg., 7: 35–51.

Melzack, R. and Wall, P.D. (1965) Pain mechanisms: a new theory. Science, 150: 971–979.

Menetrey, D., Giesler, Jr., G.J. and Besson, J.-M. (1977) Analysis of response properties of spinal cord dorsal horn neurones to nonnoxious and noxious stimuli in the spinal rat. Exp. Brain Res., 27: 15–33.

Picaza, J.A., Cannon, B.W., Hunter, S.E., Boyd, A.S., Guma, J. and Maurer, D. (1975) Pain suppression by peripheral nerve stimulation. Surg. Neurol., 4: 105–114.

Schmidt, R.F. (1971) Presynaptic inhibition in the vertebrate central nervous system. Ergebn. Physiol., 63: 20–101.

Schouenborg, J. and Sjölund, B.H. (1983) Activity evoked by A- and C-afferent fibers in rat dorsal horn neurones and its relation to a flexion reflex. J. Neurophysiol., 50: 1108–1121.

Sjölund, B.H. and Eriksson, M.B.E. (1979) Naloxone-reversible depression of C-fiber evoked flexion reflex in low spinal cats after conditioning electrical stimulation of primary afferents. Neurosci. Lett. Suppl., 3: 264.

Sjölund, B.H. and Eriksson, M.B.E. (1980) Stimulation techniques in the management of pain. In H. Kosterlitz, and L. Terenius (Eds.), Pain and Society, Verlag Chemie GmbH, Weinheim pp. 415–430.

Sjölund, B.H. (1985) Peripheral nerve stimulation suppression of C-fiber-evoked flexion reflex in rats: Part 1: Parameters of continuous stimulation. J. Neurosurg., 63: 612–616.

Sjölund, B.H. (1988) Peripheral nerve stimulation suppression of C-fibre evoked flexion reflex in rats. Part II: Parameters of low rate train stimulation of skin and muscle afferents. J. Neurosurg., in press.

Wall, P.D. and Sweet, W.H. (1967) Temporary abolition of pain in man. Science, 155: 108–109.

R. Dubner, G.F. Gebhart & M.R. Bond (Eds.)
Proceedings of the Vth World Congress on Pain
© 1988 Elsevier Science Publishers BV (Biomedical Division)

CHAPTER 67

Opposing actions of norepinephrine and clonidine on single pain-modulating neurons in rostral ventromedial medulla

M.M. Heinricher, C.M. Haws and H.L. Fields

University of California at San Francisco, Departments of Neurology and Physiology, San Francisco, CA, USA

Summary

On- and off-cells are putative nociceptive modulating neurons in the rat rostral ventromedial medulla. Using single unit recording and iontophoretic techniques, we examined the responses of these cells to norepinephrine and the selective alpha-2 receptor agonist clonidine. On-cells, but not off-cells, are responsive to these substances. Iontophoretically applied norepinephrine facilitates, while clonidine suppresses, on-cell activity. These observations are consistent with an important facilitatory effect of on-cells on nociceptive transmission at the level of the spinal cord.

Introduction

The rostral ventromedial medulla (RVM), a region that includes the nucleus raphe magnus and adjacent reticular formation, has been implicated in a descending nociceptive modulating system which projects to the spinal cord via the dorsolateral funiculus. Fields et al. (1983a) have characterized two classes of neurons in the RVM of the lightly anesthetized rat that show changes in firing rate closely correlated with the occurrence of the tail flick response (TF), a nocifensive reflex evoked by application of noxious heat to the tail. Cells of one class, on-cells, accelerate and cells of the second class, off-cells, pause just prior to the TF. Cells of a third class, neutral cells, show no change in activity at the time of the TF.

Drugs that produce behavioral antinociception consistently affect the activity of on-cells and off-cells in RVM. Spontaneous discharge and the TF-related burst of on-cells are suppressed, while off-cells show an increase in spontaneous activity and blockade of the TF-related pause. Neutral cells are unaffected by such manipulations. Thus, systemic administration of morphine (Fields et al., 1983b; Barbaro et al., 1986) and microinjection of morphine (Cheng et al., 1986) or GABA receptor antagonists (Moreau and Fields, 1986) in the PAG all suppress TF-related changes in activity while inhibiting on-cells and exciting off-cells. This suggests a role for both classes of cells in nociceptive modulation.

The neural inputs controlling the activity of these putative nociceptive modulating neurons in RVM are not known. There is evidence that noradrenergic inputs contribute to control of nociception by an action on RVM neurons. The RVM receives a noradrenergic input (Fuxe, 1965; Hammond et al.,

Correspondence: Mary M. Heinricher, Ph.D., University of California at San Francisco, Department of Neurology S-784, San Francisco, CA 94143, USA.

1980), and microinjection of agents acting at noradrenergic receptors alters nociceptive responsiveness (Hammond et al., 1980; Sagen and Proudfit, 1985). Thus, local application of the alpha-2 receptor agonist clonidine produces an increase in TF latency, whereas microinjection of the alpha-1 receptor agonist phenylephrine produces hyperalgesia. The present experiments examine the role of noradrenaline in controlling the activity of the proposed nociceptive modulating neurons in the RVM. We used extracellular single unit recording and iontophoretic techniques to investigate the effects of norepinephrine and clonidine on the activity of on-, off- and neutral cells in the RVM.

Methods

Male Sprague-Dawley rats (250–300 g) were initially anesthetized with pentobarbital (60 mg/kg, i.p.) and a catheter was inserted into an external jugular vein. The animals were then placed in a stereotaxic apparatus, a small craniectomy performed and the underlying dura removed. Following surgery, the animals were allowed to recover from the initial anesthetic until a TF could be elicited. They were then maintained in a lightly anesthetized state by a continuous infusion of methohexital at a rate (15–30 mg/kg/h, i.v.) that allowed a stable TF latency and was sufficient to prevent signs of discomfort.

Five-barrel glass micropipettes, each barrel with an integral fiber to aid filling, were broken back to an overall tip diameter of 4–5 μm. A 3 M NaCl solution was used to fill the central recording barrel and one of the outer barrels for automatic current compensation. Each of the three remaining barrels was filled with one of the following solutions: norepinephrine hydrochloride (NE, 0.2 M, pH 4.4–4.7), clonidine hydrochloride (CLON, 0.1 M, pH 4.4–4.7), yohimbine hydrochloride (YOH, 0.01 M, pH 4.1–4.7) or prazosin hydrochloride (PRAZ, 0.01 M, pH 4.1–4.4). Drugs were dissolved in distilled water and the pH adjusted appropriately by the addition of 0.1 M HCl. Fresh solutions were prepared at the beginning of each experiment. Positive currents of 5–20 nA were generally used for drug ejection and negative retaining currents of 10–15 nA were applied to each solution between ejection periods to minimize spontaneous leakage of active substances from the electrode.

RVM neurons were isolated and classified as on-, off- or neutral cells according to the system of Fields et al. (1983a). The characterized cell was then tested for responses to iontophoretic application of NE (generally 10–20 nA, 1–2 min pulses) or the alpha-2 receptor agonist CLON (5–20 nA, 3–5 min

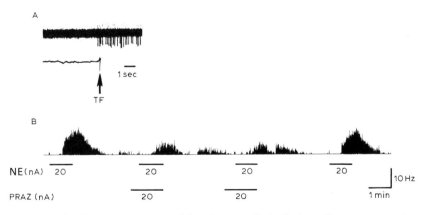

Fig. 1. NE facilitates spontaneous activity of an on-cell. A. Single oscilloscope sweep shows typical on-cell burst (upper trace) just preceding the TF (lower trace). Tail heating starts at the beginning of the trace; sweep length is 10 s. B. Rate-meter record showing facilitation of on-cell discharge by NE applied for 1 min. This effect was greatly attenuated by application of PRAZ beginning 30 s prior to NE.

pulses). In some experiments, the effectiveness of PRAZ and/or YOH (10–20 nA) in blocking agonist-induced changes in firing rate were tested.

The TF was evoked using a projector lamp focused on the blackened ventral surface of tail. A thermistor probe placed in contact with the tail surface provided a signal for feedback control of the heat stimulus.

Recording sites were marked by deposition of Pontamine Sky Blue dye.

Results

Iontophoretic application of NE produced a dose-related facilitation of on-cell activity (Fig. 1). Effects were relatively rapid in onset (25–45 s from beginning of ejection) and typically outlasted the period of drug application by 60–90 s. The activation produced by NE could be reversed by iontophoretic application of the alpha-1 receptor antagonist PRAZ, but not the alpha-2 receptor antagonist YOH. The effects of NE were not mimicked by equivalent current or pH controls.

In contrast with its facilitation of on-cell discharge, iontophoretic application of NE failed to affect off-cell (Fig. 2) or neutral cell activity.

Iontophoretic application of clonidine con-

sistently produced a long-lasting inhibition of on-cell discharge. The effect was quite slow in onset, with a gradual decrease in firing rate beginning 2–3 min after CLON ejection was begun. Full recovery of spontaneous activity was prolonged, requiring anywhere from 15 to 30 min. The inhibitory effects of CLON were greatly attenuated by iontophoresis of YOH (Fig. 3).

Like NE, CLON had no effect on the activity of off-cells or neutral cells.

Discussion

These observations demonstrate that iontophoretically applied norepinephrine and clonidine selectively modify the activity of only one RVM cell class, on-cells, and have little or no effect on either off-cells or neutral cells. On-cells were excited by norepinephrine, and this facilitatory effect was reversed by the selective alpha-1 receptor antagonist, prazosin, but not by the alpha-2 receptor antagonist, yohimbine. This suggests that the excitation is mediated by activation of alpha-1 adrenergic receptors. On-cells were inhibited by iontophoresis of the selective alpha-2 receptor agonist, clonidine, an effect that could be attenuated by the alpha-2 receptor antagonist, yohimbine. This result provides evi-

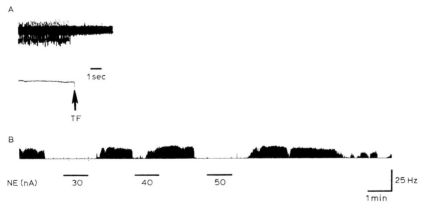

Fig. 2. NE has no effect on the spontaneous activity of an off-cell. A. Single oscilloscope sweep showing off-cell pause, which occurs approximately 500 ms before the tail-flick (lower trace). B. Rate-meter record showing that NE applied for 1 min has no effect on the spontaneous activity of an off-cell, even when high currents were used.

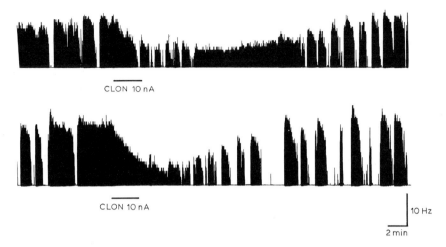

CLON 10 nA

CLON 10 nA

10 Hz

2 min

Fig. 3. Clonidine-induced inhibition of spontaneous on-cell activity. Rate-meter record shows the reproducible supression of spontaneous activity of an on-cell by clonidine (10 nA) applied over a period of 3 min. The effect is slow in onset (approximately 1 min after the onset of clonidine application) and recovery is seen approximately 20 min after drug application.

dence that the receptor mediating the suppressive effect is of the alpha-2 subtype. Thus, alpha-1 and alpha-2 adrenergic receptors mediate opposing actions on this class of RVM neurons.

In the awake rat, microinjection of an alpha-1 receptor agonist into the RVM reduces, whereas administration of an alpha-2 receptor agonist prolongs, TF latency (Sagen and Proudfit, 1985). Previous explanations of these observations focused on the possibility that NE depresses the activity of inhibitory output neurons in the RVM through a post-synaptic action at the alpha-1 receptor. Clonidine was postulated to act at presynaptic alpha-2 receptors to block release of NE. However, both excitatory and inhibitory effects of iontophoretically applied norepinephrine in RVM have been reported (Behbehani et al., 1981; Wessendorf and Anderson, 1981; Willcockson et al., 1983), making this proposal unlikely. Our data suggest that the opposing behavioral effects of microinjected alpha-1 and alpha-2 receptor agonists may be explained by their opposing actions on one physiologically identified class of RVM neurons, on-cells.

There is a good deal of evidence indicating that the off-cell is the RVM neuron that inhibits nociceptive transmission at spinal levels (Fields and Heinricher, 1985). The function of the on-cell is less

clear, particularly if one assumes that the RVM has only an inhibitory influence on nociceptive transmission. The fact that on-cells show an abrupt increase in firing beginning just prior to the TF makes it unlikely that cells of this class have a significant inhibitory effect on the reflex. Moreover, on-cell activity is completely suppressed following administration of morphine in doses sufficient to inhibit the TF (Barbaro et al., 1986; Cheng et al., 1986). These properties are, in fact, consistent with a facilitatory role for the on-cell. The data presented here support this proposal. On-cell enhancement of spinal nociceptive transmission could be due to an indirect effect mediated predominantly at the level of the RVM (i.e., the on-cell could modify off-cell activity). It would also be possible for on-cells to exert a direct facilitatory action, as on-cells are known to project to the spinal cord (Vanegas et al., 1984).

In summary, we have shown that on-cells, but not off-cells or neutral cells, are responsive to iontophoretically applied alpha-1 and alpha-2 adrenergic receptor agonists. These observations are consistent with an important facilitatory modulating effect of on-cells at the level of the spinal cord, and would imply that RVM neurons exert a bidirectional, rather than purely inhibitory control over nociceptive transmission.

Acknowledgements

We wish to thank Pat Littlefield for histology and Annette Lowe for artwork. This work was supported by PHS grants DA 01949 and NS21445, and a grant from the Migraine Foundation. MMH was supported by NIH fellowship NS07442.

References

Barbaro, N., Fields, H.L. and Heinricher, M.M. (1986) Putative pain modulating neurons in the rostral ventral medulla: reflex-related activity predicts effects of morphine. Brain Res., 366:203–210.

Behbehani, M.M., Pomeroy, S.L. and Mack, C.E. (1981) Interaction between central gray and nucleus raphe magnus: role of norepinephrine. Brain Res. Bull., 6:361–364.

Cheng, Z.-F., Fields, H.L. and Heinricher, M.M. (1986) Morphine microinjected into the periaqueductal gray has differential effects on 3 classes of medullary neurons. Brain Res., 375:57–65.

Fields, H.L., Bry, J., Hentall, I.D. and Zorman, G. (1983a) The activity of neurons in the rostral medulla of the rat during withdrawal from noxious heat. J. Neurosci., 3:2545–2552.

Fields, H.L., Vanegas, H., Hentall, I.D. and Zorman, G. (1983b) Evidence that disinhibition of brainstem neurons contributes to morphine analgesia. Nature, 306:684–686.

Fields, H.L. and Heinricher, M.M. (1985) Anatomy and physiology of a nociceptive modulatory system. Phil. Trans. R. Soc. London B, 308:361–374.

Fuxe, K. (1965) Evidence for the existence of monoamine neurons in the central nervous system. Acta Physiol. Scand., 52, Suppl. 247: 37–84.

Hammond, D.L., Levy, R.A. and Proudfit, H.K. (1980) Hypoalgesia following microinjection of noradrenergic antagonists in the nucleus raphe magnus. Pain, 9:85–101.

Moreau, J.-L. and Fields, H.L. (1986) Evidence for GABA involvement in midbrain control of medullary neurons that modulate nociceptive transmission. Brain Res., 397:37–46.

Sagen, J. and Proudfit, H.K. (1985) Evidence for pain modulation by pre- and postsynaptic noradrenergic receptors in the medulla oblongata. Brain Res., 331:285–293.

Vanegas, H., Barbaro, N.M. and Fields, H.L. (1984) Tail-flick related activity in medullospinal neurons. Brain Res., 321:135–141.

Wessendorf, M.W. and Anderson, E.G. (1983) Single unit studies of identified bulbospinal serotonergic units. Brain Res., 279:93–103.

Willcockson, W.S., Gerhart, K.D., Cargill, C.L and Willis, W.D. (1983) Effects of biogenic amines on raphe-spinal tract cells. J. Pharmacol. Exp. Ther., 225:637–645.

R. Dubner, G.F. Gebhart & M.R. Bond (Eds.)
Proceedings of the Vth World Congress on Pain
© 1988 Elsevier Science Publishers BV (Biomedical Division)

CHAPTER 68

Evaluation of analgesic effect of PAG stimulation using a new rat model for tonic pain

H. Jokura[1], T. Otsuki[3], H. Nakahama[2], H. Niizuma[1], J. Suzuki[1] and S. Saso[3]

Divisions of [1]Neurosurgery and [2]Neurophysiology, Institute of Brain Diseases, Tohoku University School of Medicine, and [3]Neurological Research Center, Miyagi National Hospital, Miyagi, Japan

Summary

The analgesic effect of electrical stimulation in the periaqueductal gray (PAG) was evaluated using a new rat model for tonic pain. Monosodium urate crystals were injected into one of the knee joint cavities and, by measuring the pressure which the animal put on the contralateral paws, the analgesic effects of various treatments could be evaluated quantitatively and objectively. It was found that electrical stimulation in the PAG can produce strong analgesia, which was not antagonized by systemic naloxone administration.

Introduction

It is now well accepted that electrical stimulation of several deep brain structures produces strong analgesic effects. This phenomenon can be used as a tool for elucidating the physiology of pain, but most experimental results using deep brain stimulation are obtained from tests which use acute painful stimuli. Recently, several reports using chronic or tonic pain animal models have indicated that the neural mechanisms concerning the transmission and control of chronic or tonic pain may be different from those of acute pain. We have previously described a new rat tonic pain model in which the analgesic effect of various methods can be evaluated objectively and quantitatively (Okuda et al., 1984; Otsuki et al., 1986). In this study, we re-evaluated the analgesic effects of periaqueductal gray (PAG) stimulation using this model.

Materials and methods

Male Sprague-Dawley rats weighing 200–300 g were used. Under pentobarbital anesthesia, a single bipolar stimulating microelectrode was stereotaxically implanted into the PAG using the atlas of Fifkova and Marsala (1967). Electrodes were constructed of insulated stainless-steel wires (0.1 mm outer diameter), which were cut and placed with the tips vertically separated by 0.5 mm.

One week after the implantation surgery, the rats were observed in a freely moving state within a transparent cage during electrical brain stimulation. Biphasic, rectangular pulse pairs, each pulse lasting 50 μ s and separated by a 100 μ s interval, were delivered at 20 Hz. Stimulation was begun at a peak-to-peak amplitude of 200 μA and was increased stepwise to 10 mA. When rats showed behavioral changes due to stimulation, the stimula-

Correspondence: T. Otsuki, Neurological Research Center, Miyagi National Hospital, Kassenhara-100, Takase, Yamamoto, Watari, Miyagi 989–22, Japan.

tion was stopped. Similar trials were repeated three times and the weakest of the three thresholds not producing behavioral changes was used subsequently to test the analgesic effects of brain stimulation. The next day 6 mg of monosodium urate crystals in 0.05 ml of saline containing 10% Tween 80 were injected into the knee joint cavity of the rat's hind leg under light ether anesthesia.

Four hours later, when rats showed consistent behavioral changes, such as severe limping, measurement of the pressure of the hind paws was performed using pressure transducers with the rat held in a gently restraining apparatus. The mean paw pressures over a period of 1 min for the injected and non-injected hind paws were obtained by microcomputer and the ratio between them was calculated (the paw pressure ratio). The paw pressure ratio was measured at 5-min intervals several times prior to, during and following PAG stimulation. The PAG stimulation was performed for 15 min and, if

the stimulation caused the ratio to increase more than 2-fold, the stimulation was judged effective.

In effective cases, a similar experiment was then performed and naloxone (1 mg and, subsequently, 10 mg/kg i.p.) was administered systemically 5 min after the start of brain stimulation.

Upon completion of the experiments the rats were killed with an overdose of pentobarbital. Small electrolytic lesions for determination of the location of the electrode tips were then made and the rats were perfused with saline and 10% formalin containing 1% potassium ferrocyanide.

Results

Behavioral changes caused by PAG electrical stimulation in a free-moving state were mainly classified as hyper- or hypoactivity. In the former case, sniffing, respiratory acceleration and exploratory be-

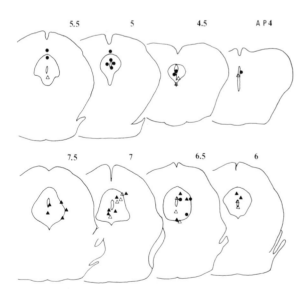

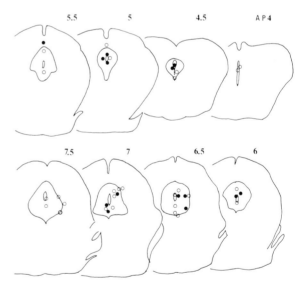

Fig. 1. Location of electrode tips in relation to stimulation-produced behavioral changes. Solid circles, electrode placements where stimulation induced hypoactivity; open triangles, stimulation-induced hyperactivity, without exploratory behavior; solid triangles, stimulation-induced hyperactivity with exploratory behavior. There was a tendency for hypoactivity to be produced at rostral locations and hyperactivity at caudal locations.

Fig. 2. Location of electrode tips. Solid circles, electrode placements where electrical stimulation produced strong analgesia, i.e., a paw pressure ratio during stimulation/prestimulation greater than 2. Open circles, electrode placements where stimulation produced no or weak analgesia (<2). Effective points are found to be scattered and not localized to the ventro-caudal part of the PAG.

havior with an increase of locomotion were observed. In contrast, in the latter case, the rats showed decreased locomotion and sometimes catatonic postures with tail stiffness. Hyperactivity was observed mostly in the caudal part of the PAG, whereas hypoactivity was elicited in rostral PAG regions (Fig. 1).

Fourteen of 41 electrodes in the PAG were found to produce significant analgesic effects (Fig. 2). The effective stimulation sites were scattered throughout almost the entire PAG with no apparent ventro-dorsal differences. Rostral PAG stimulation had a tendency to produce more analgesic effects compared to the caudal PAG.

Naloxone was administered systemically in 7 of the 14 rats which showed significant analgesic effects. In all cases, however, administration not only of 1 mg but also subsequently of 10 mg/kg of naloxone did not antagonize the analgesic effects of PAG stimulation (Fig. 3).

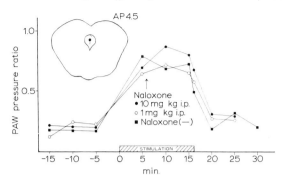

Fig. 3. A typical example of an effective case. The paw pressure ratio increased from about 0.2 to 0.7 during stimulation. Just after stimulation it is still high but returned to the prestimulation level after 5 min. Systemic administration of naloxone (1 mg and subsequently 10 mg/kg i.p.) had no effect on the stimulation-produced analgesia.

Discussion

In the present experiment, it was found that PAG electrical stimulation can produce significant analgesic effects using our tonic pain model, which was originally developed in order to evaluate, objectively and quantitatively, the effects of various analgesic methods on clinically related spontaneous and tonic pain. It was also shown that the analgesic effect produced by PAG stimulation was not antagonized by naloxone (1–10 mg/kg), which often has an antagonistic effect on PAG stimulation analgesia when evaluated by the tail-flick test.

Electrical stimulation of the PAG can produce aversive behavior in animals, which is known often to produce stress-induced analgesia. We therefore carefully determined the intensity of the stimulation current so that it caused no apparent behavioral changes in a freely moving state.

Recently, with our tonic pain model, we observed that there is a difference in the mechanism of pain modulation between the PAG and nucleus raphe magnus (NRM) as far as antinociception produced by microinjection of serotonin is concerned (Inase et al., 1987). It was also found that destruction of the NRM (Abbott et al., 1982; Abbott and Melzack, 1983) or the dorsolateral funiculus of the spinal cord (Ryan et al., 1985), both of which are considered to play an essential role in the descending pain inhibitory system, has no effect on PAG stimulation-produced analgesia or on the analgesic effect of systemic morphine, when evaluated by the formalin test.

Therefore, it was concluded that, as far as tonic pain is concerned, the analgesic effects of electrical PAG stimulation might be mediated by a neural mechanism which is different from the intrinsic pain-modulating neural systems which are mediated by opioid transmitters.

References

Abbott, F.V., Melzack, R. and Samuel, C. (1982) Morphine analgesia in the tail-flick and formalin test is mediated by different neural systems. Exp. Neurol., 75: 644–651.

Abbott, F.V. and Melzack, R. (1983) Dissociation of the mechanisms of stimulation-produced analgesia in tests of tonic and phasic pain. In J.J. Bonica et al. (Eds.), Advances in Pain and Therapy, Vol. 5, Raven Press, New York, pp. 401–409.

Fifkova, E. and Marsala, J. (1967) Stereotaxic atlases for the cat, rabbit and rat. In J. Bures, M. Petran and J. Zachar. (Eds.), Electrophysiological Methods in Biological Research, Academic Press, New York, pp. 653–731.

Inase, M., Nakahama, H., Otsuki, T. and Fang, J. (1987) Analgesic effects of serotonin microinjection into nucleus raphe magnus and raphe dorsalis evaluated by the monosodium urate (MSU) tonic pain model in the rat. Brain Res., 426: 205–211.

Okuda, K., Nakahama, H., Miyakawa, H. and Shima, K. (1984)

Arthritis induced in cat by sodium urate: a possible animal model for tonic pain. Pain, 18: 287–297.

Otsuki, T., Nakahama, H., Niizuma, H. and Suzuki, J. (1986) Evaluation of analgesic effects of capsaicin using a new rat model for tonic pain. Brain Res., 365: 235–240.

Ryan, S.M., Watkins, L.R. and Maier, S.F. (1985) Spinal pain supression mechanisms may differ from phasic and tonic pain. Brain Res., 334: 172–175.

R. Dubner, G.F. Gebhart & M.R. Bond (Eds.)
Proceedings of the Vth World Congress on Pain
© 1988 Elsevier Science Publishers BV (Biomedical Division)

CHAPTER 69

Tolerance to stimulation-produced analgesia from the periaqueductal grey of freely moving rats and its mediation by μ opioid receptors

M.J. Millan*, A. Członkowski and A. Herz

Department of Neuropharmacology, Max-Planck-Institut für Psychiatrie, Am Klopferspitz 18a, D-8033 Planegg-Martinsried, FRG

Summary

Electrical stimulation of the ventral periaqueductal grey (PAG) of freely moving rats elicited an antinociception as evaluated in the tail-flick test to noxious heat. Intravenous perfusion (via minipumps) with a low dose of naloxone (NLX), which is selective for μ opioid receptors, blocked this stimulation-produced analgesia (SPA). Following removal of pumps after 1 week of perfusion, SPA was potentiated; this reflects a supersensitivity of μ receptors. Recurrent stimulation led to a progressive decline in SPA: this could be reinstated in an NLX-reversible manner by an increase in current intensity. Tolerance did not reflect generalized behavioural deficits, depletion of CNS pools of endogenous opioid peptides or conditioning. In fact, tolerant rats showed a 'cross-tolerance' to the μ opioid agonist, morphine, consistent with a pharmacological tolerance at the level of the opioid receptor. We conclude that the SPA that is elicited from the ventral PAG of freely moving rats is mediated by μ opioid receptors and that a 'genuine' pharmacolog-
ical-like tolerance thereby develops upon recurrent stimulation.

Electrical stimulation of the periaqueductal gray (PAG) of the rat reproducibly evokes an antinociception, in the mediation of which an opioidergic mechanism is considered to play a role (Mayer and Hayes, 1975; Akil et al., 1976; Cannon et al., 1982). There is, however, a multiplicity both of opioid peptides and opioid receptor types in the mammalian CNS. The three peptide families are represented by β-endorphin, dynorphin and met-enkephalin and the three major receptor types are μ, δ and κ (Millan, 1986). We have previously provided evidence that an activation of PAG pools of β-endorphin may generate stimulation-produced analgesia (SPA) (Millan et al., 1986, 1987c). In the current studies, we attempted to elucidate the identity of the opioid receptor type responsible. In addition, we evaluated the nature and mechanisms underlying the 'tolerance' to SPA which appears to develop upon recurrent stimulation of the PAG (Millan et al., 1987 a, b).

As described in detail elsewhere (Millan et al., 1986), this work was performed on male rats bearing a single chronic, stereotaxically implanted electrode in the ventral PAG in the region of the dorsal raphé. Nociception was determined by use of the

---

*To whom correspondence should be addressed.
Abbreviations: NLX, naloxone: SPA, stimulation-produced analgesia

tail-flick test to noxious heat. Rats were stimulated for 10 min at 350 μA in a modified Skinner Box via a flexible cable allowing for 'free' behaviour.

Stimulation evokes an antinociception, maximal in intensity immediately after termination of stimulation (at which time rats were tested), and subsiding over 20 min. Placement in the box in the absence of stimulation is ineffective. We have recently characterized a procedure whereby, via intravenous perfusion of a low dose of naloxone (0.5 mg/kg/h) from osmotic minipumps, it is possible to selectively block μ opioid receptors (Millan and Morris, in preparation). In the presence of such a dose of naloxone, 3 days after implantation of pumps, SPA was almost entirely blocked (Fig. 1). It is, further, well-known that long-term occupation of opioid receptors by an antagonist leads to their up-regulation (Schulz et al., 1979; Zukin and Tempel, 1986); this is functionally expressed in a supersensitivity to the agonist. After 1 week of perfusion with naloxone, pumps were removed and rats displayed a facilitation in SPA (Fig. 1). In a parallel experiment it

was shown that perfusion with this dose of naloxone likewise blocked the antinociception produced by the μ receptor agonist, morphine, but not that by the κ receptor agonist, U50,488H (not shown). Following removal of the pumps the effect of morphine, but not U50,488H, was potentiated. Evidently, the data speak strongly for a mediation of SPA by μ receptors.

We wished to further pursue this issue in studies addressing the nature of the tolerance which develops to SPA. It may be seen from Fig. 2 that the magnitude of the SPA seen is proportional to current intensity. In rats which were stimulated twice daily at a current of 350 μA for 1 week, this no longer induced an antinociception. Indeed, the entire dose–response curve was shifted to the right and parallel to that of naive animals. Further, it could be shown that the SPA reinstated by increasing current intensity was sensitive to naloxone (Fig. 2). These data demonstrate that the tolerance which develops to SPA closely resembles that which develops to opioids, such as morphine, and that it fulfills the criteria of a pharmacological tolerance.

We found that this tolerance could not be accounted for in terms of psychological models of tolerance (Baker and Tiffany, 1985). For example, it recovered spontaneously, could not be extinguished

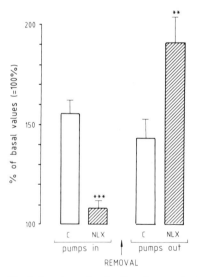

Fig. 1. In rats perfused with naloxone at a dose of 0.5 mg/kg/h, the antinociceptive action of stimulation (350 μAs) is blocked. Removal of pumps (after 7 days) leads to a supersensitivity to the actinociceptive effects of stimulation. Mean $\pm$ SEM shown. $n \geq$ six per column. Asterisks indicate significance of naloxone vs. Control differences. **$P \leq 0.01$; ***$P \leq 0.001$ (Student's two-tailed t-test).

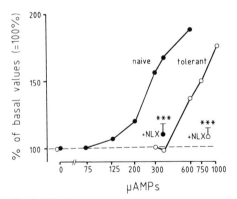

Fig. 2. The 'dose-response' curve for induction of antinociception is shifted to the right in recurrently-stimulated (tolerant) as compared to naive rats. Perfusion of rats with naloxone (0.5 mg/kg/h) blocks antinociception in both naive and 'tolerant' rats. Mean or mean $\pm$ SEM depicted. $N \geq$ four per point. Asterisks indicate significance of effect of naloxone. ***$P \leq 0.01$ (Student's two-tailed t-test).

by negative conditioning and rats exposed to cues of stimulation showed no (compensatory) hyperalgesia (Millan et al., 1987b). Further, an extensive examination of endocrinological, physiological and behavioural parameters revealed no indications of stress or debilitation in animals stimulated acutely or chronically (Millan et al., 1987b). There were no signs of significant tissue damage at the site of the electrode tip. These observations suggest that the tolerance does not reflect any generalized deficits.

An additional possibility is that recurrent stimulation may lead to a depletion of pools of endogenous opioid peptides mediating SPA. Of special pertinence in this regard are PAG pools of β-endorphin. We have observed that acute stimulation results in a rapid depletion of β-endorphin in the PAG, as determined by radioimmunoassay, presumably reflecting its release (Millan et al., 1987c). In fact, in rats allowed to rest for 24 h following chronic stimulation, we saw no significant alteration in levels of β-endorphin in the PAG or elsewhere in brain and the pituitary. Dynorphin and met-enkephalin were also found not to be affected in either the PAG or other discrete regions of the CNS (Millan et al., 1987b). These data suggest that a depletion of endogenous opioids does not underlie this tolerance.

A final experiment shed light on this issue and also provided further evidence for the mediation of SPA by μ opioid receptors. This was the observation, depicted in Fig. 3, that rats tolerant to SPA displayed a cross-tolerance to the μ receptor agonist, morphine, but not the κ receptor agonist, U50,488H. The present data are complemented by the previous observation that SPA is attenuated in rats rendered tolerant to morphine (Mayer and Hayes, 1975; Mayer and Murgin, 1976). There is, thus, bilateral cross-tolerance between SPA and the anti-nociception produced by morphine. In the light of the above results, the most reasonable explanation for the observed tolerance to SPA is that recurrent stimulation is associated with the repetitive release of the opioid mediating SPA; this leads to a tolerance at the level of the (μ) receptor and coupled post receptor processes in a fashion analo-

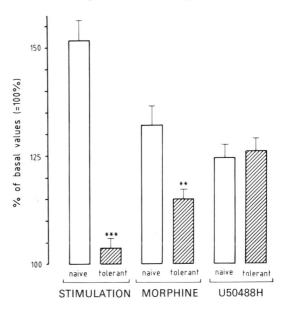

Fig. 3. The antinociceptive actions of stimulation and morphine, but not U50,488H are attenuated in (tolerant) rats which have been exposed to recurrent stimulation. Rats were stimulated on seven occasions at 350 μA over 4 days in the 'tolerant' group and not stimulated in the naive group. One day later, rats were stimulated again, or were treated with morphine (0.75 mg/kg, s.c.) or U50,488H (7.50 mg/kg, s.c.). Mean $\pm$ SEM shown. $N \geq$ six per column. Asterisks indicate significance of tolerant vs. naive values. **$P \leq 0.01$; ***$P \leq 0.001$ (Student's two-tailed t test).

gous to morphine.

We previously indicated that this opioid may be β-endorphin (Millan, et al., 1986). Clearly, there arise two interrelated questions: what is the location of this μ opioid receptor and does β-endorphin act directly thereon? There are reasons to believe that the simplest explanation, that β-endorphin acts via μ opioid receptors in the PAG, may be the correct one (see Millan et al., 1987a). However, there is *no* evidence which directly proves this assertion. Indeed, it has even been speculated that β-endorphin acts via a particular (ε) receptor and that its actions are indirectly mediated via a (naloxone-sensitive) μ receptor at the spinal level (Tseng et al., 1976; Schulz et al., 1981; Tseng and Fujimoto, 1984). This intriguing hypothesis requires further examination.

In conclusion, the present study indicates that the

SPA which can be elicited from the ventral PAG is mediated via μ opioid receptors and that upon recurrent stimulation a genuine tolerance develops thereto in freely moving rats.

References

Akil, H., Mayer, D.J. and Liebeskind, J.C. (1976) Antagonism of stimulation-produced analgesia by naloxone, a narcotic antagonist. Science, 191:961–962.

Baker, T.B. and Tiffany, S.T. (1985) Morphine tolerance as habituation. Psychol. Rev., 92:78–108.

Cannon, J.T., Prieto, G.J., Lee, A. and Liebeskind, J.C. (1982) Evidence for opioid and non-opioid forms of stimulation-produced analgesia in the rat. Brain Res., 243:315–321.

Mayer, D.J. and Hayes, R.L. (1975) Stimulation-produced analgesia: development of tolerance and cross-tolerance to morphine. Science, 188:941–943.

Mayer, D. and Murgin, R. (1976) Stimulation-produced analgesia (SPA) and morphine analgesia (MA): cross-tolerance from application at the same brain site. Fed. Proc., 35:385.

Millan, M.H., Millan, M.J. and Herz, A. (1986) Depletion of central β-endorphin blocks midbrain stimulation-produced analgesia in the rat. Neuroscience, 18:641–649.

Millan, M.J. (1986) Multiple opioid systems and pain. Pain, 27:303–347.

Millan, M.J., Członkowski, A. and Herz, A. (1987a) Evidence that μ-opioid receptors mediate midbrain 'Stimulation-produced analgesia' in the rat. Neuroscience, 22: 885–896.

Millan, M.J., Członkowski, A. and Herz, A. (1987b) An analysis of the 'tolerance' which develops to analgetic electrical stimulation of the periaqueductal grey of freely-moving rats. Brain Res., 435: 97–111.

Millan, M.J., Członkowski, A., Millan, M.H. and Herz, A., (1987c) Activation of periaqueductal grey pools of β-endorphin by electrical stimulation in the rat. Brain Res., 407:199–203.

Schulz, R., Wüster, M. and Herz, A. (1981) Pharmacological characterization of the ε-opiate receptor. J. Pharmacol. Exp. Ther., 216:604–616.

Schulz, R., Wüster, M. and Herz, A. (1979) Supersensitivity to opioids following the chronic blockade of endorphin action by naloxone. Naunyn-Schmiedeberg's Arch. Pharmacol., 306:93–96.

Tseng, L.-F. and Fujimoto, J.M. (1984) Evidence that spinal endorphin mediates intraventricular β-endorphin induced tail-flick inhibition and catalepsy. Brain Res., 302:231–237.

Tseng, L.-F., Loh, H.H. and Li, C.H. (1976) β-Endorphin: cross-tolerance to and cross-physical dependence on morphine. Proc. Natl. Acad. Sci. USA, 73:4187–4189.

Zukin, R.S. and Tempel, A. (1986) Neurochemical correlates of opiate receptor upregulation. Biochem. Pharmacol. 35:1623–1627.

Acknowledgement

We thank A. Huber for excellent technical assistance.

Author index

Subject index

Prepared by H. Kettner, M.D., Middelburg, The Netherlands